Musculoskeletal Essentials

Applying the Preferred Physical Therapist Practice Patterns℠

Musculoskeletal Essentials

Applying the Preferred Physical Therapist Practice Patterns℠

Editor
Marilyn Moffat, PT, DPT, PhD, FAPTA, CSCS
Professor, Physical Therapy Department
New York University
New York, New York

Associate Editors
Elaine Rosen, PT, DHSc, OCS, FAAOMPT
Associate Professor
Hunter College Schools of the Health Professions
New York, New York
Partner
Queens Physical Therapy Associates
Forest Hills, New York

Sandra Rusnak-Smith, PT, DHSc, OCS
Partner
Queens Physical Therapy Associates
Forest Hills, New York

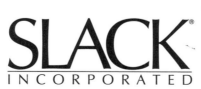

SLACK®
INCORPORATED

Delivering the best in health care information and education worldwide www.slackbooks.com

ISBN-10: 1-55642-667-4
ISBN-13: 978-1-55642-667-4

The procedures and practices described in this book should be implemented in a manner consistent with the professional standards set for the circumstances that apply in each specific situation. Every effort has been made to confirm the accuracy of the information presented and to correctly relate generally accepted practices. The authors, editor, and publisher cannot accept responsibility for errors or exclusions or for the outcome of the material presented herein. There is no expressed or implied warranty of this book or information imparted by it. Care has been taken to ensure that drug selection and dosages are in accordance with currently accepted/recommended practice. Due to continuing research, changes in government policy and regulations, and various effects of drug reactions and interactions, it is recommended that the reader carefully review all materials and literature provided for each drug, especially those that are new or not frequently used. Any review or mention of specific companies or products is not intended as an endorsement by the author or publisher.

SLACK Incorporated uses a review process to evaluate submitted material. Prior to publication, educators or clinicians provide important feedback on the content that we publish. We welcome feedback on this work.

Published by: SLACK Incorporated
                 6900 Grove Road
                 Thorofare, NJ 08086 USA
                 Telephone: 856-848-1000
                 Fax: 856-853-5991
                 www.slackbooks.com

Contact SLACK Incorporated for more information about other books in this field or about the availability of our books from distributors outside the United States.

Library of Congress Cataloging-in-Publication Data

Musculoskeletal essentials: applying the preferred physical therapist practice patterns / editor, Marilyn Moffat; associate editors, Elaine Rosen, Sandra Rusnak-Smith.
    p. ; cm. -- (Essentials in physical therapy)
    Includes bibliographical references and index.
    ISBN-13: 978-1-55642-667-4 (alk. paper)
    ISBN-10: 1-55642-667-4 (alk. paper)
    1. Musculoskeletal system--Diseases--Physical therapy. 2. Musculoskeletal system--Diseases--Patients--Rehabilitation.   I. Moffat, Marilyn. II. Rosen, Elaine. III. Rusnak-Smith, Sandra. IV. Series.
    [DNLM: 1. Musculoskeletal Diseases--rehabilitation. 2. Physical Therapy Modalities--standards. 3. Case Reports. 4. Musculoskeletal Manipulations--methods. 5. Patient Care Planning. WE 140 M9846 2006]
    RC925.5M8785 2006
    616.7--dc22

Printed in the United States of America.

Last digit is print number: 10 9 8 7 6 5 4 3 2 1

Dedication

Undertaking a task of this magnitude is never possible without the utmost support of many individuals to whom
I am deeply indebted. Thus this book is dedicated to: all of my Moffat and Salant families;
physical therapy colleagues; APTA staff; faculty, support staff, and students at New York University;
and all of my patients and clients who made this endeavor possible.

—MM

This book would not be possible without the untiring support of
my wonderfully patient and understanding husband, Jed.
Much appreciation to my patients, family, and colleagues
who have all helped me grow and learn throughout the years.

—ER

I would like to thank my husband, Peter; my daughter, Rachel; and my son, Andrew
for their encouragement and understanding throughout this endeavor.
I would also like to acknowledge my colleagues, friends, family, and patients
who have all contributed in some way to making this book possible.

—SRS

Contents

Acknowledgments

This edited book is one of a series of four books that would not have been possible without the dedication, incredibly hard work, and generosity of so many individuals. I am eternally indebted to each of the following outstanding physical therapists for their willingness to share their expertise, their enthusiasm, and their unbelievable patience in seeing this work come to fruition:

- Associate Editors:
  - Elaine Rosen, PT, DHSc, OCS, FAAOMPT
  - Sandra Rusnak-Smith, PT, DHSc, OCS
- Contributing Authors:
  - Suzanne R. Babyar, PT, PhD
  - Marc Campolo, PT, PhD, SCS, ATC, CSCS
  - S. Betty Chow, PT, MA, OCS
  - Joshua A. Cleland, PT, DPT, PhD, OCS
  - Susan Collura Schiliro, PT, DPT, CHT
  - Marie Corkery, PT, MHS, FAAOMPT
  - Karen A. Fritzsche, PT
  - Matthew B. Garber, PT, DSc, OCS, FAAOMPT
  - Tom Holland, PT, PhD
  - Lorna King, MSc, PT, MTC
  - Gary Krasilovsky, PT, PhD
  - Bella J. May, PT, EdD, FAPTA
  - Elaine Rosen, PT, DHSc, OCS, FAAOMPT
  - Sandra Rusnak-Smith, PT, DHSc, OCS
  - Roslyn Sofer, MA, PT, OCS
  - Mary Ann Wilmarth, PT, DPT, MS, OCS, MTC, Cert. MDT

The putting together of a book requires the astute skills of both editorial and publishing staff. Working with colleagues and associates at SLACK Incorporated has indeed been a pleasure, and I am indebted to them for their perceptive reviews and their continued encouragement provided along the way. To the following individuals I owe my thanks:

- Carrie Kotlar, who first approached me with the idea of doing this book and stood by throughout the process with unwavering support
- John Bond, who jumped in whenever we needed support from the top
- Jennifer Cahill and Kimberly Shigo, who had the editorial tasks of making our manuscripts into a published book

And last, but not least, are so many who have influenced my life, have challenged me to strive to do the best that I am able, and have supported and encouraged me along the way. My heartfelt thanks are extended to:

- My mother, for her unconditional support
- My father and my husband who were always there for me, were both the epitomy of role models, and were both taken from me too early in life
- My sister and brother-in-law, my stepdaughter, and my grandchildren for always reminding me of what is important in life
- All of my physical therapy colleagues, who have been such an integral part of my life

♦ The staff at the American Physical Therapy Association, who continually supported me throughout the years and who sometimes met unbelievable demands to see the *Guide* project reach the format it is today

♦ The faculty and support staff at New York University, my students, and my patients who have taught me so much and made me realize what insight and passion mean in realizing one's goals

Setting an example is not the main means of influencing others; it is the only means—Albert Einstein

—MM

We would like to thank Greg Gao MD, PT, for his creative illustration.

—ER and SRS

About the Editors

Marilyn Moffat, PT, DPT, PhD, FAPTA, CSCS, a recognized leader in the United States and internationally, is a practitioner, a teacher, a consultant, a leader, and an author. She received her baccalaureate degree from Queens College and her physical therapy certificate and PhD degrees from New York University. She is a Full Professor of Physical Therapy at New York University, where she directs both the professional doctoral program (DPT) and the post-professional graduate master's degree program in pathokinesiology. She has been in private practice for more than 40 years and currently practices in the New York area.

Dr. Moffat was one of the first individuals to speak and write about the need for a doctoral entry-level degree in physical therapy. Her first presentation on this topic was given to the Section for Education in 1977.

Dr. Moffat completed a 6-year term as the President of the American Physical Therapy Association (APTA) in 1997. Prior to that she had served on the APTA Board of Directors for 6 years and also as President of the New York Physical Therapy Association for 4 years. During her term as President of the APTA, she played a major role in the development of the Association's *Guide to Physical Therapist Practice* and was project editor of the Second Edition of the *Guide*. Among her many publications is the *American Physical Therapy Association's Book of Body Maintenance and Repair*. As part of her commitment to research, Dr. Moffat is currently a member of the Board of Trustees of the Foundation for Physical Therapy, was a previous member of the Financial Advisory Committee, and has done major fundraising for them over the years.

She is currently on the Executive Committee of the World Confederation for Physical Therapy (WCPT) as the North American/Caribbean Regional Representative, and she was a member of the WCPT Task Force to develop an international definition of physical therapy. She coordinated the efforts to develop international guidelines for physical therapist educational programs around the world. She has given more than 800 professional presentations throughout her practice lifetime, and she has taught and provided consultation services in Taiwan, Thailand, Burma, Vietnam, Panama City, Hong Kong, and Puerto Rico.

Her diversified background is exemplified by the vast number of APTA and New York Physical Therapy Association committees and task forces on which she has served or chaired. She has served as Editor of *Physical Therapy*, the official publication of the Association. She was also instrumental in the early development of the TriAlliance of Rehabilitation Professionals, composed of the APTA, the American Occupational Therapy Association, and the American Speech-Language-Hearing Association. She has been an Associate of the Council of Public Representatives of the National Institutes of Health.

Dr. Moffat is a Catherine Worthingham Fellow of the APTA. She has been the recipient of APTA's Marilyn Moffat Leadership Award; the WCPT's Mildred Elson Award for International Leadership; the APTA's Lucy Blair Service Award; the Robert G. Dicus Private Practice Section APTA Award for contributions to private practice; Outstanding Service Awards from the New York Physical Therapy Association and from the APTA; the Ambassador Award from the National Strength and Conditioning Association; the Howard A. Rusk Humanitarian Award from the World Rehabilitation Fund; the United Cerebral Palsy Citation for Service; the Sawadi Skulkai Lecture Award from Mahidol University in Bangkok, Thailand; New York University's Founders Day Award; the University of Florida's Barbara C. White Lecture Award; the Massachusetts General's Ionta Lecture Award; the Chartered Society of Physiotherapist's Alan Walker Memorial Lecture Award; the APTA Minority Affairs Diversity 2000 Award; and the Section of Health Policy's R. Charles Harker Policy Maker Award. In addition, the New York Physical Therapy Association also named its leadership award after her. She was the APTA's 2004 Mary McMillan Lecturer, the Association's highest award. Dr. Moffat has been listed in *Who's Who in the East*, *Who's Who in American Women*, *Who's Who in America*, *Who's Who in Education*, *Who's Who in the World*, and *Who's Who in Medicine and Healthcare*.

She is also currently on the Board of Directors of the World Rehabilitation Fund and is a member of the Executive Committee. In addition to her professional associations, she was elected to be a member of Kappa Delta Pi and Pi Lambda Theta.

Dr. Moffat has served on a Citizen's Advisory Council of the New York State Assembly Task Force on the Disabled, has been a member of the State Board for Physical Therapy in New York, has served as a consultant to the New York City Police Department, and has been a member of the Boards of Trustees of Children's Village and the Four Oaks Foundation. The Nassau County Fine Arts Museum, the Howard A. Rusk Rehabilitation Medicine Campaign Committee, Saint John's Church of Lattingtown, and the Nassau County American Red Cross have been the recipients of her volunteer services.

Elaine Rosen, PT, DHSc, OCS, FAAOMPT, received her BS in Physical Therapy from Hunter College in 1973, Master in Science in Work Physiology from Long Island University in 1977 and Doctor of Health Science in Orthopaedic Physical Therapy from the University of St. Augustine in 1998. Dr. Rosen is an associate professor at Hunter College Program in Physical Therapy in New York City. She is also a partner in Queens Physical Therapy Associates in Forest Hills, New York. She has been in practice for more than 30 years.

Dr. Rosen served as Director of the Orthopaedic Section of the American Physical Therapy Association from 1994 through 1999. She has served in many other capacities on the state and local levels of the APTA.

Dr. Rosen has authored *Musculoskeletal Examination* published by Blackwell Publishing in 1996 and 2002. She has also authored chapters and articles in other professional books and journals. Over her career she has given many professional presentations and has taught in Puerto Rico and Israel. She has served as a guest lecturer at New York University and Touro College.

Dr. Rosen was the recipient of Distinguished Alumni Award, Hunter College, Schools of the Health Professions, April 22, 2004. She was awarded the 2003 James A. Gould Award for Excellence in Teaching Orthopaedic Physical Therapy given by the Orthopaedic Section of the APTA. She has been listed in *Who's Who in American Women* and *Who's Who in Medicine and Healthcare.*

Sandra Rusnak-Smith, PT, DHSc, OCS, received her Certificate in Physical Therapy from Hunter College in 1976, Master in Art from New York University in 1994, and Doctor of Health Science in Orthopaedic Physical Therapy from the University of St. Augustine in 2002. Dr. Rusnak-Smith has been an adjunct assistant professor at Hunter College, Touro College, Downstate, and Long Island University. She is also a partner in Queens Physical Therapy Associates in Forest Hills, New York. She has been in practice for more than 30 years.

Dr. Rusnak-Smith has served in many capacities on the state and local levels of the APTA and has been the recipient of the Outstanding Service Award from New York Chapter.

Dr. Rusnak-Smith has authored a chapter on the Thoracic Spine and published in the *Journal of Orthopaedic and Sports Physical Therapy.* Over her career she has given many professional presentations.

Contributing Authors

Suzanne R. Babyar, PT, PhD
Assistant Professor
Physical Therapy Program
Hunter College Schools of the Health Professions
New York, New York

Marc Campolo, PT, PhD, SCS, ATC, CSCS
Chair, Department of Physical Therapy
and Sports Science
Seton Hall University
South Orange, New Jersey

S. Betty Chow, PT, MA, OCS
Staff Physical Therapist
Hospital for Special Surgery
New York, New York

Joshua A. Cleland, PT, DPT, PhD, OCS
Assistant Professor
Franklin Pierce College
Concord, New Hampshire
Physical Therapist
Rehabilitation Services of Concord Hospital
Concord, New Hampshire

Susan Collura Schiliro, PT, DPT, CHT
Owner, Susan Collura Schiliro, PT, DPT,
CHT, PC
Forest Hills, New York

Marie Corkery, PT, MHS, FAAOMPT
Associate Clinical Specialist
Department of Physical Therapy
Bouvé College of Health Sciences
Northeastern University
Boston, Massachusetts

Karen A. Fritzsche, PT
Clinical Supervisor of Education
Hospital for Special Surgery
New York, New York

Matthew B. Garber, PT, DSc, OCS,
FAAOMPT
Assistant Chief, Physical Therapy Service
Assistant Professor, US Army-Baylor
University Postprofessional
Doctoral Program in Orthopaedic Manual
Physical Therapy
Brooke Army Medical Center
Fort Sam Houston, Texas

Tom Holland, PT, PhD
Assistant Professor
Hunter College Schools of the Health Professions
New York, New York

Lorna King, MSc, PT, MTC
Staff Physical Therapist
Chelsea Community Hospital
Chelsea, Missouri

Gary Krasilovsky, PT, PhD
Associate Professor and Director
Physical Therapy Program
Hunter College Schools of the Health Professions
New York, New York

Bella J. May, PT, EdD, FAPTA
BJM Enterprises
Dublin, California

Marilyn Moffat, PT, DPT, PhD, FAPTA, CSCS
Professor, Physical Therapy Department
New York University
New York, New York

Elaine Rosen, PT, DHSc, OCS, FAAOMPT
Associate Professor
Hunter College Schools of the Health Professions
New York, New York
Partner
Queens Physical Therapy Associates
Forest Hills, New York

Sandra Rusnak-Smith, PT, DHSc, OCS
Partner
Queens Physical Therapy Associates
Forest Hills, New York

Roslyn Sofer, MA, PT, OCS
Assistant Professor
Touro College School of Health Sciences
Bay Shore, New York
Clinical Assistant Professor
Health Science Center at Brooklyn,
SUNY Downstate
Brooklyn, New York
Director, Community Physical Therapy
Rego Park, New York

*Mary Ann Wilmarth, PT, DPT, MS, OCS,
MTC, Cert. MDT*
Director, Transitional DPT Program
Bouvé Institute
Department of Physical Therapy
Northeastern University
Boston, Massachusetts
Independent Study Course Editor
Orthopaedic Section, APTA, Inc

Preface

Musculoskeletal Essentials: Applying the Preferred Physical Therapist Practice Patterns[SM] is part of a series of four books (*Musculosketelal Essentials, Neuromuscular Essentials, Cardiovascular Essentials,* and *Integumentary Essentials*) aimed at promoting an understanding of physical therapist practice and challenging the clinical thinking and decision making of our practitioners. In this book, 17 distinguished contributors have written chapters to take the *Guide to Physical Therapist Practice* to the next level of practice. Each chapter provides the relevant information for the pattern described by the *Guide* and emphasizes the process through which a physical therapist goes to take the patient from the examination to discharge. The Introduction to this book describes what each chapter contains.

It has been a goal of this entire series, and certainly is a strong hope of each of us involved in editing this series, that these *Essentials* will provide students and practitioners with a valuable reference for physical therapist practice.

As a way of introduction to the *Guide to Physical Therapist Practice*, the information below provides a brief overview of its development. Since I was involved in each step of the entire process, I know the unbelievable amount of work done by so many to see that landmark work reach fruition.

DEVELOPMENT OF THE *GUIDE*

The *Guide to Physical Therapist Practice* was developed based on the needs of membership by the American Physical Therapy Association (APTA) under my leadership as President of the Association. As an integral part of all of the groups responsible for writing the *Guide* and as one of three Project Editors for the latest edition of the *Guide*, I was delighted when SLACK Incorporated approached me to take the *Guide* to the next step for students and clinicians.

HISTORY

In the way of history, the development of the *Guide* began in 1992 with a Board of Directors-appointed task force upon which I served and which culminated in the publication of *A Guide to Physical Therapist Practice, Volume I: A Description of Patient Management* in the August 1995 issue of *Physical Therapy*. The APTA House of Delegates approved the development of Volume II, which was designed to describe the preferred patterns of practice for patient/client groupings commonly referred for physical therapy.

In 1997, Volume I and Volume II became Part One and Part Two of the *Guide*, and the first edition of the *Guide* was published in the November 1997 issue of *Physical Therapy*. In 1998, APTA initiated Parts Three and Four of the *Guide* to catalog the specific tests and measures used by physical therapists in the four system areas and the areas of outcomes, health-related quality of life, and patient/client satisfaction. Additional inclusions in the *Guide* were standardized documentation forms and templates that incorporated the patient/client management process and a patient/client satisfaction instrument.

A CD-ROM version of the *Guide* was developed that included not only Part One and Part Two, but also the varied tests and measures used in practice along with their reliability and validity.

FIVE ELEMENTS OF PATIENT/CLIENT MANAGEMENT

The patient/client management model includes the five essential elements of examination, evaluation, diagnosis, prognosis, and intervention that result in optimal outcomes. The patient/client management process is dynamic and allows the physical therapist to progress the patient/client in the process, return to an earlier element for further analysis, or exit the patient/client from the process when the needs of the patient/client cannot be addressed by the physical therapist. The patient/client management process incorporates the disablement model (pathology/pathophysiology, impairments, functional limitations) throughout the five elements and outcomes, but also includes all aspects of risk reduction/prevention; health, wellness, and fitness; societal resources; and patient/client satisfaction. This is the physical therapist's clinical decision-making model.

APPLICATION OF THE *GUIDE* TO CLINICAL PRACTICE

The *Guide* has its practice patterns grouped according to each of the four systems—musculoskeletal, neuromuscular, cardiovascular/pulmonary, and integumentary. Thus, this *Essentials* series continues where the *Guide* leaves off and brings the *Guide* to meaningful, clinically based examples of each of the patterns. In each chapter in each system area, an overview of the pertinent anatomy, physiology, pathophysiology, imaging, and pharmacology is presented; then three to five cases are presented for each pattern. Each case initially details the physical therapist examination, including the history, systems review, and tests and measures selected for that case. Then the evaluation, diagnosis, and prognosis and plan of care for the case are presented. Prior to the specific interventions for the case is the rationale for the interventions based on the available literature, thus ensuring that, when possible, the interventions are evidence-based. The anticipated goals and expected outcomes for the interventions are put forth as possible in functional and measurable terms. Finally, any special considerations for reexamination, discharge, and psychological aspects are delineated.

Foreword
to the *Essentials in*
Physical Therapy Series

There are many leaders, many educators, and some visionaries, but only a very special few individuals have all three characteristics. The Editor of this series of books, Dr. Marilyn Moffat, certainly has demonstrated these traits and is again helping to guide the profession of physical therapy, as well as all therapists, to a new level of cognitive analysis when implementing and effectively using the *Guide to Physical Therapist Practice*.

Dr. Moffat's dream was for the American Physical Therapy Association to develop the original *Guide*. She nurtured its birth, as well as its development. In 2001, the second edition and evolution of additional practice patterns was introduced to the profession. Although the *Guide* lays the foundation for the entire diagnostic process used by a physical therapist as a movement specialist, many colleagues have difficulty bridging the gap between this model for the entire patient management process and its application to an individual consumer of physical therapy services. Through Dr. Moffat's vision, she recognized this gap and has again tried to link the highest standard of professional process to the patient/client and his or her specific needs.

When you take the leadership of the Editor and combine that with the expertise and clinical mastery of the various chapter authors, the quality of these texts already sets the highest standard of literary reference for an experienced, novel, or student physical therapist.

There are few individuals who could or would take on this dedicated process that will widen the therapist's comprehension of a very difficult and complex process. Dr. Moffat has again contributed, in her typical scholarly fashion, to the world of physical therapy literature and to each practitioner's role as a service provider of health care around the world.

—*Darcy Umphred, PT, PhD, FAPTA*
University of the Pacific
Stockton, California

Foreword
to *Musculoskeletal Essentials*

The *Guide to Physical Therapist Practice*, first published in 1995, is a landmark consensus-based document written for those within and outside of our profession. This inclusive overview of physical therapist and physical therapist assistant practice includes the elements of the patient/client management, patient data collection tools, clinical outcome measures, practice patterns, standards of practice, and guides to professional conduct, all presented within the context of the disablement and evidenced-based practice models. In essence, this document presents who we are and what we subscribe to be as health care professionals. The five essential elements of the patient/client management model—examination, evaluation, diagnosis, prognosis, and intervention—provide a framework for physical therapist practice from initial visit through patient discharge or discontinuation.

Since 1995, the physical therapy profession has needed a publication that "brings the *Guide* alive" from a clinical perspective, in particular, the Preferred Practice Patterns. The Preferred Practice Patterns are meant to describe what is considered to be "best practice," based on what clinical experts consider to the most used or most appropriate interventions. This is in contrast to clinical guidelines whose foundations are based on evidence that speaks to the efficacy and effectiveness of interventions. Practice patterns can form the basis for future clinical guidelines, but must undergo appropriate validation scrutiny to do so. Dr. Marilyn Moffat's timely offering of the *Essentials in Physical Therapy* series of books, including *Musculoskeletal Essentials*, not only expertly fills the void in physical therapy literature related to the practical application of the *Guide,* but also begins the validation process.

Dr. Moffat, Dr. Elaine Rosen, and Dr. Sandra Rusnak-Smith have recruited an outstanding group of expert clinicians and educators for *Musculoskeletal Essentials*. The selected practice patterns are clearly described with relevant anatomy, physiology, and pathophysiology information providing the backdrop for the patient cases that follow. Case after patient case is presented providing varied clinical scenarios that will inform and challenge the student as well as the experienced clinician. The authors draw on their extensive patient care and post-professional educational experiences to illustrate clinical decision making at its best. Upon completion of the book, the reader will be well-versed in the patient/client management, disablement, and evidenced-based practice models as they apply to patient populations with primary orthopedic conditions. Drs. Moffat, Rosen, and Rusnak-Smith and the contributing authors are to be commended. Their efforts will advance the practice and education of physical therapists, helping make the American Physical Therapy Association Vision 2020 a reality.

—*William Boissonnault, PT, DHSc, FAAOMPT*
University of Wisconsin
Madison, Wisconsin

Introduction

The chapters in *Musculoskeletal Essentials* take the *Guide to Physical Therapist Practice*[1] to the next level and parallel the patterns in the *Guide*.

INTRODUCTORY INFORMATION

In each case, where appropriate, a review of the pertinent anatomy, physiology, pathophysiology, imaging, and pharmacology is provided as a means of background material.

PHYSICAL THERAPIST EXAMINATION

Each pattern details three to five case studies appropriate to that pattern in *Guide* format. Thus, the case begins with the physical therapist examination, which is divided into the three parts of the examination—the history, the systems review, and the specific tests and measures selected for that particular case.

HISTORY

The history provides the first information that will be obtained from the patient/client. The history is a crucial first step in the clinical decision-making process as it enables the physical therapist to form an early hypothesis that helps guide the remainder of the clinical examination. The interview with the patient/client and a review of other available information provide the initial facts upon which further testing will be done to determine the concerns, goals, and eventual plan of care.

SYSTEMS REVIEW

After the history has been completed, the next aspect of the examination is the systems review, which is comprised of a quick screen of the four systems areas and a screen of the communication, affect, cognition, language, and learning style. The cardiovascular/pulmonary review includes assessment of blood pressure, edema, heart rate, and respiratory rate. The integumentary review includes assessing for the presence of any scar formation, the skin color, and the skin integrity. The musculoskeletal review includes assessment of gross range of motion, gross strength, gross symmetry, height, and weight. The neuromuscular review consists of an assessment of gross coordinated movements (eg, balance, locomotion, transfers, and transitions). The screen for communication, affect, cognition, language, and learning style includes an assessment of the patient's/client's ability to make needs known, consciousness, expected emotional/behavioral responses, learning preferences, and orientation.

TESTS AND MEASURES

The specific tests and measures to be selected for the patient/client are based upon the results found during the history taking and during the systems review. These latter two portions of the examination identify the clinical indicators for pathology/pathophysiology, impairments, functional limitations, disabilities, risk factors, prevention, and health, wellness, and fitness needs that will enable one to select the most appropriate tests and measures for the patient/client.

EVALUATION, DIAGNOSIS, AND PROGNOSIS AND PLAN OF CARE

The next step in the patient/client management model is evaluation. All of the data obtained from the examination (history, systems review, and tests and measures) are analyzed and synthesized to determine the diagnosis, prognosis, and plan of care for the patient/client. Then, once the evaluation has been completed and all data have been analyzed, the diagnosis for the patient/client and the pattern(s) into which the patient/client fits are determined.

After a review of the prognosis statement, of the expected range of number of visits per episode, and of the factors that may modify the frequency of visits for the pattern in the *Guide*, the prognosis is determined. Mutually established outcomes and the interventions for the patient/client are determined.

In each case the *Guide* has set the expected course of visits for the patient/client (see Expected Range of Number of Visits Per Episode of Care in each pattern in the *Guide*). This range should be appropriate for 80% of the population. Any additional impairment(s) found during the examination may or may not increase the number of expected visits. There are many factors that may modify the frequency or duration of visits. These may include: the patient's/client's adherence to the program set by the physical therapist, the type and amount of social support and caregiver expertise, the patient's/client's level of impairment, the patient's/client's health insurance plan, and the patient's/client's overall health status. Each patient/client must be looked at individually when determining the frequency and duration of visits.

INTERVENTIONS

Through all the information gathered in the examination and evaluation and with the diagnosis, prognosis, and plan of care in place, the specific interventions for this patient are selected. Whenever possible, interventions that have been shown to be effective through high-quality scientific research are utilized. At the end of all of the interventions is a composite section on anticipated goals and expected outcomes.

REEXAMINATION AND DISCHARGE

Reexamination will be performed throughout the episode of care, particularly as the setting of care changes. Discharge will occur when anticipated goals and expected outcomes have been attained.

PSYCHOLOGICAL ASPECTS

For each case, psychological aspects are important to consider when attempting to motivate patients/clients to comply with a long-range intervention program of exercise and functional training. Among these considerations for all patterns are:

- ◆ Behavior is governed by expectancies and incentives
- ◆ The likelihood that people adopt a health behavior depends on three perceptions:
  - • The perception that health is threatened
  - • The expectancy that their behavioral change will reduce the threat
  - • The expectancy that they are competent to change the behavior

It is necessary for physical therapists to understand reasons for noncompliance and formulate intervention plans accordingly. The number one indicator of future noncompliance is past poor compliance. Any psychological considerations beyond these in a particular case will be further detailed in that case.

PATIENT/CLIENT SATISFACTION

And finally for each case, the patient/client satisfaction with the physical therapy management would be determined by using the standard Patient/Client Satisfaction Questionnaire found in the back of the *Guide*.

REFERENCES

1. American Physical Therapy Association. Guide to physical therapist practice. 2nd ed. *Phys Ther*. 2001;81:9-744.

CHAPTER ONE

Primary Prevention/ Risk Reduction for Skeletal Demineralization (Pattern A)

S. Betty Chow, PT, MA, OCS

Marilyn Moffat, PT, DPT, PhD, FAPTA, CSCS

ANATOMY

The human skeleton is composed of 206 bones that form a structural framework that offers the body several basic functions: protection, mobility, and metabolism. The skull and thorax provide protection by encasing the internal organs of the head and trunk. Contractions of muscles attached to the skeleton provide for movement of the joints. In addition, at the microscopic level, the skeletal system serves as a reservoir for ions (calcium, phosphorus, magnesium, and sodium) and serves as an environment for this reservoir to maintain serum homeostasis.[1] The anatomy and physiology of bone are also detailed in Pattern G: Impaired Joint Mobility, Muscle Performance, and Range of Motion Associated With Fracture.

BONE COMPOSITION

Bone is a form of specialized connective tissue that is composed primarily of an extracellular matrix that consists of one-third part organic matrix referred to as osteoid and two-thirds mineral crystals. Of this extracellular matrix, 90% to 95% of it consists of collagen. The collagen in its uncalcified state will mineralize to become bone. The remaining portion of the extracellular matrix consists of fluid and a gelatinous ground substance of proteoglycans ([PGs] chondroitin sulfate and hyaluronic acid) that acts as a cementing substance between layers of mineralized collagen. The inorganic component of bone consists primarily of calcium and phosphate in the form of small crystals known as hydroxyapatite $Ca_{10}(PO_4)_6(OH)_2$ that are embedded in the protein collagen fibers. The rigid nature of bone is due to the deposition of these minerals. Other inorganic components include carbonate, magnesium, potassium, and sodium ions. Water is mostly found around the collagen fibers, the ground substance, and the hydration shells around the bone crystals. The remainder of water resides in the canals of the bony structures (haversian and Volkmann's).[1,2]

Macroscopic Structure

Bone is classified into two types: cortical and cancellous. Both types are found in each bone, however, the quantity of each type will vary within a particular bone.[3] Cortical bone, also referred to as compact or dense bone, is the solid outer shell and makes up 80% of the skeleton.[3] It is found in the long bone shafts and on the surfaces of the skull, the pelvis, and other flat bones.[1] Cancellous bone, also referred to as trabecular or spongy bone, is formed by the thin trabecular plates within the cortical shell and makes up 20% of the skeleton. It is found at the ends of long bones, within the vertebrae, and inside of the skull, pelvis, and other flat bones.[1] Certain bones, such as the distal radius, the vertebral body, and the proximal femur, have the greatest proportions of cancellous bone.[3] It is at these sites that bone loss due to osteopenia and osteoporosis most commonly occur. Surface area is one factor influencing bone loss. While cortical bone has four times the mass of cancellous bone, cancellous bone has eight times greater surface area[4]—the greater the surface area, the greater the metabolic turnover rate.[3] Hence, bones with higher content of cancellous bone, such as the distal radius, vertebral body, and proximal femur, are more metabolically active and are sites where bone loss will occur.

The periosteum is a fibrous membrane that covers the bones except at the articulating surfaces. The outer layer of the periosteum is composed of collagenous tissue and some fat cells, and the inner layer is composed of elastic fibers. The periosteum allows for the passage of nerve and blood vessels into haversian canals and contains an osteogenic layer of osteoblasts that are responsible for bone growth and repair. The inner layer, the endosteum, is a thin membrane lining the medullary (central) canal and contains both osteoblasts and osteoclasts. Within the medullary canal is the yellow marrow that consists of mainly fatty tissue.[1,2]

Microscopic Structure

The basic unit of cortical bone is an osteon that consists of lamellae and a central channel. Within this structure, blood vessels and nerves are situated longitudinally along the length of the bone. Collagen fibers are deposited concentrically in a layer-to-layer orientation around the blood vessels and nerves. This is known as the lamella, and the canal that is formed by the lamella around the blood vessels and nerves is the haversian canal. In between the lamellae, there are small cavities called lacunae. Osteocytes, which are osteoblasts with maintenance duties, are found in the lacunae. These lacunae are connected to the central haversian canal via canaliculi. The haversian canals of each osteon are connected by Volkmann's canals.[1,5]

In cancellous bone, instead of the lamellae being deposited in a concentric manner, they are deposited in parallel.[5] There are no osteons in cancellous bone. It consists of an irregular latticework of thin bone known as trabeculae. Lacunae and osteocytes are also found within the trabeculae. Nourishment is received directly from the blood vessels of the periosteum that penetrate through the trabeculae.[1,6]

PHYSIOLOGY

The pertinent bone physiology for this pattern relates to bone growth or bone modeling and bone remodeling. Three different types of bone cells are involved with bone modeling and bone remodeling: osteoblasts, osteocytes, and osteoclasts. Osteoblasts are known as bone-forming cells since they produce substances for the extracellular matrix where ossification and calcification occur.[4] When the osteoblast is surrounded by extracellular matrix and is in a state of

low level/decreased activity, it is known as an osteocyte. The exact function of osteocytes is not known, but it is believed that they play a role in transmitting information for bone resorption and formation.[3,4] In contrast to bone formation, bone resorption is the function of osteoclasts.

Prior to maturation of the skeleton, bone modeling occurs to promote skeletal growth. During childhood and teenage years, new bone is added faster than old bone is removed. As a result, bones become larger, heavier, and denser. Bone formation continues at a pace faster than resorption until peak bone mass (maximum bone density and strength) is reached around age 30. In reality, only a small increase in bone mass is experienced by most after the age of 20.[7] The process of bone remodeling occurs in the matured adult skeleton. This process attempts to balance the activities of bone resorption (breakdown) and bone formation (rebuilding).[3]

In addition to its role in skeletal integrity, remodeling is important for mineral homeostasis. The bones serve as stores of calcium, magnesium, phosphorous, and sodium and regulate the blood levels of these substances. The regulation of these minerals involves complex processes that rely on interdependent feedback mechanisms. Multiple compounds in the body can control the activity of bone cells and/or the intestine and kidneys that will directly affect the concentration of the minerals circulating in the body. Of these compounds, there are three main hormones identified: calcitonin, parathyroid hormone (PTH), and vitamin D. Each hormone influences the level of plasma calcium. Normal serum levels of calcium have a narrow range between 9 and 11 mg/100 mL and are under the control of the nervous system. In the state of hypercalcemia, when levels are greater than 11 mg, cells in the thyroid gland release calcitonin.[1,2] The calcitonin then stimulates calcium salt deposit (hydroxyapatite) into the osteoid and inhibits osteoclastic resorption.[3] In the state of hypocalcemia when levels fall below 9 mg, the parathyroid releases PTH that activates osteoclasts to degrade the matrix and release calcium into the blood. PTH also increases plasma calcium levels by resorption of calcium in the kidneys. Vitamin D, which is now considered a hormone, in its active form allows for calcium absorption through the small intestine; thus elevating plasma calcium levels. For vitamin D to be turned into its active form, it is converted first by skin via ultraviolet light after it is ingested in the body and then by the liver and kidneys.[1,2]

Other hormones, such as growth hormones, glucocorticosteroids, estrogen, and progesterone, affect bone metabolism, but they are not controlled by the feedback mechanisms of calcium levels in the plasma. Of these other hormones, glucocorticoids and estrogen affect bone formation, glucocorticoids will decrease osteoblastic activity, and estrogen will decrease osteoclastic activity.[3]

PATHOPHYSIOLOGY

Osteoporosis has been defined by the National Institutes of Health (NIH) in the following way: "Osteoporosis, or porous bone, is a disease characterized by low bone mass and structural deterioration of bone tissue, leading to bone fragility and an increased susceptibility to fractures of the hip, spine, and wrist."[8] According to the World Health Organization (WHO), the definition of osteoporosis and osteopenia are based on bone mineral density (BMD) at any skeletal site in white women. The BMD is used as a predictor of future fractures. The BMD is expressed as a t score (in standard deviations) that is the comparison of BMD to young normal adults. The following are the definitions established by WHO:

♦ Normal is less than 1 standard deviation (SD) above or below peak mean.

♦ Osteopenia is 1 SD below peak mean, but not more than 2.5 SD.

♦ Osteoporosis is more than 2.5 SD below peak mean.

♦ Severe osteoporosis is more than 2.5 SD below peak mean with sustained fracture.[9]

Since this definition is based on the comparison to young normal female adults (reference population), there are limitations of defining osteoporosis and osteopenia in this manner. This definition cannot account for men, younger people before the acquisition of peak bone mass, and non-white individuals. In addition, BMD values do not provide information regarding bone geometry, bone quality, and the time when peak bone mass was achieved.[10]

After age 30, the approximate age when peak bone mass is attained, regardless of sex, bone resorption slowly begins to exceed bone formation. The effect is loss of bone mass. Hence, this loss of bone mass is an age-related phenomenon. Osteoporosis develops when bone resorption occurs too quickly or if replacement occurs too slowly. It is more likely to develop if one did not reach optimal bone mass during the bone-building years.[8] In females, bone loss is most rapid in the first few years after menopause but persists into the postmenopausal years.[11]

Thinning of the bone matrix in osteoporosis occurs as a result of the changes in the activity of the cells that are responsible for maintaining the physiology of bone. Factors that affect cell activity are hormones and age. In Type I, or postmenopausal osteoporosis, the decrease in estrogen levels increases osteoclastic activity. Osteoclasts will decrease matrix thickness and calcification especially in cancellous bone. Sites of trabecular bone loss include the vertebral body, distal forearm, ankle, mandible, and maxilla, resulting in tooth loss.[12] Type I osteoporosis usually occurs 15 to 20 years after menopause.[12] Type II or age-related (senile) osteoporosis begins in the third decade with bone density changes usually occurring at osteopenic/osteoporotic levels above the age of 70.[4] It occurs in both genders but it is twice as common in women.[12] The gradual loss of bone is due to the drop in vitamin D synthesis (leads to lack of calcium absorption) or increased parathyroid activity (increases osteoclastic activity).[2] Bone loss occurs in both cortical and cancellous bone.[12] Common fracture sites associated with Type II osteoporosis occur at the hip, pelvis, proximal humerus, and/or proximal tibia.[12]

Secondary osteoporosis occurs as a result of specific, defined clinical disorders, such as hypogonadism, celiac disease, and inflammatory bowel disease, or from the effects of glucocorticoid medications.[8,10]

The NIH no longer considers osteoporosis to be age or gender dependent. Previous studies focused on the postmenopausal female population; however, increasing research has been published on men. One in eight men over the age of 50 years experiences an osteoporosis-related fracture in his lifetime. Men account for 30% of all hip fractures, and they lose BMD at a rate of up to 1% per year with advancing age.[13]

IMAGING

All of the methods used to assess BMD measure the bones' ability to absorb the radiation and/or sound waves to determine their density. The density is measured via the grams of calcium hydroxyapatite per square centimeter. The following imaging techniques may be used for BMD screening according to the National Osteoporosis Foundation.[14] All of the following techniques are considered to be good indicators of future fracture.

♦ DXA or DEXA=Dual energy x-ray absorptiometry measures the spine, hip, or wrist; measures area bone density, gold standard

♦ pDXA=Peripheral dual energy x-ray absorptiometry measures the forearm, finger, or heel

♦ SXA=Single energy x-ray absorptiometry measures the forearm, finger, or heel

♦ QCT=Quantitative computed tomography most commonly used to measure the trabecular bone density at the spine, but can be used at other sites; measures volumetric bone density, higher levels of radiation

♦ pQCT=Peripheral quantitative computed tomography measures the wrist

♦ US densiometry=Ultrasound densiometry uses sound waves to measure density at the calcaneus, tibia, and patella

In addition to BMD tests, metabolic evaluations may be necessary to investigate possible secondary causes of osteoporosis. One such common test is the urine N-telopeptide analysis (NTX). It is used as a marker of bone breakdown and indicates current levels of bone loss (ie, it tells about bone resorption). In certain individuals where bone loss occurs in atypical clinical presentations (eg, multiple fractures with normal/near normal bone density), a bone biopsy is used to rule out other metabolic bone disorders such as osteomalacia and mastocytosis. A bone biopsy provides information regarding the pathophysiology of bone loss.[15]

PHARMACOLOGY

The following pharmacological agents are recommended by the National Osteoporosis Foundation for the management of patients/clients who are at risk of skeletal demineralization.[14]

- Bis- (or di-) phosphonates (antiresorptive meds)[14]
  - Examples: Alendronate (Fosamax), Risedronate (Actonel)
  - Actions: Impair osteoclast function and thus reduce bone resorption, and inhibit osteoclastic activity. Have been shown to increase BMD and reduce fracture risk
  - Administered: By mouth
  - Studies: Over 3 to 4 years bisphosphonate use led to:
    - Increased BMD in hip by 5% and spine by 7%
    - Reduced risk of vertebral fracture by 48%
    - Reduced loss of height and progression of vertebral deformities
    - Reduced hip and wrist fractures by 50%
  - Side effects: Nausea, abdominal pain, dyspepsia, esophagitis, esophageal or gastric ulcer
- Calcitonin[14]
  - Example: Salmon calcitonin (Miacalcin)
  - Action: Is an antiresorptive agent that targets osteoclasts directly
  - Administered: As a nasal spray or subcutaneous injection
  - Studies:
    - Decreases vertebral fracture rate between 21% and 54%
  - Side effects: Rhinitis and rarely epistaxis
- Estrogen/hormone therapy (ET/HT)[14]
  - ET examples: Climara, Estrace, Estraderm, Estratab, Ogen, Ortho-Est, Premarin, Vivelle
  - Action: Antiresorptive agent
  - Administered: By mouth or patch
  - Studies:
    - Reduced risk of vertebral fractures and hip fractures by 34%
  - Side effect: May increase risk of breast cancer[16]
- PTH[14]
  - Example: Forteo
  - Action: Is an anabolic agent

- Administered: By subcutaneous injection
- Studies: After 18 months of use
  - Decreases risk of vertebral fractures by 65%
  - Decreases risk of nonvertebral fractures by 54%
- Side effects: Not known in humans; in rats caused increased incidence of osteosarcoma
- Raloxiphene[14]
  - Example: Evista
  - Actions: Is a bone anabolic agent; has ability to inhibit the death of osteoblasts
  - Administered: By mouth
  - Studies:
    - Noted 15% to 40% increases in vertebral bone mass over 2 years
  - Side effects: Increases risk of deep vein thrombosis (DVT) and increases hot flashes

In addition, the following drugs that the patient/client may be taking or may have been taking may lead to osteoporosis.

- Aluminum[14]
  - Examples: Aluminum-containing antacids
  - Results of use:
    - May lead to deposits of aluminum in bone preventing normal deposition of calcium
  - Used for treatment of: Gastrointestinal problems, excessive hydrochloric acid secretion
- Anticonvulsants[14]
  - Examples: Phenytoin (Dilantin) and phenobarbital
  - Results of use:
    - Cause bone loss
  - Used for treatment of: Seizure disorders
- Glucocorticosteroids (corticosteroids, steroids)[14]
  - Examples: Cortisone, hydrocortisone, prednisone, prednisolone, methylprednisolone, dexamethasone
  - Results of use:
    - Decrease amount of calcium absorbed from food and increase loss of calcium in urine
    - Suppress numbers, lifespan, and function of osteoblasts
    - Decrease bone formation, decrease the number of osteoid seams, lower mineral apposition rate, and reduce trabecular thickness[17]
    - Estimated that up to 50% of longer term users of glucocorticoids (greater than 1 year) have osteoporosis and a large proportion of them will suffer from fractures[18]
  - Used for treatment of: Rheumatoid arthritis (RA), respiratory conditions, gastrointestinal disorders, thyroid conditions, multiple myeloma
- Thyroxine[14]
  - Examples: Thyroid hormones

- Results of use:
  - Excessive amounts cause bone removal to exceed bone formation
  - Decrease bone mass
- Used for treatment of: Underactive thyroid conditions
- Cytoxic drugs[14]
  - Examples: Methotrexate, Adriamycin
  - Results of use:
    - Cause bone loss because of toxic effects on bone-forming cells
  - Used for treatment of: Cancer and immune disorders
- Immunosuppressants
  - Example: Cyclosporine A
  - Results of use:
    - Leads to bone loss
    - Often used in conjunction with glucocorticoids, which may lead to increased bone loss
  - Used for treatment of: Patients who have undergone transplants and patients with autoimmune diseases
- Heparin[14]
  - Examples: Calciparine, Liquaemin
  - Results of use:
    - Believed to increase the rate of bone breakdown and impair bone formation
  - Used for treatment of: Clotting disorders
- Cholestyramine and colestipol[14]
  - Example: Questran
  - Results of use:
    - Decreases absorption of vitamin D and may lead to reduced calcium absorption
  - Used for treatment of: High blood cholesterol levels

Case Study #1: Osteopenia

Mrs. Mary Garcia is a 49-year-old healthy female, menopausal, previous smoker (one to two packs per day for 20 years), non-exerciser. DEXA reveals t score of -1.0 SD at the femoral neck and -2.0 SD at the lumbar spine.

PHYSICAL THERAPIST EXAMINATION

HISTORY

- General demographics: Mrs. Garcia is a 49-year-old Hispanic female whose primary language is English and her native language is Spanish. She is right-hand domi-

nant. She is a college graduate.
- Social history: Mrs. Garcia is married and is the mother of a son, age 26, and a daughter, age 24.
- Employment/work: She is a third-grade teacher in a local elementary school.
- Living environment: She lives on the seventh floor of an apartment with an elevator.
- General health status
  - General health perception: Mrs. Garcia reports the status of her health to be good.
  - Physical function: Her reported physical function is normal for her age.
  - Psychological function: Normal.
  - Role function: Teacher, wife, mother.
  - Social function: She is involved in tutoring children with English as a second language and in church activities. She enjoys reading and knitting.
- Social/health habits: Mrs. Garcia was a smoker for 20 years at one to two packs/day. She stopped 10 years ago.
- Family history: Her mother had osteoporosis with a history of three spinal fractures.
- Medical/surgical history: Mrs. Garcia's menopausal symptoms started at the age of 47. There was no other significant medical or surgical history.
- Prior hospitalizations: She was hospitalized for the birth of each child.
- Preexisting medical and other health-related conditions: Noncontributory. No history of falls.
- Current condition(s)/chief complaint(s): Mrs. Garcia does not want to sustain the same fractures her mother did as a result of osteoporosis. She wants to avoid a rounded back.
- Functional status and activity level: She is totally independent in all activities of daily living (ADL) and instrumental activities of daily living (IADL). She has been a non-exerciser.
- Medications: Mrs. Garcia is taking 1000 mg of calcium/day.
- Other clinical tests: Written DEXA report revealed t score of -1.0 SD at the femoral neck and -2.0 SD at the lumbar spine.

SYSTEMS REVIEW

- Cardiovascular/pulmonary
  - Blood pressure (BP): 130/82 mmHg
  - Edema: None
  - Heart rate (HR): 70 bpm
  - Respiratory rate (RR): 13 bpm
- Integumentary
  - Presence of scar formation: None

- Skin color: Within normal limits (WNL)
- Skin integrity: WNL

♦ Musculoskeletal
- Gross range of motion: Limited (from upper quarter screen)
- Gross strength: Limited (from upper and lower quarter screens)
- Gross symmetry: Symmetrical
- Height: 5'2" (1.57 m)
- Weight: 110 lbs (49.9 kg)

♦ Neuromuscular
- Balance: Minimally unsteady
- Locomotion, transfers, and transitions: WNL

♦ Communication, affect, cognition, language, and learning style: WNL
- Communication, affect, and cognition: Alert and able to communicate needs
- Learning preferences: Visual learner

TESTS AND MEASURES

♦ Aerobic capacity/endurance
- Rockport Walking test (1-mile walk as fast as possible) revealed fitness category at lower end of average (walked 1 mile in 19 minutes with a heart rate of 146) (Norms for ages 40 to 49: high=heart rate of 100 to 200 in 10 to 15 minutes, average=heart rate of 100 to 200 in 17.5 to 19.5 minutes, low=heart rate of 130 to 200 in over 22 minutes)[19]

♦ Anthropometric characteristics
- Body mass index (BMI)=705 x (body weight [in pounds] divided by height[2] [in inches]). Mrs. Garcia's BMI was 20.17 (WHO normal standard for women=19.1 to 25.8)[20,21]
- Skin fold thickness subscapular and suprailiac: Percentage of body fat was 20.3% and 21% respectively (16% to 25% is ideal for women)

♦ Arousal, attention, and cognition
- Outcome Expectations for Exercise (OEE)[22] indicated awareness of exercise benefits

♦ Environmental, home, and work barriers: None

♦ Ergonomics and body mechanics
- Analysis of body mechanics during self-care, home management, work, community, and leisure actions, tasks, and activities revealed difficulty with overhead activities, prolonged standing activities, and altered posture during all activities, poor spinal proprioception (ie, postural awareness)

♦ Gait, locomotion, and balance
- One-Legged Stance test revealed ability to maintain one-legged stance for only three (norm=five) of the 30-second trials[23]

♦ Motor function
- Observation of dexterity, coordination, and agility revealed activities WNL

♦ Muscle performance
- Dynamometry revealed grip strength of 18 kg (normal 23 kg) of dominant side (R)[24,25]
- Manual muscle testing (MMT) revealed the following deviations from normal:
  - Thoracic spine extension=3/5
  - Lower abdominals=2/5
  - Scapular adduction R=3/5, L=3/5
  - Scapula depression R=3/5, L=3/5
  - Upper extremity (UE) shoulder flexion R and L=4/5
  - UE shoulder extension R and L=4/5
  - UE shoulder abduction R and L=4/5
  - UE shoulder external rotators R and L=4/5
  - Lower extremity (LE) hip abductors R and L=4/5
  - LE hip extensors R and L=4+/5

♦ Posture
- Observational assessment and grid photographs revealed:
  - Forward head
  - Moderately increased thoracic spine kyphosis
  - Slightly decreased lumbar spine lordosis
  - Slight scapular abduction
  - Genu recurvatum 2 degrees on right
  - Bilateral hallux valgus
  - Pes planus bilaterally

♦ Range of motion
- Joint active and passive movement
  - Cervical spine range of motion (ROM) (cervical range of motion device [CROM])
    ▸ Flexion=0 to 45 degrees
    ▸ Extension=0 to 50 degrees
    ▸ Rotation=R 0 to 48 degrees and L 0 to 44 degrees
    ▸ Lateral flexion=R 0 to 20 degrees and L 0 to 22 degrees
  - Thoracic spine ROM (inclinometer)
    ▸ Flexion=0 to 44 degrees
    ▸ Extension=0 degrees
  - Lumbar spine ROM (inclinometer)
    ▸ Flexion=0 to 45 degrees
    ▸ Extension=0 to 15 degrees
    ▸ Lateral flexion=R 0 to 20 degrees and L 0 to 22 degrees
  - Apley's scratch test using distance between second fingers was 9 inches with right upper extremity (RUE) flexion and 11 inches with left upper

extremity (LUE) flexion
- ■ Shoulder ROM (goniometer)
  - ▸ Flexion=R 0 to 150 degrees and L 0 to 155 degrees
  - ▸ Extension=R 0 to 40 degrees and L 0 to 35 degrees
  - ▸ Abduction=R 0 to 145 degrees and L 0 to 150 degrees
  - ▸ External rotation (ER)=R 0 to 70 degrees and L 0 to 65 degrees
  - ▸ Internal rotation (IR)=R 0 to 70 degrees and L 0 to 68 degrees
- ■ Hip ROM (goniometer)
  - ▸ Extension=0 degrees
  - ▸ Flexion, abduction, adduction, and external and internal rotation: WNL
- ● Muscle length, soft tissue extensibility
  - ■ Thomas test revealed bilateral minimal hip flexor tightness=R 4 degrees and L 5 degrees
  - ■ Straight leg raise (SLR) test=R 0 to 60 degrees and L 0 to 68 degrees
  - ■ Prone knee flexion: Tight right rectus femoris=0 to 100 degrees
- ◆ Self-care and home management
  - ● Interview concerning ability to safely perform self-care and home management actions, tasks, and activities revealed that they could be done, but difficulty was noted with overhead activities, forward bending, and heavy tasks
- ◆ Work, community, and leisure integration or reintegration
  - ● Interview concerning ability to safely manage work, community, and leisure actions, tasks, and activities revealed that they could be done, but difficulty was noted with overhead activities, forward bending, and heavy tasks

EVALUATION

Mrs. Garcia's history and risk factors previously outlined indicated that she is a menopausal female, previous smoker, non-exerciser, and has a family history of osteoporosis. Her aerobic fitness is only fair. She has poor balance; faulty posture; decreased muscle performance in her thoracic spine, scapula, and UE muscles; and decreased ROM in her spine and UEs and LEs. She also has difficulty with overhead activities, forward bending, and heavy tasks during her ADL and IADL.

DIAGNOSIS

Mrs. Garcia is a client at risk of skeletal demineralization that may lead to osteoporosis. She has impaired: aerobic capacity/endurance; ergonomics and body mechanics; bal-

ance; muscle performance; posture; and range of motion. She is functionally limited in self-care and home management and in work, community, and leisure actions, tasks, and activities. These findings are consistent with placement in Pattern A: Primary Prevention/Risk Reduction for Skeletal Demineralization. The identified impairments and functional limitations will be addressed in determining the prognosis and the plan of care.

PROGNOSIS AND PLAN OF CARE

Over the course of the visits, the following mutually established outcomes have been determined:
- ◆ Ability to perform physical actions, tasks, and activities related to self-care, home management, work, community, and leisure is improved with improved body mechanics
- ◆ Aerobic capacity and endurance are increased
- ◆ Balance is improved
- ◆ Energy expenditure per unit of work is decreased
- ◆ Fitness is improved
- ◆ Knowledge of behaviors that foster healthy habits, wellness, and prevention is increased
- ◆ Muscle performance is increased
- ◆ Physical capacity is improved
- ◆ Postural control/spinal proprioception is improved
- ◆ Risk factors (decreased physical activity, balance, ROM, muscle performance) are reduced
- ◆ Risk of secondary impairment (such as altered posture, increase risk of falls, fracture) is reduced
- ◆ ROM is increased

To achieve these outcomes, the appropriate interventions for this client are determined. These will include: coordination, communication, and documentation; patient/client-related instruction; therapeutic exercise; functional training in self-care and home management; and functional training in work, community, and leisure integration or reintegration.

Based on the diagnosis and the prognosis, Mrs. Garcia is expected to require six visits over 8 weeks. Mrs. Garcia has good social support, is motivated, and follows through with her home exercise program. She is not severely impaired and is healthy.

INTERVENTIONS

RATIONALE FOR SELECTED INTERVENTIONS

Therapeutic Exercise

Exercise is the choice of physical therapist intervention for individuals with osteoporosis or osteopenia. Exercise is not only an intervention that may maximize bone mass, but it may also address other impairments associated with the condition.

Kyphotic postural change is the "most physically disfiguring and psychologically damaging effect of osteoporosis."[26] Progressive kyphotic postural changes may predispose an individual to back pain, increase the risk of falls, alter balance sway, increase the chance of vertebral fractures, and alter respiratory function.[26-28] It has also been found that back extensor strength was negatively correlated with the number of vertebral compression fractures.[29]

Disuse results in bone mass loss. Sedentary individuals in general have less bone mass than exercising individuals. Exercise prevents or slows the gradual loss of BMD occurring after the 40th year and the more rapid loss in women at menopause. Exercise leads to: 1) increased osteoblastic activity, 2) increased muscle mass and strength, 3) endogenous electrical activity inducing bone formation, and 4) increased serum osteocalcin. Exercise promotes growth hormone release from the pituitary gland, which in turn increases bone formation.[30,31]

Weightbearing is essential for increasing bone mineralization. Activities with high skeletal impact (walking, running, aerobics, dancing) are usually recommended. Wolff's law states that "the bone elements place or displace themselves in the direction of functional forces, and increase or decrease their mass to reflect the amount of the functional forces."[32]

Huddleston found high BMD in the dominant arm of lifetime tennis players as compared to the nondominant control arm, a finding that supported a regional effect of exercise on bone.[33] Studies have analyzed BMD following strenuous physical activity, aerobic activity, and weight training. Higher bone density was found in active individuals, especially those engaging in strong skeletal loading.[34-36]

Grove and Londeree looked at high vs low impact exercise and found little difference in BMD between groups. Both groups did better than non-exercising controls.[37]

Bassey and Ramsdale studied two groups of premenopausal women who exercised weekly in class and daily at home for 1 year. The experimental group did intermittent high-impact exercise, and the control group did low-impact exercise. At 6 months, the experimental group had an increase of 3.4% in trochanteric bone density. At 6 months, the groups changed programs. At the end of 1 year, the original control group had a significant increase of 4.1% in trochanteric density, while the other group maintained their improvement relative to baseline.[38]

The use of a weighted vest was found to significantly decrease pain, improve physical functioning, and increase bone density by 1%. Women with osteoporosis were found to have significantly lower back extensor strength than normal women, and the weighted vest improved function.[39] The weighted vest was also found to prevent hip bone loss in postmenopausal women.[40]

Wolff in a meta-analysis of randomized control trials found that exercise training programs prevented or reversed bone loss of almost 1% per year at the lumbar spine and femoral neck as compared with controls in both pre- and postmenopausal women. The exercise training program for subjects with osteopenia included several types of exercises: endurance, strength, and high-impact.[41] Kemmler also noted increased bone density of the lumbar spine and increased isometric maximum strength (trunk, hips, elbows, and grip) in women with osteopenia after 14 months of an exercise program performed twice per week at home and twice per week in a clinic. The exercise program consisted of endurance exercises, jumping, strength training, and stretching.[42]

Exercises that do not impact directly on bone are also of significant value for fracture risk reduction.[8] Women with osteoporosis and kyphotic postures improved on balance scores measured on computerized posturography with balance exercises and back extensor strengthening exercises.[29] Sinaki and associates studied the relationship between back extensor strength and posture. They concluded that back extensor strength correlated negatively with thoracic kyphosis,[43] and, in addition, back extensor strength was negatively correlated with the number of vertebral compression fractures.[29]

In addition to exercises, client education that serves the purpose of reducing negative emotions associated with osteoporosis is important. This is critical since there is a significant level of fear and anxiety that develops after an individual is diagnosed with osteoporosis.[26,27] Gold suggested that "long-term management of the anxiety associated with osteoporosis should include at least three components: education, exercise, and empowerment."[28]

COORDINATION, COMMUNICATION, AND DOCUMENTATION

Communication will occur with Mrs. Garcia and her family members to engender support for her exercise program. All elements of the client's management will be documented. A referral to a nutritionist/dietitian will be made to ensure an appropriate diet for enhancing bone density.

PATIENT/CLIENT-RELATED INSTRUCTION

The client will be instructed in the risk factors related to osteopenia and osteoporosis, the importance of exercise, the need to continue to eliminate smoking, and the appropriateness of diet modifications. Mrs. Garcia's family will understand the importance of exercise especially as osteoporosis may be a familial risk, the exercise routine, the need to provide support for the client, ways of providing reminders to the client to ensure that her interventions are done, and ways of participating in the client's physical therapy program.

Mrs. Garcia will also understand the need for stress management.[44,45] Particular emphasis will be placed upon the following as they relate to potential alteration in BMD as a result of increased stress:

♦ Stress creates a drain on the adrenal glands
♦ Adrenalin production is increased
♦ Metabolism is increased
♦ Calcium depletion occurs
♦ Phosphorous and potassium depletion occurs
♦ Vitamin B and C depletion occurs

Potential information related to diet modification that may be given to Mrs. Garcia may include the following:

♦ Eliminate the negatives (eg, sugar, caffeine, alcohol)
♦ Eat foods high in calcium (eg, milk products, yogurt, cheese, beans, cauliflower, kale, almonds, walnuts, carrots, figs, shellfish, spinach, turnips)
♦ Recommended calcium supplements[14,46]:
  • Women 51 to 70 years: 1200 mg (safe upper limit 2500 mg/day)
  • Women over 70 years: 1200 mg (safe upper limit 2500 mg/day)

Supplement Form	% Elemental Calcium
Calcium carbonate	40%
Calcium phosphate/tribasic	39%
Calcium phosphate/dibasic	30%
Calcium citrate	21%
Calcium lactate	13%
Calcium gluconate	9%

  • To be effective, it is important that a calcium supplement break up rapidly. If the pill passes whole into the intestine, its benefit will be lost. To test, place the pill in a glass of warm water or vinegar and stir every few minutes. If the pill is not at least 75% broken up within 30 minutes, it probably is not delivering its full measure of calcium[47]
  • Antacids as a source of calcium: Be careful of the amount of aluminum rather than calcium in the antacid that may lead to an increased loss of calcium through the kidney[48]
  • Believed that majority of calcium supplements are most effective when taken with meals or at bed time[47]
  • Recommended to not take more than 500 to 600 mg of calcium at one time, but taking it all at once is better than not taking the calcium[47]
  • Drink a glass of liquid with each supplement to promote disintegration and absorption
  • Possibility that high intake of calcium may contribute to kidney stones in those susceptible to the problem. Have client consult physician[49]
♦ Take 400 to 800 international units (IU) of vitamin D daily that may be combined with the calcium supplement or may be taken separately

THERAPEUTIC EXERCISE

♦ Aerobic capacity/endurance conditioning
  • Parameters for aerobic capacity/endurance conditioning[50-53]
    ■ Mode
      ‣ Aerobic
      ‣ Use of large muscles
      ‣ Continuous or for prolonged period
      ‣ Examples: Weightbearing, walking, treadmill, climbing machine, elliptical trainer, hiking, aerobics classes, jump rope
    ■ Duration
      ‣ Minimum of 20 to 30 minutes before any other parameters are altered
      ‣ Increase duration progressively
      ‣ Goal is a minimum of 40 to 50 minutes
    ■ Intensity
      ‣ Determine the training intensity: For example, usually 60%, 70%, or 80% of the target heart rate (THR), but may be much lower depending on fitness level
      ‣ Determine the maximum heart rate (MHR): 220 minus the age
      ‣ Determine the THR: THR=MHR minus the resting heart rate (RHR) times the training intensity (%) plus the RHR
      ‣ Teach client to count pulse at rest and during exercise
      ‣ Determine appropriate perceived exertion: Borg Scale (10-point non-linear scale)[54]
        ○ 0=Nothing at all
        ○ 0.5=Very, very light/weak (just noticeable)
        ○ 1=Very light/weak
        ○ 2=Light/weak
        ○ 3=Moderate
        ○ 4=Somewhat heavy/strong
        ○ 5=Heavy/strong
        ○ 6
        ○ 7=Very heavy/strong
        ○ 8
        ○ 9
        ○ 10=Extremely heavy/strong (almost maximal)
        ○ Maximal
      ‣ Determine lactate threshold: Talk test—Begin aerobic exercise (treadmill, bicycle, jump rope, etc) slowly; increase intensity while carrying on a conversation until it is difficult to speak; take pulse; slow down until can carry on conversation again; repeat three times and divide by three to get lactate threshold[55]

- Frequency
  - ▸ Start with three to four times per week unless period of exercise is less than 15 minutes
  - ▸ Progress to six times a week (ideally). If walking program is selected, strive for 3 miles in 45 minutes, 5 to 6 days/week
- Maintenance
  - ▸ When achieved desired fitness level: Three to four times per week

♦ Balance, coordination, and agility training
- Balance for as long as possible while standing bilaterally and unilaterally eyes open and eyes closed, and while standing bilaterally and unilaterally in plantarflexion and dorsiflexion eyes open and eyes closed
- Standing balance on increasingly softer foam surfaces
- Balance exercises in quadruped, kneeling, or standing on Both Sides Up Balance Trainer (BOSU)
- Balance exercises lying or standing on foam rollers incorporating arm and leg movements
- Exercise ball: Balance training
- Yoga "tree" posture with increasing difficulty with foot placement on opposite leg
- High step march in place
- Tandem walking: Walking down a hallway placing the heel of the advancing foot directly in front of the toes of the supporting foot
- Side stepping: Down a hallway
- Carioca: Going down a hallway by side stepping right, crossing left in back of right, side stepping right, crossing left in front of right; then return side stepping left, crossing right in back of left, side stepping left, crossing right in front of left

♦ Body mechanics and postural stabilization: Decrease forward head and rounded shoulders, thoracic kyphosis, increase abdominal and back extensor tone
- Body mechanics training
  - Chin in, stomach in, lower scapula borders pinched together
  - Instructions in sitting, standing, ADL, IADL especially bending and lifting
  - Special instructions for computer use
- Postural control training and postural stabilization exercises: Axial extension of head, slight scapula retraction, abdominal contraction throughout all exercises
  - Elbow press back: Sitting or standing against wall
  - Elbow press down: Supine with forearms up
  - Flexion, abduction, IR/ER UEs
  - Abdominal strengthening (avoid thoracic flex-

ion): Isometrics, on Styrofoam rollers building to core stabilization coordinated with arm and leg movements, sitting knees up and 1/2 lower downs (eccentric contractions keeping spine straight)
  - Bridging: Add leg movement
  - Quadruped: Neutral spine, coordinate with arm and leg movements
  - Prone (if possible): On elbows, press up
  - Prone: Plank position, modified push-ups
  - Sitting: Stomach in, chin in; arms up; elbow press back; pectoralis stretch
  - Exercise ball: Arm and leg exercises with trunk stabilization
  - Standing: Posture, arm pull downs
  - Standing: "W" position of arms, wall slide
  - Postural alignment during gait: Book or pillow on top of head
- Posture awareness training
  - Notes all around home, car, office
  - Use mirror for visual input of appropriate alignment

♦ Flexibility exercises
- Stretching exercises should be done after warming up, using a slow and steady stretch accompanied by deep breathing, and building hold up to 30 to 60 seconds
- Neck ROM
- Trunk ROM (avoid excessive flexion)
- Hamstring stretch: Supine, sitting (keeping trunk straight, hinging at the hips and not rounding the spine)
- Hip flexor stretch
- Quadriceps/rectus femoris stretch
- Apley's position for flexibility
- Wall stretch anterior chest

♦ Relaxation
- Breathing exercises
- Breathing while stretching and exercising
- Relaxation techniques (eg, Jacobson's)
- Complementary exercise approaches (eg, yoga relaxation techniques)

♦ Strength, power, and endurance training
- Begin with mat progressive resistive exercise (PRE) (arm press ups, flys, overheads, scapula adduction and depression) for UE and trunk strengthening
- UE weight training program with free weights, elastic bands, or machines (eg, overhead press, row, shrugs, flexion, abduction, elbow flexion and extension, wrist flexion and extension, press ups, flys, French curls, latissimus, scapula adduction)
- LE weight training program with free weights, elastic

bands, or machines (eg, squats, lunges, hip flexion, hip extension, hip abduction, hip adduction, hip external and internal rotation, heel rises)

- Progress to quadruped
- Core stabilization of abdominals and back extensors (including use of foam rollers)
- Seated push-ups
- Wall slides
- Plank (yoga position): Straight line push-up position (stomach and chin in strongly)
- Downward dog (yoga position)
- Weighted vest: With removable weights; determine comfortable weight that can be worn for 5 minutes and gradually build up time wearing the vest and then the weight that is worn

Maintenance of a regular exercise program must be instilled in this client. To do this there are several keys that may be helpful in achieving an exercise program that the client will do on a life-long basis. These tips may be included in part of the patient/client-related instruction and may include any or all of the following:

- Establish a variety of enjoyable activities and alternating activities when possible
- Establish a realistic time frame for exercise
- Make exercise a family experience when possible
- Add exercise to one's weekly schedule (walk to work if possible, climb up and down several flights of stairs in her apartment building instead of taking the elevator, wear a weighted vest while at home)
- Find activities that may be done during work hours (climb stairs while she is at work)
- Find activities that may be done after work
- Find fun alternative activities for weekends
- Allow flexibility
- If a scheduled exercise time is missed, work into schedule at another time during the day or week
- Use entertainment whenever possible
  - Music when doing weight exercises or while walking outside
  - TV while on treadmill
  - Books on tape at anytime
- Keep exercise schedule or log

FUNCTIONAL TRAINING IN SELF-CARE AND HOME MANAGEMENT

- Self-care and home management
  - Review all actions, tasks, and activities and postural alignment for self-care and home management
  - Walk to supermarket and carry things evenly weighted in both hands or carry load close to body to reduce the lever arm

- Consider buying aerobic exercise equipment and weights for home
  - One-time expense
  - May be used by other family members
  - Convenient

FUNCTIONAL TRAINING IN WORK, COMMUNITY, AND LEISURE INTEGRATION OR REINTEGRATION

- Work
  - Review all actions, tasks, and activities and postural alignment for work
  - Walk from home, subway, or train station to school
  - Take stairs instead of the elevator
  - Walk down the hall to speak to someone instead of using the phone
  - Stay at hotels with fitness centers
  - Take elastic band and jump rope when traveling
- Leisure
  - Be active and have fun at the same time
  - Plan family outings and vacations to include physical activity

ANTICIPATED GOALS AND EXPECTED OUTCOMES

- Impact on pathology/pathophysiology
  - Osteogenic effects of exercise are maximized.
- Impact on impairments
  - Aerobic capacity is increased to point where the client's HR is lowered and time to complete 1 mile is decreased.
  - Lactate threshold is improved.
  - Balance is improved so that the client can stand on one leg for all five trials.
  - Muscle length is elongated to within functional limits (WFL).
  - Muscle performance is increased to WNL.
  - Postural control is improved, and the client is able to demonstrate proper posture during sitting and standing activities.
  - ROM is increased to WNL.
  - Weightbearing status is improved.
- Impact on functional limitations
  - Ability to perform physical actions, tasks, and activities related to self-care, home management, work, community, and leisure is improved.
  - Client is able to demonstrate proper body mechanics during bending and lifting activities.
  - Client is independent in performance of exercise program.

- Risk reduction/prevention
  - Client is able to verbalize risk factors for skeletal demineralization.
  - Risk factors are reduced.
- Impact on health, wellness, and fitness
  - Behaviors that foster healthy habits, wellness, and prevention are acquired.
  - Fitness is improved.
  - Health status is improved.
  - Physical function is improved.
- Impact on societal resources
  - Documentation occurs throughout the client management and follows APTA's *Guidelines for Physical Therapy Documentation*.[56]
- Patient/client satisfaction
  - Client and family knowledge and awareness of the diagnosis, prognosis, interventions, and anticipated goals and expected outcomes are increased.
  - Sense of well-being is improved.

REEXAMINATION

Reexamination is performed throughout the episode of care.

DISCHARGE

Mrs. Garcia is discharged from physical therapy after a total of six physical therapy sessions and attainment of her goals and expectations. These sessions have covered her entire episode of care. She is discharged because she has achieved her goals and expected outcomes.

Case Study #2: Osteopenia

Mr. Joseph Smith is a 50-year-old healthy male who has been on medications for asthma since childhood. DEXA reveals a t score of -1.5 SD at the lumbar spine.

PHYSICAL THERAPIST EXAMINATION

HISTORY

- General demographics: Mr. Smith is a 50-year-old white male whose primary language is English. He is right-side dominant. He graduated from technical training school.

- Social history: He is married with three children, two sons, ages 10 and 15, and one daughter, age 12.
- Employment/work: Mr. Smith is an aviation mechanic. He works full-time, 5 to 6 days per week, 6 to 8 hours per day.
- Living environment: He lives in a one-level home.
- General health status
  - General health perception: Mr. Smith reports his health status to be good.
  - Physical function: His reported physical function is normal for his age.
  - Psychological function: Normal.
  - Role function: Mechanic, husband, father.
  - Social function: He is involved in Little League Baseball as a coach and is active in the Rotary Club.
- Social/health habits: Mr. Smith smoked one pack per day for 10 years. He is a social drinker (one to five alcoholic beverages per week).
- Family history: His father had a stroke in his late 70s.
- Medical/surgical history: He has had asthma since childhood and pollen allergies.
- Prior hospitalizations: Two hospitalizations as a child for an asthmatic attack.
- Preexisting medical and other health-related conditions: He has a 45-year history of asthma that has been treated with various forms of asthmatic medication.
- Current condition(s)/chief complaint(s): Mr. Smith was diagnosed with osteopenia. He is concerned about the health of his bones and wishes to learn exercises to address this. He also indicated that only his wife and health care professionals know of his condition, a "woman's problem" from his perception.
- Functional status and activity level: He is independent in all ADL, IADL, and able to perform all work-related physical activities without problems. Mr. Smith has no formal exercise program. He occasionally plays ball with his children.
- Medications: Flovent (inhaler), history of Medrol (an oral anti-inflammatory corticosteroid) and Allegra.
- Other clinical tests: The DEXA test revealed a t score of -1.5 SD at the lumbar spine.

SYSTEMS REVIEW

- Cardiovascular/pulmonary
  - BP: 120/76 mmHg
  - Edema: None
  - HR: 72 bpm
  - RR: 14 bpm
- Integumentary
  - Presence of scar formation: None
  - Skin color: WNL

- Skin integrity: WNL
- ◆ Musculoskeletal
  - Gross range of motion: Limited (from lower quarter screen)
  - Gross strength: WNL (from upper and lower quarter screens)
  - Gross symmetry: Symmetrical
  - Height: 5'11" (1.8 m)
  - Weight: 170 lbs (77.1 kg)
- ◆ Neuromuscular
  - Balance: No unsteadiness based on observation
  - Locomotion, transfers, and transitions: WNL
- ◆ Communication, affect, cognition, language, and learning style: WNL
  - Communication and cognition: Alert and able to communicate needs
  - Expected emotional/behavioral responses: Uneasy with discussions about osteopenia/osteoporosis based on Mr. Smith's belief that it is a "woman's problem"
  - Learning preferences: Visual learner

TESTS AND MEASURES

- ◆ Aerobic capacity/endurance
  - Rockport Walking test (1-mile walk as fast as possible) revealed his fitness category to be average (walked 1 mile in 20 minutes with a HR of 135) (Norms for ages 50 to 59: high=HR of 100 to 180 in 10 to 14 minutes, average=HR of 100 to 200 in 17 to 21 minutes, low=HR of 140 to 200 in over 22 minutes)[19]
- ◆ Anthropometric characteristics
  - BMI=23.7 (see Case Study #1)[21]
- ◆ Arousal, attention, and cognition
  - OEE[22] indicated awareness of exercise benefits
- ◆ Environmental, home, and work barriers: None
- ◆ Ergonomics and body mechanics
  - Analysis of body mechanics during self-care, home management, work, community, and leisure actions, tasks, and activities revealed altered posture during all activities, poor spinal proprioception (ie, postural awareness)
- ◆ Gait, locomotion, and balance
  - Able to maintain balance in work-simulated positions (ie, half-kneel and kneeling)
  - One-Legged Stance test revealed ability to maintain one-legged stance for five 30-second trials[23]
- ◆ Motor function
  - Observation of dexterity, coordination, and agility revealed activities to be WNL
- ◆ Muscle performance
  - MMT revealed 5/5 for BUEs and BLEs (bilateral)

- MMT scores were 5/5 for upper and lower abdominals and 4/5 for back extensors
- ◆ Posture
  - Observational assessment and grid photographs revealed:
    - Slight forward head
    - Moderately increased thoracic spine kyphosis
    - Slightly decreased lumbar spine lordosis
    - Slight scapular abduction bilaterally
- ◆ Range of motion
  - Cervical spine ROM (CROM)
    - Flexion=0 to 30 degrees
    - Extension=0 to 40 degrees
    - Rotation=R 0 to 45 degrees and L 0 to 45 degrees
    - Lateral flexion=R 0 to 20 degrees and L 0 to 25 degrees
  - Thoracic spine ROM (inclinometer)
    - Flexion=0 to 44 degrees
    - Extension=0 to 5 degrees
  - Lumbar spine ROM (inclinometer)
    - Flexion=0 to 30 degrees
    - Extension=0 to 10 degrees
    - Lateral flexion=R 0 to 15 degrees and L 0 to 15 degrees
  - Hip ROM (goniometer)
    - Extension=0 degrees bilaterally
    - Flexion=110 degrees bilaterally
    - External rotation=R 0 to 35 degrees, L 0 to 40 degrees
    - Internal rotation=R 0 to 10 degrees, L 0 to 15 degrees
  - Apley's scratch test using distance between second fingers was 4 inches with RUE flexion and 6 inches with LUE flexion
  - Shoulder ROM: WNL
  - Thomas test revealed bilateral hip flexor tightness=R 8 degrees, L 5 degrees
  - SLR test=R 0 to 65 degrees and L 0 to 65 degrees
  - Prone knee flexion: Tight rectus femoris=R 0 to 95 degrees, L 0 to 105 degrees
  - Ober test revealed bilateral tensor fascia lata/iliotibial band tightness
- ◆ Self-care and home management
  - Interview concerning ability to safely perform self-care and home management actions, tasks, and activities revealed that they could be performed without difficulty
- ◆ Work, community, and leisure integration or reintegration
  - Interview and observation of body mechanics/move-

ment patterns required for work revealed use of poor mechanics for bending and sitting

EVALUATION

Mr. Smith's history indicates the use of glucocorticoid steroid as a risk factor for skeletal demineralization. He has faulty ergonomics and body mechanics while bending and sitting, poor muscle performance in his back extensor muscles, faulty posture, and decreased ROM in his spine and LEs. In addition to these physical findings, Mr. Smith feels that his condition is not socially acceptable for men.

DIAGNOSIS

Mr. Smith is a client at risk of skeletal demineralization. He has impaired: ergonomics and body mechanics; muscle performance; posture; and range of motion. He is functionally limited in work, community, and leisure actions, tasks, and activities. These findings are consistent with placement in Pattern A: Primary Prevention/Risk Reduction for Skeletal Demineralization. The identified impairments and functional limitations will be addressed in determining the prognosis and the plan of care.

PROGNOSIS AND PLAN OF CARE

Over the course of the visits, the following mutually established outcomes have been determined:

♦ Ability to perform physical actions, tasks, and activities related to self-care, home management, work, community, and leisure is improved with improved body mechanics

♦ Fitness is improved

♦ Knowledge of behaviors that foster healthy habits, wellness, and prevention is increased

♦ Muscle performance is increased

♦ Postural control/spinal proprioception is improved

♦ Risk factors (decreased physical activity, ROM, muscle performance, and impaired posture/body mechanics) are reduced

♦ Risk of secondary impairment (such as increased risk of falls, fracture) is reduced

♦ ROM is increased

To achieve these outcomes, the appropriate interventions for this client are determined. These will include: coordination, communication, and documentation; patient/client-related instruction; therapeutic exercise; and functional training in work, community, and leisure integration or reintegration.

Based on the diagnosis and the prognosis, Mr. Smith is expected to require four visits over a 4-week period of time. Mr. Smith has good social support, is motivated, and follows through with his home exercise program. He is not severely impaired and is healthy.

INTERVENTIONS

RATIONALE FOR SELECTED INTERVENTIONS

See Case Study #1 for rationale for exercises.

COORDINATION, COMMUNICATION, AND DOCUMENTATION

Communication will occur with Mr. Smith and his family members to engender support for his exercise program. All elements of the client's management will be documented. A referral to a support group to address Mr. Smith's perception of his current condition as a "woman's problem" will be suggested. In addition, a referral to nutritionist/dietitian will be made to ensure appropriate diet for enhancing bone density.

PATIENT/CLIENT-RELATED INSTRUCTION

The client will be instructed in the risk factors related to osteopenia and osteoporosis, the importance of exercise, and the appropriateness of diet modifications. Mr. Smith will receive instructions in posture and body mechanics, risk factors, and a health/wellness/fitness program. Instructions related to potential effects of stress (refer to Case Study #1) and diet modification will be given to Mr. Smith (refer to Case Study #1). Additional information related to diet modification that may be given to Mr. Smith may include the following:

♦ Recommended calcium supplements[57,58]:

  • Men 25 to 64 years: 1000 mg

  • Men 65+ years: 1500 mg

THERAPEUTIC EXERCISE

♦ Aerobic capacity/endurance conditioning

  • Parameters for aerobic capacity/endurance conditioning (see Case Study #1)[50-53]

    ▪ Mode

      ‣ Aerobic

      ‣ Use of large muscles

      ‣ Continuous or for prolonged period

      ‣ Examples: Weightbearing, walking, treadmill, climbing machine, elliptical trainer, hiking, aerobics classes, jump rope

    ▪ Duration

      ‣ Minimum of 20 to 30 minutes before any other parameters are altered

      ‣ Increase duration progressively

      ‣ Goal is a minimum of 40 to 50 minutes

- Intensity
  - Determine THR: THR=(MHR-RHR) x % + RHR
  - Use 60%-70%-80% of the THR
  - Teach to count pulse at rest and during exercise
  - Determine appropriate perceived exertion
  - Perceived exertion: Borg scale[54] (see Case Study #1)
  - Talk test[55] (see Case Study #1)
- Frequency
  - Start with three to four times per week unless period of exercise is less than 15 minutes
  - Progress to six times a week (ideally). If walking program is selected, strive for 3 miles/hour for 45 minutes, 5 to 6 days/week
- Maintenance
  - When achieved desired fitness level: Three to four times per week
- Body mechanics and postural stabilization
  - Postural control training and postural stabilization activities
    - Decrease forward head and rounded shoulders, thoracic kyphosis, increase abdominal and back extensor tone (see Case Study #1)
    - Abdominal isometric contraction in various positions (supine, quadruped, sitting, and standing)
    - Cervical retraction exercises in sitting and standing
    - Squats, cable column with UE resistance to simulate lifting
    - Weight-shifting of LE in half-kneeling
    - Diagonal UE movement patterns in kneeling
    - Resistive scapular retraction
    - Body Blade exercises
- Flexibility exercises
  - Stretching exercises should be done after warming up, using a slow and steady stretch accompanied by deep breathing, and building hold up to 30 to 60 seconds
  - Hamstring stretch
  - Hip flexor stretch
  - Knee extensors (rectus femoris) stretch
  - Iliotibial band stretch
  - Pectoralis muscle group stretch
  - Neck ROM (all ranges)
  - Trunk ROM (avoid excessive flexion)
- Relaxation
  - Relaxation exercises: Imagery
  - Breathing exercises
  - Breathing while stretching and exercising

- Complementary exercise approaches (eg, yoga relaxation techniques)
- Strength, power, and endurance training (see Case Study #1)

Maintenance of a regular exercise program must be instilled in this client. To do this there are several keys that may be helpful in achieving an exercise program that the client will do on an life-long basis. These tips are included in Case Study #1.

FUNCTIONAL TRAINING IN WORK, COMMUNITY, AND LEISURE INTEGRATION OR REINTEGRATION

- Work
  - Review all actions, tasks, and activities and postural alignment for work
  - Walk from home, subway, or train station to work
  - Take stairs instead of the elevator
  - Walk down the hall to speak to someone instead of using the phone
  - Stay at hotels with fitness centers
  - Take elastic band and jump rope when traveling
- Leisure
  - Be active and have fun at the same time
  - Plan family outings and vacations to include physical activity

ANTICIPATED GOALS AND EXPECTED OUTCOMES

- Impact on pathology/pathophysiology
  - Osteogenic effects of exercise are maximized.
- Impact on impairments
  - Aerobic capacity is increased.
  - Muscle performance of back extensors is increased to 5/5.
  - Postural control is improved.
  - ROM is improved 10% to 15%.
  - Weightbearing status is improved.
- Impact on functional limitations
  - Ability to perform physical actions, tasks, and activities related to self-care, home management, work, community, and leisure is improved.
  - Client is able to demonstrate proper body mechanics during bending and lifting activities.
  - Client is independent in performance of exercise program.
- Risk reduction/prevention
  - Client is able to verbalize risk factors for skeletal demineralization.
  - Risk factors are reduced.

♦ Impact on health, wellness, and fitness
  • Behaviors that foster healthy habits, wellness, and prevention are acquired.
  • Fitness is improved.
  • Health status is improved.
  • Physical function is improved.
♦ Impact on societal resources
  • Documentation occurs throughout the client management and follows APTA's *Guidelines for Physical Therapy Documentation*.[56]
♦ Patient/client satisfaction
  • Client and family knowledge and awareness of the diagnosis, prognosis, interventions, and anticipated goals and expected outcomes are increased.
  • Sense of well-being is improved.

REEXAMINATION

Reexamination is performed throughout the episode of care.

DISCHARGE

Mr. Smith is discharged from physical therapy after a total of four physical therapy sessions and attainment of his goals and expectations. These sessions have covered his entire episode of care. He is discharged because he has achieved his goals and expected outcomes.

Case Study #3: Osteopenia

Ms. Amy Jones is a 25-year-old healthy female marathon runner. DEXA reveals a t score of -1.5 and -2.0 SD at the right and left femoral necks respectively.

PHYSICAL THERAPIST EXAMINATION

HISTORY

♦ General demographics: Amy is a 25-year-old white female whose primary language is English. She is right-side dominant.
♦ Social history: Amy is a graduate student and is currently studying international business.
♦ Employment/work: She is a full-time student.
♦ Living environment: She is living at home with her parents during the summer break.

♦ General health status
  • General health perception: Amy reports the status of her health to be good.
  • Physical function: Her reported physical function is normal for her age.
  • Psychological function: Normal.
  • Role function: Daughter, student.
  • Social function: Student.
♦ Social/health habits: Amy is a competitive marathon runner. She has never smoked. She occasionally has a glass of beer with friends.
♦ Family history: Noncontributory.
♦ Medical/surgical history: Noncontributory.
♦ Prior hospitalizations: None.
♦ Preexisting medical and other health-related conditions: She has had chronic ankle sprains on the left and amenorrhea (last menstrual cycle was 1 year ago).
♦ Current condition(s)/chief complaint(s): Amy reports that she has become deconditioned since spraining her left ankle 2 months ago when she stepped on a small rock while hiking. Because of the pain in her left ankle/foot, she saw her orthopedist who diagnosed a fifth metatarsal (MT) stress fracture. Her fracture is healed and her goal is for a speedy recovery so that she can train again. She also reports that a DEXA was performed a month ago since her doctor was "concerned with the bone strength."
♦ Functional status and activity level: Amy discontinued using crutches and an ankle-foot orthosis 1 week ago. She is independent in all ADL and IADL. She is a full-time graduate student and a competitive marathon runner. Amy ran 5 to 7 days per week. Distance varied from 50 to 90 miles per week depending on training schedule.
♦ Medications: None.
♦ Other clinical tests: Radiographic films of the left foot/ankle revealed a healed fifth MT fracture with good callus formation. DEXA test report revealed t scores of -1.5 and -2.0 SD at the right and left femoral necks respectively.

SYSTEMS REVIEW

♦ Cardiovascular/pulmonary
  • BP: 105/66 mmHg
  • Edema: None
  • HR: 65 bpm
  • RR: 10 bpm
♦ Integumentary
  • Presence of scar formation: None
  • Skin color: WNL
  • Skin integrity: WNL

♦ Musculoskeletal
  • Gross range of motion: Limited in ankle (from lower quarter screen)
  • Gross strength: Limited in ankle (from lower quarter screen)
  • Gross symmetry: Asymmetrical stance
  • Height: 5'6" (1.68 m)
  • Weight: 112 lbs (50.8 kg)
♦ Neuromuscular
  • Balance: No unsteadiness based on observation, but uneven weightbearing
  • Locomotion, transfers, and transitions: WNL
♦ Communication, affect, cognition, language, and learning style: WNL
  • Communication and cognition: Alert and able to communicate needs
  • Expected emotional/behavioral responses: May avoid discussion or acceptance of risk factors of osteopenia/osteoporosis
  • Learning preferences: Visual learner

TESTS AND MEASURES

♦ Aerobic capacity/endurance
  • 1 Mile Walk test[59] (walk 1 mile as quickly as possible; norms are established based on sex and heart rate[60]); heart rate was 110 and her time was 17:08 minutes indicating high fitness level
♦ Anthropometric characteristics
  • BMI=18.1 (underweight)[21] (see Case Study #1)
♦ Arousal, attention, and cognition
  • OEE[22] indicated awareness of exercise benefits
♦ Environmental, home, and work barriers: None
♦ Ergonomics and body mechanics
  • Normal body mechanics during self-care, home management, work, community, and leisure actions, tasks, and activities
♦ Gait, locomotion, and balance
  • She is full weightbearing
  • One-Legged Stance test[23] revealed ability to maintain one-legged stance for five 30-second tries on the right lower extremity (RLE) and only for 10 seconds for each of the five trials on the left lower extremity (LLE)
  • Gait observation revealed decreased stance phase and decreased push-off on the LLE
♦ Motor function
  • Observation of dexterity, coordination, and agility revealed activities to be WNL
♦ Muscle performance
  • MMT revealed 5/5 for bilateral LEs except left plantarflexion, eversion, inversion 4/5, and dorsiflexion 4+/5

  • MMT scores were 5/5 for upper abdominals, lower abdominals, and trunk extensors
♦ Posture
  • No deviations noted on observational assessment
♦ Range of motion
  • Thoracic spine ROM (inclinometer)
    ▪ Flexion=0 to 40 degrees
    ▪ Extension=0 to 20 degrees
  • Lumbar spine ROM (inclinometer)
    ▪ Flexion=0 to 40 degrees
    ▪ Extension=0 to 30 degrees
    ▪ Lateral flexion R=0 to 30 degrees and L=0 to 30 degrees
  • Ankle ROM (goniometer)
    ▪ Dorsiflexion R=30 degrees, L=10 degrees
    ▪ Plantarflexion R=60 degrees, L=30 degrees
    ▪ Eversion R=30 degrees, L=10 degrees
    ▪ Inversion R=40 degrees, L=40 degrees
♦ Self-care and home management
  • Interview concerning ability to safely perform self-care and home management actions, tasks, and activities revealed that they could be performed without difficulty
♦ Work, community, and leisure integration or reintegration
  • Interview concerning ability to safely manage work, community, and leisure actions, tasks, and activities revealed that they could be done without difficulty. However, Amy realizes that her current impairments restrict her from returning to marathon running at this time

EVALUATION

Amy's history and risk factors previously outlined indicated that she is a high intensity physically active female with either primary or secondary amenorrhea, a stress fracture, and low BMI suggests that she exhibits components of the Female Athlete Triad syndrome (consisting of disordered eating, amenorrhea, and osteoporosis).[61] In addition, the examination demonstrates signs that the healing tissues due to the ankle sprain and fifth MT stress fracture are competent to withstand loading forces. However, impairments exist. She has poor balance, decreased muscle performance in her left ankle muscles, and decreased ROM in her LLE. These impairments limit her ability to return to running.

DIAGNOSIS

Amy is a client at risk of further skeletal demineralization. She has impaired: gait, locomotion, and balance; muscle performance; and range of motion. She is functionally limited in work, community, and leisure actions, tasks, and activities. These findings are consistent with placement in Pattern A: Primary Prevention/Risk Reduction for Skeletal Demineralization. The identified impairments and functional limitations will be addressed in determining the prognosis and the plan of care.

PROGNOSIS AND PLAN OF CARE

Over the course of the visits, the following mutually established outcomes have been determined:

♦ Ability to perform physical actions, tasks, and activities related to self-care, home management, work, community, and leisure is improved
♦ Balance is increased
♦ Knowledge of behaviors that foster healthy habits, wellness, and prevention is increased
♦ Muscle performance is increased
♦ Risk factors (decreased physical activity, balance, ROM, muscle performance) are reduced
♦ Risk of secondary impairment (such as increased risk of falls, fracture) is reduced
♦ ROM is increased

To achieve these outcomes, the appropriate interventions for this client are determined. These will include: coordination, communication, and documentation; patient/client-related instruction; therapeutic exercise; and functional training in work, community, and leisure integration or reintegration.

Based on the diagnosis and the prognosis, Amy is expected to require 12 visits over a 12-week period of time.[26] Additional visits may be required to address the additional impairments related to the ankle sprain and fifth MT fracture. Amy has good social support, is motivated, and follows through with her home exercise program. She is not severely impaired and is healthy, but has the additional problem related to her fracture.

INTERVENTIONS

RATIONALE FOR SELECTED INTERVENTIONS

See Case Study #1 for rationale for interventions related to skeletal demineralization.

COORDINATION, COMMUNICATION, AND DOCUMENTATION

Communication will occur with Amy. All elements of the client's management will be documented. A referral to nutritionist/dietitian will be made to ensure appropriate diet

for enhancing bone density and to increase client's weight to normalize BMI. Communication with the physician(s) will include discussions regarding the cause of Amy's report of amenorrhea (diagnostic tests) and current interventions.

PATIENT/CLIENT-RELATED INSTRUCTION

The client will be instructed in the risk factors and consequences related to osteopenia and osteoporosis, the importance of exercise, the need for an appropriate training schedule, the need to avoid overtraining, and the appropriateness of diet modifications.

In addition, Amy will also understand the need for stress management.[45,46] Information related to diet modification may be given to Amy as it relates to her osteopenia (see Case Study #1), and she will be referred to a nutritionist for her low BMI and possible disordered eating. She will also understand the importance of seeing her physician concerning her amenorrhea.

THERAPEUTIC EXERCISE

♦ Aerobic capacity/endurance conditioning
  • Parameters for aerobic capacity/endurance conditioning (see Case Study #1)[51-54]
    ▪ Mode, duration, intensity, and frequency will incorporate aerobic capacity/endurance conditioning activities to return her to her marathon running
♦ Balance, coordination, and agility training
  • Balance/proprioception board
  • Balance machine (eg, Kinesthetic Ability Trainer [KAT])
  • Carioca
  • Box jumps
♦ Flexibility exercises
  • Stretching exercises should be done after warming up, using a slow and steady stretch accompanied by deep breathing, and building hold up to 30 to 60 seconds
  • Calf stretches
  • PROM (passive), AAROM (active-assistive), and AROM (active) of left ankle for all motions of ankle, subtalar, metatarsophalangeal (MTP), and phalangeal joints
  • Balance board
♦ Gait and locomotion training
  • Forward treadmill walking: Begin at 2.5 to 3.0 mph and increase as tolerated to running speed
  • Retro treadmill walking: Begin at 1.7 mph and increase as tolerated
  • Walk/jog program
♦ Relaxation
  • Breathing exercises

- Breathing while stretching and exercising
- Relaxation techniques (eg, Jacobson's)
- Complementary exercise approaches (eg, yoga relaxation techniques)

♦ Strength, power, and endurance training
- PREs left ankle with weighted boot
- Bilateral and unilateral plantarflexion and dorsiflexion
- Balance board
- Elastic bands
- Mini squats
- Plyometrics

FUNCTIONAL TRAINING IN WORK, COMMUNITY, AND LEISURE INTEGRATION OR REINTEGRATION

♦ Leisure
- Review training guidelines for running
- Review proper form for running

ANTICIPATED GOALS AND EXPECTED OUTCOMES

♦ Impact on pathology/pathophysiology
- Osteogenic effects of exercise are maximized.

♦ Impact on impairments
- Aerobic capacity is increased, and the client returns to running 4 miles a day, three times a week.
- Balance is improved so that the client is able to maintain one-legged stance for five 30-second tries on LLE.
- Muscle performance of left ankle plantarflexion, eversion, inversion, and dorsiflexion are 5/5.
- Postural control is improved.
- ROM of left ankle is increased so that dorsiflexion is 30 degrees, plantarflexion is 60 degrees, and eversion is 30 degrees.
- Weightbearing status is improved.

♦ Impact on functional limitations
- Ability to perform physical actions, tasks, and activities related to self-care, home management, work, community, and leisure is improved.
- Client is able to demonstrate proper body mechanics during bending and lifting activities.
- Client is independent in performance of exercise program.

♦ Risk reduction/prevention
- Risk factors are reduced.
- Client is able to verbalize risk factors for skeletal demineralization.

♦ Impact on health, wellness, and fitness

- Behaviors that foster healthy habits, wellness, and prevention are acquired.
- Fitness is improved.
- Health status is improved.
- Physical function is improved.

♦ Impact on societal resources
- Documentation occurs throughout the client management and follows APTA's *Guidelines for Physical Therapy Documentation.*[56]

♦ Patient/client satisfaction
- Client and family knowledge and awareness of the diagnosis, prognosis, interventions, and anticipated goals and expected outcomes are increased.
- Sense of well-being is improved.

REEXAMINATION

Reexamination is performed throughout the episode of care.

DISCHARGE

Amy is discharged from physical therapy after a total of 12 physical therapy sessions and attainment of her goals and expectations. These sessions have covered her entire episode of care. She is discharged because she has achieved her goals and expected outcomes.

REFERENCES

1. Johnson LR, ed. *Essential Medical Physiology.* 3rd ed. New York, NY: Elsevier Academic Press; 2003.
2. Guyton AC, Hall JE. *Textbook of Medical Physiology.* 10th ed. Philadelphia, Pa: WB Saunders Co; 2000.
3. Lundon K. *Orthopedic Rehabilitation Science: Principles for Clinical Management of Bone.* Woburn, Mass: Butterworth-Heinemann; 2000.
4. Salter RB. *Textbook of Disorders and Injuries of the Musculoskeletal System.* 3rd ed. Baltimore, Md: Lippincott; 1999.
5. Baron RE. Anatomy and ultrastructure of bone. In: Favus MJ, ed. *Primer on the Metabolic Bone Diseases and Disorders of Mineral Metabolism.* 3rd ed. Philadelphia, Pa: Lippincott-Raven; 1996.
6. Tortora GJ, Anagonostakos NP. *Principles of Anatomy and Physiology.* 5th ed. New York, NY: Harper & Row; 1987.
7. Beck BR, Shoemaker MR. Osteoporosis: understanding key risk factors and therapeutic options. *The Physician and Sports Medicine.* 2000;28(2):67-81.
8. National Institutes of Health, National Resource Center. *Osteoporosis and Related Bone Disease.* Bethesda, Md: National Institutes of Health; 2003.
9. Kanis JA, Melton LJ, Christiansen C, et al. The diagnosis of osteoporosis. *J Bone Miner Res.* 1994;9(8):1137-1141.
10. Marcus R, Majumder S. The nature of osteoporosis. In: Marcus R, Feldman D, Kesley J, eds. *Osteoporosis.* Vol 2. 2nd

ed. San Diego, Calif: Academic Press; 2001:3-16.

11. Meunier PJ, Delmas PD, Easstell R, et al. Diagnosis and management osteoporosis in postmenopausal women; clinical guidelines: International Committee for Osteoporosis Clinical Guidelines. *Clin Ther.* 1999;21(6):1025-1044.

12. Riggs L, Khosla S, Melton LJ. The Type I/Type II Model for Involuntional Osteoporosis: update and modification based on new observations. In: Marcus R, Feldman D, Kesley J, eds. *Osteoporosis.* Vol 2. 2nd ed. San Diego, Calif: Academic Press; 2001:49-57.

13. Amin S, Felson DT. Osteoporosis in men. *Rheum Dis Clin North Am.* 2001;27(1);19-48.

14. National Osteoporosis Foundation. *Physician's Guide to Prevention and Treatment of Osteoporosis.* Washington, DC: National Osteoporosis Foundation; 2003.

15. Chavassieux P, Arlot M, Meunier PJ. In: Marcus R, Feldman D, Kesley J, eds. *Osteoporosis.* Vol 2. 2nd ed. San Diego, Calif: Academic Press; 2001:501-508.

16. Lindsay R, Cosman F. In: Marcus R, Feldman D, Kesley J, eds. *Osteoporosis.* Vol 2. 2nd ed. San Diego, Calif: Academic Press; 2001:577-595.

17. Lane NE. An update on glucocorticoid-induced osteoporosis. *Rheum Dis Clin North Am.* 2001;27(1):235-254.

18. Leong GM, Center JR, Henderson NK, Eisman JA. In: Marcus R, Feldman D, Kesley J, eds. *Osteoporosis.* Vol 2. 2nd ed. San Diego, Calif: Academic Press; 2001:169-185.

19. Heywood VH. *Advanced Fitness Assessment & Exercise Prescription.* 3rd ed. Champaign, Ill: Human Kinetics; 1998.

20. World Health Organization. *Preventing and Managing the Global Epidemic of Obesity: Report of the World Health Organization Consultation of Obesity.* Geneva, Switzerland: WHO; 1997.

21. USDA Center for Nutrition Policy and Promotion. Body Mass Index and Health. *Nutrition Insights.* 2000;March.

22. Resnick B, Zimmerman S, Orwig D, Furstenberg AL, Magaziner J. Model testing for reliability and validity of the Outcome Expectations for Exercise Scale. *Nurs Res.* 2001;50(5):293-299.

23. Giogetti MM, Harris BA, Jette A. Reliability of clinical balance outcome measures in the elderly. *Physiother Res Int.* 1998;3(4):274-283.

24. Mathiowetz V, Kashman N, Volland G, Weber K, Dowe M, Rogers S. Grip and pinch strength: normative data for adults. *Arch Phys Med Rehabil.* 1985;66:69-74.

25. Crosby CA, Wehbe MA, Mawwr B. Hand strength: normative values. *J Hand Surg.* 1994;19A:665-670.

26. Gold DT, Bates CW, Lyles KW, et al. Treatment of osteoporosis: the psychological impact of a medical education program on older patients. *J Am Geriatr Soc.* 1989;37:417.

27. Lydick E, Zimmerman SI, Yawn B, et al. Development and validation of a discriminative quality of life questionnaire for osteoporosis (the OPTQoL). *J Bone Miner Res.* 1997;12:456.

28. Gold DT. The nonskeletal consequences of osteoporotic fractures: psychological and social outcomes. *Rheum Dis Clin North Am.* 2001;27(1):255-262.

29. Sinaki M, Wollan PC, Scott RW, et al. Can strong back extensors prevent vertebral fractures in women with osteoporosis? *Mayo Clin Proc.* 1996;71:951-956.

30. Snow-Harter C, Bouxsein ML, Lewis BT, et al. Effects of resistance and endurance exercise on bone mineral status of young women: a randomized exercise intervention trail. *J Bone Miner Res.* 1992;7(7):761-769.

31. Margulies JY, Simkin A, Leichter I, et al. Effect of intense physical activity on the bone mineral content in the lower limbs of young adults. *J Bone Joint Surg.* 1986;68(7):1090-1093.

32. Wolff J. *Gesetz der transformation der knochen.* Berlin, Germany: Springer-Verlag; 1892.

33. Huddleston AL, Rockwell D, Kulund DN, et al. Bone mass in lifetime tennis athletes. *JAMA.* 1980;244(10):1107-1109.

34. Leichter I, Simkin A, Margulies JY, et al. Gain in mass density of bone following strenuous physical activity. *J Orthop Res.* 1989;7(1):86-90.

35. Friedlander AL, Genant HK, Sadowsky S, et al. A two-year program of aerobics and weight-training enhances BMD of young women. *J Bone Miner Res.* 1995;10(4):574-585.

36. Pruitt LA, Jackson RD, Bartels RL, et al. Weight-training effects on bone mineral density in early postmenopausal women. *J Bone Miner Res.* 1992;7(2):179-185.

37. Grove KA, Londeree BR. Bone density in postmenopausal women: high impact vs low impact exercise. *Med Sci Sports Exerc.* 1992;24(11):1190-1194.

38. Bassey EJ, Ramsdale SJ. Increase in femoral bone density in young women following high impact exercise. *J Bone Miner Res.* 1992;7:761-769.

39. Shaw JM, Snow CM. Weighted vest exercise improves indices of fall risk in older women. *J Gerontol Biol Sci Med.* 1998;53(1):M53-M58.

40. Snow CM, Shaw JM, Winters KM, Witzke KA. Long-term exercise using weighted vests prevents hip bone loss in post-menopausal women. *J Gerontol Biol Sci Med.* 2000;55(9): M489-M491.

41. Wolff I, van Croonenborg J, Kemper HCG, et al. The effect of exercise training programs on bone mass: a meta-analysis of published controlled trials in pre- and postmenopausal women. *Osteoporos Int.* 1999;9:1-12.

42. Kemmler W, Engelke K, Weineck J, et al. The Erlangen fitness osteoporosis prevention study: a controlled exercise trial in early postmenopausal women with low bone density-first-year results. *Arch Phys Med Rehabil.* 2003;84:673-682.

43. Sinaki M, Itoi E, Rodgers JW, et al. Correlation of back extensor strength with thoracic kyphosis and lumbar lordosis in estrogen-deficient women. *Am J Phys Med Rehabil.* 1996;75(5):370-374.

44. Chrousos G P, Loriaux DL, Gold PW. The concept of stress and its historical development. In: Mechanisms of Physical and Emotional Stress. *Adv Exp Med Biol.* 1988;245:3-7.

45. Michelson D, Stratakis C, Hill L, Galliven E, et al. Bone mineral density in women with depression. *N Engl J Med.* 1996;335:1176-1181.

46. Institute of Medicine. *Dietary Reference Intakes for Calcium, Phosphorous, Magnesium, Vitamin D, and Fluoride.* Washington, DC: National Academy Press; 1999.

47. Osteoporosis Report. *Quarterly Membership Report.* Washington, DC: National Osteoporosis Foundation; Spring 1999.

48. Spencer H, Kramer L. Antacid-induced calcium loss. *Arch Intern Med.* 1983;143(4):657-659.

49. McArdle WD, Katch FI, Katch VL. *Sports and Exercise Nutrition.* Philadelphia, Pa: Lippincott Williams & Wilkins;

1999.

50. Popock NA, Eisman JA, Yeates MG, et al. Physical fitness is a major determinant of femoral neck and lumbar spine bone density. *J Clin Invest.* 1986;78(3):618-621.

51. Kelley GA. Aerobic exercise and bone density at the hip in postmenopausal women: a meta-analysis. *Prev Med.* 1998;27(6):798-807.

52. Todd JA, Robinson RJ. Osteoporosis and exercise. *Postgrad Med J.* 2003;79:320-323.

53. Dilsen G, Berker C, Oral A. The role of physical exercise in prevention and management of osteoporosis. *Clin Rheumatol.* 1989;8(Suppl 2):S70-S75.

54. Borg G. *Borg's Perceived Exertion and Pain Scales.* Champaign, Ill: Human Kinetics; 1998.

55. Dehart-Beverley MM, Foster C, Porcari JP, et al. Relationship between the talk test and ventilatory threshold. *Clinical Exercise Physiology.* 2000;2:343-38.

56. American Physical Therapy Association. Guide to physical therapist practice. 2nd ed. *Phys Ther.* 2001;81:9-744.

57. Optimal calcium intake: NIH consensus panel. *JAMA* 1994;272:1942-1948.

58. http://static.highbeam.com/g/geriatrics/august011994/nihincreasedailycalciumrequirementstolowerosteopor/. Accessed May 25, 2004.

59. Cureton KJ, Sloniger MA, O'Bannon JP, Black DM, McCormack WP. A generalized equation for prediction of V–O$_2$ peak from 1-mile run/walk performance. *Med Sci Sports Exerc.* 1995;27(3):445-451.

60. http://www.hooah4health.com/toolbox/targetingfitness/charts/chartsOneMileWalk.htm. Accessed August 5, 2004.

61. Otis CL, Drinkwater B, Johnson M, Loucks A, Wilmore J. American College of Sports Medicine Position Stand. The female athlete triad. *Med Sci Sports Exerc.* 1997;29:i-ix.

CHAPTER TWO

Impaired Posture
(Pattern B)

Elaine Rosen, PT, DHSc, OCS, FAAOMPT
Sandra Rusnak-Smith, PT, DHSc, OCS

ANATOMY

OVERVIEW OF POSTURE

Posture has been defined as a "composite of the positions of all the joints of the body at any given moment"[1] or as "a situation when the center of gravity of each body segment is placed vertically above the segment below."[2] "Standard"[1] or "ideal"[3] posture is a state of muscular and skeletal balance that should be maintained with minimal stress or strain on the body without deviations and can be used as the basis for comparison when evaluating skeletal alignment.[1,3] Normal muscle tone is needed to sustain "standard" posture, and the upright position is maintained by postural muscles working synergistically against gravity as influenced by the motor control system. Detailed description of the motor control process is beyond the scope of this chapter and is described in more detail in Pattern C: Impaired Muscle Performance and *Neuromuscular Essentials: Applying the Preferred Physical Therapist Practice Patterns.*[SM]

Posture can be described as either static or dynamic. In static posture, the body is maintained in a particular position. In dynamic posture, the body is moving. During the course of the day we constantly adjust the position of our bodies to respond to the environment and ergonomic demands and to maintain a level of comfort.[4] Posture is most commonly evaluated in either the standing or sitting positions. It has been suggested that posture should also be evaluated in the positions or movements that a person most often assumes.[5]

Most commonly, clinicians assess posture without the use of an objective measure.[6] The plumb line is one method that can be used to objectify postural measurements.[7] Hickey and associates[8] used the plumb line measuring technique and found higher intra- and intertester reliability measurements when compared to the CROM. The plumb line establishes a line of reference that corresponds to the midline of the body passing through particular anatomical landmarks on the body allowing for equal weight distribution and joint stability. In the lateral view, the plumb line should ideally pass though specific anatomical and surface landmarks. The anatomical landmarks include the external auditory meatus, the dens, the bodies of the cervical vertebrae, the bodies of the lumbar vertebrae, the sacral promontory, slightly posterior to the center of the hip joint, slightly anterior to the center of the knee and the lateral malleolus, and through the calcaneocuboid joint.[1] The surface landmarks include: the ear lobe, the shoulder joint, midway between the front and back of the chest, midway between the back and the abdomen, the greater trochanter, and slightly anterior to the midline of the knee and the lateral malleolus.[1] In the posterior

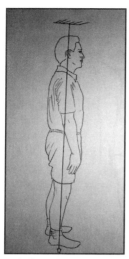

Figure 2-1. Plumb line for normal postural alignment. Artwork by Greg Gao, MD, PT.

view the plumb line passes through the midline of the body. The degree of deviation is detected by clinical observation and is recorded as slight, moderate, or marked[1] (Figure 2-1). Deviations from the norm may be an indication of a series of imbalances and abnormal strains on the musculoskeletal system.[9] The earlier the postural faults are recognized and addressed, the greater the possibility of a successful outcome from the physical therapy interventions. If these postural faults go uncorrected for a prolonged period of time, multiple structural adaptations and compensations may occur.

Additional devices that can be used to quantify postural faults are more costly to purchase and can be more difficult to use. In most cases only a limited number of postural deviations can be assessed. These devices include but are not limited to inclinometers,[10] photography, standing radiography, force plates, and three-dimensional computer analysis.[6]

When performing a postural examination, a comprehensive approach should be taken. The clinician should observe the patient from all perspectives in an unobstructed area having the patient appropriately exposed. Care should be given to have proper lighting so that shadows do not create false illusions and that lines on the floor or on the wall do not influence the examiner's perception of alignment. The clinician should observe the patient's body type; note the presence of muscle atrophy or hypertrophy; note any change in contour of muscles, joints, or bones; and note the presence of any scars. Although the physical therapist compares side to side for symmetry, one must recognize that the human body is not perfectly symmetrical. Care should be given to the accuracy of hand placement, since deviations of the angle and location from side to side can alter findings.

From a posterior standing view, the following structures are observed:

- Distribution of the weight on both feet
- Alignment of the feet, heels, arches, heights of the lateral malleoli, and positions of the Achilles tendons
- Heights of the fibula heads
- Heights of the popliteal fossae
- Alignment of the gluteal folds, ischial tuberosities, posterior superior iliac spines (PSIS)
- Greater trochanters and iliac crests
- Leg lengths (measure if necessary)
- Presence of a lateral shift
- Alignment of the vertebrae (note scoliosis and side of convexity), ribs, rib angles (note protrusion), intercostals spaces
- Position of the scapulae (note winging or elevation)
- Distance of the UEs from the trunk
- Comparison of shoulder levels
- Alignment of the head (normal midline, tilted, or rotated)

From a lateral standing view, the following structures are observed:

- Weight distribution on anterior and posterior aspects of the feet
- Alignment of the feet
- Alignment of the knees (note recurvatum or excessive flexion)
- Position of the hips
- Alignment of the curves of each spinal region (including lumbar lordosis—normal, flattened, or exaggerated; thoracic kyphosis—normal, flattened, increased, or Dowager's hump; cervical lordosis—normal, flattened, or forward)
- Diameter of the anterior-posterior thoracic cage
- Alignment of the shoulders (normal or rounded)

From an anterior standing view, the following structures are observed:

- Alignment of the toes, feet, arches, and heights of the lateral malleoli
- Alignment of the tibias (note bowing)
- Heights of fibula heads
- Alignment of the knees (note genu varum or valgum)
- Position of the patellae
- Levels of greater trochanters, anterior superior iliac spines (ASIS), and iliac crests
- Configuration and symmetry of the thoracic cage
- Position of the sternum
- Rib symmetry (note any protrusions)
- Distance of the UEs from the trunk
- Carrying angle of each elbow
- Level of the shoulders
- Alignment of the clavicles and the sternoclavicular (SC) and acromioclavicular (AC) joints

♦ Alignment of the head (normal mid-line, tilted, or rotated)

Poor posture may be caused by poor habits, muscle imbalances, adaptive soft tissue shortening, and pain. Anatomical factors that may alter posture include ligamentous tightness or laxity, bony anomalies, muscle tightness, or elongation.[11] The ability to maintain normal posture may progressively deteriorate with aging. Common postural deformities include:

♦ Forward head posture (FHP) is excessive anterior position of the head and neck

♦ Kyphosis is increased posterior curvature of the spine which results in excessive flexion of the involved segments of the spine

♦ Dowager's hump is anterior wedging of the thoracic vertebral bodies usually secondary to degenerative changes and osteoporosis

♦ Lordosis is increased anterior curvature of the spine which results in hyperextension of the involved area of the spine

♦ Scoliosis is a lateral curvature of the spine, can be in the shape of a "C" or "S" curve (rotolateral curvature of the spine)

♦ Sway back is hyperextension of the spine at the lumbosacral angle

♦ Flat back is decreased lumbar lordosis and posterior pelvic rotation

♦ Coxa valga is an increase in the medial angulation between the neck and shaft of the femur

♦ Coxa vara is a decrease in the medial angulation between the neck and shaft of the femur

♦ Genu valgum is also referred to as "knock knees" and results when the medial tibiofemoral angle is greater than 185 degrees causing increased tensile forces on the medial condyle[12]

♦ Genu varum is also referred to as "bow legs" and results when the medial tibiofemoral angle is 175 degrees or less causing tensile forces on the lateral tibial condyle[12]

♦ Genu recurvatum is hyperextension of the knee

♦ Forefoot varus is an inversion deviation of the forefoot on the hind foot when the subtalar joint is in the neutral position

♦ Hind foot valgus is an eversion deviation of the calcaneus when the subtalar joint is in the neutral position; it is often associated with tibia valgus

♦ Hallux valgus is medial deviation of the head of the first MT bone in relation to the center of the body and lateral deviation of the head of the first MT bone in relation to the center of the foot

♦ Pes planus is excessive valgus of the hind foot. The everted position creates (or is a result of) a medial rotatory stress on the leg. This abnormality may cause structural deviations of the knee joint, including excessive angulation of the patellar tendon.[12] This deviation of the calcaneus may result in lowering of the arch of the foot, a functional leg length difference, and increased tension of the plantar ligaments and the plantar aponeurosis. Prolonged stress of these structures can result in microtears, pain, and inflammation referred to as plantar fasciitis (see Pattern E: Impaired Joint Mobility, Motor Function, Muscle Performance, and Range of Motion Associated With Localized Inflammation).

The specific anatomy of all of the joints related to the study of posture is quite extensive and beyond the scope of this chapter. Individual joint anatomy of the foot will be discussed in this chapter. Anatomy of the cervical, thoracic, and lumbar spines and the pelvic girdle is discussed in Pattern F: Impaired Joint Mobility, Motor Function, Muscle Performance, Range of Motion, and Reflex Integrity Associated With Spinal Disorders. Anatomy of the shoulder, hip, knee, metacarpophalangeal (MCP), and basal joints is discussed in Pattern H: Impaired Joint Mobility, Motor Function, Muscle Performance, and Range of Motion Associated With Joint Arthroplasty.

THE FOOT

The foot can functionally be divided into three parts: the hind foot, the midfoot, and the forefoot. The hind foot is made up of the talus and the calcaneus. The calcaneus is the largest of the tarsal bones and is located inferior to the talus. It allows for the attachment of muscles, tendons, and the plantar fascia. The talus has a head, a body, and a neck. The head and neck of the talus are supported by the sustentaculum tali, located on the anteromedial aspect of the calcaneus. The wedge-shaped superior surface of the talus is referred to as the trochlea. The head articulates with the navicular and the sustentaculum tali. The body articulates with the inferior surface of the tibia and the medial and lateral malleoli.[13,14]

The joints that make up the hind foot are the distal tibiofibular joint, the talocrural joint, and the subtalar joint. The distal tibiofibular joint is a syndesmosis and therefore allows for very little movement. The talocrural joint is a synovial hinge joint consisting of the body of the talus that is situated between the distal end of the tibia and the fibula malleoli. The fibula malleolus is posterior to the tibial malleolus and extends inferiorly along the entire length of the lateral aspect of the talus. The talocrural joint allows for both dorsiflexion and plantarflexion. During dorsiflexion, the fibula malleolus moves laterally, the tibia and fibula separate, and the wider anterior aspect of the talus moves posteriorly. The primary function of this joint is to maintain stability.[13,14]

The subtalar joint is a synovial joint at the articulation between the talus and the calcaneus that allows for gliding and inversion/eversion. The talus articulates with the navicular and the calcaneus articulates with the cuboid. The posterior articulation between the talus and the calcaneus is concave superiorly (talus) and convex inferiorly (calcaneus) and the antero-medial articulation is convex superiorly (talus) and concave inferiorly (calcaneus).[15] When the talus is fixed, the major motions are calcaneal abduction (valgus) and adduction (varus). The combined motions of these joints create inversion and eversion. Inversion is produced by calcaneal adduction, navicular cranial rotation, and glide of the talus. Eversion is comprised of the opposite movements.[16]

The midfoot consists of the navicular, cuboid, and the cuneiform bones. The navicular is the most medial and is located between the head of the talus and the cuneiforms. In some individuals, there may be a facet for articulation with the cuboid. The navicular assists in preserving the longitudinal arch. The cuboid is located between the calcaneus and the fourth and fifth MTs. It also articulates with the lateral cuneiform and the navicular. There are three cuneiform bones that are wedge shaped and articulate with the navicular and the bases of the first to third MTs. The medial cuneiform is the largest. The joints of the midfoot include the talocalcaneonavicular joint, the cuneonavicular joint, the cuboideonavicular joint, the intercuneiform joints, the cuneocuboid joint, and the calcaneocuboid joint. The talocalcaneonavicular joint is a ball and socket synovial joint, which allows for gliding and rotation. The cuneonavicular joint is a plane synovial joint that allows for minimal gliding and rotation. The cuboideonavicular joint is fibrous and allows slight gliding and rotation. The intercuneiform joints and the cuneocuboid joint are plane synovial joints allowing minimal glide and rotation. The calcaneocuboid joint is saddle shaped and allows gliding with conjunct rotation.[11,13]

The forefoot consists of the five MTs and 14 phalanges. The first MT is the largest and bears the greatest amount of weight. Each MT has a head that articulates with its proximal phalanx and a base that articulates with the corresponding tarsal bone. The joints of the forefoot are the tarsometatarsal (TMT) joints, the intermetatarsal joints, the MTP joints, and the interphalangeal (IP) joints. The TMT joints and the intermetatarsal joints are plane synovial joints that allow for gliding. The MTP joints are condyloid synovial joints that allow for flexion, extension, abduction, and adduction. The IP joints are synovial hinge joints that allow for flexion and extension.[13,14]

PHYSIOLOGY

The many causes of poor posture may include poor habits, repetitive movements, muscle imbalances, bony abnormalities, soft tissue restrictions, fatigue, and pain. Postural abnormalities originate when muscles and associated structures have difficulty maintaining postural control. Excessive stresses may be exerted on joints and periarticular structures causing them to become overstretched or injured.[17] Hickey and Hukins[7] reported that if overstretched ligaments exceeded 4% of their resting length, irreversible damage can result. Recurring microtrauma leads to loss of elasticity and

decreased ROM. According to Twomey and Taylor,[4] maintaining static erect posture causes postural fatigue resulting in an increase in the lumbar lordosis, extension of the lumbar spine, and a slow creep of the soft tissue. Creep can be defined as the progressive deformation of a structure under constant load.

Deviation from normal posture can create changes in muscle length. Depending on the position of the trunk and extremities, muscles may become shortened or lengthened. The shortened position may result in a loss of sarcomeres. Muscles subsequently become tightened and lose their elasticity. The lengthened position may result in an increase in sarcomeres, altering the length-tension properties.[5,18]

Postural deviations may occur secondary to muscle imbalances. Tight muscles have a propensity to pull on the structures to which they are attached allowing the antagonist muscle to become elongated and weak. Imbalances are the basis of increased tissue strain and decreased efficiency of the involved area.

Deformation of cartilage and subsequent nutritional changes can occur secondary to increased weightbearing stresses on the joints. These may lead to impaired circulation and increased accumulation of waste products resulting in fatigue and pain. These changes may also lead to degenerative changes in the joints, thus creating inflammation.[19]

Aging alters the elastic properties of connective tissue, causing a loss of muscle and joint flexibility, strength, and ROM. Muscle strength may decrease with age secondary to disuse and overall reduced exercise.[4] Muscle mass may also decrease leading to atrophy and a decrease in muscle performance.[5] These factors contribute to the deterioration of postural alignment and alteration of the spinal curves.

PATHOPHYSIOLOGY

Poor posture can change normal anatomical relationships. The joints in the kinematic chain may become compromised resulting in modification of the gait pattern. Alteration of foot biomechanics may alter the entire kinetic chain leading to dysfunctions of the ankle, knee, hip, sacroiliac, and shoulder joints and the lumbar, thoracic, and cervical spines. Each joint has a direct influence on its surrounding counterpart.

POSTURAL SYNDROME

Deviations from normal anatomy may cause increased stress on the soft tissue, ligaments, fascia, muscles, and tendons that may result in musculoskeletal pain and movement impairments.[5] Prolonged stress on these structures may result in microtears and overuse of the involved muscles resulting in pain and inflammation. This chain of events culminates in swelling of the surrounding structures, loss of elasticity, reduction of the ROM, and pain. Repetitive stresses may erode the articular surfaces of the involved joints yielding osteophyte formation and may result in muscle ischemia, changes in the characteristics of collagen, disc degeneration, and possible disc herniation.

SCHEUERMANN'S DISEASE

Impaired posture can also arise from diseases such as Scheuermann's disease (Figure 2-2). Scheuermann's disease (juvenile kyphosis, vertebral epiphysitis, vertebral osteochondritis) is a disease of unknown etiology. Scheuermann believed that the cause of the kyphosis was an avascular necrosis of the vertebral ring apophysis.[20] The disease appears to have a genetic component with an autosomal dominant mode of inheritance.[21] Other theories regarding the pathogenic mechanisms of Scheuermann's kyphosis include endocrine abnormalities, increase in growth hormone,[21] hereditary abnormalities, vitamin deficiency, juvenile osteoporosis,[22,23] malnutrition, and mechanical factors.[22,24] Muller and Gschwend found a relationship between Turner's syndrome and Scheuermann's disease.[20] Studies have shown defective cartilage in the vertebral growth plate and the end plate, decreased vertical growth of the anterior vertebral body, and abnormal collagen-proteoglycan ratios in the vertebral body endplates.[23]

Abnormalities in the matrix of the cartilaginous end plate have been found that would interfere with vertical growth.[24] Schmorl discussed herniation of the intervertebral disc material through the growth plate with subsequent loss of disc height as the cause of the kyphosis.[20,24]

The disease manifests itself as a degeneration of the vertebral body resulting in a structural sagittal plane kyphosis in the thoracic or the thoracolumbar spine.[25] The kyphosis is created by a wedging of more than 5 degrees of the anterior aspect of three or more thoracic vertebrae with vertebral end plate irregularities.[21,25-27] The diagnosis can be made with the presence of wedging of more than 5 degrees of a single vertebrae.[25] Schmorl's nodes and decreased intervertebral disc space height are commonly seen. Widened laminas, thickened transverse processes, and short, downward-sloping spinous processes (SPs) have been noted in surgical patients.[28] Compression of the spinal cord may occur with subsequent manifestation of neurological symptoms.

IMAGING

POSTURAL SYNDROME

Plain films are used to determine the presence of postural deviations in patients that have alterations in bony alignment and degenerative changes creating spinal and joint abnormalities. It is useful to have anteroposterior (A/P), lateral, and oblique views.

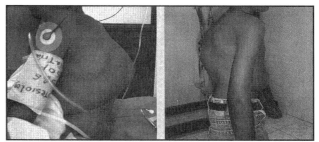

Figure 2-2. Scheuermann's disease. Reprinted with permission of Dr. Andrew Moulton.

SCHEUERMANN'S DISEASE

The diagnosis of Scheuermann's disease is confirmed by measuring the amount of kyphosis utilizing the Cobb method in a standing lateral radiograph of the spine. Findings on x-rays characteristic of Scheuermann's disease include vertebral wedging, irregular vertebral end plates, Schmorl's nodes, and decreased vertebral height.[22,26] Other common radiographic findings include narrowing of the intervertebral disc spaces, three or more vertebrae wedged 5 degrees or more, and an increase in normal thoracic kyphosis greater than 45 degrees.[20]

Magnetic resonance imaging (MRI) may be used to determine both soft tissue and bony alignment, discal protrusion, degeneration, and tears of ligament and tendons. Patients who are diagnosed with Scheuermann's disease may demonstrate protrusion of disc material into the vertebral body on MRI.

Bone density studies may be used to give information regarding demineralization. Additional details regarding these studies can be found in Pattern A: Primary Prevention/ Risk Reduction for Skeletal Demineralization.

PHARMACOLOGY

The following pharmacological agents are utilized in the management of patients with postural disorders: anti-inflammatories to decrease inflammation of joints or soft tissue (see Pattern E: Impaired Joint Mobility, Motor Function, Muscle Performance, and Range of Motion Associated With Localized Inflammation for additional details), analgesics for pain relief (see Pattern D: Impaired Joint Mobility, Motor Function, Muscle Performance, and Range of Motion Associated With Connective Tissue Dysfunction for additional details), and drugs to facilitate bone regeneration in patients who present with skeletal demineralization (see Pattern A: Primary Prevention/Risk Reduction for Skeletal Demineralization for additional information).

Case Study #1: Postural Dysfunction

Dr. Thomas Schoenberg is a 46-year-old male dentist with complaints of progressively deteriorating posture.

PHYSICAL THERAPIST EXAMINATION

HISTORY

- General demographics: Dr. Schoenberg is a 46-year-old white male whose primary language is English. He is right-hand dominant.
- Social history: Dr. Schoenberg is married and has three children, two daughters ages 21 and 19 and a son, age 17.
- Employment/work: He is actively practicing as a general dentist.
- Living environment: He lives with his wife and family in a private colonial style house in the suburbs.
- General health status
  - General health perception: He reports that the status of his health is good.
  - Physical function: He reports that he functions well for his age.
  - Psychological function: Normal.
  - Role function: Dentist, husband, father.
  - Social function: He enjoys playing on the computer and reading.
- Social/health habits: He reports that he smoked one pack of cigarettes a day for 5 years and stopped smoking at the age of 25.
- Family history: His mother had osteoporosis.
- Medical/surgical history: He has hypercholesterolemia.
- Prior hospitalizations: He was hospitalized for a tonsillectomy at age 5.
- Preexisting medical and other health-related conditions: Noncontributory.
- Current condition(s)/chief complaint(s): Dr. Schoenberg is complaining of increasingly poor posture. He is concerned about the pain in his neck and upper back with occasional radiation down the right arm.
- Functional status and activity level: He is totally independent in all ADL and IADL. He reports that he likes to walk. He has been following a gentle self-designed exercise program for many years.
- Medications: He is presently taking Lipitor to regulate his cholesterol level.
- Other clinical tests: Radiographs revealed mild narrowing of the disc spaces and minimal osteophytes in the cervical spine.

SYSTEMS REVIEW

- Cardiovascular/pulmonary
  - BP: 130/80 mmHg
  - Edema: None noted
  - HR: 85 bpm
  - RR: 15 bpm
- Integumentary
  - Presence of scar formation: None
  - Skin color: WNL
  - Skin integrity: WNL
- Musculoskeletal
  - Gross range of motion: Restricted in cervical and thoracic spines and shoulders bilaterally as ascertained from the upper quarter exam
  - Gross strength: Decreased in cervical flexors and extensors, shoulder flexors and abductors, scapula adductors and depressors, and thoracic extensors as ascertained from the upper quarter exam
  - Gross symmetry: Severe forward head
  - Height: 5'8" (1.727 m)
  - Weight: 180 lbs (81.684 kg)
- Neuromuscular
  - Balance: WNL
  - Locomotion, transfers, and transitions: WNL
- Communication, affect, cognition, language, and learning style
  - Communication, affect, and cognition: WNL
  - Learning preferences: Visual leaner

TESTS AND MEASURES

- Anthropometric characteristics
  - BMI=705 x (body weight [in pounds] divided by height^2 [in inches])
  - Dr. Schoenberg's BMI=27.4
  - BMI values between 25 and 30 are considered to be overweight[29]
- Ergonomics and body mechanics
  - Analysis of body mechanics during self-care, home management, work, community, and leisure actions, tasks, and activities revealed altered posture during all activities
  - Dr. Schoenberg leans forward for prolonged periods of time while working on his patients in the dental chair
  - He slumps in his computer chair especially when he gets involved surfing the Internet
  - He tends to slouch when reading novels in his favorite recliner
- Joint integrity and mobility
  - Joint integrity and mobility assessment entails not only the osteokinematic and arthrokinematic analy-

sis but also the structural integrity of the joint

- This includes special tests designed to assess ligamentous stability, compression, distraction tests, impingement tests, and joint play[30-33]
- Cervical spine
  - Flexion: Passive physiological intervertebral mobility (PPIVM) testing was moderately restricted with firm and ligamentous end feel
  - Extension: Posteroanterior (P/A) glide was mildly restricted with hard end feel
  - Sidebending: Side glide intervertebral mobility was moderately restricted bilaterally with hard end feel, PPIVM testing moderately restricted bilaterally
  - Rotation: PPIVM for rotation was mildly restricted bilaterally with firm end feel
  - Distraction of cervical spine was mildly restricted
- Thoracic spine
  - Flexion: PPIVM testing was WNL, firm and ligamentous end feel
  - Extension: P/A glide on SPs was moderately restricted throughout thoracic spine, firm end feel
  - Sidebending: PPIVM was WNL
  - Rotation: PPIVM testing was mildly restricted bilaterally, lateral glide on SPs was mildly restricted with firm end feel
- Shoulder complex
  - Glenohumeral (GH) joint
    - Flexion: Distraction was mildly restricted, A/P glide was moderately restricted
    - Extension: P/A glide was WNL
    - Abduction: Lateral distraction was mildly restricted, inferior glide was mildly restricted
    - ER: P/A glide was mildly restricted
    - IR: A/P glide was WNL
  - Scapulothoracic (ST) joint
    - Distraction was mildly restricted
    - Upward rotation was mildly restricted
    - Retraction was moderately restricted
  - AC joint
    - Anterior glide was WNL
    - Posterior glide was mildly restricted
  - SC joint
    - Superior glide was WNL
    - Inferior glide was mildly restricted
    - Anterior glide was WNL
    - Posterior glide was mildly restricted
- ◆ Motor function
  - Observation of dexterity, coordination, and agility revealed activities WNL

- ◆ Muscle performance
  - Dynamometry revealed a right grip strength of 140 lbs (normal mean for patient's age is 116.8 lbs), left grip strength 125 lbs (normal mean 112.8)[34]
  - MMT revealed the following deviations from normal:
    - Cervical spine extension=3/5
    - Cervical spine flexion=3+/5
    - Thoracic spine extension=3/5
    - Scapula adduction R=3/5, L=3/5
    - Scapula depression R=3/5, L=3/5
    - UE shoulder flexion R=4/5, L=4/5
    - UE shoulder abduction R=4/5, L=4/5
  - Muscle tension (palpation)
    - Spasm
      - Upper trapezius R>L
      - Bilateral middle trapezius
      - Scaleni bilaterally
      - Sternocleidomastoid (SCM) bilaterally
      - Suboccipital muscles R>L
      - Rhomboids R>L
- ◆ Pain
  - Numeric pain rating scale ([NPS] 0=no pain and 10=worst possible pain)
    - Pain of 4/10 on the NPS in the cervical spine, 3/10 across the thoracic spine, especially between the scapulae, and 3/10 across the low back
    - Downie and associates[35] described a high degree of agreement between the visual analog scale (VAS), NPS, and the simple descriptive scale (SDS), although they reported that the NPS performed better
    - Jensen[36] found the NPS to be the most practical tool for pain assessment
  - Neck Disability Index[37]
    - Dr. Schoenberg scored 16/50 or 32% on the Neck Disability Index
    - This indicates a mild to moderate degree of dysfunction
    - The Neck Disability Index has been shown to have stable psychometric properties
    - It is an objective method of measuring pain in patients with neck disability
    - It has a high correlation to scores on the visual analogue scale (0.60) and the McGill Pain Questionnaire (0.69 to 0.70)[38]
- ◆ Posture
  - Observational assessment done from all perspectives, and grid photographs and plumb line were used
    - Lateral view: Severe FHP, thoracic kyphosis, protracted shoulders, internally rotated UEs

- ■ Posterior view: Elevated left shoulder girdle, abducted scapulae
- ■ Anterior view: Severe FHP, elevated left shoulder girdle, protracted shoulders, internally rotated UEs
- ◆ Range of motion
  - ● Functional ROM: Decreased ability to elevate both UEs to end range, decreased ability to look up to the ceiling, decreased ability to look over either shoulder
  - ● Joint active and passive movement
    - ■ Cervical spine ROM was measured using the CROM instrument
      - ‣ Intratester reliability was found to be high (ICC=0.93)[39] and intertester reliability was found to be moderate (ICCs=0.83, 0.775)[8,39] for CROM measurements
      - ‣ Hickey found moderate intertester reliability for both the CROM and the plumb line technique[8]
      - ‣ The validity of the CROM measurement was compared to a radiographic measurement, and the Pearson's r correlation was very high between the two methods (flexion r=0.97, P<0.001, extension r=0.98, P<0.001)[40]
      - ‣ Flexion=60 degrees
      - ‣ Extension=40 degrees
      - ‣ Lateral flexion=20 degrees bilaterally
      - ‣ Rotation R=50 degrees and L=45 degrees
    - ■ Thoracic spine (inclinometry)
      - ‣ Flexion=60 degrees
      - ‣ Extension=0 degrees
      - ‣ Lateral flexion=15 degrees bilaterally
      - ‣ Rotation=30 degrees
    - ■ Shoulder (goniometry)
      - ‣ Active flexion R=0 to 160 degrees and L=0 to 157 degrees
      - ‣ Active abduction R=0 to 160 degrees and L=0 to 155 degrees
      - ‣ Active ER R=0 to 60 degrees and L=0 to 60 degrees
  - ● Muscle tightness
    - ■ Pectoral tightness bilaterally
- ◆ Reflex integrity
  - ● Deep tendon reflexes (DTRs) or myotatic reflexes: Right brachioradialis reflex=1+
  - ● All other reflexes WNL
- ◆ Sensory integrity
  - ● Patient perceives a greater decrease in pinprick on the right as compared to the left on the lateral forearm
- ◆ Self-care and home management

- ● Interview concerning ability to safely perform self-care and home management actions, tasks, and activities found they could be done WNL despite mild discomfort
- ◆ Work, community, and leisure integration or reintegration
  - ● Interview concerning ability to safely manage work, community, and leisure actions, tasks, and activities revealed that they could be done, but pain was experienced with reaching forward and lifting heavy objects

EVALUATION

Dr. Schoenberg's history and risk factors previously outlined indicated that he is a 46-year-old male dentist, previous smoker, overweight, non-vigorous exerciser, with hypercholesterolemia, and a family history of osteoporosis. He has faulty postural alignment; decreased strength in his cervical and thoracic spines, scapula, and UE muscles; and decreased ROM in his spine and UEs. He has difficulty with overhead activities, reaching forward, and heavy tasks during his ADL and IADL. He also experiences pain in his thoracic spine and pain radiating down his RUE while performing tasks at work.

DIAGNOSIS

Dr. Schoenberg is a patient who has impaired posture with pain. In addition, he has impaired: ergonomics and body mechanics, joint integrity and mobility, muscle performance, and range of motion. He is functionally limited in self-care, home management, work, community, and leisure actions, tasks, and activities. These findings are consistent with placement in Pattern B: Impaired Posture. The identified impairments and functional limitations will be addressed in determining the prognosis and the plan of care.

PROGNOSIS AND PLAN OF CARE

Over the course of the visits, the following mutually established outcomes have been determined:
- ◆ Ability to perform physical actions, tasks, and activities related to self-care, home management, work, community, and leisure is improved
- ◆ Fitness is improved
- ◆ Knowledge of behaviors that foster healthy habits, wellness, and prevention is increased
- ◆ Muscle length is increased
- ◆ Muscle performance is increased
- ◆ Muscle spasm is decreased
- ◆ Physical capacity is improved

♦ Physical function is improved
♦ Postural control is improved
♦ Risk factors are reduced
♦ Risk of secondary impairment is reduced
♦ ROM is increased
♦ Stress is decreased

To achieve these outcomes, the appropriate interventions for this patient are determined. These will include: coordination, communication, and documentation; patient/client-related instruction; therapeutic exercise; functional training in self-care and home management; functional training in work, community, and leisure integration or reintegration; manual therapy techniques; electrotherapeutic modalities; and physical agents and mechanical modalities.

Based on the diagnosis and the prognosis, Dr. Schoenberg is expected to require 12 to 14 visits over 12 to 14 weeks. Dr. Schoenberg has good social support, is motivated, and follows through with his home exercise program. He is not severely impaired and is healthy.

INTERVENTIONS

RATIONALE FOR SELECTED INTERVENTIONS

Visser and Straker[41] studied 26 dental assistants and 28 dental therapists and demonstrated that both groups experienced pain in the back, neck, and shoulder areas that was related to their work. They indicated an increase in discomfort throughout the working day. They described the typical working position where the dental operator is positioned at 11 o'clock on the right side of the patient's head. In order to achieve manual access to the patient's oral cavity, the dental operator must flex the trunk, while rotating left and sidebending right. In order to gain visual access, the operator must position him- or herself in full cervical flexion with some additional sidebending or rotation. Maintenance of these asymmetrical postures while working creates stress on spinal structures and static muscle contraction is required in the back and shoulders. Finsen and associates[42] utilized a questionnaire to determine risk factors related to musculoskeletal disorders inherent in the practice of dentistry. They found that there was a high static load on the muscles in the neck and shoulder region secondary to sustained work postures necessary to perform job tasks. They concluded that variation in work posture and decreasing static muscle activity may have the benefit of decreasing musculoskeletal problems for this population. Valachi and Valachi[43] noted that flexibility and core strength played a role in maintaining balance of the musculoskeletal system in dentists.

McKenzie[17] believes that an individual begins to experience pain as soon as "mechanical deformation of innervated

structures" is sufficient to irritate free nerve endings. This mechanical deformation from prolonged stretch also causes stress and subsequent pain in the ligaments, the apophyseal joint capsules, and the annulus fibrosus. For additional information regarding the McKenzie approach, the reader is referred to Pattern F: Impaired Joint Mobility, Motor Function, Muscle Performance, Range of Motion, and Reflex Integrity Associated With Spinal Disorders.

Individuals who perform repeated activities over a prolonged period of time are susceptible to the development of shortened muscles, connective tissues, ligaments, and tendons. In order to compensate for the shortened position, in this case the head and neck posture, the body adapts in the adjacent structures. In this case, where a dentist is sitting with a FHP throughout the work day, shortening of the posterior cervical musculature will develop with concurrent weakness of the anterior musculature. The thoracic spine will develop an increased kyphosis to accommodate for the FHP. Tightness will be noted in the anterior chest musculature including the pectoral muscles subsequently pulling the shoulder girdle internally. This shortened position leads to soft tissue restrictions requiring the use of stretching exercises to increase flexibility, using techniques such as contract-relax.[44,45]

Therapeutic Exercise

Exercise is an important choice of physical therapist interventions for individuals with postural abnormalities. Exercise is not only an intervention that may maximize muscle capability to align posture, but it may also address other impairments associated with this condition. Exercise in this situation will help to improve the flexibility of the muscles, increase ROM of joints, improve postural alignment, and thereby decrease pain. Movement will help the remodeling process.[17] Exercise conditions muscles and leads to increased muscle strength, power, and endurance. It leads to better core and therefore postural stabilization allowing for better awareness of position and movement.[46,47]

Improper posture of the head, neck, and shoulders has been recognized as a contributing factor to cervical pain and myofascial pain syndromes.[6,9,48] Changes in sitting posture may have an affect on head and neck position. Black and associates[49] measured the sitting angles of 30 healthy patients using the Metrecom and found that different sitting postures created changes in both the upper and lower cervical spines. They found that as the lumbar spine moved toward extension the cervical spine moved toward flexion and exactly the opposite occurred in lumbar flexion. The FHP requires the individual to flex the lower cervical spine and extend the upper cervical spine.[9] FHP increases the strain on the posterior cervical muscles, ligaments, and apophyseal joints.[50] Neck pain may occur secondary to overstretching of the soft tissues created by positions that maintain prolonged loading.[17] Valachi and Valachi[43] noted that appropriate adjustments to ergonomic equipment are vital in order to prevent musculoskeletal disorders in the dental population.

Many postural deviations may occur secondary to muscle imbalances.[51] Tight muscles have a propensity to pull on the structures to which they are attached allowing the antagonist muscle to become weak. Imbalances may cause increased tissue strain and decreased efficiency of the involved area and decreased ROM. Swank and associates[52] investigated utilizing weights as a means of enhancing a stretching program in a group of 43 subjects ranging in age from 55 to 83 years. They concluded that an exercise program of modest intensity may have a significant positive impact on joint ROM and flexibility. McCarthy and associates[44] performed a single blind trial design study on 40 asymptomatic subjects utilizing cervical contract-relax stretching exercises and found an increase in cervical ROM while the subjects continued with the exercise program. They noted that the ROM reverted back to the pre-study level after 7 days when the exercise program was discontinued.

Electromyography (EMG) studies have shown that there is an increase in tension in the upper trapezius muscles in the presence of FHP[50,53,54] and conversely decreased muscle activity in both axial extension and the neutral position of the cervical spine.[53] Muscles that have both cervical spine and shoulder girdle attachments are affected by altered shoulder posture. Carlson and associates[55] demonstrated decreased muscle tension and less EMG activity in the trapezius muscle after a controlled study using stretching procedures in relaxation training.

Abnormalities in scapula position may also have an affect on muscle tension, altering muscle strength and shoulder stability. The scapula musculature is responsible for positioning the glenoid that in turn allows for efficient glenohumeral movement. Scapulohumeral (SH) rhythm is adversely affected by weak or fatigued scapula muscles.[56,57] Wang and associates[58] performed a study on 20 asymptomatic subjects with forward shoulder posture. The subjects performed stretching of the pectoral muscles and resistive strengthening exercises of the scapula retractors, elevators, glenohumeral abductors, and external rotators. They concluded that muscle strength, posture, scapula stability, and SH rhythm were improved. Closed-kinetic-chain (CKC) activities have been documented as being the most physiological way of retraining scapula firing patterns. CKC exercises create higher compressive forces, greater joint congruity, decrease shear, and stimulate the proprioceptors allowing for greater dynamic stabilization.[59,60]

The shortened position created by FHP may result in a loss of sarcomeres causing muscles to become tightened and lose their elasticity. On the contralateral side, lengthening may result in an increase in sarcomeres altering the length-tension properties.[5,18] Deformation of the cartilage and subsequent nutritional changes may occur secondary to the increased weightbearing stresses that are placed on the joints. This may lead to impaired circulation and increased accumulation of waste products. Ultimately, these changes may also lead to degenerative changes in the joints leading to inflammation. These conditions may lead to fatigue and pain.[19] Ylinen and associates[61] demonstrated that chronic neck pain was decreased with isometric strength training and dynamic endurance training in a study of 180 female office workers. Chronic or frequent neck problems may be improved with the use of proprioceptive exercises and dynamic resisted strengthening exercises of the neck-shoulder musculature.[62]

Poor posture may be secondary to sustained loading of the soft tissues that surround the involved area. This static position, if maintained for extended periods of time, which some authors report may be as little as 1 minute,[19] causes pain secondary to mechanical deformation of the involved tissues. The tissues over time become overstretched leading to minor trauma and decreased elasticity. Postural pain is usually positional and not related to movement. The pain is generally caused by the poor posture and will be alleviated when the position is altered. The patient's complaint of pain is intermittent in nature and is alleviated when the sustained load is removed. Sitting for too long at a computer or in a car or working in prolonged standing positions may cause pain of postural origin. Evans and associates,[63] in a randomized clinical trial of 191 patients with chronic neck pain, concluded that exercise and spinal manipulation are valuable tools for intervention with patients with this diagnosis.

Strengthening exercises should be directed to the elongated and weakened muscles. Stretching should be utilized to elongate the shortened structures. Mobilization should be directed at hypomobile joint capsules. Long-term improvement of posture will only be possible following the balancing of all the surrounding structures and alleviation of external stresses. A comprehensive approach addressing both soft tissue and bony structures will allow for better balancing of length and strength and ultimately for the resumption of full or functional ROM of the involved joints.[51]

Manual Therapy Techniques

Manual techniques include the use of skilled hands to enhance tissue extensibility, joint mobility, modulate pain, decrease spasm, and reduce soft tissue swelling. Improvements in ROM, pain, and function have been demonstrated with manual physical therapy interventions for painful, stiff spines and extremity joints.[30-33,45,63,64]

Muscle tightness leading to shortened positions and soft tissue restrictions require the use of soft tissue massage and myofascial release.[65]

Prolonged shortening of the soft tissues ultimately leads to joint hypomobility. Mobilization techniques that are directed toward the restricted motion may be applied to the cervical and thoracic spines and shoulder girdle. In addition,

Grades I and II oscillation techniques[30] may be applied to the same joints with pain relief as the desired goal.[32,64] Wyke[66] noted that pain relief may be produced through stimulation of the Types I and II joint receptors located in the ligaments and joint capsule.

Patients receiving spinal manipulation as part of their care required less anti-inflammatory and analgesic medications.[67] Patients who received manual therapy as part of their treatment protocol demonstrated more rapid and greater improvement in their physical performance.[68,69] A systematic review of 36 randomized controlled studies did not support the efficacy of manipulation.[68] Indications were noted that manipulation might be effective for certain types of patients.[70] Bronfort and associates[71] found that exercise in addition to spinal manipulation was more beneficial for patients with chronic neck pain than spinal manipulation alone.

Electrotherapeutic Modalities

This patient may benefit from the use of transcutaneous electrical nerve stimulation (TENS). The major physiological and therapeutic effect of TENS is the reduction of pain. This is thought to occur by triggering and modulating the peripheral and central nervous systems through a series of neurohormonal, neurophysiological, and cognitive systems.[72] With appropriate application of the TENS unit, the patient's treatment may be augmented and facilitated with reduced pain.

Treatment for this patient may also be augmented with the use of electrical muscle stimulation (EMS). EMS may be used to reduce soft tissue edema by creating a pumping effect through repeated muscle contraction. Muscle spasm may be reduced by producing a tetanizing effect of the muscle. Studies demonstrating this effect have only been performed in the levator ani muscle. Some evidence indicates that EMS may increase blood flow in the muscles following repetitions of muscle contraction.[72]

Physical Agents and Mechanical Modalities

Ultrasound may be incorporated as an adjunct in the treatment of this patient to introduce a thermal effect, decrease the inflammatory response, decrease pain, and enhance tissue healing. The thermal effect may be produced when the sound wave passes through the involved tissue, since vibration is initiated by cycles of high pressure. A simultaneous mechanical effect occurs secondary to cavitation in the tissues that disrupts the cell membrane, thus enhancing skin permeability and decreasing the inflammatory response and concurrent pain.[72]

Hot packs may also be incorporated into this patient's treatment to promote tissue healing, decrease joint stiffness, and ultimately create relaxation of the tissues with a subsequent reduction of pain.[72]

Intermittent mechanical traction may benefit this patient by maximizing the opening between the cervical vertebrae.

In the classic study by Colachis and Strohm,[73] the patient should be placed in supine with the neck at a 24-degree angle for maximal posterior separation. The force should be low (approximately 10 lbs) initially and gradually increased to achieve optimal symptom relief. An occipital halter is recommended to avoid any undue pressure on the temporomandibular joint (TMJ).[74] Traction may be a beneficial adjunct to manual therapy for this patient's cervical radicular complaints.

COORDINATION, COMMUNICATION, AND DOCUMENTATION

Communication will occur with Dr. Schoenberg and his family members to engender support for his exercise program. All elements of the patient's management will be documented. A referral to a nutritionist/dietitian for weight control guidelines will be made to ensure an appropriate diet and weight loss. A plan of care will be developed and discussed with the patient.

PATIENT/CLIENT-RELATED INSTRUCTION

Education regarding his current condition, impairments, and functional limitations will be discussed. The patient will be instructed in appropriate body mechanics, proper posture, and core stabilization. Risk factors will be discussed including a discussion concerning weight management and the influence that poor posture may have on aerobic capacity and functional activities. A nutritional referral will be made. Ergonomic instruction for work and use of the computer will be provided. Body mechanics for work and leisure activities will be addressed.

It is critical for patients to receive education regarding appropriate seating. Dentists should use adjustable height seats with variable angles. Exercise breaks are essential in risk reduction for possible work-related injuries.[19] It is suggested that preventative instructions should be included in entry-level dental education, as well as in continuing education.[41]

THERAPEUTIC EXERCISE

♦ Aerobic capacity/endurance conditioning
  ● Although the patient was not tested for aerobic capacity, it is appropriate for this patient to participate in some type of aerobic training
♦ Body mechanics and postural stabilization
  ● Body mechanics training
    ▪ Appropriate sitting posture for work and leisure activities
    ▪ Appropriate use of body mechanics while utilizing dental tools, including retrieving tools
    ▪ Appropriate lifting and carrying instructions
    ▪ Appropriate bending instructions
  ● Postural control training

- Proper alignment of head, cervical spine and thoracic spine, and shoulders
- Axial extension to achieve position of no more than 2 inches from the deepest portion of the cervical lordosis to the apex of the thoracic kyphosis[75]
- Scapula retraction and depression
- Chicken wing position (hands behind head, horizontal abduction of shoulders)
- Corner stretch
- Transition of position from supine to sitting, standing, and walking
- Transition of position to functional activities at work
- Transition of position to functional activities at leisure, including driving the car
- Postural stabilization activities[76]
  - Eye movements laterally to elicit muscle contraction
  - Tongue movements behind maxillary teeth to elicit muscle contraction
  - Axial extension starting in supine and progressing to sitting and upright
  - Maintenance of axial extension position with bilateral arm raises
  - Maintenance of axial extension position with arm raises with addition of weights, starting, for example, with a low weight for 8 to 12 reps and increasing accordingly
  - Glut sets
  - Bridging
  - Unilateral bridging
  - Maintain bridge and add hip flexion right and then left
  - Maintain bridge and add knee extension right and then left
  - Decrease base of support
  - Utilize ball for supine exercises
  - Prone glut sets
  - Arm raises unilateral and then bilateral in prone, progressing to quadruped and then over the exercise ball
  - Leg raises unilateral prone, progressing to quadruped
  - Bilateral leg raises over the exercise ball
  - Alternate opposite arm and leg
  - Incorporate the use of the foam roller and unstable surfaces like wobble board or foam rubber cushion in sitting and standing with bilateral and unilateral stance
  - Utilize balance beam

- Challenge patient out of center of gravity/base of support
- Postural awareness training
  - Use of mirror for visual input of appropriate alignment
  - Notes all around home, car, office
- Flexibility exercises
  - Stretching exercises should be done after warming up, using a slow and steady stretch accompanied by deep breathing, and building hold up to 30 to 60 seconds
  - Cervical ROM in all directions
  - Shoulder ROM in all directions
  - Scapula ROM in all directions including diagonals
  - Anterior chest wall stretching
  - Thoracic extension
- Strength, power, and endurance training
  - Cervical isometric exercises in all directions using a ball between the head and the wall[77]
  - UE weight training for shoulder flexion, abduction, IR, and ER, for example, starting with a low weight for 8 to 12 reps and progressing according to patient's tolerance, being sure that good postural alignment is maintained
  - Seated push-ups
  - Wall push-ups
  - Wobble board with clockwise and counterclockwise circles of UEs
  - Fitter for UEs forward and back and sideways
  - Plyometrics with a variety of weighted balls

Maintenance of a regular exercise program must be instilled in this patient. To do this there are several keys that may be helpful in achieving an exercise program that the patient will do on a life-long basis. These tips may be included in part of the patient-related instruction and may include any or all of the following:

- Establish a variety of enjoyable activities and alternating activities when possible
- Establish a realistic time frame for exercise
- Make exercise a family experience when possible
- Add exercise to one's weekly schedule (walk to work if possible, climb up and down several flights of stairs in his office building instead of taking the elevator, wear a weighted vest while at home)
- Find activities that may be done during work hours (climb stairs while he is in office)
- Find activities that may be done after work
- Find fun alternative activities for weekends
- Allow flexibility
- If a scheduled exercise time is missed, work into schedule at another time during the day or week

- ◆ Use entertainment whenever possible
  - Play music when performing weight exercises or while walking outside
  - Watch TV while on the treadmill
  - Use books on tape at anytime

FUNCTIONAL TRAINING IN SELF-CARE AND HOME MANAGEMENT

- ◆ Self-care and home management
  - Review all actions, tasks, and activities and postural alignment for self-care and home management

FUNCTIONAL TRAINING IN WORK, COMMUNITY, AND LEISURE INTEGRATION OR REINTEGRATION

- ◆ Work
  - Simulation of the work environment including sitting on high rolling stool
  - Simulation of work tasks involved in dentistry and modifications to improve body mechanics and awareness of movement
  - Training in simulated tasks
  - Work training using the drill, cavitron, and other tools, and positioning himself appropriately while taking x-rays
- ◆ Community
  - Simulation of tasks needed to work as a volunteer in his synagogue running raffles and organizing the bazaar
- ◆ Leisure
  - Instruction and simulation of appropriate reading positions emphasizing correct cervical posture
  - Awareness of body position while using the computer
- ◆ Injury prevention or reduction
  - Awareness of safety precautions involved with work

MANUAL THERAPY TECHNIQUES

- ◆ Massage
  - Connective tissue massage/myofascial release[65]
    - To anterior chest wall, anterior shoulder, and posterior cervical and thoracic spine musculature
- ◆ Mobilization/manipulation
  - Soft tissue
    - Cervical and thoracic paraspinal muscles
    - Suboccipital muscles
    - Upper trapezius, scaleni, SCM
    - Rhomboids and middle trapezius
  - Spinal and peripheral joints[30-33]
    - Manual cervical distraction to increase interverte-

bral space and improve intervertebral mobility
- Passive accessory intervertebral mobility (PAIVM) to increase axial extension of the cervical spine
- P/A glide of SPs/bilateral transverse processes of thoracic spine to decrease kyphosis and increase mobility
- Longitudinal and lateral distraction of the GH joint to increase joint space and ROM in flexion and abduction
- P/A glide of GH joint to increase anterior capsule length and increase ROM in ER
- Scapula distraction, depression, and adduction to increase mobility

ELECTROTHERAPEUTIC MODALITIES

- ◆ EMS or TENS to decrease pain and spasm

PHYSICAL AGENTS AND MECHANICAL MODALITIES

- ◆ Sound agents
  - Ultrasound to decrease the pain and enhance tissue perfusion and oxygenation
- ◆ Thermotherapy
  - Hot packs to increase muscle extensibility and decrease spasm in cervical and thoracic spine muscles
- ◆ Traction device
  - Intermittent/sustained, as indicated, cervical traction to increase intervertebral joint space and open nerve root foramen

ANTICIPATED GOALS AND EXPECTED OUTCOMES

- ◆ Impact on pathology/pathophysiology
  - Joint restriction is reduced by 10% to 15%.
  - Muscle spasm is eliminated.
  - Neural compression is decreased.
  - Nutrient delivery to tissue is increased.
  - Pain is decreased from a 4/10 to a 1-2/10.
  - Soft tissue restriction in shoulders, scapula, and cervical spine and thoracic spine is reduced.
  - Tissue perfusion and oxygenation is increased.
  - Tissue restriction is normalized.
- ◆ Impact on impairments
  - Joint mobility of shoulder, scapula, and cervical spine and thoracic spine is improved by 10% to 15%.
  - Muscle length of the pectoralis is elongated by 10%.
  - Muscle performance including strength, power, and endurance is increased in cervical spine extension and flexion, thoracic spine extension, scapula adduc-

tion and depression to 4/5, and shoulder flexion and abduction 4+/5.

- Postural alignment, control, and awareness for work (dentist, caring for patients) and leisure (reading, computer) actions, tasks, and activities are improved.
- Posture while working and reading is appropriately maintained.
- Quality of movement is improved.
- Relaxation is increased.
- ROM in cervical spine and thoracic spine and shoulder girdle is improved to WNL.

◆ Impact on functional limitations
  - Ability to perform physical actions, tasks, and activities or ADL and IADL with or without devices and equipment related to self-care, home management, work (dentist, caring for patients), community, or leisure (reading, computer) is achieved.
  - Tolerance of positions and actions, tasks, and activities required for work (dentistry) and leisure (at computer) is improved.

◆ Risk reduction/prevention
  - Communication enhances risk reduction and prevention of complications.
  - Risk factors are decreased.
  - Risk of recurrence of present condition is decreased.
  - Risk of secondary impairment is decreased.
  - Safety is improved.
  - Self-management of symptoms is improved.

◆ Impact on health, wellness, and fitness
  - Behaviors that promote healthy nutrition, physical activity, and wellness are promoted. BMI is improved to 26.8.
  - Fitness is improved.
  - Health status is improved.
  - Physical function is improved.

◆ Impact on societal resources
  - Documentation occurs throughout patient management and across all settings and follows APTA's *Guidelines for Physical Therapy Documentation.*[78]
  - Utilization of physical therapy services is optimized.

◆ Patient/client satisfaction
  - Care is coordinated with patient, family, and other professionals.
  - Client and family knowledge and awareness of the diagnosis, prognosis, interventions, and anticipated goals and expected outcomes are increased.
  - Interdisciplinary collaboration occurs through case conferences.
  - Patient satisfaction is achieved.
  - Sense of well-being is improved.

REEXAMINATION

Reexamination is performed throughout the episode of care.

DISCHARGE

Dr. Schoenberg is discharged from physical therapy after a total of 14 physical therapy sessions and attainment of his goals and expectations. These sessions have covered his entire episode of care. He is discharged because he has achieved his goals and expected outcomes.

Case Study #2:
Pronated Feet

Mrs. Hui Sing (Emily) Chen is a 51-year-old female with complaints of pain in her lower extremities, especially in her knees and feet and in her low back.

PHYSICAL THERAPIST EXAMINATION

HISTORY

◆ General demographics: Emily Chen is a 51-year-old Asian female whose primary language is Chinese. Her English comprehension is good, however, her spoken English is at a basic level. She is right-hand dominant.

◆ Social history: Emily Chen is a widow and has four grown children, three sons ages 25, 23, 20, and a daughter, age 27, and two grandchildren.

◆ Employment/work: She is a homemaker and a part-time dressmaker who still does larger jobs for former customers on special request.

◆ Living environment: She lives by herself in a walk-up apartment.

◆ General health status
  - General health perception: She reports that the status of her health is fair.
  - Physical function: She reports that she is starting to have more difficulty getting around, particularly with the stairs.
  - Psychological function: Normal.
  - Role function: Dressmaker, mother, grandmother.
  - Social function: She enjoys sewing and also takes pride in cooking for her family.

◆ Social/health habits: She reports that she is a non-smoker.

◆ Family history: Her father had osteoarthritis (OA), scoliosis, and hypertension (HTN).

- Medical/surgical history: HTN, hypothyroidism, OA.
- Prior hospitalizations: She was hospitalized for the delivery of her four children.
- Preexisting medical and other health-related conditions: Noncontributory.
- Current condition(s)/chief complaint(s): Emily Chen is presently complaining of pain in both of her feet for the past several months and more recently pain in her knees. She is experiencing more difficulty climbing the stairs. She also reports achy sensations across her low back that increase when she stands or walks for a prolonged period of time.
- Functional status and activity level: She is totally independent in all ADL and IADL. She reports that she likes to walk but has been forced to limit the distance because of increased symptoms.
- Medications: Lopressor, Synthroid, Celebrex, Actonel.
- Other clinical tests: Bone density studies of her hips and spine reveal normal bone density.

SYSTEMS REVIEW

- Cardiovascular/pulmonary
  - BP: 140/85 mmHg
  - Edema: Minimal edema noted in the right knee, otherwise WNL
  - HR: 80 bpm
  - RR: 14 bpm
- Integumentary
  - Presence of scar formation: None
  - Skin color: WNL
  - Skin integrity: WNL
- Musculoskeletal
  - Gross range of motion: Limited in cervical, thoracic, and lumbar spines and shoulders, hips, knees, and ankles bilaterally as ascertained by the upper and lower quarter exams
  - Gross strength: Limited in cervical extensors, thoracic extensors, abdominals, shoulder flexors and abductors, hip extensors, knee extensors, and ankle dorsiflexors and invertors as ascertained by the upper and lower quarter exams
  - Gross symmetry: Slight asymmetry due to mild scoliosis
  - Height: 5'1" (1.549 m)
  - Weight: 140 lbs (63.504 kg)
- Neuromuscular
  - Balance: Loses her balance easily with pertubations
  - Locomotion, transfers, and transitions: WNL
- Communication, affect, cognition, language, and learning style
  - Communication, affect, and cognition: WNL
  - Learning preferences: Auditory learner

TESTS AND MEASURES

- Anthropometric characteristics
  - BMI=705 x (body weight [in pounds] divided by height^2 [in inches])
  - BMI=26.52
  - BMI values between 25 and 30 are considered to be overweight[29]
  - Girth: ½-inch increase in circumference of the right knee secondary to edema, ¼-inch decrease in girth 3 inches above the patella secondary to muscle atrophy
- Cranial and peripheral nerve integrity
  - Sensation: WNL in all four extremities
- Ergonomics and body mechanics
  - Analysis of body mechanics during self-care, home management, work, community, and leisure actions, tasks, and activities revealed that Mrs. Chen leans forward and often kneels while measuring hems on pants and skirts
  - She often sits for long periods of time
- Gait, locomotion, and balance
  - Nudge/Push test rated fair for posterior perturbations[79]
- Joint integrity and mobility
  - Joint integrity and mobility assessment entails not only the osteokinematic and arthrokinematic analysis but also the structural integrity of the joint
  - This includes special tests designed to assess ligamentous stability, compression, distraction tests, impingement tests, and joint play[30-33]
  - Cervical spine
    - Flexion: PPIVM testing revealed minimal restriction with firm and ligamentous end feel
    - Extension: P/A glide was moderately restricted with hard end feel
    - Sidebending: Side glide PPIVM testing was minimally restricted bilaterally with hard end feel
    - Rotation: PPIVM was minimally restricted bilaterally with firm end feel
    - Distraction of cervical spine mildly restricted
  - Thoracic spine
    - Flexion: PPIVM testing was WNL with firm and ligamentous end feel
    - Extension: P/A glide on SPs was moderately restricted throughout with firm end feel
    - Rotation: PPIVM testing was minimally restricted bilaterally, lateral glide on SPs minimally restricted with firm end feel
    - Sidebending: Moderately restricted L, minimally restricted R
  - Lumbar spine

- Flexion: PPIVM was mildly restricted
- Extension: P/A on SPs was mildly restricted
- Sidebending: Prone hip abduction PPIVM sidebending was more restricted on R than L
- Rotation: Prone lifting of iliac crest revealed mild restriction bilaterally
- Shoulder complex
  - GH joint
    ▸ Flexion: Distraction was minimally restricted bilaterally, A/P glide was minimally restricted bilaterally
    ▸ Extension: P/A glide was WNL
    ▸ Abduction: Lateral distraction was minimally restricted bilaterally, inferior glide was minimally restricted bilaterally
    ▸ ER: P/A glide was minimally restricted bilaterally
    ▸ IR: A/P glide was WNL
  - AC joint
    ▸ Anterior glide: WNL
    ▸ Posterior glide: Minimally restricted bilaterally
  - SC joint
    ▸ Superior glide: WNL
    ▸ Inferior glide: Minimally restricted bilaterally
    ▸ Anterior glide: WNL
    ▸ Posterior glide: Minimally restricted bilaterally
  - ST joint
    ▸ Distraction: Minimally restricted bilaterally
    ▸ Upward rotation: Minimally restricted bilaterally
    ▸ Retraction: Minimally restricted bilaterally
- Hip
  - Longitudinal distraction: Minimally restricted R>L
  - Lateral distraction: Minimally restricted R>L
  - A/P glide of the femur: Moderately restricted R>L
- Knee
  - Distraction: Minimally restricted R>L
  - A/P glide tibia: Minimally restricted R>L
  - P/A glide tibia: Moderately restricted R>L
  - P/A glide fibula head: Minimally restricted R>L
  - Medial glide tibia: Mildly hypermobile R>L
  - Lateral glide tibia: Moderately restricted R>L
- Ankle
  - Distraction: R was moderately restricted, L minimally restricted
  - Anterior glide tibia on talus: R was moderately restricted, L minimally restricted
  - Calcaneal rock: Bilaterally moderately restricted R>L in inversion
  - Superior glide navicular on talus: R was severely restricted, L moderately restricted
  - Great toe
    - Distraction: First MTP joint was moderately restricted bilaterally
- ◆ Motor function
  - Observation of dexterity, coordination, and agility revealed activities WNL
- ◆ Muscle performance
  - Dynamometry revealed a right grip strength of 45 lbs (normal mean for patient's age is 42.6 lbs), left grip strength 40 lbs (normal mean 37.6)[34]
  - MMT revealed the following deviations from normal:
    - Cervical spine extension=3/5
    - Thoracic spine extension=3/5
    - Scapula depression R=3/5, L=3/5
    - Shoulder flexion R=4/5, L=4/5
    - Shoulder abduction R=4/5, L=4/5,
    - Hip flexion R=3/5, L=4/5
    - Hip extension R=3/5, L=4/5
    - Knee extension R=3+/5, L=4/5
    - Knee flexion bilaterally=4+
    - Ankle inversion R=3/5, L=4/5
    - Great toe abduction bilaterally=3
  - Muscle tension (palpation)
    - Spasm
      ▸ Upper trapezius L>R
      ▸ Lumbar paraspinals L>R
      ▸ Right buttock
- ◆ Pain
  - Pain using the NPS (0=no pain and 10=the worst possible pain) was 6-7/10 in both knees and ankles and 3/10 across her low back
  - Mrs. Chen scored 35/50 on the Oswestry Low Back Pain Disability Questionnaire (ODQ) indicating a moderate degree of disability
    - The ODQ has been shown to be an instrument with high internal consistency[80]
- ◆ Posture
  - Observational assessment done from all perspectives, and grid photographs and plumb line used
    - Lateral view: Revealed forward head, thoracic kyphosis, increased in the upper thoracic spine, decreased lordosis, mildly flexed hips and knees with R>L, pes planus R third degree, L first degree

- Posterior view: Revealed mild scoliosis, mildly elevated right shoulder, inferior right iliac crest, genu valgus R>L
- Anterior view: Revealed mild scoliosis, mildly elevated right shoulder, inferior right iliac crest, genu valgus R>L, bilateral hallux valgus

◆ Range of motion
  - Functional range
    - Decreased ability to elevate both UEs to end range
    - Decreased ability to look up to the ceiling
    - Decreased ability to look over either shoulder
    - Decreased lumbar flexion, extension, and bilateral lateral flexion
    - Decreased R hip ER and IR
    - Decreased knee flexion bilaterally
    - Decreased R knee extension
    - Decreased R ankle dorsiflexion
    - Decreased R ankle inversion
    - Decreased large toe abduction
  - Joint active and passive movement
    - Cervical spine ROM was measured using the CROM instrument. Intratester reliability was found to be high (ICC=0.93)[39] and intertester reliability was found to be moderate (ICCs=0.83, 0.775)[8,39] for CROM measurements
    - Hickey found moderate intertester reliability for both the CROM and the plumb line technique[8]
    - The validity of the CROM measurement was compared to a radiographic measurement, and the Pearson's r correlation was very high between the two methods (flexion r=0.97, P<0.001, extension r=0.98, P<0.001)[40]
      ‣ Cervical spine (CROM)
        ○ Flexion=45 degrees
        ○ Extension=20 degrees
        ○ Lateral flexion=15 degrees bilaterally
        ○ Rotation=R 35 degrees, L 38 degrees
      ‣ Thoracic spine (inclinometry)
        ○ Flexion=30 degrees
        ○ Extension=0 degrees
        ○ Lateral flexion=10 degrees bilaterally
        ○ Rotation=25 degrees
      ‣ Lumbar spine (inclinometry)
        ○ Flexion=25 degrees
        ○ Extension=10 degrees
        ○ Lateral flexion=10 degrees
        ○ Rotation=3 degrees
      ‣ Shoulder (goniometry)
        ○ Flexion R=0 to 150 degrees and L=0 to 153 degrees

○ Abduction R=0 to 150 degrees and L=0 to 153 degrees
○ ER R=50 degrees and L=55 degrees
‣ Hip (goniometry)
  ○ Flexion=WNL
  ○ Extension=R=0 degrees and L=5 degrees
  ○ Abduction=R=0 to 20 degrees and L=25 degrees
  ○ Adduction=WNL
  ○ IR=0 to 10 degrees bilaterally
  ○ ER=WNL
‣ Knee (goniometry)
  ○ Flexion=0 to 120 degrees bilaterally
  ○ Extension R=-7 degrees and L=-5 degrees
‣ Ankle (goniometry)
  ○ Dorsiflexion=R=0 to 5 degrees and L=0 to 10 degrees
  ○ Plantarflexion=WNL
  ○ Inversion=R=0 to 15 degrees and L=0 to 25 degrees
  ○ Eversion=WNL
- Muscle length
  - Tight pectoralis bilaterally
  - Tight cervical extensors
  - Tight scaleni
  - Tight lumbar extensors
  - Tight hip flexors bilaterally
  - Tight hip external rotators
  - Tight hamstrings bilaterally
  - Tight ankle evertors bilaterally
  - Tight heel cords bilaterally
  - Tight toe flexors and arch bilaterally

◆ Reflex integrity
  - DTRs or myotatic reflexes: Brisk and symmetrical (1+) x 4

◆ Self-care and home management
  - Interview concerning ability to safely perform self-care and home management actions, tasks, and activities revealed that they could be accomplished with mild discomfort, but pain was experienced with climbing stairs, kneeling, squatting, and walking and with prolonged standing

◆ Work, community, and leisure integration or reintegration
  - Interview concerning ability to safely manage work, community, and leisure actions, tasks, and activities revealed that they could be performed for short periods of time but with discomfort. Pain was noted during climbing stairs, kneeling, squatting, walking, and prolonged standing

EVALUATION

Mrs. Chen's history and risk factors previously outlined indicated that she is a 51-year-old Asian female retired seamstress, non-smoker, non-exerciser, with HTN, hypothyroidism, OA, and a family history of OA, HTN, and scoliosis. She has faulty postural alignment; poor body mechanics; decreased joint mobility; decreased muscle strength in her cervical, thoracic, and lumbar spines and LE muscles; and decreased ROM in her spine, UEs, and LEs. She has difficulty with overhead activities, reaching forward, kneeling, squatting, and climbing stairs during her ADL and IADL. She has pain at a level of 6-7/10 in her knees and ankles and 3/10 across her low back.

DIAGNOSIS

Mrs. Chen is a patient with faulty alignment of her feet and pain in her knees and low back that have caused postural dysfunctions throughout her LEs, pelvis, low back, and thoracic and cervical spines. She has impaired: ergonomics and body mechanics; gait, locomotion, and balance; joint integrity and mobility; muscle performance; posture; and range of motion. She is functionally limited in self-care and home management and in work, community, and leisure actions, tasks, and activities. These findings are consistent with placement in Pattern B: Impaired Posture. The identified impairments and functional limitations will then be addressed in determining the prognosis and the plan of care.

PROGNOSIS AND PLAN OF CARE

Over the course of the visits, the following mutually established outcomes have been determined:
- Ability to perform physical actions, tasks, and activities related to self-care, home management, work, community, and leisure is improved with improved body mechanics
- Balance is improved
- Joint integrity and mobility are improved
- Joint swelling, inflammation, and restriction are reduced
- Knowledge of behaviors that foster healthy habits, wellness, and prevention is increased
- Muscle length is increased
- Muscle performance is increased
- Muscle spasms are decreased
- Muscle strength is increased
- Pain is decreased
- Physical capacity is improved
- Physical function is improved
- Postural control is improved

- Risk factors are reduced
- Risk of secondary impairment is reduced
- ROM is improved
- Stress is decreased

To achieve these outcomes, the appropriate interventions for this patient are determined. These will include: coordination, communication, and documentation; patient/client-related instruction; therapeutic exercise; functional training in self-care and home management; functional training in work, community, and leisure integration or reintegration; manual therapy techniques; prescription, application, and, as appropriate, fabrication of devices and equipment; electrotherapeutic modalities; and physical agents and mechanical modalities.

Based on the diagnosis and the prognosis, Mrs. Chen is expected to require 18 to 20 visits over 16 to 18 weeks. Mrs. Chen has good social support, is motivated, and follows through with her home exercise program. She is not severely impaired and is fairly healthy.

INTERVENTIONS

RATIONALE FOR SELECTED INTERVENTIONS

Poor posture may result in changes of normal anatomical relationships. The joints in the kinematic chain may become compromised resulting in a modification of the gait pattern. Alteration in foot biomechanics may lead to dysfunctions of the ankle, knee, hip, sacroiliac, and shoulder joints and the lumbar, thoracic, and cervical spines. Each joint has a direct influence on its surrounding counterpart. For example, if the subtalar joint is held in pronation, a medial rotatory force is exerted on the leg causing medial rotation at the knee and/or hip joint. The pronated position of the foot may result in lowering of the arch, creating a functional leg length difference. A pelvic obliquity or a scoliosis may then develop, ultimately leading to postural faults at the shoulder girdle and the cervical/thoracic spine.

CKC mechanics occur when the LE is in a weightbearing position. The calcaneus is capable of inversion and eversion; however, the foot is unable to perform dorsiflexion/plantarflexion or abduction/adduction. Inversion/eversion do not occur as isolated movements but rather as combined motions at the proximal talar joint. In weightbearing, the talus moves in the opposite direction of the calcaneus. During closed chain subtalar supination, the calcaneus inverts. Given that the calcaneus cannot adduct or plantarflex in weightbearing, abduction and dorsiflexion must occur at the talus. The talus abducts carrying the tibia and fibula with it. This motion creates lateral rotation of the leg and relative knee extension. During closed chain subtalar pronation the calcaneus everts, and the talus plantarflexes and adducts in relation to the calcaneus. This motion creates adduction of the talus causing medial rotation of the leg and relative knee flexion. In non-weightbearing mechanics, the motions of the subtalar joint and the leg occur independently of each other.[12]

Pronation and supination twists of the TMT joints occur when the transverse tarsal joint is unable to counter-rotate or when compensation for the position of the hind foot is needed. When the entire forefoot sustains an inversion rotation around a hypothetical axis at the second ray it is referred to as a supination twist of the TMT joints. A supination twist occurs when the hind foot pronates in weightbearing and the transverse tarsal joint supinates to allow for counter-rotation of the forefoot. If the range of transverse tarsal supination is not adequate to counter the pronating force, the medial forefoot will press into the ground and the lateral side will be lifted. In order to maintain contact with the ground, the first and second rays will dorsiflex while the fourth and fifth rays will plantarflex. This motion is associated with inversion.[12]

Pronation twist occurs when both the hind foot and the transverse tarsal joints are supinated. When the hind foot supinates, the forefoot becomes elevated on its medial side and presses into the ground on the lateral side. A pronation twist occurs at the forefoot, with eversion and plantarflexion at the first and second rays and dorsiflexion at the fourth and fifth rays.[12]

Therapeutic Exercise

Exercise is an important choice of physical therapist interventions for individuals with postural abnormalities. Exercise is not only an intervention that may maximize muscle capability to align posture, but it may also address other impairments associated with this condition. Many postural deviations may occur secondary to muscle imbalances.[51] The reader is referred to Case Study #1 for additional rationale for therapeutic exercise.

Manual Therapy Techniques

Bang and Deyle[64] and others[30,65] have demonstrated improvements in ROM, pain, and function associated with manual physical therapy interventions used in the management of patient populations with painful stiff spines and extremity joints.[30-33] Manual therapy techniques include the use of skilled hands to enhance tissue extensibility, joint mobility, modulate pain, decrease spasm, and reduce soft tissue swelling. The reader is referred to Case Study #1 for additional information on rationale on manual therapy.

Electrotherapeutic Modalities

Electrotherapeutic modalities have been documented to decrease pain, muscle spasm, and relax the soft tissue structures. The reader is referred to the rationale for these modalities in Case Study #1 for additional information on rationale for electrotherapeutic modalities.

Physical Agents and Mechanical Modalities

Thermotherapy includes the use of moist heat to enhance tissue perfusion and oxygenation[72] and cryotherapy to decrease pain, joint swelling, and inflammation.[72] The reader is referred to the rationale for these modalities in Case Study #1 for additional information on rationale for physical agents and mechanical modalities.

COORDINATION, COMMUNICATION, AND DOCUMENTATION

Communication will occur with Mrs. Chen. All elements of the patient's management will be documented. Referrals for weight loss and nutritional programs are appropriate. A plan of care will be developed and discussed with the patient.

PATIENT/CLIENT-RELATED INSTRUCTION

Education regarding her current condition, impairments, and functional limitations will be discussed. The patient will be instructed in appropriate body mechanics, proper posture, flexibility, mobility, ROM, strengthening, core stabilization, and balance activities. Risk factors will be discussed including being overweight and the influence that poor posture can have on aerobic capacity and functional activities. A nutritional referral will be made. Ergonomic instruction for work as a dressmaker will be provided.

THERAPEUTIC EXERCISE

♦ Aerobic capacity/endurance conditioning
  • Although the patient was not tested for aerobic capacity, it is appropriate for this patient to participate in some type of aerobic training (eg, recumbent bicycle)
♦ Balance, coordination, and agility training
  • Sitting on exercise ball in front of a mirror
  • Bouncing on exercise ball
  • Unilateral stance on stable surface with pertubations
  • Bilateral standing on foam rubber cushion
  • Unilateral standing on foam rubber cushion
  • Side gliding
  • Braiding
  • Standing on foam roller
  • Balance beam
  • Obstacle course
♦ Body mechanics and postural stabilization
  • Body mechanics training
    ▪ Appropriate sitting posture for work and leisure actions, tasks, and activities
    ▪ Appropriate use of body mechanics while dressmaking

- Appropriate lifting and carrying instructions
- Appropriate bending instructions
- Postural control training
  - Proper alignment of head and cervical, thoracic, and lumbar spines
  - Axial extension to achieve position of no more than 2 inches from the deepest portion of the cervical lordosis to the apex of the thoracic kyphosis[75]
  - Scapula retraction and depression
  - Chicken wing position (hands behind head, horizontal abduction of shoulders)
  - Proper postural position during transition:
    - From supine to sitting, standing, and walking
    - From sit to kneel
    - From 1/2 kneel to stand
    - To functional activities at work
    - To functional activities at leisure
- Postural stabilization activities[76]
  - Axial extension starting in supine and progressing to sitting and upright
  - Maintenance of axial extension position with bilateral arm raises
  - Maintenance of axial extension position with arm raises with addition of weights, starting, for example, with a low weight for 8 to 12 reps and increasing accordingly
  - Glut sets
  - Bridging
  - Unilateral bridging
  - Maintain bridge and add hip flexion right and then left
  - Maintain bridge and add knee extension right and then left
  - Prone glut sets
  - Utilize ball for supine exercises
    - Arm raises in supine over ball
    - Knee extension in supine over exercise ball
  - Alternate opposite arm and leg
  - Incorporate use of the ball for prone exercises
  - Incorporate the use of the foam roller and unstable surfaces like wobble board or foam rubber cushion in sitting and standing with bilateral and unilateral stance
  - Decrease base of support
  - Utilize balance beam
  - Challenge patient out of center of gravity/base of support
- Postural awareness training
  - Use of mirror for visual input of appropriate alignment

- Notes all around home, car, office
- Flexibility exercises
  - Stretching exercises should be done after warming up, using a slow and steady stretch accompanied by deep breathing, and building hold up to 30 to 60 seconds
  - Cervical ROM in all directions both AROM and AAROM
  - Shoulder ROM in flexion, abduction, and ER
  - Thoracic ROM extension, rotation and lateral flexion
  - Lumbar ROM in all directions
  - Hip ROM for extension, abduction, and IR
  - Knee ROM in all directions
  - Ankle ROM: Hind foot eversion, dorsiflexion, inversion
  - Cervical flexion and lateral flexion stretching
  - Anterior chest wall and shoulder stretching
  - Hamstring stretching
  - Quadriceps stretching
  - Hip flexor stretching
  - Heel cord stretching
  - Corner stretch
- Strength, power, and endurance training
  - UE weight training for shoulder flexion, abduction, IR, and ER starting, for example, with a low weight, 8 to 12 reps and progressing according to patient's tolerance, being sure that good postural alignment is maintained
  - LE weight training for hip and knee flexion and extension and ankle inversion starting, for example, with a low weight, 8 to 12 reps and progressing according to patient's tolerance
  - Seated push-ups
  - Wall push-ups and push-up plus[81]
  - Stool rolling forward and backward
  - Plyometrics with a variety of weighted balls

Maintenance of a regular exercise program must be instilled in this patient. To do this there are several keys that may be helpful in achieving an exercise program that the patient will do on an life-long basis. These are included in Case Study #1.

FUNCTIONAL TRAINING IN SELF-CARE AND HOME MANAGEMENT

- Self-care and home management
  - Review all actions, tasks, and activities and postural alignment for self-care and home management

FUNCTIONAL TRAINING IN WORK, COMMUNITY, AND LEISURE INTEGRATION OR REINTEGRATION

- ◆ Work
  - Simulation of the work environment including sitting at the sewing machine
  - Simulation of work tasks involved in hemming clothes, sewing buttons, etc and modifications to improve body mechanics and awareness of movement
  - Training in simulated tasks
- ◆ Community
  - Simulation of tasks needed for her church activities
- ◆ Leisure
  - Instruction and simulation of appropriate positions for reading, sewing, and watching television emphasizing correct cervical posture
- ◆ Injury prevention or reduction
  - Awareness of safety precautions involved with work

MANUAL THERAPY TECHNIQUES

- ◆ Massage
  - Connective tissue massage/myofascial release[65]
    - To plantar fascia, hamstrings, and paraspinal muscles
- ◆ Mobilization/manipulation
  - Soft tissue
    - Anterior chest wall
    - Anterior shoulder capsule
    - Cervical, thoracic, and lumbar paraspinal muscles
    - Suboccipital muscles
    - Upper trapezius, scaleni, SCM
    - Rhomboids and middle trapezius
    - Hip flexors
    - Hamstrings
    - Quadriceps
    - Gastroc-soleus
    - Lateral aspect of both knees
    - Plantar fascia
  - Spinal and peripheral joints[30-33]
    - Manual distraction to cervical, thoracic, and lumbar spines to increase intervertebral space and improve intervertebral mobility
    - Longitudinal and lateral distraction of the GH joint to increase joint space and ROM in flexion and abduction
    - Distraction of the tibia to increase joint space and increase ROM of the knee
    - Distraction of the talocrural joint to increase joint space and increase ROM of ankle dorsiflexion and inversion
  - Grades III and IV mobilizations performed in the resting position, progressing the physiological position of the joint to follow the pathological end range until patient reaches the anatomical limit
    - P/A glide of GH joint to increase anterior capsule length and increase ROM in ER
    - PAIVM to increase axial extension of the cervical spine
    - PAIVM to increase thoracic extension and lumbar flexion and extension
    - P/A glide of SPs/bilateral transverse processes of thoracic spine to decrease kyphosis and increase mobility
    - P/A glide of SPs/bilateral transverse processes of lumbar spine to decrease lordosis and increase mobility
    - Lateral distraction of femur to increase length of capsule and increase ROM in abduction and IR
    - Ventral glide of the femur to increase hip extension
    - Posterior glide of the tibia to increase knee flexion
    - Anterior glide of the tibia to increase knee extension
    - Posterior glide of the talus to increase ankle dorsiflexion
    - Calcaneal rock to increase calcaneal inversion

PRESCRIPTION, APPLICATION, AND, AS APPROPRIATE, FABRICATION OF DEVICES AND EQUIPMENT

- ◆ Orthotic device
  - The patient will be referred to a podiatrist for evaluation and fabrication of an appropriate foot orthotic device

ELECTROTHERAPEUTIC MODALITIES

- ◆ EMS and TENS to decrease pain and spasm

PHYSICAL AGENTS AND MECHANICAL MODALITIES

- ◆ Sound agents
  - Ultrasound to increase tissue perfusion, oxygenation, and nutrient delivery to the tissues
- ◆ Thermotherapy
  - Hot packs to increase muscle extensibility and decrease spasm in cervical and thoracic spine muscles

♦ Traction device
  ● Intermittent/static, as indicated, cervical traction to increase intervertebral joint space and open nerve root foramen

ANTICIPATED GOALS AND EXPECTED OUTCOMES

♦ Impact on pathology/pathophysiology
  ● Edema is decreased to ¼ inches around right knee.
  ● Joint restriction is reduced by 10% to 15%.
  ● Muscle spasm is eliminated.
  ● Neural compression is decreased.
  ● Nutrient delivery to tissue is increased.
  ● Pain is decreased from 6-7/10 to 4-5/10 in knees and ankles and from 3/10 to 1/10 across the low back. Oswestry was reduced from 35/50 to 25/50.
  ● Soft tissue restriction is reduced in cervical, thoracic, and lumbar spines; shoulders; hips; knees; and ankles.
  ● Tissue perfusion and oxygenation are increased.
  ● Tissue restriction is normalized.
♦ Impact on impairments
  ● Balance is improved from fair to good on the Nudge/Push test for posterior perturbations.
  ● Joint mobility of shoulder, hips, knees, ankles, feet, and cervical, thoracic, and lumbar spines is improved by 10% to 15%.
  ● Joint stability is improved.
  ● Muscle length is elongated in the pectorals, cervical extensors, scaleni, lumbar extensors, hip flexors and external rotators, hamstrings, ankle evertors, heel cords, and toe flexors by 10%.
  ● Muscle performance including strength, power, and endurance is increased in cervical spine extension, thoracic spine extension, scapula depression to 4/5, shoulder flexion and abduction to 4+/5, hip flexion and extension to 4/5 on the right and 4+/5 on the left, knee flexion to 5/5, knee extension to 4/5 on the right and 4+/5 on the left, ankle inversion to 4/5 on the right and 4+/5 on the left, and great toe abduction to 4/5.
  ● Optimal joint alignment and loading of the foot are improved.
  ● Postural alignment, control, and awareness during actions, tasks, and activities within the home (homemaker) and during work (dressmaker) and leisure are improved. FHP and thoracic kyphosis are minimally improved.
  ● Quality of movement is improved.
  ● Relaxation is increased.
  ● ROM is WFL in cervical (extension, rotation, and sidebending), thoracic (extension), and lumbar (flexion, extension, sidebending, and rotation) spines; shoulders (flexion and abduction); hips (extension, abduction, and IR); knees (flexion and extension); ankles (dorsiflexion and inversion); feet; and toes.
♦ Impact on functional limitations
  ● Ability to perform physical actions, tasks, and activities related to self-care, home management (homemaker), work (dressmaker), community, and leisure is improved.
  ● Tolerance of positions and actions, tasks, and activities required for work (sitting at the sewing machine) and leisure is improved.
♦ Risk reduction/prevention
  ● Communication enhances risk reduction and prevention of complications.
  ● Risk factors are decreased.
  ● Risk of recurrence of present condition is decreased.
  ● Risk of secondary impairment is decreased.
  ● Safety is improved.
  ● Self-management of symptoms is improved.
♦ Impact on health, wellness, and fitness
  ● Behaviors that promote healthy nutrition, physical activity, and wellness are promoted.
  ● Fitness is improved.
  ● Health status is improved.
  ● Physical function is improved.
♦ Impact on societal resources
  ● Documentation occurs throughout patient management and across all settings and follows APTA's *Guidelines for Physical Therapy Documentation.*[78]
♦ Patient/client satisfaction
  ● Patient and family knowledge and awareness of the diagnosis, prognosis, interventions, and anticipated goals and expected outcomes are increased.
  ● Patient satisfaction with program is achieved.
  ● Sense of well-being and control are improved.
  ● Stressors are decreased.

REEXAMINATION

Reexamination is performed throughout the episode of care.

DISCHARGE

Mrs. Chen is discharged from physical therapy after a total of 18 physical therapy sessions and attainment of her goals and expectations. These sessions have covered her entire episode of service. She is discharged because she has achieved her goals and expected outcomes.

Case Study #3: Scheuermann's Disease

Joe Brown is a 20-year-old male who has a thoracic kyphosis and has been diagnosed with Scheuermann's disease.

PHYSICAL THERAPIST EXAMINATION

HISTORY

♦ General demographics: Joe Brown is a 20-year-old black American male whose primary language is English. He is right-hand dominant. He is presently a college student.

♦ Social history: He is single.

♦ Employment/work: He is a student in his junior year at an out-of-town college.

♦ Living environment: He lives in off-campus housing with several friends.

♦ General health status
  • General health perception: Joe reports that he is in good health.
  • Physical function: He perceives that he functions normally for his age.
  • Psychological function: Normal.
  • Role function: Student.
  • Social function: He is involved in clubs and some non-contact sports at school. He particularly enjoys playing tennis.

♦ Social/health habits: Joe does not smoke and likes to drink beer on the weekends.

♦ Family history: His mother has HTN.

♦ Medical/surgical history: Joe was diagnosed with Scheuermann's disease at age 15 with a 68-degree kyphosis as measured using Cobb's angle. He wore an orthosis to correct his scoliosis for 18 months full-time from the time of diagnosis and then for 6 months part-time. His current curve is 50 degrees.[24]

♦ Prior hospitalizations: None.

♦ Preexisting medical and other health-related conditions: Noncontributory.

♦ Current condition(s)/chief complaint(s): Joe is concerned about his appearance. He is concerned that his posture and his ability to perform activities might deteriorate now that he is not wearing an orthosis.

♦ Functional status and activity level: He is totally independent in all ADL and IADL. He exercises as part of his gym class, walks regularly, and plays tennis.

♦ Medications: He only takes over-the-counter (OTC) vitamins.

♦ Other clinical tests: Plain films reveal kyphosis (Cobb method) of 50 degrees[20] with vertebral wedging, irregular vertebral end plates, Schmorl's nodes, and decreased vertebral height.[22,26] Narrowing of the intervertebral disc spaces and three wedged vertebrae were also noted.[24] His MRI reveals protrusion of discal material into the vertebral bodies at T4-7. His bone density test was normal.

SYSTEMS REVIEW

♦ Cardiovascular/pulmonary
  • BP: 118/76 mmHg
  • Edema: None
  • HR: 70 bpm
  • RR: 10 bpm

♦ Integumentary
  • Presence of scar formation: None
  • Skin color: WNL
  • Skin integrity: WNL

♦ Musculoskeletal
  • Gross range of motion: Restricted in cervical, thoracic, and lumbar spines; both shoulders; bilateral SLR; bilateral hip extension
  • Gross strength: Limited in scapula retractors, extensors (cervical, thoracic, and lumbar), and hip extensors
  • Gross symmetry
    ▪ Mild forward head
    ▪ Moderate thoracic kyphosis
    ▪ Scoliosis
    ▪ Anterior pelvic tilt
    ▪ Moderate lumbar lordosis[82]
  • Height: 6'3" (1.905 m)
  • Weight: 180 lbs (81.648 kg)

♦ Neuromuscular
  • Balance: WNL
  • Locomotion, transfers, and transitions: WNL

♦ Communication, affect, cognition, language, and learning style
  • Communication, affect, and cognition: WNL
  • Learning preferences: Auditory learner

TESTS AND MEASURES

♦ Anthropometric characteristics
  • BMI=705 x (body weight [in pounds] divided by height^2 [in inches])
  • BMI=22.56
  • BMI between 18.5 and 24.9 is considered to be normal[29]

♦ Cranial and peripheral nerve integrity
  • Sensation: WNL in all four extremities

- ◆ Ergonomics and body mechanics
  - Analysis of body mechanics during self-care, home management, work, community, and leisure actions, tasks, and activities revealed altered posture during all activities
  - Joe tends to slump forward as he takes notes in class and also while spending long hours in the library studying
  - He also tends to slouch as he plays tennis
- ◆ Joint integrity and mobility
  - Joint integrity and mobility assessment entails not only the osteokinematic and arthrokinematic analysis but also the structural integrity of the joint
  - This includes special tests designed to assess ligamentous stability, compression, distraction tests, impingement tests, and joint play[30-33]
  - Cervical spine
    - Flexion: PPIVM testing was mildly restricted with firm and ligamentous end feel
    - Extension: PPIVM testing was mildly restricted with firm and ligamentous end feel
  - Lumbar spine
    - Flexion: PPIVM testing was moderately restricted throughout the lumbar spine
    - Extension: PPIVM using P/A pressure on SPs was WNL
  - Shoulder complex
    - GH joint
      - ▸ Flexion: Distraction was minimally restricted bilaterally, A/P glide was minimally restricted bilaterally
      - ▸ Extension: P/A glide was WNL
      - ▸ Abduction: Lateral distraction was minimally restricted bilaterally, inferior glide was minimally restricted bilaterally
      - ▸ ER: P/A glide was minimally restricted bilaterally
      - ▸ IR: A/P glide was WNL
    - AC joint
      - ▸ Anterior glide was WNL
      - ▸ Posterior glide was minimally restricted bilaterally
    - SC joint
      - ▸ Distraction was minimally restricted bilaterally
      - ▸ Superior glide was WNL
      - ▸ Inferior glide was minimally restricted bilaterally
      - ▸ Anterior glide was WNL
      - ▸ Posterior glide was minimally restricted bilaterally
    - ST joint

- ▸ Distraction was minimally restricted bilaterally
- ▸ Upward rotation was minimally restricted bilaterally
- ▸ Retraction was moderately restricted bilaterally
  - Hip
    - Longitudinal and lateral distraction were minimally restricted bilaterally
    - Anterior glide of the femur was moderately restricted bilaterally
- ◆ Motor function
  - Observation of dexterity, coordination, and agility revealed activities WNL
- ◆ Muscle performance
  - Dynamometry revealed a right grip strength of 135 lbs (normal mean for patient's age is 121 lbs), left grip strength 125 lbs (normal mean 104.5 lbs)[34]
  - MMT revealed the following:
    - Cervical spine extension=4/5
    - Thoracic spine extension=3/5
    - Abdominals=3/5
    - Lumbar extension=4/5
    - Scapula adduction=R 3/5 and L 3/5
    - Scapula depression=R 3/5 and L 3/5
    - Shoulder flexion=R 4/5 and L 4/5
    - Hip extension=4/5
  - Muscle tension (palpation)
    - Spasm
      - ▸ Paraspinals along thoracic kyphosis
      - ▸ Rhomboids and middle trapezeii
- ◆ Pain
  - Using the NPS (0=no pain and 10=the worst possible pain), pain of 4/10 at the apex of the thoracic kyphosis and 2/10 at the lumbar spine
  - Downie and associates[35] described a high degree of agreement between the VAS, NPS, and SDS although they report that the NPS performed better
  - Jensen[36] found the NPS to be the most practical tool
- ◆ Posture
  - Observational assessment and grid photographs were used
    - Lateral view: FHP, thoracic kyphosis, protracted shoulders, internally rotated UEs, anterior pelvic tilt, increased lumbar lordosis
    - Posterior view: Scoliosis, internally rotated UEs, protracted shoulders
    - Anterior view: Scoliosis, internally rotated UEs
- ◆ Range of motion
  - Functional range: Decreased ability to elevate and

abduct both UEs to end range, decreased ability to extend trunk and stand erect

- Joint active and passive movement
  - Shoulder (goniometry)
    - Flexion=R 0 to 150 degrees and L 0 to 155 degrees
    - Abduction=R 0 to 150 degrees and L 0 to 155 degrees
    - ER=R 0 to 50 degrees and L 0 to 50 degrees
  - Hip (goniometry)
    - SLR=R 0 to 50 degrees and L 0 to 52 degrees
  - Cervical spine ROM was measured using the CROM instrument. Intratester reliability was found to be high (ICC=0.93)[39] and intertester reliability was found to be moderate (ICCs=0.83, 0.775)[8,39] for CROM measurements
  - Hickey found moderate intertester reliability for both the CROM and the plumb line technique[8]
  - The validity of the CROM measurement was compared to a radiographic measurement, and the Pearson's r correlation was very high between the two methods (flexion r=0.97, P<0.001, extension r=0.98, P<0.001)[40]
    - Flexion=80 degrees
    - Extension=70 degrees
    - Lateral flexion=25 degrees bilaterally
    - Rotation=R 70 degrees and L 70 degrees
  - Thoracic spine (inclinometry)
    - Flexion=50 degrees
    - Extension=0 degrees
    - Lateral flexion=15 degrees bilaterally
    - Rotation=30 degrees bilaterally
  - Lumbar spine (inclinometry)
    - Flexion=45 degrees
    - Extension=10 degrees
    - Lateral flexion=10 degrees bilaterally
    - Rotation=WNL
- Muscle tightness
  - Tightness in pectorals bilaterally
  - Tightness in horizontal abduction bilaterally
  - Tightness in hip flexors bilaterally
  - Tightness in hamstrings bilaterally
- Reflex integrity
  - DTRs or myotatic reflexes: Brisk and symmetrical in all four extremities
- Self-care and home management
  - Interview concerning ability to safely perform self-care and home management actions, tasks, and activities found they could be done within normal limits despite mild discomfort
- Work, community, and leisure integration or reintegration

- Interview concerning ability to safely manage work, community, and leisure actions, tasks, and activities revealed that they could be done, but pain was experienced with prolonged standing

EVALUATION

Joe Brown's history and risk factors previously outlined indicated that he is a 20-year-male student, exerciser, with Scheuermann's disease and a family history of HTN. He has thoracic kyphosis; altered muscle strength in his thoracic and lumbar spines, scapula, and UE muscles; and decreased ROM throughout his spine, shoulders, and with straight leg raising. He has difficulty with overhead activities, prolonged flexed postures, and extending his thoracic spine, especially during tennis and heavy tasks during his ADL and IADL. He also experiences pain at the apex of his kyphosis and across his low back.

DIAGNOSIS

Joe Brown is a patient who has been diagnosed with Scheuermann's disease with pain in his thoracic and lumbar spines. He has impaired: ergonomics and body mechanics; joint integrity and mobility; muscle performance; posture; and range of motion. He is minimally functionally limited in self-care and home management and in work, community, and leisure actions, tasks, and activities. These findings are consistent with placement in Pattern B: Impaired Posture. The identified impairments and functional limitations will be addressed in determining the prognosis and the plan of care.

PROGNOSIS AND PLAN OF CARE

Over the course of the visits, the following mutually established outcomes have been determined:

- Ability to perform physical actions, tasks, and activities related to self-care, home management, school, community, and leisure is improved
- Knowledge of behaviors that foster healthy habits, wellness, and prevention is increased
- Muscle length is increased
- Muscle performance is increased
- Muscle spasms are decreased
- Physical capacity is improved
- Physical function is improved
- Postural control is improved
- Risk factors are reduced
- Risk of secondary impairment is reduced
- ROM is increased
- Stress is decreased

To achieve these outcomes, the appropriate interventions for this patient are determined. These will include: coordination, communication, and documentation; patient/client-related instruction; therapeutic exercise; functional training in self-care and home management; functional training in work, community, and leisure integration or reintegration; and manual therapy techniques.

Based on the diagnosis and the prognosis, Joe is expected to require 10 to 14 visits over 12 to 14 weeks. He has good social support, is motivated, and follows through with his home exercise program. He is not severely impaired and is healthy.

INTERVENTIONS

RATIONALE FOR SELECTED INTERVENTIONS

Therapeutic Exercise

Exercise is an important choice of physical therapist interventions for individuals with Scheuermann's disease. Exercise is not only an intervention that may maximize muscle capability to align posture, but it may also address other impairments associated with this condition. Patients with the diagnosis of Scheuermann's disease may have pain in the area of their kyphosis and pain and stiffness compensatory to the disease process above and below the affected area. Hyperlordosis of the lumbar spine and FHP may be present.[24] Approximately one-third of the patients have a mild to moderate scoliosis.[24] Patients may also have tightening of the shoulder horizontal adductors, hip flexors, and knee flexors and weakness in the thoracic spine extensors, lumbar extensors, and hip extensors. There is evidence that the untreated kyphosis in an adult may progress. Travaglini and Conte found that 80% of 43 patients followed for 25 years demonstrated increased kyphosis.[24] Emphases on postural awareness and stabilization, body mechanics, and appropriate ergonomic adaptations are appropriate to allow for maximizing this patient's function in the future. The reader is referred to the rationale for inventions in Case Study #1.

This patient may benefit from a combination of instructions on modification of behaviors and a comprehensive program of strengthening, stretching, and manual techniques.[20,82,83]

Manual Therapy Techniques

Manual techniques include the use of skilled hands to enhance tissue extensibility, increase joint mobility, modulate pain, decrease spasm, and reduce soft tissue swelling. Improvements in ROM, pain, and function have been demonstrated with manual physical therapy interventions for painful, stiff spine and extremity joints.[30-33,65] Despite a thorough search in the literature, there is not any evidence to validate the use of mobilization of the thoracic spine in patients diagnosed with Scheuermann's disease. However, manual therapy has been shown to reduce pain in the treatment of mechanical thoracic pain.[84] Patients with Scheuermann's disease have compensatory changes in their spine above and below the primary area of involvement and also in their proximal extremity joints. The treatment of these joint and soft tissue restrictions should be addressed. Secondary muscle spasm may develop and should be addressed with soft tissue techniques and myofascial release.[65] Refer to Case Study #1 for additional rationale regarding manual therapy.

COORDINATION, COMMUNICATION, AND DOCUMENTATION

Communication will occur with Joe Brown. All elements of the patient's management will be documented. A plan of care will be developed and discussed with the patient.

PATIENT/CLIENT-RELATED INSTRUCTION

Education regarding his current condition, impairments, and functional limitations will be discussed. The patient will be instructed in appropriate stretching and strengthening exercises, body mechanics, proper posture, and core stabilization. A discussion will occur regarding the patient's diagnosis, possible progressions of the disease with scenarios describing increased symptoms, and the influence that poor posture can have on aerobic capacity and functional activities. Ergonomic instruction for school and use of the computer will be provided. Body mechanics will be discussed relating to his work, community, and leisure actions, tasks, and activities.

THERAPEUTIC EXERCISE

- Aerobic capacity/endurance conditioning
  - Although the patient was not tested for aerobic capacity, it is appropriate for this patient to participate in some type of aerobic training
- Body mechanics and postural stabilization
  - Body mechanics training
    - Appropriate sitting posture for work and leisure activities
    - Appropriate lifting and carrying instructions
    - Appropriate bending instructions
  - Postural control training
    - Proper alignment of head; cervical, thoracic, and lumbar spines; and shoulders
    - Axial extension to achieve position of no more than 2 inches from the deepest portion of the cervical lordosis to the apex of the thoracic kyphosis[75]
    - Shoulder and scapula retraction and depression

- Chicken wing position (hands behind head, horizontal abduction of shoulders)
- Corner stretch
- Proper postural position during transition:
  - From supine to sitting, standing, and walking
  - To functional activities at work
  - To functional activities at leisure including driving a car
- Postural stabilization activities[76]
  - Axial extension starting in supine and progressing to sitting and upright
  - Maintenance of axial extension position with bilateral arm raises
  - Maintenance of axial extension position with arm raises with addition of weights, starting, for example, with low weights for 8 to 12 reps and increasing accordingly, being sure that good postural alignment is maintained
  - Glut sets
  - Bridging
  - Unilateral bridging
  - Maintain bridge and add hip flexion right and then left
  - Maintain bridge and add knee extension right and then left
  - Ball exercises for postural control in sitting progressing to weights with UEs and LEs, for example, starting with low weights for 8 to 12 reps and progressing in accordance with patient's tolerance, being sure that good postural alignment is maintained
  - Ball exercises in quadruped progressing to prone with emphasis on thoracic extension
  - Push-ups from quadruped on the ball progressing to military push-up position
  - Wall push-ups
  - Pilates extension exercises
  - Plank (yoga position): Straight line push-up position (stomach and chin in strongly)
  - Pelvic stabilization on mat with arm raises
  - Pelvic stabilization on mat with leg raises
  - Pelvic stabilization on mat alternating opposite arm and leg
  - Incorporate the use of the foam roller and unstable surfaces like wobble board or foam rubber cushion in sitting and standing with bilateral and unilateral stance
  - Decrease base of support during exercises
  - Utilize balance beam
  - Challenge patient out of center of gravity/base of support

- Postural awareness training
  - Use of mirror for visual input of appropriate alignment
  - Notes all around home, car, office
- Flexibility exercises
  - Stretching exercises should be done after warming up, using a slow and steady stretch accompanied by deep breathing, and building hold up to 30 to 60 seconds
  - Cervical extension
  - Thoracic extension
  - Lumbar flexion
  - Anterior chest wall and shoulder stretching
  - Hamstring stretching
  - Hip flexor stretching
  - Heel cord stretching
- Strength, power, and endurance training
  - UE weight training for shoulder flexion, abduction, IR, and ER, for example, starting with low weights for 8 to 12 reps and progressing to patient's tolerance, being sure that good postural alignment is maintained
  - Seated push-ups
  - Wall push-ups and push-ups plus (push-up with scapular protraction)[81]
  - Wobble board with clockwise and counterclockwise circles for UEs
  - Fitter for UEs forward and back and sideways
  - Plyometrics with a variety of weighted balls

Maintenance of a regular exercise program must be instilled in this patient. To do this there are several keys that may be helpful in achieving an exercise program that the patient will do on a life-long basis. These tips may be included in part of the patient-related instruction and may include any or all of the following:

- Establish a variety of enjoyable activities and alternating activities when possible
- Establish a realistic time frame for exercise
- Add exercise to one's weekly schedule (walk to school if possible, climb up and down several flights of stairs in his dormitory instead of taking the elevator, wear a weighted vest while at home)
- Find activities that may be done during school hours (climb stairs while he is in school in between classes)
- Find activities that may be done after school
- Find fun alternative activities for weekends
- Allow flexibility
- If a scheduled exercise time is missed, work into schedule at another time during the day or week
- Use entertainment whenever possible
  - Listen to music when performing weight exercises or

while walking outside
- Watch TV while on treadmill
- Use books on tape at anytime

FUNCTIONAL TRAINING IN SELF-CARE AND HOME MANAGEMENT

♦ Self-care and home management
  - Review all actions, tasks, and activities and postural alignment for self-care and home management

FUNCTIONAL TRAINING IN WORK, COMMUNITY, AND LEISURE INTEGRATION OR REINTEGRATION

♦ Work
  - Education, guidelines, and simulation of the school environment including sitting at a desk and in a lecture hall
  - Education regarding appropriate placement of computer monitor and keyboard to maximize ergonomic function
  - Training in simulated tasks
♦ Community
  - Training in postural position for tutoring underprivileged children in the neighborhood
♦ Leisure
  - Instruction and simulation of appropriate reading positions emphasizing correct cervical posture
  - Awareness of body position while playing tennis
  - Training in simulated tennis movements
♦ Injury prevention or reduction
  - Awareness of safety precautions involved with school and leisure actions, tasks, and activities

MANUAL THERAPY TECHNIQUES

♦ Massage
  - Connective tissue massage/myofascial release[65]
    - To anterior chest wall, anterior shoulder, and posterior cervical and thoracic spines
♦ Mobilization/manipulation
  - Soft tissue
    - Cervical and thoracic paraspinal muscles
    - Suboccipital muscles
    - Rhomboids and middle trapezius
  - Spinal and peripheral joints[30-33]
    - Manual cervical distraction to increase intervertebral space and improve intervertebral mobility
    - PAIVM to increase axial extension of the cervical spine
    - P/A glide of SPs of the lumbar spine to decrease lordosis and increase mobility
    - Longitudinal and lateral distraction of the GH joint to increase joint space and ROM in flexion and abduction
    - P/A glide of GH joint to increase anterior capsule length and increase ROM in ER
    - Longitudinal and lateral distraction of the hip joint to increase joint space and ROM in extension

ANTICIPATED GOALS AND EXPECTED OUTCOMES

♦ Impact on pathology/pathophysiology
  - Joint restriction in shoulders, hips, and cervical, thoracic, and lumbar spines is reduced by 10% to 15%.
  - Muscle spasm is alleviated.
  - Pain is reduced from 4/10 to 2/10 in the thoracic spine and from 2/10 to 1/10 in the lumbar spine.
♦ Impact on impairments
  - Joint mobility in the cervical, thoracic, and lumbar spines secondary to reduction of pain is improved by 10% to 15%.
  - Muscle flexibility is increased in the pectoral muscles bilaterally, hip flexors and knee flexors by 10%.
  - Muscle performance including strength, power, and endurance is increased in cervical spine extension to 4/5, thoracic spine extension to 4/5, lumbar extension to 5/5, abdominals to 4/5, scapula adduction and depression to 4/5, shoulder flexion to 4+/5, and hip extension 4+/5.
  - Postural control and awareness is improved especially when at school and when using computer.
  - Quality of movement is improved.
  - Relaxation is increased.
  - ROM is improved in:
    - All shoulder movements by 10 degrees
    - SLR to 60 degrees
    - Cervical, thoracic, and lumbar spines by 10%
♦ Impact on functional limitations
  - Ability to perform pain-free physical actions, tasks, and activities related to self-care, home management, work (student), community, and leisure (tennis and using computer) is achieved.
  - Tolerance of positions required for school and leisure is improved.
♦ Risk reduction/prevention
  - Communication enhances risk reduction and prevention of complications.
  - Risk of deterioration of present condition is decreased.
  - Risk of secondary impairment is decreased.

- Safety is improved.
- Self-management of symptoms is improved.
♦ Impact on health, wellness, and fitness
  - Behaviors that promote healthy nutrition, physical activity, and wellness are promoted.
  - Fitness is improved.
  - Physical function is improved.
♦ Impact on societal resources
  - Documentation occurs throughout patient management and across all settings and follows APTA's *Guidelines for Physical Therapy Documentation.*[78]
  - Utilization of physical therapy services is optimized.
♦ Patient/client satisfaction
  - Care is coordinated with patient, family, and other professionals.
  - Communication and coordination of care is acceptable to the patient.
  - Interdisciplinary collaboration occurs through case conferences.
  - Patient and family knowledge and awareness of the diagnosis, prognosis, interventions, and anticipated goals and expected outcomes are increased.
  - Patient perceives that services are available and acceptable.
  - Patient satisfaction with physical therapy program is achieved.
  - Sense of well-being is improved.
  - Stressors are decreased.

REEXAMINATION

Reexamination is performed throughout the episode of care.

DISCHARGE

Mr. Brown is discharged from physical therapy after a total of 12 physical therapy sessions and attainment of his goals and expectations. These sessions have covered his entire episode of care. He is discharged because he has achieved his goals and expected outcomes.

REFERENCES

1. Kendall FP, McCreary EK, Provance PG. *Muscles Testing and Function.* 4th ed. Baltimore, Md: Williams & Wilkins; 1993.
2. Watson AWS, Macdonncha C. A reliable technique for the assessment of posture: assessment criteria for aspects of posture. *J Sports Med Phys Fitness.* 2000;40:260-270.
3. Posture Committee of the American Academy of Orthopedic Surgeons. Posture and its relationship to orthopedic disabilities: a report of the Posture Committee of the American Academy of Orthopedic Surgeons. Evanston, Ill: American Academy of Orthopedic Surgeons; 1947:1.
4. Twomey LT, Taylor JR. *Physical Therapy of the Low Back.* 2nd ed. New York, NY: Churchill Livingstone; 1994.
5. Hall CM, Thein Brody L. *Therapeutic Exercise Moving Toward Function.* Philadelphia, Pa: Lippincott Williams & Wilkins; 1999.
6. Braun BL, Amundson LR. Quantitative assessment of head and shoulder posture. *Arch Phys Med Rehabil.* 1989;70:322-329.
7. Hickey ER, Hukins. Relationship between the structure and function of the annulus fibrosus and the function and failure of the intervertebral disc. *Spine.* 1980;5(2):106.
8. Hickey ER, Rondeau MJ, Corrente JR, Abysalh J, Seymour CJ. Reliability of the cervical range of motion (CROM) device and plumb-line techniques in measuring resting head posture (RHP). *Journal of Manual and Manipulative Therapy.* 2000;8(1):10-17.
9. Griegel-Morris P, Larson K, Mueller-Klaus K, Oatis CA. Incidence of common postural abnormalities in the cervical, shoulder, and thoracic regions and their association with pain in two age groups of healthy subjects. *Phys Ther.* 1992;72(6):425-431.
10. Crowell R, Cummings G, Walker JR, Tillman L. Intratester and intertester reliability and validity of measures of innominate bone inclination. *J Orthop Sports Phys Ther.* 1994;20(2):88-97.
11. Magee DJ. *Orthopaedic Physical Assessment.* 4th ed. Philadelphia, Pa: WB Saunders; 2002.
12. Levangie PK, Norkin CC. *Joint Structure and Function.* 4th ed. Philadelphia, Pa: FA Davis Co; 2005.
13. Moore KL, Dalley AF. *Clinically Oriented Anatomy.* 4th ed. Philadelphia, Pa: Lippincott Williams & Wilkins; 1999.
14. Donatelli R. *The Biomechanics of the Foot and Ankle.* Philadelphia, Pa: FA Davis Co; 1990.
15. Hertling D, Kessler RM. *Management of Common Musculoskeletal Disorders.* 3rd ed. Philadelphia, Pa: Lippincott; 1996.
16. DiGiovanna EL, Schiowitz S. *An Osteopathic Approach to Diagnosis and Treatment.* Philadelphia, Pa: JB Lippincott Co; 1991.
17. McKenzie RA. *The Cervical and Thoracic Spine.* Waikanae, New Zealand: Spinal Publications; 1990.
18. Williams PE, Goldspink G. Longitudinal growth of striated muscle fibers. *J Cell Sci.* 1971;9:751-767.
19. James CPA, Harburn KL, Kramer JF. Cumulative trauma disorders in the upper extremities: reliability of the postural and repetitive risk factors index. *Arch Phys Med Rehabil.* 1997;78(8):860-866.
20. Ali RM, Green DW, Patel TC. Scheuermann's kyphosis. *Curr Opin Pediatr.* 1999;11(Feb):70-75.
21. Goodman CC, Glanzman A. Genetic and developmental disorders. In: Goodman CC, Fuller KS, Boissonnault WG, eds. *Pathology Implications for the Physical Therapist.* Philadelphia, Pa: Saunders; 2003:829-870.
22. Bradford DS, Moe JH. Scheuermann's juvenile kyphosis. *Clinical Orthopaedics.* 1975;(110):45-53.
23. Wenge D, Frick S. Scheuermann's kyphosis. *Spine.* 1999;24(24):2630-2639.
24. Lowe T. Current concepts review Scheuermann's disease. *J Bone Joint Surg.* 1990;72-A(6):940-945.

25. Weinstein S, Buckwalter J. *Turek's Orthopedic Principles and Their Application.* 5th ed. Philadelphia, Pa: JB Lippincott Co; 1994.

26. Sorensen KH. *Scheuermann's Juvenile Kyphosis. Clinical Appearances, Radiography, Aetiology, and Prognosis.* Copenhagen: Munksgaard; 1964.

27. Flynn TW. *The Thoracic Spine and Rib Cage.* Boston, Mass: Butterworth-Heinemann; 1996.

28. Sturm PF, Dobson JC, Armstrong GW. The surgical management of scheuermann's disease. *Spine.* 1993;18(6):685-691.

29. USDA Center for Nutrition Policy and Promotion. Body mass index and health. *Nutrition Insight.* 2000;March.

30. Maitland GD. *Peripheral Manipulation.* 3rd ed. London, England: Butterworth-Heinemann; 1991.

31. Maitland GD, Hengeveld E, Banke K, English K. *Maitland's Vertebral Manipulation.* 6th ed. Oxford, England: Butterworth-Heinemann; 2001.

32. Kaltenborn F. *The Spine: Basic Evaluation and Mobilization Techniques.* Minneapolis, Minn: Olaf Norlis Bokhandel; 1993.

33. Kaltenborn F. *Manual Mobilization of the Joints.* 5th ed. Minneapolis, Minn: Olaf Norlis Bokhandel; 1999.

34. Mathiowetz B, Kashman N, Volland G, et al. Grip and pinch strength, normative data for adults. *Arch Phys Med Rehabil.* 1995;66:71-72.

35. Downie W, Leatham PA, Rhind VM, et al. Studies with pain rating scales. *Ann Rheum Dis.* 1978;37:378-38.

36. Jensen MP, Karoly P, Braver S. The measurement of clinical pain intensity: a comparison of six methods. *Pain.* 1986;27(1):117-126.

37. Hains F, Waalen J, Mior S. Psychometric properties of the neck disability index. *J Manipulative Physiol Ther.* 1998;21(2):75-80.

38. Vernon H, Mior S. The neck disability index: a study of reliability and validity. *J Manipulative Physiol Ther.* 1991;14(7):409-415.

39. Garrett TR, Youdas JW, Madson TJ. Reliability of measuring forward head posture in a clinical setting. *J Orthop Sports Phys Ther.* 1993;17(3):155-160.

40. Tousignant M, de Bellefeuille L, O'Donoughue S, Grahovac S. Criterion validity of the cervical range of motion (CROM) goniometer for cervical flexion and extension. *Spine.* 2000;25(3):324-330.

41. Visser J, Straker L. An investigation of discomfort experienced by dental therapists and assistants at work. *Aust Dent J.* 1994;39(1):39-44.

42. Finsen L, Christensen H, Bakke M. Musculoskeletal disorders among dentists and variation in dental work. *Appl Ergon.* 1998; 29(2):119-125.

43. Valachi B, Valachi K. Preventing musculoskeletal disorders in clinical dentistry: strategies to address the mechanisms leading to musculoskeletal disorders. Second in a two-part series. *J Am Dent Assoc.* 2003;134(12):1604-1612, 1641-1644.

44. McCarthy P, Olsen J, Smeby I. Effects of contract-relax stretching procedures on active range of motion of the cervical spine in the transverse plane. *Clin Biomech.* 1997;12(2):136-138.

45. Nicholson GG. The effects of passive joint mobilization on pain and hypomobility associated with adhesive capsulitis. *J Orthop Sports Phys Ther.* 1985;6:238-246.

46. Akuthota V, Nadler S. Core strengthening. *Arch Phys Med Rehabil.* 2004;85(3 Suppl 1):S86-S92.

47. Stanton R, Reaburn P. The effect of short-term swiss ball training on core stability and running economy. *J Strength Cond Res.* 2004;18(3):522-528.

48. Harrison AL, Barry-Greb T, Wojtowicz G. Clinical measurement of head and shoulder posture. *J Orthop Phys Sports Ther.* 1996;23(6):353-361.

49. Black KM, McClure P, Polansky M. The Influence of different sitting positions on cervical and lumbar posture. *Spine.* 1996;21(1):65-70.

50. Wright EF, Domenech MA, et al. Usefulness of posture training for patients with temporomandibular disorders. *J Am Dent Assoc.* 2000;131:202-210.

51. Sahrmann SA. *Diagnosis and Treatment of Movement Impairment Syndromes.* St. Louis, Mo: Mosby; 2002.

52. Swank AM, Funk DC, Durham MP, Roberts S. Adding weights to stretching exercise increases passive range of motion for healthy elderly. *J Strength Cond Res.* 2003;17(2):374-378.

53. Enwemeka CS, Bonet IM, Ingle JA, Prudhithumrong S, Ogbahon FE, Gbenedio NA. Postural corrections in persons with neck pain, II. Integrated electromyography of the upper trapezius in three simulated neck positions. *J Orthop Sports Phys Ther.* 1986;8(5):240.

54. Schuldt K, Ekholm J, Harms-Ringdahl K, Nemeth G, Arborelius UP. Effects of changes in sitting work posture on static neck and shoulder muscle activity. *Ergonomics.* 1986;29:1525-1537.

55. Carlson C, Collins F, Nitz A, Sturgis E, Rogers J. Muscle stretching as an alternative relaxation training procedure. *J Behav Ther Exp Psychiatry.* 1990;21(1):29-38.

56. Voight ML, Thomson BC. The role of the scapula in the rehabilitation of shoulder injuries. *Journal of Athletic Training.* 2000;35(3):364-372.

57. Chen S, Simonian PT, Wickiewicz TL, Otis JC, Warren RF. Radiograftic evaluation of glenohumeral kinematics: a muscle fatigue model. *J Shoulder Elbow Surg.* 1999;8(1):49-52.

58. Wang C, McClure P, Pratt N, Nobilini R. Stretching and strengthening exercises: their effect on three-dimensional scapula kinematics. *Arch Phys Med Rehabil.* 1999;80(8):923-929.

59. Kibler WB. The role of the scapula in athletic shoulder function. *Am J Sports Med.* 1998;26(2):325-337.

60. Lephart SM, Henry TJ. The physiological basis for open and closed kinetic chain rehabilitation for the upper extremity. *Journal of Sport Rehabilitation.* 1996;5:71-87.

61. Ylinen J, Takala EP, Nykänen M, et al. Active neck muscle training in the treatment of chronic neck pain in women. *JAMA.* 2003;289:2509-2516.

62. Sarig-Bahat H. Evidence for exercise therapy in mechanical neck disorders. *Man Ther.* 2003;8(1):10-20.

63. Evans R, Bronfort G, Nelson B, Goldsmith C. Two-year follow-up of a randomized clinical trial of spinal manipulation, two types of exercise for patients with chronic neck pain. *Spine.* 2002;27(21):2383-2389.

64. Bang MD, Deyle GD. Comparison of supervised exercise with and without manual physical therapy for patients with shoulder impingement. *J Orthop Sports Phys Ther.* 2000;30:126-137.

65. Cantu RI, Grodin AJ. *Myofascial Manipulation, Theory*

and Clinical Application. 2nd ed. Gaithersburg, Md: Aspen Publishers; 2001.

66. Wyke B. Articular neurology: a review. *Physiotherapy.* 1972;58:94-99.

67. Andersson GB, Lucente T, Davis AM, et al. A comparison of osteopathic spinal manipulation with standard care for patients with low back pain. *N Engl J Med.* 1999;341(19):1426-1431.

68. Koes BW, Bouter LM, van Mameren H, et al. Randomised clinical trial of manipulative therapy and physiotherapy for persistent back and neck complaints: results of a one year follow up. *BMJ.* 1992;304(6827):601-605.

69. Hoving JL, Koes BW, de Vet HC, et al. Manual therapy, physical therapy, or continued care by a general practitioner for patients with neck pain. A randomized, controlled study. *Ann Intern Med.* 2002;136(10):713-722.

70. Koes BW, Assendelft WJJ, van der Heijden GJMG, Bouter LM. Spinal manipulation for low back pain an undated systematic review of randomized clinical trials. *Spine.* 1996;21(24):2860-2873.

71. Bronfort G, Evans R, Nelson B, Aker P, Goldsmith C, Vernon H. A randomized clinical trial of exercise and spinal manipulation for patients with chronic neck pain. *Spine.* 2001;26(7):788-799.

72. Belánger AY. *Evidence-Based Guide to Therapeutic Physical Agents.* Philadelphia, Pa: Lippincott Williams & Wilkins; 2002.

73. Colachis SC, Strohm BR. Cervical traction relationship of time to varied tractive force with constant angle of pull. *Arch Phys Med Rehabil.* 1965;46:815-819.

74. Camerson MH. *Physical Agents in Rehabilitation from Research to Practice.* St. Louis, Mo: Elsevier Science; 2003.

75. Rocabado M. Course notes: temporomandibular joint assessment and treatment, 1982.

76. Morgan D. Concepts in functional training and postural stabilization for the low-back injured. *Topics in Acute Care and Trauma Rehabilitation.* 1988;April:8-17.

77. Axen K, Haas F, Schicchi J, Merrick J. Progressive resistance neck exercises using a compressible ball coupled with an air pressure gauge. *J Orthop Sports Phys Ther.* 1992;16(6):275-279.

78. American Physical Therapy Association. Guide to physical therapist practice. 2nd ed. *Phys Ther.* 2001;81:9-744.

79. Umphred DA. *Neurological Rehabilitation.* 3rd ed. St. Louis, Mo: Mosby-Yearbook Inc; 1995.

80. Tibbles AC, Waalen JK, Hains F. Response set bias, internal consistency and construct validity of the oswetry low back pain disability questionnaire. *J Can Chiropr Assoc.* 1998;42(3):141-149.

81. Moseley JB Jr, Jobe FW, Pink M, et al. EMG analysis of the scapular muscles during a shoulder rehabilitation program. *Am J Sports Med.* 1992;20(2):128-134.

82. Tribus CB. Scheuermann's kyphosis in adolescents and adults: diagnosis and management. *J Am Acad Orthop Surg.* 1998;6(1):36-43.

83. Soo CL, Noble FC, Esses SI. Scheuermann kyphosis: long-term follow-up. *Spine J.* 2003;2:49-56.

84. Schiller L. Effectiveness of spinal manipulative therapy in the treatment of mechanical thoracic spine pain: a pilot randomized clinical trial. *J Manipulative Physiol Ther.* 2001:24(6):394-401.

BIBLIOGRAPHY

Aufdermaur M. Juvenile kyphosis (Scheuermann's disease): radiography, histology, and pathogenesis. *Clin Orthop.* 1981;154(Jan-Feb):166-174.

Bickley LS. *Bate's Guide to Physical Examination and History Taking.* 8th ed. Philadelphia, Pa: Lippincott Williams & Wilkins; 2003.

Brooks VB. The Neural Basis of Motor Control. New York, NY: Oxford University Press; 1986.

Evcik D, Aksoy O. Correlation of tempomandibular joint pathologies, neck pain and postural differences. Journal of Physiological Therapeutic Science. 2000;12(2):97-100.

Goodman CC, Snyder TEK. Differential Diagnosis in Physical Therapy. Philadelphia, Pa: WB Saunders Co; 2000.

Hanten WP, Olson SL, Russell JL, et al. Total head excursion and resting head posture: normal and patient comparisons. Arch Phys Med Rehabil. 200;81(1):62-66.

McArdle WD, Katch FI, Katch VL. *Exercise Physiology.* 4th ed. Baltimore, Md: Williams & Wilkins; 1996.

McPoil TG, Hunt GC. Evaluation and management of foot and ankle disorders: present problems and future directions. *J Orthop Sports Phys Ther.* 1995;21(6):381-388.

Nordin M, Frankel VH. *Basic Biomechanics of the Musculoskeletal System.* 3rd ed. Philadelphia, Pa: Lippincott Williams & Wilkins; 2001.

Raine S, Twomey LT. Head and shoulder posture variations in 160 asymptomatic women and men. Arch Phys Med Rehabil. 1997;78(11):1215-1223.

Robison R. The new back school prescription: stabilization training part I. Occupational Medicine. 1992;7(1):17-31.

Sahrmann S. Does postural assessment contribute to patient care? J Orthop Sports Phys Ther. 2002;32(8):376-379.

Saidoff DC, McDonough AL. Critical Pathways in Therapeutic Intervention Extremities and Spine. St. Louis, Mo: Mosby, Inc; 2002.

Salter RB. *Textbook of Disorders and Injuries of the Musculoskeletal System.* 3rd ed. Baltimore, Md: Williams & Wilkins; 1999.

Scoles PV, Latimer BM, DiGiovanni BF, et al. Vertebral alterations in Scheuermann's kyphosis. *Spine.* 1991;16(5):509-515.

Voss D, Ionta MK, Myers BJ. *Proprioceptive Neuromuscular Facilitation: Patterns and Techniques.* 3rd ed. Philadelphia, Pa: Lippincott Williams & Wilkins; 1985.

Wadsworth CT, Krishnan R, Sear M, Harrold J, Nielsen DH. Intrarater reliability of manual muscle testing and hand-held dynametric muscle testing. Phys Ther. 1987;67:1342-1347.

Wilford CH, Kisner C, Glenn TM, et al. The interaction of wearing multifocal lenses with head posture and pain. J Orthop Sports Phys Ther. 1996;23(3):194-199.

CHAPTER THREE

Impaired Muscle Performance (Pattern C)

Suzanne R. Babyar, PT, PhD

Gary Krasilovsky, PT, PhD

ANATOMY

GROSS STRUCTURE OF SKELETAL MUSCLE

Skeletal muscles are made up of individual muscle fibers that are 0.01 to 0.10 mm in diameter. Their length can vary from 2 to 12 cm or longer. One fiber may run the entire length of a skeletal muscle. There are four layers of fascia that surround and compartmentalize all skeletal muscle. These fascial layers (Figure 3-1) include the epimysium, which separates the muscle from surrounding structures and runs the entire length of the muscle; the perimysium, which separates the individual bundles of muscle fibers (called fascicles); the endomysium, which separates each individual muscle fiber from adjacent fibers; and the sarcolemma, which is beneath the endomysium and surrounds each muscle fiber.[1]

MICROSCOPIC STRUCTURE OF MUSCLE

Skeletal muscle is comprised primarily of water and 20% protein. Approximately 5% consists of various minerals including potassium, sodium, and calcium. Proteins include actin, myosin, troponin, and tropomyosin. Muscle fibers are highly vascular in order to provide adequate blood supply during any level of physical activity.[2]

The relationship of skeletal muscle components are illustrated by size in Figure 3-2 as entire muscle –> muscle fascicles –> muscle fibers –> myofibrils –> sarcomeres –> actin, myosin, tropomyosin, troponin complex, and other contractile proteins.

Each muscle contains bundles of muscle fascicles, and each fascicle contains many muscle fibers. The muscle fiber is the structural unit of skeletal muscle. One muscle fiber has thousands of myofibrils. The myofibrils are the functional units of a muscle fiber and are parallel to the long axis of the muscle. Myofibrils are like a long train of boxcars, with each boxcar being a sarcomere, which is the contractile unit of the myofibril. Each sarcomere contains myofilaments, the contractile mechanism, which consists of strands of actin (thin filaments) and myosin (thick filaments) proteins[2] (Figure 3-3). A network of sarcoplasmic reticulum surrounds the sarcomeres. The sarcoplasmic reticulum carries and releases the ions needed for chemical excitation of a muscle contraction.

One myofibril that is 15 mm long will have 6000 sarcomeres joined end to end. The average muscle fiber contains 4500 sarcomeres and a total of 16 billion myosin and 64 billion actin filaments.[2] The number of total sarcomeres in a muscle fiber is proportional to the length of the muscle fiber.

Microscopically, muscle fibers appear to have light and dark bands that give skeletal muscle its striated appearance (see Figure 3-3). The lighter area is known as the I-band,

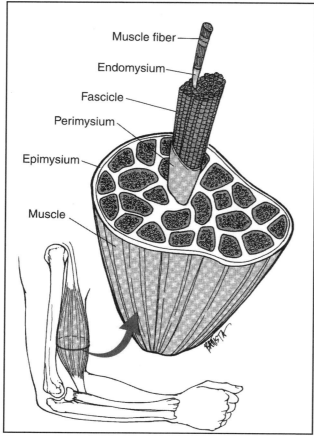

Figure 3-1. Successive connective tissue sheaths within muscle. Reprinted with permission from Oatis CA. *Kinesiology: The Mechanics and Pathomechanics of Human Movement.* Philadelphia, Pa: Lippincott Williams & Wilkins; 2004:47.

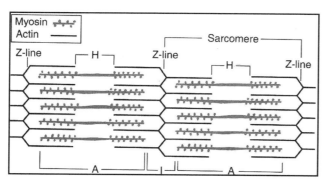

Figure 3-3. Actin-myosin organization of two successive sarcomeres showing A, H, and I bands as well as Z-lines. Reprinted with permission from Oatis CA. *Kinesiology: The Mechanics and Pathomechanics of Human Movement.* Philadelphia, Pa: Lippincott Williams & Wilkins; 2004:46.

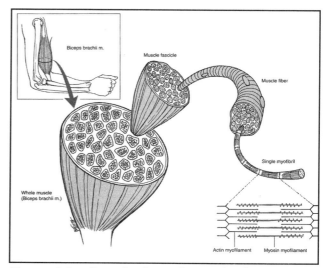

Figure 3-2. Organization of muscle from macroscopic to microscopic levels. Reprinted with permission from Oatis CA. *Kinesiology: The Mechanics and Pathomechanics of Human Movement.* Philadelphia, Pa: Lippincott Williams & Wilkins; 2004:46.

which contains only actin (thin) filaments. The darker area is the A-band, which contains alternating actin and myosin (thick) filaments. The Z-line consists of a connective tissue network that bisects the I-band, anchors the thin filaments, and provides structural integrity to the sarcomere. The H-zone, located in the middle of the A-band, is the region of thick filaments not overlapped by thin filaments. The M-band bisects the H-zone and represents the middle of the sarcomere. The M-band consists of protein structures that support the arrangement of the myosin filaments. During muscle contraction, the sarcomere I-band and H-zone decrease in length while the length of the A-band remains constant.[2,3]

THE MUSCLE SPINDLE

The muscle spindle is a long, thin structure located adjacent and parallel to muscle fibers and is composed of multiple components that have both afferent and efferent innervation (Figures 3-4a and 3-4b). The muscle spindle functions as a stretch receptor and responds to static and dynamic length changes of skeletal muscle.[4-6] This complex receptor is found in all muscles, primarily in extremity, intercostal, and cervical muscles.

Anatomical Structures of the Spindle Apparatus

♦ Intrafusal muscle fibers are generally only 2 to 4 mm in length. They are fusiform in shape, widest in the center and tapered at ends. These fibers are composed of two types of fibers:

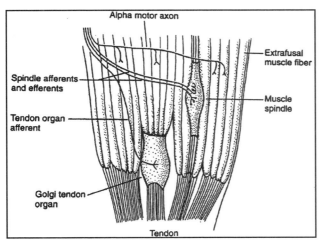

Figure 3-4a. Muscle spindle within a muscle belly. Reprinted with permission from Soderberg GL. *Kinesiology: Application to Pathological Movement.* 2nd ed. Baltimore, Md: Lippincott Williams & Wilkins; 1997:62.

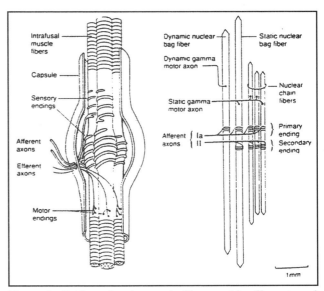

Figure 3-4b. Intrafusal muscle fibers with afferent and efferent innervation. Reprinted with permission from Soderberg GL. *Kinesiology: Application to Pathological Movement.* 2nd ed. Baltimore, Md: Lippincott Williams & Wilkins; 1997:63.

- Nuclear bag fibers are the thickest and longest and are organized in rows two to four deep.
- Nuclear chain fibers occur in a single row, aligned down the center.

♦ Afferent innervation
  - Annulospiral endings, also referred to as primary nerve endings, encircle the central region of the nuclear bag and nuclear chain fibers. The annulospiral endings are innervated by fast-conducting Type Ia afferent nerves, which synapse directly with the alpha motor neuron of the skeletal muscle in which these receptors are located.
  - Secondary endings are mainly located near the ends of nuclear chain fibers. The secondary endings are innervated by Type II afferent nerves that are slower conducting and synapse via an interneuron with the alpha motor neuron of the skeletal muscle in which they are located.

♦ Efferent innervation occurs through gamma efferent nerves to the contractile elements in the polar regions of the nuclear bag and nuclear chain fibers. The gamma efferents are considered a component of the extrapyramidal system.[3,5]

The gamma efferents that innervate the contractile fibers of the intrafusal muscle fibers produce a contraction in the polar region of the nuclear bag and nuclear chain fibers. This contraction stretches the equatorial region of the spindle, which causes depolarization of the primary (annulospiral) afferents and secondary endings. Intrafusal fibers do not change the length or tension of the entire extrafusal muscle, they simply produce changes in the sensitivity of the annulospiral endings.[3,5]

Muscle Spindles: Functional Implications

The gamma motor system controls the length and velocity sensitivity of the primary (annulospiral) endings and the length sensitivity of the secondary endings of the muscle spindles. In order to increase the discharge rate of the spindle apparatus, contraction of the intrafusal muscle fibers or stretching of the extrafusal muscle is necessary. To decrease the discharge of the spindle apparatus, one must produce intrafusal relaxation and/or extrafusal shortening.

♦ Quick stretch of a muscle increases firing of the primary and secondary endings, which facilitates contraction of the skeletal muscle being stretched.

♦ Intrafusal fiber contraction, caused by quick icing (which stimulates gamma efferent discharges), creates a stretch on the nuclear bag and nuclear chain fibers, resulting in an increase in discharge from the annulospiral and secondary endings. This creates increased muscle activation of the extrafusal (skeletal) muscle.

♦ Passively placing a muscle on slack will temporarily decrease all annulospiral and secondary ending discharges.[3]

EXTRAFUSAL MUSCLE FIBER TYPES

Limb muscles in humans consist of a combination of slow and fast twitch muscle fibers. Fiber typing is based upon their metabolic and force production properties. All the muscle fibers of one motor unit ([MU] described below) have the same fiber typing or histochemical composition.

Nerve types closely match muscle types, for example, fast conducting nerves innervate fast twitch muscles.[2,4,5]

♦ Type I: Aerobic metabolism, generating adenosine tri-phosphate (ATP)
  • Slow twitch, oxidative (SO) fibers: Burn fats with oxygen (oxidative)
  • Slow conducting nerve axons
  • Highly resistant to fatigue. They are designated as red due to high number of mitochondria and amount of myoglobin that stores oxygen
  • No lactic acid build-up occurs with repeated contractions
  • Tonic work, light loads
  • Twitch contraction time 73 ms
  • Maximum tension is 8 g of force
  • Low threshold for sustained contraction. Low amplitude action potentials, slow conduction velocity
  • These are the smallest MUs

♦ Type IIa: Aerobic metabolism, generating ATP
  • Moderately fast twitch, oxidative, glycolytic (FOG) fibers: Use both oxidative and glycolytic pathways for energy
  • Fast conducting nerve axons
  • Fatigue-resistant. They are red due to an intermediate number of mitochondria and amount of myoglobin
  • Moderate loads, very efficient in athletes
  • Twitch time is 41 ms
  • Maximum tension is 29 g of force

♦ Type IIb: Anaerobic metabolism
  • Fast, glycolytic (FG) fibers: Burn glycogen for fast release of energy
  • Fast conducting nerve axons
  • Fatigue easily. They are white with few mitochondria and little myoglobin
  • Repeated contraction results in lactic acid build-up
  • Heavy loads, phasic work
  • Twitch contraction time is 35 ms
  • Maximum tension is 75 g of force
  • Large amplitude action potentials, fast conduction velocity
  • These are the largest MUs

INNERVATION OF SKELETAL MUSCLE

The motor unit, or MU, is the functional unit for muscle contraction. A MU is composed of an anterior horn cell (AHC) in the spinal cord, the nerve axon, and all the muscle fibers innervated by that AHC. Each MU consists of strictly one type of muscle fiber, as previously described. The designation of muscle fiber type is controlled by the rate of stimulation by the AHC innervating that particular muscle fiber.[2]

Innervation ratio refers to the average size of an MU and is a ratio of the number of muscle fibers innervated by one motor neuron (AHC and axon). This ratio varies greatly depending upon the function of each particular MU.[7]

♦ Extraocular muscles—1 motor neuron : 5 muscle fibers
♦ Intrinsic hand muscles—1 motor neuron : 100 muscle fibers
♦ Anterior tibialis—1 motor neuron : 600 muscle fibers
♦ Gastrocnemius—1 motor neuron : 2000 muscle fibers

The territory of a single MU[7] covers an area that varies between the size of approximately 0.03 to 3.4 cubic millimeters. There are overlapping territories for a few MUs clustered in one region of a skeletal muscle. The number of MUs is estimated to range from 34 to 93 in some intrinsic hand muscles to 129 in the biceps brachii to almost 600 in the gastrocnemius.[7]

The neuromuscular junction is the site of transmission of the action potential from the motor nerve axon to the muscle fibers. Acetylcholine (ACh) is the neurotransmitter that facilitates the transmission of this action potential and acetylcholinesterase is the enzyme that neutralizes the ACh to cease the muscle contraction.

Few disorders affect the neuromuscular junction. These include botulism poisoning and myasthenia gravis. Botulism poisoning occurs from underprepared canned foods allowing botulism spores to reproduce. The botulism toxin blocks the ACh receptor sites. Honey also has a relatively high susceptibility to survival of botulism spores. The medical community recommends that infants under 1 year of age not be fed honey due to this potential risk.[8]

Myasthenia gravis is a disorder of the neuromuscular junction characterized by fatigue that worsens as the day progresses. In myasthenia gravis, the number of ACh receptor sites is decreased, and some of the remaining receptor sites are blocked. This results in undue fatigue. Ptosis (difficulty keeping the upper eyelid elevated) is one sign commonly associated with myasthenia gravis.

ANATOMY OF THE PELVIC FLOOR MUSCLES

The pelvic floor is primarily composed of a broad deep muscle, the levator ani muscle (Figures 3-5a and 3-5b), that has three bilateral divisions based on their muscular attachments: the iliococcygeus, the pubococcygeus, and the ischiococcygeus.[9-11] In addition, the puborectalis part of the levator ani muscle attaches from the pubic ramus to the rectum.[10] Posterior and superior to the levator ani is the coccygeus that attaches from the coccyx and fifth segment of the sacrum to the ischial spine and sacrospinous ligament.[9,11] The two levator ani and the two coccygeus muscles constitute the pelvic diaphragm.[11] Contraction of these muscles will raise the pelvic floor cranially and provide compression around the urethra.

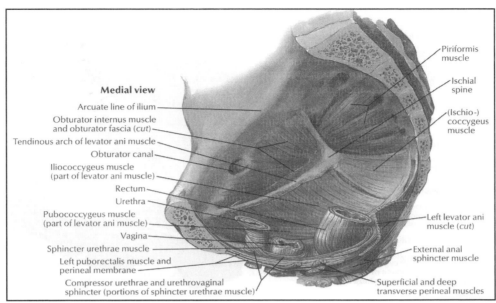

Figure 3-5a. Pelvic diaphragm of a female consisting of levator ani (with iliococcygeus and pubococcygeus divisions illustrated) and coccygeus muscle. Reprinted with permission from Netter FH. *Atlas of Human Anatomy*. 2nd ed. Summit, NJ: Ciba-Geigy Corp; 1989:Plate 333.

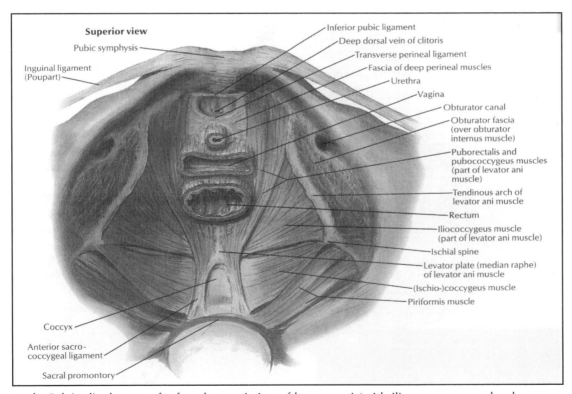

Figure 3-5b. Pelvic diaphragm of a female consisting of levator ani (with iliococcygeus and pubococcygeus divisions illustrated) and coccygeus muscle. Reprinted with permission from Netter FH. *Atlas of Human Anatomy*. 2nd ed. Summit, NJ: Ciba-Geigy Corp; 1989:Plate 333.

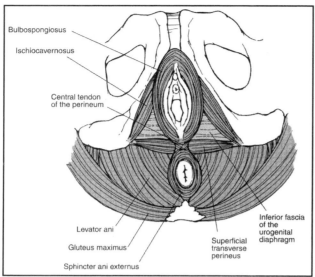

Figure 3-6. Superficial muscles of the urogenital diaphragm of a female. Reprinted with permission from Oatis CA. *Kinesiology: The Mechanics and Pathomechanics of Human Movement.* Philadelphia, Pa: Lippincott Williams & Wilkins; 2004:635.

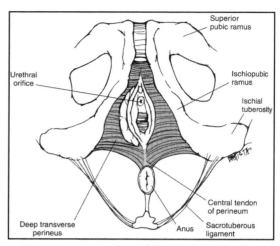

Figure 3-7. Deep muscles of the urogenital diaphragm of a female. Reprinted with permission from Oatis CA. *Kinesiology: The Mechanics and Pathomechanics of Human Movement.* Philadelphia, Pa: Lippincott Williams & Wilkins; 2004:636.

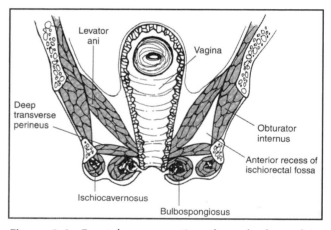

Figure 3-8. Frontal cross-section through the pelvic and urogenital diaphragms of a female at the level of the vagina. Reprinted with permission from Oatis CA. *Kinesiology: The Mechanics and Pathomechanics of Human Movement.* Philadelphia, Pa: Lippincott Williams & Wilkins; 2004:636.

Superficial to the levator ani are five paired muscles with gender-specific differences in size and orientation: the superficial muscles include the bulbospongiosus, superficial transverse perineal, and ischiocavernosus and the deeper muscles include the sphincter urethrae and deep transverse perineal muscles[9] (Figure 3-6). The external anal sphincter muscle also surrounds the anus in this layer.[11] The deep transverse perineal muscle and the sphincter urethrae (Figures 3-7 and 3-8) are referred to as the urogenital diaphragm. Both the pelvic and urogenital diaphragms can be subject to stretch and injury during pregnancy and childbearing. Authors vary in what is regarded as the pelvic floor musculature. Moore[11] suggested that the pelvic diaphragm is the main pelvic floor and the urogenital diaphragm is the subfloor.

PHYSIOLOGY

Muscle contraction is an active process that lasts 5 to 10 milliseconds. A depolarization wave leaves the AHC and travels to the neuromuscular junction causing the release of acetylcholine. ACh reacts with receptor sites to increase muscle membrane permeability allowing ions to move into the muscle cell via the transverse tubular system that transmits the action potential. This action potential signals the sarcoplasmic reticulum to release calcium ions. Binding of calcium to troponin-tropomyosin removes the inhibitory effect troponin has on preventing actin-myosin interaction. Actin is now free to combine with myosin, and muscle force is created along with splitting of ATP for energy. Actin-

myosin bonds are broken and reformed, allowing sliding of the thick and thin filaments, resulting in muscle shortening. During contraction, a single fiber may shorten 40% of its length. As the muscle contracts, the width of A-bands remains the same, the I-bands become narrower, and the H-zone in A-band is obliterated.[2,3]

FACTORS INFLUENCING MUSCLE FORCE PRODUCTION

When a single MU is fired, the force produced reaches its maximum value almost immediately. The pattern of the force generated is a reflection of the very rapid formation of many actin and myosin cross-bridges within the muscle followed by a gradual reduction in cross-bridges as calcium is returned into the sarcoplasmic reticulum. The functional force measured over time in response to a single activation of muscle is called the isometric twitch. (Refer back to structure and function of extrafusal fibers for comparative twitch times and force produced for each muscle type.) Often, a series of muscle action potentials is produced. The first action potential produces a twitch-like contraction. If a second action potential is delivered before all the calcium released by the first action potential is resequestered, more calcium is released from the sarcoplasmic reticulum, and the actin-myosin cross-bridging cycling is allowed to continue. As a result, the force measured from the activated muscle segment rises again. With higher frequencies of firing, eventually a smooth, strong, continuous force generation occurs.[3]

Additional factors associated with force output are:

♦ Prior training and type of training affect muscle fiber typing.[12] Specificity of training is an important concept for improving performance. Prolonged endurance training increases the percentage of Type I MUs and is necessary to improve endurance.[2] Weight lifters and sprinters have a greater percentage of Type II MUs with resultant increases in force production or speed, but not endurance.[5]

♦ A faster firing frequency of an MU will generate a stronger contraction, as indicated above. Training improves efficiency of MU recruitment.

♦ Muscle length affects the degree of force generated during a contraction. Maximum force output is produced at approximately 110% of the resting length.[5]

♦ Speed of shortening dictates how quickly a contraction force can be generated. The slower the velocity of a muscle contraction, the higher the force that can be generated.

♦ Muscle size and architecture affect force production for any muscle.

♦ Type of muscle contraction influences force production with eccentric contractions generating more force than isometric contractions which, in turn, are stronger than concentric contractions.[13]

♦ Muscle fatigue becomes evident with repeated contractions. Decreased force production is a common method of confirming fatigue.

♦ Health status, age, and level of motivation all influence force production.

TYPES OF MUSCLE CONTRACTION

Force production is achieved through muscle contraction. There are two basic types of muscle contractions: dynamic and static. Dynamic contractions include concentric (shortening) and eccentric (lengthening) contractions. Sarcomeres shorten via overlap and bonding of the actin-myosin complex during concentric contractions whereas actin-myosin bonds are broken during eccentric contractions. Static contractions occur when force production is achieved, but no joint movement or length changes occur in the actin-myosin complex.[13]

Most functional activities require a combination of static and dynamic muscle contractions. Static muscle contractions, or isometrics, serve as stabilizers. Dynamic muscle contractions may include reciprocal movements or concentric-eccentric activity by the same muscle group. Combining concentric and eccentric exercises provides the best functional carryover for all ADL. Because many activities require lowering a weight, or bending, squatting, and/or decelerating a limb during movement, eccentric training is a vital component of therapeutic exercise. However, eccentric loading on muscle places it at risk for injury, and the faster the eccentric movements the greater this risk. During eccentric contractions, muscle fibers and all connective tissue sheaths must elongate. Warm-up exercises prior to higher velocity eccentrics are recommended to prevent injury. In addition, individuals should train at slower speeds initially and gradually build toward higher speed eccentric work.[13]

MUSCLE RELAXATION

Muscle depolarization only lasts 5 to 10 msec. Intracellular concentration of calcium drops rapidly, possibly due to a calcium pump forcing calcium back into storage sites in the sarcoplasmic reticulum. Relaxation occurs when the calcium concentration returns to its "resting" level. This return of calcium to the sarcoplasmic reticulum frees troponin to inhibit actin-myosin interaction.[2]

MOTOR UNIT RECRUITMENT PATTERNS

The sequence of MU recruitment is dependent upon the speed and type of muscle contraction and is based upon the size principle of the AHC of the MUs.[7,14] Going from low force production requirements to greater force production requirements, the MUs to be recruited are:

♦ First: Type I are the smallest in size and have a low threshold of activation. Their firing rate is 8 to 10 per second. These MUs produce low levels of force, but have the capacity for sustained contractions.

♦ Second: Type IIa are intermediate in size and have a moderate threshold for activation. These MUs are activated with a rapid vigorous contraction and fire in short, irregular bursts at 16 to 50 per second. These MUs have lower thresholds for fatigue.

◆ Third: Type IIb are the largest size MUs and have the highest threshold for activation. Their frequency of firing is similar to Type IIa MUs. These MUs produce the highest level of force, but fatigue rapidly. With sustained muscle activity, some Type II MUs will "drop out" secondary to fatigue. These will be replaced as other Type II MUs are recruited. This dropping out and replacement continues until fatigue is reached in most muscle fibers and/or the activity is completed.[7,14]

Normal MU recruitment not only refers to the type of MUs and the order of recruitment, but also the frequency of firing of each MU. With low levels of force production, the frequency of firing of a MU may start at 5 to 7 Hz.[7] As slightly more force is required, the rate of firing is increased up to a maximum of 50 Hz. If force production requirements continue to rise, additional MUs of the same type are recruited at low frequencies. The frequency of firing of these MUs will also begin to increase.[14] The number of MUs and rate of discharge continues to increase, as greater force production is required. Eventually, additional types of MUs are also recruited and the cycle continues.

As the amount of force generated decreases from a high intensity contraction, the reduction in MU discharge occurs in sequence with the last to fire being the first to cease firing. Based on the above example, Type IIb MUs are the last to be recruited and the first to stop contracting as the intensity of the muscle contraction begins to subside. Therefore, one should note that the first MUs recruited for low intensity ADL are the Type I MUs, and with minimal effort required, Type II (a and b) MUs will not be activated. A patient who has a history of decreased use, weakness, and generalized deconditioning will have greater weakness in both Type II MUs because they have not been used. An exercise program that selectively targets Type IIb MUs may help to reverse disuse weakness more effectively than retraining in ADL. In order to selectively exercise Type II MUs, higher levels of force production and higher speeds of contraction than those encountered in ADL must be required of the patient.

Fast, quick movements result in early recruitment of phasic MUs Type II (a and b).[2] One method to selectively recruit (exercise) Type II MU is to require the patient to perform high speed resistive exercises. The patient will be able to produce moderate amounts of tension in the muscle being targeted, but they will fatigue faster, with fewer repetitions, than when the patient does slow, steady resisted exercises that first target Type I MUs.[2]

MECHANISMS OF FATIGUE

Fatigue has different meanings to different individuals. One common method of defining fatigue is a decrease in force production capability during a sustained or repetitive activity.[15,16] In isokinetic terms, fatigue is typically defined as a 50% decline in peak torque production. Fatigue may be observed in patients as a decrease in coordination, inability to perform another repetition of an exercise, or the patient stating they are too tired to continue with an exercise. There are three major anatomical sites potentially related to muscle fatigue: 1) the muscle, 2) the peripheral nerve and the neuromuscular junction, and 3) the central nervous system (CNS).[17]

Muscle

Muscle is the most common location for fatigue,[18] but the etiology is not exactly known. Several hypotheses include:

◆ During prolonged exercise (>60 minutes), depletion of glycogen is a key factor in the onset of muscle fatigue. Exercise of high intensity but low duration (10 to 20 sec) is associated with rapid force production loss secondary to depletion of phosphocreatine[18] that is stored within the muscle and rapidly converted into energy.

◆ The muscle fiber action potential may not be propagated correctly.

◆ Failure of the contractile machinery may occur in muscle, possibly due to a calcium deficit.

◆ Lactic acid buildup drops the pH that then interferes with protein function.

Neuromuscular Junction

The neuromuscular junction is rarely the site of fatigue, except experimentally. When fatigue has been induced experimentally, the frequency of stimulation exceeded the normal frequency of MU discharge. The normal neuromuscular system operates at frequencies of MU firing just below those at which the neuromuscular transmission fails. Research has confirmed that as fatigue is becoming apparent in a subject, electrical stimulation at the neuromuscular junction will result in full, normal MU recruitment[3] indicating that ACh reserves are adequate.

Hypothetically, diminished ACh availability may cause fatigue, as seen in myasthenia gravis.[7] Alternatively, fatigue may be due to a change in sensitivity of the post-synaptic membrane or a failure of the neuromuscular junction.[2] The exact mechanism has not been proven.

Psychological Failure or Central Fatigue

A well-trained and motivated subject can generate force equal to that produced with electrical stimulation. Therefore, central fatigue probably does not occur physiologically, but fatigue may occur secondary to decreased effort and motivation.[19,20]

PATHOPHYSIOLOGY

Pathologies listed under Pattern C in the *Guide to Physical Therapist Practice*[21] are quite diverse. In this chapter, a representative sample of case studies is included. The first case study refers to a child with Duchenne muscular dystrophy

(DMD) representing a primary disorder of muscle. The second case study relates to muscle weakness and loss of supporting ability of the pelvic floor muscles (PFM) in a middle-age female. The final case study represents a long-standing endocrine problem, Type 2 diabetes mellitus (DM).

DUCHENNE MUSCULAR DYSTROPHY

Muscular dystrophy is a disease associated with progressive weakness and spontaneous degeneration of skeletal muscle fibers. The age of onset, clinical manifestation, and progression of weakness for any of the muscular dystrophies are determined by the exact defect responsible for the disorder. DMD is the most common X-linked, recessive lethal disease,[22] and about one-third of those affected are due to spontaneous genetic mutations. In DMD a deficit in the particular gene (Xp21) on the X chromosome results in a failure to produce the protein dystrophin. Muscle cell destruction and increased permeability of the cell occurs. Calcium levels within the muscle rise, proteolytic enzymes are activated, and cell destruction results.[22]

Creatinine phosphokinase (CK) is a muscle enzyme that is markedly elevated when the muscle membrane is unstable and allows CK to exit the muscle. CK blood values of 50 to 100 times normal (normal is <235 U/L for males) are common with this diagnosis.[23,24]

MUs become smaller in size due to loss of muscle fibers, resulting in MUs electrically and functionally smaller than normal. This results in short duration and low amplitude MUs.[7] Force production capability is also decreased, resulting in the need to recruit many more MUs than normal for most ADL. This overuse of MUs is the framework for the onset of overwork weakness. Overwork weakness refers to a decrease in muscle strength that does not recover with rest. Muscles that are most susceptible to overwork weakness are in MUs previously affected by a disease process that greatly reduces force production capacity of that muscle. The remaining MUs are often "overworked" chronically, resulting in the risk for early "death" of the MU. This results in further weakness that does not recover with rest.[25]

There are other common findings associated with DMD. These include cardiomyopathy and average intelligence quotient falling one standard deviation below the mean.[22] The incidence of DMD is estimated to be one in every 3,500 to 5,000 boys.[26]

STRESS URINARY INCONTINENCE

Stress urinary incontinence (SUI) is one of four categories of urinary incontinence characterized by "loss of urine during activities that increase intra-abdominal pressure,"[27] such as during lifting, coughing, sneezing, or laughing.[27,28] Genuine stress incontinence is involuntary loss of urine when intravesical pressure exceeds that of the urethral sphincter that is proven through urodynamic testing.[29] SUI

coupled with urge incontinence is labeled mixed incontinence. Urge incontinence is characterized by sudden urge to urinate and uncontrolled urine loss.[27,28] Individuals with SUI seek advice from gynecologists, urologists. or urogynecologists. Prior to diagnosing SUI, these physicians must rule out bladder cancer, urinary tract infection, or diabetes as the source of the problem.[27,30]

Ordinarily, the PFM should quickly develop a strong contraction to increase intraurethral pressure just prior to the increase in intra-abdominal pressure from a cough or sneeze.[31] Kegel[32] reported that childbirth may overstretch pelvic floor musculature (and attached nerves) thus inducing tears in the muscle fibers and significantly reducing PFM function. Aging causes the PFM to lose muscle tone and strength.[27] When muscle fibers are not intact or when muscle tone and strength are inadequate, the PFM and the urinary sphincter are not able to hold back urine when bladder pressure (caused by increased intra-abdominal pressure) exceeds a critical level.[29,31] Other causes of SUI include pudendal nerve damage (often caused by childbirth or during surgery)[27] and damage to the supporting structures for the bladder and urethra (as with multiple pregnancies or prolapse of the bladder or uterus).[27,28] Associated factors include constipation, obesity, and smoking.[27,28] Some medications predispose individuals to SUI.[27,28]

Incidence of Stress Urinary Incontinence

The incidence of SUI among men and women is difficult to define because people afflicted with SUI withhold reporting it to their physicians. A 1996 estimate by the Agency for Health Care Policy and Research reported an incidence of urinary incontinence of 10% to 30% in women and 1.5% to 5% in men.[33] The current estimate is that 20% to 50% of adults with SUI actually seek help.[34,35] Although men and women experience SUI, 90% of reported cases are women. A survey by the National Association for Continence (NAFC) estimated that one in four women over the age of 18 experiences SUI.[28] Age increases the incidence. Women involved in sports may have it more frequently than sedentary individuals.[36]

DIABETES MELLITUS

DM is a disease characterized by abnormal production of insulin by the pancreas or abnormal utilization of insulin by the body's tissues. Insulin is a hormone secreted by the pancreas that assists in glucose and fat metabolism and amino acid transport throughout the body.[37,38] Skeletal muscle uses insulin to assist glucose disposal from the body.[39] Three common types of diabetes exist, each with different etiologies and clinical manifestations:

♦ Type 1, formerly known as insulin-dependent diabetes mellitus or juvenile onset diabetes mellitus, results from diminished production of insulin in the islets of Langerhans of the pancreas. These cells are destroyed through either a viral or autoimmune response.[37,38] Type 1 diabetes occurs in less than 10% of the population, abruptly striking individuals who average less than 20 years of age.[38] Because endogenous insulin will not meet the metabolic demands of the patient, exogenous insulin is required. Careful management of diet, weight, and regular aerobic exercise are also needed to prevent the many cardiovascular and neurological complications of Type 1 diabetes.[40]

♦ Type 2, formerly known as non-insulin dependent diabetes mellitus or adult-onset diabetes mellitus, begins as an improper response of the body's tissues to circulating insulin. Such improper responses are commonly associated with obesity, but the exact cause of Type 2 diabetes is not known. Insulin resistance is related to impaired activation of glucose transport in muscle, possibly secondary to inhibition by free fatty acids.[41] In addition, patients with Type 2 diabetes may have insulin deficiency. The onset of Type 2 diabetes is gradual, and patients are typically older than 40 when they are first diagnosed.[38] The American Diabetes Association[42] notes that 90% to 95% of individuals in the United States with diabetes have Type 2 diabetes. Various pharmacological agents to stimulate insulin utilization in the tissues or insulin production are prescribed to control Type 2 diabetes. When needed, exogenous insulin is also prescribed. Careful control of circulating blood glucose levels through medical nutritional therapy (MNT)[43] and regular aerobic exercise[44] have been shown to prevent the many complications associated with Type 2 diabetes. Patient education and eventual patient self-management are essential to successful control of circulating blood glucose.[45]

♦ Gestational diabetes occurs during pregnancy and can gradually subside in the postpartum period. About 4% of pregnant women in the United States will have gestational diabetes.[46] The exact cause of gestational diabetes is not known, but hormones from the placenta create insulin resistance of the mother's tissues. The mother cannot secrete enough insulin in the face of this relative insulin deficiency when blood glucose levels rise.[46] The blood glucose crosses the placenta, and the baby must secrete insulin to decrease it or else store it as fat.[37] Management is through diet, weight control, exercise, and insulin injections as needed. Most women will be able to restore blood glucose levels to normal soon after delivery of the child.[37] Some women will be diagnosed with Type 1 or Type 2 diabetes if blood glucose levels do not normalize after delivery. Some women with gestational diabetes may be prone to developing Type 2 diabetes later in life because they develop insulin resistance.[46,47]

♦ Rare types of diabetes occur through genetic problems with other cells in the pancreas (beta cells), pancreatic lesions, and other endocrine disorders that affect insulin activity.[47]

Clinical Signs and Symptoms

Polydipsia (in Types 1 and 2 diabetes), polyuria (in Types 1 and 2), and polyphagia (in Type 1) are the classic signs leading to a diagnosis of diabetes. They result from excessive circulating glucose that causes a hyperosmolarity of the blood and subsequently the urine. The glucose attracts water that is eventually excreted with the glucose (polyuria) resulting in dehydration that stimulates excessive thirst (polydipsia). Excessive hunger (polyphagia) occurs in Type 1 diabetes because the lack of insulin necessitates that the cells deprived of glucose breakdown fats and proteins for fuel. These patients may also experience weight loss from the tissue breakdown and ketonuria as the metabolic by-products of tissue breakdown (ketones, among them) are excreted. These patients are in a more fragile metabolic state and may exhibit diabetic ketoacidosis (DKA) that could progress to hyperosmolar coma. Patients presenting with Types 1 and 2 diabetes may also complain of fatigue, weakness, blurred vision, and a sense of dizziness.[37,38]

Blood and urine levels of glucose are abnormal upon initial diagnosis. In addition, individuals with Type 1 diabetes may have insulin antibodies in the blood and human leukocyte antigens on specific chromosomes indicating the genetic link.[37,38,47]

Individuals with Type 2 diabetes may also initially have LE pain or paresthesias (associated with a diabetic neuropathy) and poor or delayed wound healing. They may also exhibit hyperlipidemia as an early sign of diabetes.[38]

"Tight" blood glucose control, with prepandial levels near normal at 110 mg/dL and glycosylated (HbA$_{1C}$) less than 7%, is the goal of the medical management of individuals with DM, except in cases where patients show frequent episodes of hypoglycemia.[48,49] HbA$_{1C}$ gives an indication of mean glycemia over the preceding 2 to 3 months.[40] Such control has been shown to reduce the risk of diabetic complications and delay their onset.

Hypoglycemia in a person who is exercising or has just exercised can be seen through the following signs and symptoms associated with the sympathetic nervous system (perspiration, piloerection, tachycardia, pallor, shakiness, hunger, weakness, and nervousness or irritability).[38,50,51] In addition, decreased glucose to the brain may result in headache, convulsion, blurred vision, dysarthric speech, perioral numbness, confusion, lability and coma.[38] Intake of simple sugars through glucose tablets, sugar, juice, or non-diet soda will help raise blood glucose levels. Individuals with Type 1 diabetes may require emergency injection of the hormone glucagon to restore blood sugar, especially if they are experiencing hypoglycemia unawareness.[51] Hyperglycemia can have some of the same signs and symptoms as hypoglycemia in addition to increased thirst, frequent urination, and high levels of sugar in the urine. Signs of DKA would include acetone breath, weak and rapid pulse, dehydration, and Kussmaul's breathing ("air hunger" marked by deep, gasping respiration).[37] Signs of a hyperosmolar hyperglycemic nonketotic syndrome (HHNS) include thirst, polyuria leading to volume loss, severe dehydration, seizures, and changes in mental status including lethargy, confusion, and coma. The prognosis for DKA and HHNS worsens with age. Administration of insulin and restoration of fluid and electrolyte balances are necessary in cases of DKA and HHNS.[38,52]

PHARMACOLOGY

PHARMACOLOGY FOR MUSCULAR DYSTROPHY

The pharmacological interventions for individuals with muscular dystrophy are primarily based upon management of secondary medical conditions. Corticosteroids administered daily (0.75 mg/kg) have been proven to be effective in reducing the progression of weakness associated with DMD.[53,54] This intervention does not reverse the effects of the disease, but does slow the progressive loss of muscle power, and therefore, maintains function for a longer period of time.

PHARMACOLOGY FOR DIABETES MELLITUS

The pharmacological management will vary with Type 1 and Type 2 diabetes. In each case, the physician works with the patient to carefully titrate the dosages of medications according to the metabolic demands. Often, patients benefit from more than one medication at the same time. MNT and exercise are also included in the optimal blood glucose control, and the physician must consider these factors when prescribing medication.[40]

Individuals with Type 1 diabetes will require exogenous insulin. The dosage regimen depends on the patient's age, medical status, duration of the illness, and the stability of the blood glucose level throughout the day.[38] Dosage schedules may range from once a day for a more stable patient to 4 times a day for someone with poor blood glucose control. The modes of administration are through intramuscular injection or through insulin pumps.[38,40,49,55]

Insulin preparations are classified according to the time when insulin will be available to the system: rapid-acting, short-acting, intermediate-acting, and long-acting. The rapid acting medications (eg, human analog) will be available to the system within 30 minutes and will have peak effec-

tiveness between 30 minutes to 2 hours. These will last up to 4 hours. This medication is suited for the insulin pump that delivers metered doses of insulin throughout the day. Short-acting insulin (regular insulin and semilente) takes 30 minutes to 3 hours to be available to the system with peaks between 2 and 8 hours with durations up to 16 hours (semilente). Intermediate-acting insulin (NPH, lente, isophane insulin suspension, and regular insulin) is available in 3 to 4 hours or less. Peaks range from 4 to 12 hours and duration from 24 to 48 hours. Long-acting insulin (ultralente) takes 4 to 6 hours to be available to the system with peaks at 18 to 24 hours and durations of 36 hours.[37,38,49,55]

Individuals with Type 2 diabetes may manage blood glucose levels with oral medications, although some will require regular insulin injections or pump. Four types of oral medications with different loci of control are in common use. Sulfonylureas act by stimulating cells of the islets of Langerhans in the pancreas to secrete more insulin. They also act by stimulating insulin receptor binding throughout the body. Metformin (Glucophage) works on hepatic and peripheral tissues to enhance their sensitivity to insulin thus improving the effectiveness of circulating insulin. Thiazolidinediones (pioglitazone and rosiglitazone) also work at the tissue level to reduce insulin-resistance. Acarbose works in the intestines to slow the digestion of sugars. A regimen including more than one medication is common for individuals with Type 2 diabetes.[37,38,49]

Low doses of aspirin and cholesterol-reducing medications may also be part of the total management of individuals with diabetes.[38,56] These may help reduce the risk of stroke or heart attack and the complications associated with peripheral vascular disease (PVD).[56]

MUSCLE PERFORMANCE MEASURES

OVERVIEW

Muscle performance measures can be categorized into those measuring contraction and extensibility characteristics and those measuring function. Measurement of contraction characteristics includes the ability of the muscle to contract and the strength or force-generating ability of the muscle. Simple palpation of the muscle contraction during MMT may verify that a muscle is contracting. EMG will allow more sophisticated analysis of the ability of muscle to contract, but not the force output. The force-generating ability of a muscle may be graded on an ordinal scale as in MMT (Table 3-1) or quantified using hand-held or isokinetic dynamometers to measure isometric contractions. The speed of generating peak force (timed rate of tension development) may be measured with isokinetic dynamometers that record force output from concentric (shortening) or eccentric (lengthening) contractions over a variety of joint movement velocities.

Table 3-1

MANUAL MUSCLE TESTING SCALE

	Grades		Grading Criteria
0	Zero	0	No palpable muscle contraction on command.
1	Trace	T	Palpable muscle contraction but no joint movement.
2-	Poor minus	P-	With limb positioned in a gravity-neutral (horizontal) position, palpable muscle contraction and able to move limb segment through part of the specified arc of motion.
2	Poor	P	With limb positioned in a gravity-neutral (horizontal) position, palpable muscle contraction and able to move limb segment through the specified arc of motion, but unable to counter a resistive force.
2+	Poor plus	P+	Limb positioned in a gravity-neutral (horizontal) position, palpable muscle contraction, able to move limb segment through the specified arc of motion, and able to counter a light resistive force.
3-	Fair minus	F-	Limb segment working against gravity and able to move segment through part of the specified arc of motion.
3	Fair	F	Limb segment working against gravity, able to move segment through the specified arc of motion, but unable to counter a resistive force.
3+	Fair plus	F+	Limb segment working against gravity, able to move segment through the specified arc of motion, and able to counter a light resistive force.
4-	Good minus	G-	Limb segment working against gravity, able to move segment through the specified arc of motion, and able to counter a resistive force that is between light and moderate.
4	Good	G	Limb segment working against gravity, able to move segment through the specified arc of motion, and able to counter a moderate resistive force.
4+	Good plus	G+	Limb segment working against gravity, able to move segment through the specified arc of motion, and able to counter a resistive force that is slightly more than moderate.
5	Normal	N	Limb segment working against gravity, able to move segment through the specified arc of motion, and able to counter a strong resistive force.

Adapted from Kendall FP, McCreary EK, Provance PG. *Muscles: Testing and Function.* Philadelphia, Pa: Williams & Wilkins; 1993:189.

Extensibility of muscle may be tested with flexibility or muscle length tests that require stabilization of one muscle attachment while the other is put on a stretch.[57] Goniometric measurements of the resultant joint position quantify muscle extensibility.[57] Tests for muscle extensibility will be presented in other parts of this text (see Pattern D: Impaired Joint Mobility, Motor Function, Muscle Performance, and Range of Motion Associated With Connective Tissue Dysfunction).

The balance between muscle strength and length throughout the body influences functional movement patterns. Where imbalances exist, movement impairment syndromes or musculoskeletal pain result and are perpetuated through faulty movement and altered function,[58] as found in Pattern B: Impaired Posture. Careful assessment of muscle length and strength may assist the physical therapist's decision-making about designing an optimal intervention.

Specialized functional tests (eg, Trendelenburg test) are utilized to assess specific functions of isolated contractions or stretch of individual muscles or muscle groups in order to confirm a diagnosis.[59] In other cases, the patient exhibits a pathognomonic sign (eg, Gower's sign) that illustrates poor muscle function.

EVALUATION OF MUSCLE STRENGTH

Wright and Lovett developed MMT to assess changes in patients with polio during the epidemic in the early 1900s.[60] They based the measurement system on the degree to which the muscle or muscle group could move the limb segment through a specified arc of motion and, if indicated, meet the manual resistance (counterpressure) of the examiner. A five-point ordinal scale (normal=5, good=4, fair=3, poor=2, trace=1, zero=0) was developed with each grade defined (see Table 3-1). Today, a 12-point ordinal scale is in common usage (see Table 3-1). The scoring system is based on the degree to which the subject can perform simple, cardinal plane limb segment movement against gravity (fair minus [–] or 3 to 5 and above) or with gravity minimized (poor plus [+] or 2+ to zero). When resistance is offered, it can be in the form of a holding contraction at a standardized point in the arc of motion (the "break" test)[57] or as an active resistance test at a constant velocity throughout the arc of motion.[60] Reliability and validity of MMT varies with the ability of the examiners to consistently judge resistive forces, the ability of the patients to follow commands and sustain a muscle contraction, and the consistency with which the patients generate force.[60] Reliability is better for the grades that require no resistance (fair [3/5] and below). Intratester reliability is better than intertester reliability when resistance is needed to grade strength.[61,62]

Hand-held dynamometers can provide a more objective measure of the muscle's force-generating ability. Hand-held dynamometers (Figure 3-9) have been successfully used for individuals with neurological impairments[63,64] including cerebral palsy,[65] spinal muscular atrophy,[66] stroke,[67] and spinal cord injury[68] and with patients in acute rehabilitation settings.[69] The length-tension curve for each muscle forms the basis for applying the resistance to an isometric contraction of the muscle.[70] The limb segment is positioned at the point in the arc of motion where maximal tension is normally generated and the subject is asked to match the resistive force applied by the examiner through the hand-held dynamometer. As long as the examiner keeps the resistive force perpendicular to the limb segment and uses the same point in the arc of motion and point of application of the resistive force, reliability is good. Intertester and intratester reliability was good for UE tests with a portable (hand-held) dynamometer but not for LE muscles in one study.[71] Other studies with individuals with renal disease[72] and patients in acute rehabilitation[69] verify that knee extension strength can be reliably measured by one or more examiners. More recent studies have shown that measuring LE strength with a hand-held dynamometer has good test-retest reliability[65] and interrater reliability[64] in patients with neuromuscular disorders.

Hand grip dynamometers may be used to assess functional grip strength.[73-75] Sources of error for dynamometry include the examiner's ability to apply the dynamometer appropriately and match the resistance of the patient, inadequate stabilization of the patient, inability of the patient to sustain an isometric contraction against resistance, instrument errors in reading or recording results, and motivation or fatigue issues for both the patient and the examiner.[70]

An isokinetic dynamometer fixed at 0 degrees/sec at a particular point in the arc of motion for a limb segment will yield similar results as a hand-held dynamometer if the subject generates the same force.[76] More typically, physical therapists use isokinetic dynamometers to test and train a muscle's ability to generate concentric and/or eccentric force through a specified arc of motion at a specified rate of speed.

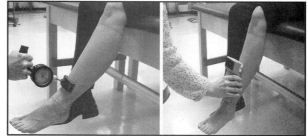

Figure 3-9. Hand-held dynamometry of knee extension with two different dynamometers.

Generally, testing reciprocal motions of the joint at slow (30 degrees/sec) and fast (120 degrees/sec) speeds serves as the baseline, although speed settings can exceed 180 degrees/sec when training elite athletes. Test-retest reliability was shown for quadriceps contractions at 30, 90, 120, and 180 degrees/sec.[76] Data generated from isokinetic testing include analysis of peak torque and timed rate of tension development, velocity spectrum analysis, and fatigue assessment. Sources of error for repeated isokinetic testing include problems with aligning the joint axis with the dynamometer axis, improper or inconsistent patient positioning and stabilization, and variations in the patient's motivation, pain, and fatigue threshold. Typically, large muscles or muscle groups are tested with isokinetic dynamometry (Figure 3-10). Training protocols with isokinetic testing vary according to the needs of the patient, nature of the injury, and desired functional outcome.

ELECTROMYOGRAPHY

In cases where the patient needs more sophisticated diagnostic testing, needle electrodes are used for EMG. When inserted into the muscle belly, these electrodes will display one or more MUs during a voluntary contraction and abnormal electrical discharges that occur in the muscle at rest. With a strong effort (35% of maximum or higher), a complete interference pattern will appear on the EMG tracing to represent MU activity.[77] In a neuropathy, an incomplete interference pattern may be seen with strong effort or a single unit interference pattern may be seen in a patient with severe nerve damage and only a few MUs remaining. The size, shape, and electrical configuration of MUs are also evaluated during diagnostic EMG. Normal MUs have a specific range of amplitude and duration. MUs that are longer in duration and/or have more phases (polyphasic) than a normal MU are indicative of nerve damage. MUs shorter in duration and lower in amplitude than normal are indicative of a myopathy. At rest, a patient with a neuropathy or myopathy may have fibrillation potentials and/or positive sharp waves due to instability of the muscle membranes. Undifferentiated waveforms seen at rest, which are reported

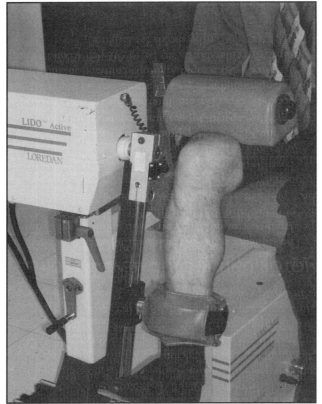

Figure 3-10. Isokinetic dynamometry of knee extension. Notice alignment of knee axis with that of dynamometer.

as increased insertional activity when the needle electrode is being inserted, may indicate pathology.[78] Sources of error include improper placement of the electrodes, incorrect interpretation of waveforms seen, and volume conduction from adjacent muscles or from other MUs of the same muscle.

Kinesiological EMG with surface or fine wire electrodes are used for movement analysis or biofeedback (Figure 3-11). Surface electrodes are secured to clean, dry skin over the muscles being evaluated. When impedance to the electrical signal from the muscle is low, muscle activity may be recorded. Kinesiological EMG may be used to study the relative timing of muscle contractions and the intensity of the contraction during a functional activity.[79,80] Sources of error for kinesiological EMG include inaccurate or inconsistent positioning of the recording electrodes, movement artifact from electrodes and wires, an improper electrode-skin interface, and volume conduction from adjacent muscles.[79,80]

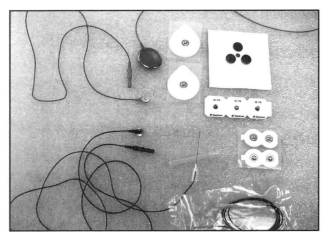

Figure 3-11. Array of surface and needle electrodes for electrodiagnosis and kinesiological electromyography.

Case Study #1: Muscular Dystrophy

Jimmy Rowe is a 7-year-old male with Duchenne muscular dystrophy.

PHYSICAL THERAPIST EXAMINATION

HISTORY

♦ General demographics: Jimmy is a 7-year-old white, English-speaking boy, who is right-hand dominant. He attends his local elementary school and is in the second grade.

♦ Social history: He lives with his parents, an older brother, and a younger sister. The parents are very supportive and concerned about meeting Jimmy's physical and emotional needs.

♦ Growth and development: His pre- and post-natal histories were unremarkable. His motor development was initially WNL but became delayed. He achieved sitting at 6 months, however, crawling was achieved at 10 months and walking at 14 months.

♦ Living environment: Jimmy and his family live in a ranch-style house with two steps to enter the front door.

♦ General health status
  • General health perception: No specific health concerns were reported by the parents, except for the implications of DMD.

- Physical function: He is less physically active, and his gait is more awkward than his peers or Jimmy's older brother at the same age.
- Psychological function: Jimmy's teachers report that he is somewhat withdrawn in class. He has not expressed concerns about his present problems; however, he has expressed thoughts about the future similar to his healthy peers.[81]
- Role function: Second-grade student.
- Social function: He has developed some close friendships in school, and these children encourage his continued participation during recess and other activities (eg, table tennis).

♦ Family history: Both parents are alive and well. His siblings have no signs of a neuromuscular disorder. Genetic testing of Jimmy's mother reveals a defect in the Xp21 region that is a deficit in the short arm of the X chromosome.[82,83]

♦ Medical/surgical history: Jimmy has no other significant medical or surgical history.

♦ Current condition(s)/chief complaint(s): He experiences weakness and reduced endurance for play. His parents report that he is having increased difficulty with ADL, such as getting up from low seats and the floor, climbing stairs, lifting objects above his head, and physical activities with his peers. His parents are concerned about maintaining Jimmy's functional level as long as possible.

♦ Functional status and activity level: He is independent in ADL. His parents report that he falls more frequently than his peers during physical play activities and is unable to participate in many physical activities. He appears awkward when he walks, climbs stairs, rises from the floor, or tries to run.

♦ Medications: Jimmy is taking corticosteroids[53] (prednisone 0.75 mg/kg) daily to assist in reducing the progression of weakness associated with DMD.[54]

♦ Other clinical tests
- Electrodiagnostic evaluation: Revealed short duration and low amplitude MUs in the proximal and distal muscles of all four extremities, with motor and sensory conduction studies WNL; a complete interference pattern was seen on early effort. These findings are consistent with myopathy.
- Laboratory tests: CK blood values of 10,000 were revealed in the initial diagnostic workup and are consistent with this diagnosis.[23,24]
- Radiological assessment of the femur and humerus: Revealed long bone atrophy and osteoporosis that increase the risk of fractures. Radiological screenings of the lumbar and thoracic spines were negative for scoliosis.
- Electrocardiogram (ECG): Revealed abnormalities in R waves and Q waves.
- Muscle biopsy required surgical removal of a small piece of skeletal muscle and examination of the muscle fibers microscopically: Revealed typical findings of increased fibrosis, small groups of basophilic fibers, and ruptured fibers.[25]

SYSTEMS REVIEW

♦ Cardiovascular/pulmonary
- BP: 111/70 mmHg
- Edema: None
- HR: 74 bpm
- RR: 14 bpm

♦ Integumentary
- Presence of scar formation: None
- Skin color: WNL
- Skin integrity: WNL

♦ Musculoskeletal
- Gross range of motion: WNL except for limitations in hip extension, adduction, and ankle dorsiflexion bilaterally
- Gross strength: Decreased in all trunk, neck, and extremity muscles, with proximal and extensor muscles more affected than distal and flexor muscles
- Gross symmetry: Present throughout except for hypertrophy of the left calf muscles and normal calf girth on the right
  - As the disease progresses, pseudohypertrophy is seen in various muscle groups, as muscle fibers are replaced by connective tissue and fat
- Height: 4'2" (1.27 m) (75th percentile for age 7)[84]
- Weight: 55 lbs (24.948 kg) (about 55th percentile for age 7)[85]

♦ Neuromuscular
- Balance is impaired during ambulation
- Gait is wide-based and slower than normal
- He has minimal difficulty with transfers

♦ Communication, affect, cognition, language, and learning style: WNL
- Communication and cognition: Alert and able to communicate needs
- Learning preferences: A visual learner who requires some repetition of information

TESTS AND MEASURES

♦ Aerobic capacity/endurance
- Endurance is reduced secondary to muscle fatigue

♦ Anthropometric characteristics
- BMI is 15.53 which is approximately the 37th percentile for boys his age[86]
  - Two considerations are important in overall

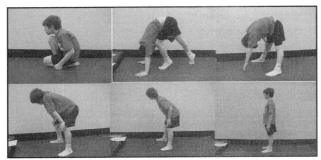

Figure 3-12. Gower's maneuver.

weight management for children with DMD: Prednisone and decreased physical activity will increase the potential for obesity[87,88]

  - ■ Obesity will also further decrease functional strength of muscles
  - ● Pseudohypertrophy of the left calf muscle
- ♦ Assistive and adaptive devices
  - ● He uses an incentive spirometer at home
  - ● Use of adaptive and assistive devices for ADL will be assessed and/or recommended, as needed, for specific ADL
- ♦ Environmental, home, and school barriers
  - ● Analysis of barriers revealed that there are two steps at the front entrance to the house
  - ● A railing presently enables Jimmy to climb the stairs when he is tired
  - ● He is presently able to manage ambulation at school, and he has been given permission to use the elevator when necessary
  - ● The school is wheelchair accessible
  - ● He avoids the use of weighted objects with ADL and IADL due to strength and fatigue issues
- ♦ Gait, locomotion, and balance
  - ● He ambulates with a wide base of support, with his left heel elevated from the floor (he bears weight on the ball of his left foot)
  - ● His feet exhibit equinovarus only during ambulation
  - ● His right hand is kept on his right iliac crest to assist in maintaining his lordotic, upright posture
  - ● He ambulates approximately 200 feet at a slow pace
  - ● He uses his hands more often (Gower's maneuver) to assist in walking, climbing stairs, rising from the floor, or running (Figure 3-12)
    - ■ Gower's maneuver is seen in children with proximal weakness, especially of the extensor muscles of the LE
    - ■ The child begins to stand from a seated position on the floor by raising his buttocks first (the "butt

first maneuver"), followed by extending his knees with the use of his hands
  - ■ From this position, he will use his hands on his thighs to help raise his upper body until he is fully upright[25]
  - ● He has difficulty with elevation activities
  - ● He has difficulty reaching overhead when standing due to balance problems
- ♦ Muscle performance
  - ● MMT results are found in Table 3-2
- ♦ Posture
  - ● Observational assessment and grid photographs revealed:
    - ■ Increased base of support, increased lumbar lordosis, and his right hand on his right iliac crest when standing
    - ■ Scapular winging bilaterally, right greater than left
- ♦ Range of motion
  - ● ROM in BUE and BLEs is WNL except for the following:
    - ■ Ankle
      - ▸ Ankle plantarflexion PROM with the knee straight is 10 to 40 degrees
      - ▸ Unable to achieve neutral talocrural position
      - ▸ With the knee flexed, passive dorsiflexion=0 to 10 degrees and plantarflexion=0 to 40 degrees
    - ■ Muscle length
      - ▸ Iliotibial band: Positive Ober test bilaterally; bilateral hip adduction 0 to 20 degrees
      - ▸ Iliopsoas: Positive Thomas test bilaterally; flexion contracture of 15 degrees bilaterally; bilateral hip flexion 15 to 115 degrees, unable to achieve neutral hip alignment
  - ● Rib cage expansion measured by tape measure at the level of T9 is 1.25 inches
- ♦ Self-care and home management
  - ● Interview concerning ability to safely perform self-care and home management actions, tasks, and activities revealed that basic self-care could be done independently, but prolonged ADL, such as dressing, feeding, and showering, revealed decreased endurance
  - ● He has minimal difficulty with transfers to and from deep chairs and low toilets
- ♦ Ventilation and respiration/gas exchange
  - ● Pulmonary function tests revealed a restrictive pattern of pulmonary impairment[89]
  - ● The following impairments would be present depending upon the severity of the disease
    - ■ Vital capacity is diminished

- Inspiratory capacity is diminished
- Expiratory reserve volume is diminished
- Total lung capacity is diminished
- Tidal volume is diminished
- Residual volume is increased
- Maximal voluntary ventilation is severely decreased
- Lungs clear
- Good diaphragmatic breathing, but inadequate use of secondary muscles of respiration
- Deep breathing and forced expiration impaired

♦ Work, community, and leisure integration or reintegration
- Interview concerning ability to safely manage school, community, and leisure actions, tasks, and activities revealed that he is able to attend school in a regular classroom, he uses a school elevator when he needs to go to the second floor of the school, and he has difficulty in participating in play activities with his classmates
- He has minimal difficulty with transfers to and from a car

Evaluation

Jimmy's history and findings are consistent with a diagnosis of DMD. He has a supportive family structure and his physical needs at home and school are presently being met. He has altered motor performance in all skeletal muscles of his neck, trunk, and extremities, with associated limitations in ROM in his LEs. He has difficulty with anti-gravity activities, such as getting up from the floor, rising from low seats or chairs, climbing stairs, and reaching overhead. He cannot handle weighted objects for performing ADL and IADL. Fatigue is apparent with prolonged duration activities, especially walking. Respiratory function is also a major concern due to involvement of the secondary muscles of respiration and the greatly increased risk of developing pneumonia as he gets older.

Diagnosis

Jimmy is a 7-year-old boy with DMD. He has impaired: aerobic capacity/endurance; anthropometric characteristics; gait, locomotion, and balance; muscle performance; posture; range of motion; and ventilation and respiration/gas exchange. He is functionally limited in self-care and home management and in school, community, and leisure actions, tasks, and activities. In addition, he is at risk for: contracture development and progression, motor weakness, declining ability to perform ADL, disuse weakness in less affected muscles, falls, and respiratory complications. These findings are consistent with placement in Pattern C: Impaired Muscle

Table 3-2
CASE STUDY #1: DUCHENNE MUSCULAR DYSTROPHY MANUAL MUSCLE TESTING RESULTS

Muscle	Right	Left
Shoulder flexors	2+	3-
Shoulder abductors	3+	3+
Shoulder IR	3	3+
Shoulder ER	3+	3+
Scapula adductors	2	2+
Serratus anterior	2-	2
Upper trapezius	4	4
Lower trapezius	2-	2-
Elbow flexors	3+	4-
Elbow extensors	3	3+
Supination	3+	3+
Pronation	3+	3+
Wrist flexion	4	4
Wrist extension	4	4
Finger flexors	4	4
Finger extension	4-	3+
Intrinsics	4	4
Neck flexors	2+	2+
Neck extensors	4-	4-
Trunk flexors	2	2
Trunk obliques	2	2
Trunk extensors	3+	3+
Hip flexors	3-	3
Hip extensors	2+	2+
Hip abductors	2+	2+
Hip adductors	3-	3-
Hip IR	3+	3+
Hip ER	3+	3+
Knee extensors	3+	3+
Knee flexion	4-	4-
Ankle dorsiflexors	4-	4-
Ankle plantarflexors	4	5
Ankle everters	4-	4-
Ankle inversion	4-	4-
Toe flexors	4-	4-
Toe extensors	3+	3+

Performance. The identified impairments will be addressed in determining the prognosis and the plan of care.

Prognosis and Plan of Care

Over the course of the visits, the following mutually established outcomes have been determined:
♦ Ability to perform ADL will be maintained

♦ Ambulation endurance shall be maintained and frequency of falls reduced or eliminated

♦ Communication between family, patient, school, and medical team will be optimized

♦ Disuse weakness will be reduced and overuse weakness prevented

♦ Educate the patient, family members, and school on risk factors associated with DMD

♦ Incentive spirometry results will reveal improved ventilatory capability

♦ Muscle contractures will be reduced

♦ Postural drainage techniques will be competently demonstrated by family members

♦ Risk factors will be reduced and risk of injury or secondary impairment will be reduced

♦ Stress management and relaxation techniques will be incorporated in daily routine

To achieve these outcomes, the appropriate interventions for this patient are determined. These will include: coordination, communication, and documentation; patient/client-related instruction; therapeutic exercise; functional training in self-care and home management; functional training in school, community, and leisure integration or reintegration; prescription, application, and, as appropriate, fabrication of devices and equipment; and airway clearance techniques.

Based on the diagnosis and prognosis, Jimmy will receive therapy twice a week for the first month, and then his home therapy will be monitored twice a month by the therapist. Over the course of a 2- to 6-month period of time, he will receive 18 visits. Jimmy has good social support, is motivated, and follows through with his home exercise program.

INTERVENTIONS

RATIONALE FOR SELECTED INTERVENTIONS

Therapeutic Exercise

Muscular dystrophy results in a slow decline in motor function, with extensor muscles more affected than flexor muscles. As motor decline continues, muscle imbalances occur. To compensate for the loss of muscle strength, postural compensations occur that result in muscle contractures and potential deformity.[25,90] Stretching and increasing muscle flexibility reduces the impact of these changes and prevents/slows down the progression of these deformities.[91] Prevention of soft tissue contractures is extremely important in this patient population.

Muscle strength declines as viable muscle fibers are lost. The resulting impairment of strength results in functional limitations in many aspects of ADL, with special atten-

tion to declining ambulatory capability.[92] This decline is further impacted by disuse weakness[93] of some muscles and overuse weakness of other muscles. Muscles that are being compensated for due to primary weakness are susceptible to disuse weakness. Proper education of the patient and family members coupled with the prescription of an appropriate exercise program helps to reduce the onset of disuse weakness. Muscles with MMT grades below 3 are also susceptible to overwork weakness. This is especially evident in frequently used muscles of the dominant extremity. Extreme care must be taken to protect these muscles from continued overwork. They must not be utilized in ADL or exercise so that the threshold for fatigue not be reached in these muscles.

Respiratory function closely corresponds to skeletal muscle function and viability. Although the diaphragm is not significantly involved, the accessory inspiratory and expiratory muscles of respiration are affected in DMD. Impaired ventilatory function leads to decreased mobility of the rib cage. Respiratory exercises can help improve some parameters of respiratory strength and function[94] and maintain rib cage mobility and lung tissue elasticity, thereby helping to maintain respiratory function.

Maintaining independent ambulation is a primary goal of the patient, family members, and the health care system. Strong clinical evidence supports that the maintenance of ambulation has many positive attributes.[25] ROM is easily maintained as long as the child is ambulatory and/or able to stand and bear weight on both LEs daily. Ambulation is also excellent for maintaining LE muscle strength. Scoliosis development is greatly controlled by the spine being in an extended posture during ambulation with an increased lumbar lordosis. The spine is intrinsically stable in an extended position. Once ambulation ability is lost, a scoliosis can progress rapidly and flexion contractures occur quickly in BLEs.[25] Strength declines due to decreased activity level, with concurrent potential for increased weight gain. Loss of ambulation and resultant wheelchair positioning tends to result in more rapid progression of a scoliosis.[95,96]

The iliotibial band, iliopsoas, and gastrocnemius muscles require early and vigorous stretching to maintain their optimal length for function. Loss of ROM leads to earlier loss of ambulation ability.[25]

Disuse weakness occurs in some muscles due to greatly reduced usage. In the case of a child with DMD, muscles less affected by the disease may become weaker due to decreased functional activity in all ADL. The muscles undergoing disuse weakness will respond to a low level of exercise.

COORDINATION, COMMUNICATION, AND DOCUMENTATION

Communication will occur with family members to gain support for his home exercise program. Communication with school personnel is needed for appropriate implementation of an individualized educational plan (IEP). Collaboration and coordination with muscular dystrophy clinic staff and family pediatrician is also needed.

PATIENT/CLIENT-RELATED INSTRUCTION

The patient and family members will be instructed in the risk factors related to DMD and the importance of maintaining functional abilities, performing a ROM program, and carrying out a home program. Jimmy's family will understand the importance of exercise, the importance of emotional support for their child, ways to monitor changes in his physical or functional status, and ways to vary his physical therapy program. They have been instructed to perform stretching exercises and request information about any additional physical therapy that may be indicated.

THERAPEUTIC EXERCISE

- ♦ Body mechanics and postural stabilization
  - Instructions for maintaining postural alignment during ADL such as sitting, reaching, bending/lifting, standing, and ambulation
  - Proprioceptive neuromuscular facilitation (PNF) techniques including individual scapular and pelvic PNF patterns against appropriate resistance
  - UE PNF patterns while holding light weights (starting at 1 lb and progressing as appropriate)
  - Real or simulated throwing exercise, passing a therapeutic ball, or working against the light resistance of therapeutic tubing or bands may be incorporated to add variety
- ♦ Flexibility exercises
  - Stretching exercises should be done after warming up, using a slow and steady stretch accompanied by deep breathing, and building hold up to 30 to 60 seconds
  - Stretching, especially of the tensor fascia latae (TFL) and iliotibial band (ITB), gastrocnemius/soleus, and hip flexor muscles[25]
    - Stretching these muscles daily is extremely important and should be performed as slow, prolonged static stretches to utilize the viscoelastic and plastic properties of connective tissue[90]
    - Proper technique requires good proximal stabilization in the following suggested positions:
      - ‣ TFL and ITB
        - ○ Sidelying on a bed with the lowermost leg flexed for stability and uppermost leg stretching into adduction, done with the hip slightly flexed and later (when hip extension increases) in hip extension
      - ‣ Gastrocnemius/soleus
        - ○ Standing with one foot behind the other,

heel of rear foot on ground, lunge forward while keeping the knee of the rear leg straight, and tracking over the second ray of the foot, hold for a slow count and relax
- ○ Then allow knee of the rear leg to bend slightly, hold again for a slow count and relax
- ○ Repeat at least three times for each leg and try to maintain a neutral position of the low back during all stretching
  - ‣ Hip flexors
    - ○ For the rectus femoris
      Lie prone with the knee in flexion while maintaining a neutral position of the low back, hold for a slow count and relax. Repeat at least three times for each leg
    - ○ For the iliopsoas muscle
      Use the Thomas test position to stretch. In supine, both knees are brought to the chest, then one leg is lowered into extension, while the other leg is held in flexion to stabilize the pelvis, hold for a slow count and relax, bring both legs up again, and repeat with the opposite leg[90]
  - Supine ROM for shoulder flexion and abduction and knee extension
- ♦ Gait and locomotion training
  - Gait training for improving heel toe gait and upright standing for prolonged weightbearing
  - Special emphasis placed on narrowing the base of support to reduce the compensatory equinovarus
- ♦ Relaxation
  - Aquatic relaxation techniques
  - Taught in a heated pool to induce muscle relaxation for overworked muscles
  - Jacobson relaxation techniques with breathing strategies
  - Gentle yoga stretches with an emphasis on deep breathing and relaxation
  - Visualization and imagery to induce total relaxation
- ♦ Strength, power, and endurance training
  - Patient should not become fatigued during these exercises, therefore, five or fewer repetitions are recommended
  - Muscles can be exercised, but exercise to fatigue increases the risk of overwork weakness
  - Active-assistive, active, and resistive exercises emphasizing low repetition strengthening of muscles weakened by the disease process. These will include[90]:
    - Hip extensors
      - ‣ Start in sidelying and progress to prone position

- ▸ Take care to maintain a neutral low back
- Knee extensors
  - ▸ In sidelying, exercise the uppermost leg as it is supported on a powder board with a very low weight
  - ▸ Progress to sitting
- Hip abductors
  - ▸ Start in supine and progress to sidelying
  - ▸ Working the uppermost leg against gravity may help reduce signs of a Trendelenburg gait
- Trunk and neck flexors
  - ▸ Start in supine with pelvic tilt exercises
  - ▸ Progress to curl-up with arms at the side
- Scapular stabilizers
  - ▸ Start in prone with simple scapular adduction held isometrically for a slow count to five
  - ▸ Progress to scapular adduction and depression that is held during bilateral GH extension
- Encourage patient to count out loud during these exercises to prevent breath-holding
- Active exercises in standing (closed chain) should emphasize appropriate postural alignment during real or simulated sports activities, such as table tennis
- Marching in place, side-stepping, and walking in circles or figures-of-eight can be incorporated for variety
- Aquatic programs
  - Allow the use of buoyancy of water for active assistive exercises of weak muscles and resistive exercises for strengthening muscles above Grade 3
  - Prevent undue stress and injury during exercise
  - Can be one of the best modes of exercise in this patient population[97]
- Ventilatory muscle exercises
  - Incentive spirometer exercises with emphasis on increasing vital capacity and rib cage mobility
  - Diaphragmatic breathing instruction
  - Resisted inspiratory exercises to improve respiratory strength and endurance in this patient[98-100]
  - Examples of basic exercises include blowing bubbles in a cup a water using a straw and making a pinwheel spin for 2, 3, or 4 seconds

FUNCTIONAL TRAINING IN SELF-CARE AND HOME MANAGEMENT

- ◆ Self-care and home management
  - A home assessment will be required to determine present and future needs for:
    - Bathing
    - Dressing
    - Grooming
  - Devices and equipment use and training
    - Wheelchair usage for long distance mobility
    - Assistive and adaptive device or equipment training during ADL and IADL, for example, a rolling backpack for carrying his schoolbooks may be easier for him to manage in school rather than a standard backpack
    - Protective or supportive device or equipment training during ADL and IADL

FUNCTIONAL TRAINING IN SCHOOL, COMMUNITY, AND LEISURE INTEGRATION OR REINTEGRATION

- ◆ School, community, and leisure
  - Training in wheelchair propulsion and safety for long distance mobility
- ◆ Injury prevention or reduction
  - Injury prevention and safety awareness education during ADL and ambulation
  - Fall prevention strategies

PRESCRIPTION, APPLICATION, AND, AS APPROPRIATE, FABRICATION OF DEVICES AND EQUIPMENT

- ◆ Adaptive devices
  - Rolling backpack for school books
  - Keep additional set of textbooks at home to lighten load
- ◆ Assistive devices
  - Long-handled reachers
  - Wheelchair
    - Prescription will include: Lightweight, folding wheelchair with solid insert seat and back; removable, adjustable height desk arms; push-to-lock brakes with brake extensions; and swinging, detachable footrests with adjustable angle footplate
    - Elevating leg rests can be ordered as needed later to prevent hamstring contractures during prolonged use
    - Ankle-foot orthoses to help control for plantarflexion contracture development may be considered in the future
- ◆ Supportive devices
  - Incentive spirometer

AIRWAY CLEARANCE TECHNIQUES

Teaching postural drainage and assistive cough techniques to patient and family members is very important.[25,100] Due to severe respiratory compromise in the later stages of the disease, knowledge of these techniques prior to the onset of a respiratory episode, such as pneumonia, reduces the stress and anxiety of performing them when the child is in respiratory distress.

ANTICIPATED GOALS AND EXPECTED OUTCOMES

- ◆ Impact on impairments
  - A 10% increase in vital capacity may be possible in 6 to 8 weeks.
  - Aerobic capacity is increased or maintained.
  - Airway clearance is improved, and he exhibits improved expiratory volume and cough after 4 weeks.
  - Endurance is improved, and he is able to walk through hallways at school without significantly elevated HR for about 200 feet.
  - Energy expenditure per unit of work is decreased.
  - Gait and locomotion are stabilized, and his base of support is progressing toward normal in 8 weeks.
  - Increased lumbar lordosis will be reduced.
  - Mobility of the rib cage is increased by 1 inch.
  - Muscle performance, especially endurance, is increased or maintained, and recent declines in MMT grades will be stabilized for 8 to 12 weeks.
  - Muscle strengthening without fatiguing is achieved.
  - Postural control is improved, and static and dynamic standing balance will be stable over the next 12 weeks.
  - Relaxation is improved.
  - Respiratory muscle function is improved.
  - ROM is improved and contractures decreased, so that PROM is improved by 10 degrees in ankle dorsiflexion and 5 degrees in hip movements within 4 weeks.
  - Ventilation and respiration/gas exchange are improved, and pulmonary function tests (PFTs) will reveal improvements in total lung capacity and vital capacity at 3-month follow-up by physician.
  - Work of breathing is decreased.
- ◆ Impact on functional limitations
  - Ability to perform and independence in physical actions, tasks, and activities related to self-care ADL, IADL, school, and play with or without devices and equipment is improved or maintained.
  - Energy conservation techniques are independently incorporated into ADL.

- Functional independence is maintained.
- Level of supervision required for task performance is decreased.
- Tolerance of positions and actions, tasks, and activities at school and play is improved.
- ◆ Risk reduction/prevention
  - Communication enhances risk reduction and prevention of complications.
  - Falls are reduced.
  - Risk factors are reduced or prevented.
  - Risk of secondary impairment is decreased.
  - Self-management of symptoms is improved.
  - Safety is improved.
- ◆ Impact on health, wellness, and fitness
  - Behaviors that promote healthy nutrition, physical activity, and wellness are acquired.
  - Health status is maintained.
  - Physical function is improved.
  - Proper nutrition to maintain ideal body weight is achieved.
- ◆ Impact on societal resources
  - Documentation occurs throughout patient management and across all settings and follows APTA's *Guidelines for Physical Therapy Documentation*.[97]
  - IEPs and mandatory communication and reporting are obtained or completed.
  - Utilization of physical therapy services is optimized.
- ◆ Patient/client satisfaction
  - Access, availability, and services provided are acceptable to patient.
  - Care is coordinated with patient, family, and other professionals.
  - Interdisciplinary collaboration occurs through case conferences.
  - Knowledge of how to utilize rehabilitation team/school personnel services appropriately is achieved.
  - Patient and family demonstrate realistic knowledge, awareness, and understanding of the disease process, diagnosis, prognosis, interventions, and anticipated goals and expected outcomes.
  - Patient satisfaction is achieved.
  - Referrals are made to other professionals or resources whenever necessary and appropriate.
  - Sense of well-being and control is improved.

REEXAMINATION

Reexamination is performed throughout the episode of care.

DISCHARGE

Jimmy is discharged from physical therapy after a total of 18 outpatient physical therapy sessions and attainment of his goals and expectations. These sessions have covered his entire episode of care. He is discharged because he has achieved his goals and expected outcomes.

Case Study #2: Stress Urinary Incontinence

Mrs. Kim is a 41-year-old woman who reports a 4-month history of urinary incontinence with coughing and sneezing.

PHYSICAL THERAPIST EXAMINATION

HISTORY

♦ General demographics: Mrs. Kim is a 41-year-old, English-speaking, Asian female. She is right-hand dominant. She is a college graduate.

♦ Social history: She lives with her husband and three young children ages 1, 3, and 5.

♦ Employment/work: Mrs. Kim teaches high school math.

♦ Living environment: She lives in a two-story walk-up apartment with nine steps to enter the building and 15 steps to get to the second level.

♦ General health status
  • General health perception: Mrs. Kim reports that she enjoys good health except for the urinary incontinence. She denies any problem with pregnancy or delivery of any child, but she notes that the last child was 8 pounds at birth.
  • Physical function: She works 5 days a week and tries to get to the gym "when she can."
  • Psychological function: The incontinence embarrasses her especially when it occurs in a work or social setting.
  • Role function: Mother, wife, teacher.
  • Social function: She enjoys spending time with her family and entertaining her large extended family.

♦ Social/health habits: She denies smoking and consumes alcohol only on special occasions.

♦ Family history: According to Mrs. Kim, her mother and older sister also experience urinary incontinence.

♦ Medical/surgical history: Mrs. Kim is premenopausal. She denies being pregnant at this time. She had an episiotomy with the vaginal delivery of each of her three children with the largest incision for the last child who weighed more than the others at birth. She had an appendectomy in 1990. She is being monitored for HTN but does not take any medication at this time.

♦ Prior hospitalizations: She was hospitalized for the appendectomy and the birth of each child.

♦ Preexisting medical and other health-related conditions: None.

♦ Current condition(s)/chief complaint(s): Mrs. Kim notes that for several months before and after the birth of her third child, she had infrequent episodes of urinary incontinence when sneezing and coughing, which subsided after about 3 months post-partum. During the past 4 months, the symptoms returned and became progressively more frequent with increasing amounts of urine leakage. She attributes the change to lifting the youngest child who now weighs 18 lbs and the middle child who weighs 30 lbs. She denies pain or other problems with sexual activity. She denies a history of sexual abuse.

♦ Functional status and activity level: She is independent in all ADL and IADL. She uses the treadmill and weight machines at the gym but manages to get there only twice a week. Her workouts do not induce stress incontinence, but she always voids before starting her workout.

♦ Medications: None.

♦ Other clinical tests
  • The urologist ruled out bladder infection and all tests for urine flow were WNL. Specialized testing included urinalysis, uroflowmetry, cystometry, and stress tests to provide differential diagnosis and to determine the exact bladder capacity associated with urine loss during coughing or stressful activities.[27,28,101] The amount of urine lost during stress incontinence can be calculated by weighing an incontinence pad after a specified period of use and comparing its weight to that of the dry pad. Forty-eight-hour pad tests[101] and stress tests with a known bladder volume and a uniform type of stress (coughing or doing jumping exercise) can be used to quantify the degree of SUI.[102] Mrs. Kim refused the 48-hour pad test and stress test at this time due to scheduling issues.
  • The gynecologist noted a slightly anteverted uterus and weakness of the PFM with a perineometer reading that showed moderate weakness. One form of perineometer for assessing PFM strength is a vaginal balloon catheter (inserted a standard of 3.5 cm inside the vagina) with a pressure transducer to record the amount of pressure (in cm H_2O) generated by the PFM during a strong contraction.[102]

SYSTEMS REVIEW

♦ Cardiovascular/pulmonary
  • BP: 125/85 mmHg
  • Edema: None
  • HR: 70 bpm
  • RR: 13 bpm
♦ Integumentary
  • Presence of scar formation: None
  • Skin color: WNL
  • Skin integrity: WNL
♦ Musculoskeletal
  • Gross range of motion: WNL throughout UEs, LEs, and spine
  • Gross strength: WNL for major muscle groups of the UEs and LEs
  • Gross symmetry: Posture appears symmetrical in standing; thoracic kyphosis appears flattened
  • Height: 5'1" (1.55 m)
  • Weight: 100 lbs (45.36 kg)
♦ Neuromuscular
  • Balance: WNL
  • Gait, locomotion, transfers, and transitions: WNL
♦ Communication, affect, cognition, language, and learning style: WNL
  • Communication and cognition: Alert and able to communicate needs
  • Learning preferences: Active learning style

TESTS AND MEASURES

♦ Aerobic capacity/endurance
  • While WFL, she has difficulty maintaining muscle control while ambulating at 3.5 mph on the treadmill
♦ Anthropometric measurements
  • BMI: 18.9 which is WNL[103]
♦ Cranial and peripheral nerve integrity
  • Cranial nerves, UE, and LE sensory and motor tests: WNL
♦ Ergonomics and body mechanics
  • Analysis of her standing posture and the physical demands of the job revealed that all were done using appropriate body mechanics
  • Analysis of her body mechanics while lifting and carrying her children revealed that she tended to lift them with appropriate body mechanics, but she supported them on her left pelvis causing a lateral shift of her trunk to the right
♦ Gait, locomotion, and balance
  • Difficulty maintaining PFM contraction on unstable surfaces

♦ Muscle performance
  • The stopwatch-timed urine stream interruption test
    ■ Two seconds elapsed before Ms. Kim was able to contract the PFM and stop the flow of urine
    ■ PFM strength is correlated to urinary continence,[104] therefore, a delayed ability to stop the urine flow indicated problems with the PFM
    ■ The urine stream interruption test was validated with an uroflowmeter and a digital measure of PFM strength and showed adequate repeatability[105,106]
    ■ Urine stream interruption has the risk of introducing bacteria into the bladder if a reflux of held urine from the distal urethra enters the proximal urethra or bladder
    ■ Patients should be reminded to void fully after completing the test
    ■ Although the test can be used to give baseline data and to monitor patient progress,[107] the monitoring should be on a monthly basis[107] to minimize the risk of urinary tract infection
  • Vaginal (digital) palpation (after securing informed consent and while using standard precautions)
    ■ The physical therapist should secure signed informed consent for the procedure which details the need for and the procedure of the examination, and the patient's right to stop the examination at any time should be emphasized[27]
    ■ A third person in the room during the vaginal palpation may be needed for medical-legal reasons[27]
    ■ The therapist should wear sterile, latex-free gloves during vaginal palpation of the PFM strength
    ■ Weakness of the muscles is evidenced by the inability to sustain a contraction longer than 5 seconds
    ■ Vaginal palpation while observing the pelvic floor tighten and move upward (inward) ensures the PFM are contracting[31,32,108,109]
    ■ Her PFM contraction was adequate to raise the pelvic floor but only for 5 seconds
    ■ Bø and Finckenhagen[110] examined the concurrent validity and interrater reliability of measuring PFM strength through vaginal palpation using the 6-point, modified Oxford scale (0=no contraction, 1=flicker, 2=weak, 3=moderate, 4=good, 5=strong). The criterion reference was vaginal squeeze pressure (cm H_2O) recorded from a vaginal balloon catheter (perineometer) connected to a microtip pressure transducer. The mean pressure readings did not differ across the six categories which casts doubt on the validity of the scale. Two examiners had adequate interrater

reliability (Spearman rho=0.7), however, their ratings systematically differed by one category for 10 of the 20 participants.[110] Isherwood and Rane[111] conducted a similar experiment with one examiner conducting both vaginal palpation (rating strength via the 6-point, Oxford scale) and perineometry (yielding a 12-point ordinal scale). Good agreement was established between vaginal palpation and perineometry to determine the strength of the PFM.[111] Vaginal palpation of the PFM contraction is an essential part of the examination because the examiner can assess the presence of a contraction and whether the patient is performing the exercise correctly. Assigning an ordinal grade to the muscle strength via vaginal palpation may not be feasible for scientific purposes or when more than one physical therapist will work with a patient[110]

- MMT revealed the following:
  - Abdominal muscles=4/5 strength
  - Back extensors=5/5
  - UEs and LEs: WNL
- Pain
  - Urinary tract or pelvic pain
    - No pain during intercourse
    - No low back or sacroiliac joint pain
- Posture
  - Observational assessment revealed:
    - Slight flattening of the thoracic kyphosis
    - When distracted, Mrs. Kim assumed a posture marked by an increased lumbar lordosis
- Range of motion
  - Spine and all extremities: WNL except
    - Bilateral hip abduction=0 to 35 degrees
    - Straight leg raise=0 to 60 degrees
  - Flexibility (muscle length)
    - Tightness of the hip adductors bilaterally
    - Tightness of the hamstrings bilaterally
- Reflex integrity
  - WNL
- Self-care and home management
  - Interview concerning ability to safely perform self-care and home management actions, tasks, and activities revealed that she was able to meet the demands of these activities, but was fatigued after busy days
  - Subjective assessment of severity of SUI using a leakage index or voiding diary[102] revealed consistent leakage with coughing and sneezing
- Sensory integrity
  - Sensation in the "saddle" area is intact
  - Sensation is WNL throughout trunk and LEs

- Work, community, and leisure integration or reintegration
  - Interview concerning ability to safely perform work, community, and leisure actions, tasks, and activities revealed that she was able to meet the demands of these activities, but was fatigued after busy days
  - Subjective assessment of severity of SUI using a social activity index[102,112] revealed no problem with social activity

EVALUATION

Mrs. Kim has a 4-month history of stress urinary incontinence that is becoming progressively worse. She has weakness and difficulty sustaining contractions of the PFM for longer than 5 seconds. She has abdominal muscle weakness and decreased flexibility of the proximal muscles of the LEs. Her body mechanics while carrying her children increased her trunk lateral shift. Sensory tests and LE muscles tests were WNL thus ruling out neurological involvement.

DIAGNOSIS

Mrs. Kim has stress urinary incontinence that has become progressively worse. She has impaired: ergonomics and body mechanics; muscle performance; posture; and range of motion. She is functionally limited in self-care and home management; and in work, community, and leisure actions, tasks, and activities. These findings are consistent with placement in Pattern C: Impaired Muscle Performance. The identified impairments will be addressed in determining the prognosis and the plan of care.

PROGNOSIS AND PLAN OF CARE

Over the course of the visits, the following mutually established outcomes have been determined:
- Ability to stand without excessive lumbar lordosis will improve
- Flexibility of the proximal LE muscles will improve
- Frequency of stress incontinence with coughing and sneezing will decrease
- Lifting and carrying techniques will improve
- Overall fitness will increase
- Performance of the PFM, including increased strength and endurance of the muscles, will improve
- Strength of the abdominal muscles will increase
- The volume of urine that leaks during stress incontinence with coughing and sneezing will decrease
- To begin a preventative and maintenance program to manage the SUI

To achieve these outcomes, the appropriate interventions for this patient are determined. These will include: coordination, communication and documentation; patient/client-related instruction; therapeutic exercise; functional training in self-care and home management; functional training in work, community, and leisure integration or reintegration; and electrotherapeutic modalities.

Based on the diagnosis and prognosis, Mrs. Kim is expected to require between 9 and 12 visits over an 8-week period of time. Mrs. Kim is a healthy, motivated individual with good social support and will follow through with her home exercise program.

INTERVENTIONS

The NAFC categorizes interventions as behavioral, pharmacological, and surgical.[113] Behavioral intervention includes patient education, exercise prescription for PFM, changes in fluid intake as indicated, and use of biofeedback or electrical stimulation to enhance PFM contraction strength.[27,28] Physical therapists play a major role in patient education, exercise prescription, and applying biofeedback or electrical stimulation. Pharmacological intervention includes changing medications that may increase urine output (eg, diuretics) because there are no approved medications for controlling SUI. Surgical intervention is indicated when the bladder and urethra need to be realigned and when support devices or tension-free tape for the pelvic floor are implanted. Other procedures include collagen implantation around the urethra and radio frequency bladder neck suspension that shrinks the tissues of the pelvic floor to lift the urethra and bladder neck into better alignment.[27,28]

RATIONALE FOR SELECTED INTERVENTIONS

Therapeutic Exercise

Mrs. Kim's primary goal is to restore the strength, power, and endurance of her PFM. She also wishes to prevent progression of the problem as she ages. The first choice of treatment for SUI is PFM training as it is effective and has no known side effects.[31] Kegel[32] introduced PFM exercise and documented an 84% cure rate.[108] Bø[31] noted that adequate PFM exercise must be specific to these muscles, without unnecessary use of abdominal, gluteal, or adductor muscles. Correct contractions must produce inward movement of the perineum.[31] Some abdominal muscle contraction may be synergistic with PFM contraction but should not be the sole contraction.[114] Training must include contractions that are stronger than those needed for normal ADL in order to progressively overload the muscle and stimulate muscle fiber regeneration.[31] Increasing the intensity and/or duration of the PFM contraction, decreasing the rest time between successive contractions, and increasing the number of repetitions performed in each exercise bout will all progressively overload the muscles and improve the training effect.[31] The need to ensure specificity and proper progression of the exercises over the average training period of 3 to 6 months necessitates frequent monitoring by the physical therapist at regular intervals.[31]

Many variations of Kegel's exercises have evolved over time. The NAFC recommends two types of contractions: prolonged holding and fast contractions. The prolonged contractions enhance recruitment of slow-twitch muscle fibers and later fast-twitch fibers. The fast contractions require recruitment of fast-twitch muscles.[27,31,115,116] Such training is presumed to help maintain PFM tone and holding during a sudden cough or sneeze.[27,31,117] Researchers have shown that daily PFM exercise produced a high cure rate among women with SUI.[32,102,117] Bø[102] demonstrated that women with SUI who responded to PFM training had a strong positive relationship between PFM strength and improvement in SUI. Bø, Talseth, and Vinsnes[118] showed that daily PFM exercise and 45-minute weekly group instruction for 6 months yielded improved quality of life and physical activities for women with SUI when compared to a control group who did not exercise. Fonda and associates[119] worked with men and women over the age of 60 and found improvement in the severity of symptoms and quality of life measures with individualized, conservative management including pelvic floor muscle exercises, bladder retraining (to normalize daily frequency of urination), and patient education and continence aids. Janssen and associates[120] showed that women with stress, urge, or mixed incontinence who received group training had an equal effect as a cohort receiving individual training for PFM exercises. Cammu, Van Nylen, and Amy[121] found that women with genuine stress incontinence, who had been successful with PFM training, had a 66% chance of continuing favorable results for at least 10 years.

Mørkved, Bø, Schei, and associates[122] worked with a large sample of pregnant women who were randomized into control and treatment groups at 18 weeks gestation to study the effect of PFM exercise on SUI during pregnancy. Women in the treatment group had 12 weekly group classes directed at PFM strengthening and practiced PFM contractions daily. The control group had usual care. Significantly fewer women in the exercise group reported urinary incontinence as the pregnancy progressed and for 3 months post-partum. In another study, Mørkved and Bø[123] followed participants in a matched control trial for 1 year post-partum and found that the group who had an 8-week PFM training program immediately post-partum had fewer episodes of SUI and better contraction of the PFM after 1 year.

Wells[124] reviewed 22 studies about the efficacy of the pelvic floor muscle training with most studies showing improvement in stress urinary incontinence and some reporting large rates of cure. More recently, Hay-Smith and associates[125] reviewed 43 studies about PFM training for SUI in women and concluded that PFM training was better than no treatment. These reviewers were not able to determine if adding electrical stimulation, vaginal cone training, or biofeedback to a PFM training protocol enhanced the effect.[125] Using a stratified, single-blind, randomized controlled trial, Bø, Talseth, and Holme[117] found that PFM exercise was superior to electrical stimulation of the muscles or to the use of vaginal cones (used as a form of resisted exercise).

An adjunct to training PFM is the use of vaginal cones or vaginal balls of increasing weights (20 to 100 g). Vaginal balls and cones are small weights made of inert materials that are tethered to a filament for ease of removal. The patient can insert one ball or cone in the vagina and hold it by a tonic PFM contraction for a specified time period, usually 15-minute sessions[126-128] twice a day[129] or as tolerated. The weighted cones serve as a form of sensory biofeedback because the woman must keep one in place without slippage during typical ADL. Increasing the weight of the cone inserted as the PFM become stronger serves as a form of progressive resistance training. Several studies found that vaginal cone training improved strength of PFM contractions in healthy women and women with SUI[128] and reduced their symptoms.[130] Herbison and associates[130] reviewed 15 studies about weighted vaginal cones and determined that training with cones alone was better than no treatment for SUI. The effectiveness of training with weighted vaginal cones may be equal to PFM training and to electrical stimulation but better designed studies are needed to confirm this trend.[130] Side effects of the use of vaginal cones may include vaginitis, bleeding, and discomfort.[117] Motivation to use vaginal cones may also be an issue for some women.[117] Arvonen and associates[126] trained two groups of women with SUI with and without weighted vaginal balls (50 and 65 g of 28-mm diameter; 80 and 100 g of 32-mm diameter). Both groups trained with similar protocols for maximal and submaximal contractions of specified durations and frequency with the experimental group incorporating vaginal balls into the training. After 4 months of training, both groups improved muscle strength and decreased urinary leakage. Improvement in urinary leakage, as measured by a pad stress test with a standardized bladder volume, was significantly better in the group training with vaginal balls than in those training with PFM alone. No side effects for the use of vaginal balls was reported in this study.[126]

Like any muscle, appropriate postural alignment will improve the tension generated. Although Mrs. Kim has adequate postural alignment, she has weak abdominal muscles and tends toward an excessive lumbar lordosis. A training program to improve strength and endurance of the abdominal musculature will be incorporated into her program. Stretching the muscles that attach to the pelvis (adductors, hamstrings, rectus femoris, and iliopsoas) is also needed to allow her to assume a relaxed but stable standing posture. Lumbar stabilization exercises and resisted exercises will be added to the program prior to discharge. The strengthening program will include lifting and carrying activities with appropriate body mechanics and training for lifting and carrying her young children. Using proper body mechanics may help reduce intra-abdominal pressure on the pelvic floor during lifting thus reducing her symptoms.[131] Self-management strategies, a home exercise program, and preventative exercise will comprise the instructions to the patient.

Improved general fitness helps maintain muscle energy use, tone, and vascularity throughout the body. In addition, aerobic exercise may mobilize the pelvis[132] to maintain joint integrity and bone strength. These aspects will be important to Mrs. Kim as she ages.

Electrotherapeutic Modalities

Biofeedback

Biofeedback is a method of enhancing the patient's awareness of the ability of the PFM to contract and to increase muscle fiber recruitment. Kegel was the first to use biofeedback with a perineometer attached to a manometer that gave visual feedback for squeeze pressure around a pneumatic vaginal chamber caused by PFM contraction.[32,108] Pages and associates[133] compared 4 weeks of intensive group physical therapy with 4 weeks of biofeedback for treating genuine stress incontinence. The biofeedback was through a pressure sensor inserted into the vagina with audible feedback when a minimal pressure of 40 cm H_2O was achieved. Participants in both groups also followed a 2-month period of unsupervised home exercise upon completion of the experimental phase. Although no control group was utilized, the participants were randomized into groups. Results showed that patients in both groups improved the quality of the PFM contractions and reduced nocturnal urinary frequency while those in the group physical therapy also reduced daytime urinary frequency. Participants in the biofeedback group had higher contraction pressures of the PFM and a better subjective outcome.[133]

Morkved, Bø, and Fjortoft[101] performed a single-blind, randomized, controlled trial with a stratified design to determine the effectiveness of 6 months of intensive, individual PFM training with and without biofeedback in women with urodynamically proven stress incontinence. A vaginal pressure probe was used for home biofeedback. Both treatment regimens were effective. Biofeedback plus PFM training did not significantly improve performance when compared to PFM training alone. The authors acknowledge that biofeedback may serve as a good motivational tool during training for some women.[101]

Surface electromyography (sEMG)-assisted biofeedback can also be used with PFM training. Aukee et al[134] examined 30 patients undergoing PFM training with and without sEMG biofeedback 20 minutes daily, 5 days per week for 12 weeks. Both groups had improved pelvic floor muscle force and decreased urine leakage after training. The only difference between groups was in the PFM force generated in the supine position for the women receiving sEMG biofeedback. Forces generated in standing were the same in both groups after training.[134]

Weatherall[135] conducted a meta-analysis of five trials and applied odds-ratio analysis to the pooled data to compare biofeedback with PFM exercise to PFM exercise alone. Biofeedback plus PFM exercise versus PFM alone had an odds-ratio of 2.1 (95% CI=0.99 to 4.4) showing that biofeedback may be an effective adjunct to PFM exercise.[135]

A protocol whereby functional electrical stimulation (FES, 24 sec duration) is followed by biofeedback (three phases totaling 32 seconds) was compared to intensive PFM exercise[136,137] and a control[137] group for women with SUI. Both experimental groups improved over the 6-week trial but the FES-biofeedback group showed significant improvement in the pressure (mmHg) measured by a vaginal perineometer when compared to PFM exercise group[136,137] and controls.[137] Quality of life also increased for the FES-biofeedback groups to a greater extent than for intensive PFM exercise group.[136]

Electrical Muscle Stimulation

Symptoms of SUI should be reduced or even cured if the strength and endurance of the PFM can be improved.[108] The training may be augmented with electrical stimulation of the affected muscles or biofeedback. Each will be tried with Mrs. Kim and she will choose the electro agent that best augments the active contractions and improves her ability to sustain the contraction for greater periods of time.[131]

EMS of the PFM has been shown to be effective in increasing strength of the muscles.[117,138] In a double-blind, controlled trial with 14 women, Blowman and associates[138] reported that the seven women in the group receiving neuromuscular stimulation did not require surgery while four of the six in the group receiving sham neuromuscular stimulation required surgical correction of genuine stress incontinence. Biphasic waveforms (80 microseconds, 10 Hz, 60 minutes per day for 4 weeks) allowing a prolonged recovery phase for repolarization were selected for this trial.[138]

Sand and associates[139] studied the effect of transvaginal neuromuscular electrical stimulation on urodynamically proven, genuine stress incontinence with 52 women in a multicenter, placebo-controlled trial. The experimental group used an electrostimulator with an insertable vaginal electrode with 2 stimulus output channels (50 cps and 12.5 cps) with a pulse duration of 0.3 msec and a current range of 0 to 100 mA. The placebo group used the same electrode and an electrostimulator that was capable of only 1 mA of current. Both groups used the devices twice daily for 12 weeks with duty cycles and treatment times increasing on

a fixed scheduled. After 2 weeks, the groups did not differ in symptoms. After 12 weeks, subjective improvement in symptoms, decreased leakage, and PFM strength measured by a perineometer were significantly improved in the experimental group but not in the control group.[139]

Several protocols compare groups of patients performing PFM exercise to those receiving electrical stimulation.[117,138] Both treatment strategies improve strength of contraction of the PFM and reduce some of the symptoms of stress urinary incontinence. Electrical stimulation and PFM appear to have similar effects with one not superior to the other when each are combined with behavioral therapy.[140] Bø, Talseth, and Holme[117] found that PFM training (8 to 12 strong contractions tid and weekly physical therapy) was superior to electrical stimulation and vaginal cones (20 minutes daily, progressing cone weight as tolerated) in relieving objective signs of genuine stress incontinence. Side effects from electrical stimulation may include discomfort or tenderness and bleeding.[117]

COORDINATION, COMMUNICATION, AND DOCUMENTATION

Communication will occur with Mrs. Kim and her gynecologist (the referring physician). Mrs. Kim does not wish to include her husband in the discussion of this problem at this time. All elements of the patient's management will be documented.

PATIENT/CLIENT-RELATED INSTRUCTION

Mrs. Kim must develop an adequate understanding of the problem and its long-term sequelae in order to commit to changing her behaviors. The physical therapist will instruct Mrs. Kim in the normal anatomy of the pelvic floor and emphasize the importance of adequate muscle tone to prevent stress incontinence. The patient will be instructed in home exercises to increase strength and endurance of the pelvic floor and abdominal muscles as detailed below. In addition, flexibility exercises for the proximal LE muscles will be instituted. Short- and long-term strategies to deal with the stress incontinence will include frequent voiding and PFM contraction prior to a sneeze or cough. Warning signs of urinary tract or bladder infection, nerve damage, or unexplained progression of SUI will be discussed along with instructions to seek the attention of the physician should these occur. A brochure entitled "You Can Do Something About Incontinence: A Physical Therapist's Perspective"[107] will be given to and reviewed with Mrs. Kim, as well as information about the NAFC website.[113]

THERAPEUTIC EXERCISE

♦ Aerobic capacity/endurance conditioning
  • Mode

- Stationary bicycle and treadmill for aerobic conditioning based upon Mrs. Kim's preference for these exercises
  - Duration
    - 20 minutes initially
    - Increase duration progressively to 30 to 45 minutes
  - Intensity
    - Moderate: Raising HR to 60% to 70% of maximum (220–age)
    - Progressing as tolerated
    - Progressing to increased speed while maintaining PFM contraction
  - Frequency
    - Initially three times a week incorporating her normal routine for the gym
- Balance, coordination, and agility training
  - Balance/proprioception board
  - Balance boards
  - Tandem walking
  - High speed balance challenges
- Body mechanics and postural stabilization
  - Body mechanics training
    - Incorporate lifting and carrying weights[131] similar to those of her children into the training
    - Emphasize body mechanics and contraction of the PFM prior to and during lifting[131]
  - Postural control training and postural stabilization exercises: axial extension of head, slight scapula retraction, abdominal contraction throughout all exercises
    - Postural awareness retraining and postural stabilization exercises will be expanded as abdominal and PFM strength improves
    - Exercises for postural stabilization using the foam roller or a therapeutic ball
    - Spinal stabilization with a contraction of abdominal muscles and back extensors in appropriate positions to allow controlled movement of the pelvic girdle during exercises (eg, quadruped exercises; treadmill walking; coordinated arm, trunk, and leg movement)[117] and during ADL
      - Maintain appropriate contractions of abdominal and back extensor muscles[117] in quadruped and alternately lifting and holding (for a count of five) one arm and the opposite leg, progress by increasing the number of repetitions
      - Practice sit to stand using appropriate contractions of abdominal and back extensor muscles, holding progressively larger weights
      - Practice reaching in all directions (either seated or standing) maintaining a neutral lumbar spine
      - Treadmill walking increasing duration and speed while maintaining a neutral lumbar spine
- Flexibility exercises[132]
  - Stretching exercises should be done after warming up, using a slow and steady stretch accompanied by deep breathing, and building hold up to 30 to 60 seconds
  - Stretching exercises for the iliopsoas, hamstrings, adductors, and rectus femoris
    - Contract-relax and/or hold-relax for the PNF LE diagonal patterns to augment the effect of static stretching of these muscles
  - Flexibility exercises for hip flexors, adductors, and hamstrings with focus on posture, contracting stabilizing muscles to achieve appropriate, prolonged (1- to 2-minute) stretch
  - Incorporate flexibility exercises in yoga stretching or as part of warm-up and cool-down for aerobic training
  - Soft tissue mobilization to affected muscles, if needed
- Strength, power, and endurance training
  - PFM (Kegel) exercises
    - Hold an active contraction of the PFM for up to 6 to 8 sec, relax completely for 10 sec and repeat 10 times, completing three sets per day[117]
    - Progress holding time and/or number of repetitions[117,124]
    - Train in a variety of functional positions and postures
    - Initially, may need to perform the exercises in a supine position
    - Later, perform holding contractions while the patient is sitting, standing, or walking
    - Practice using the contractions while lifting or reaching
    - Perform three to four fast contractions of the PFM, rest 6 sec, and repeat 10 times, at least three sets per day
    - Alternate fast contractions with holding contractions and rest[115,117,122]
    - If not making significant progress with PFM training, incorporate use of vaginal cones or balls
  - PREs
    - Abdominal muscles
      - Start in supine with arms at side, perform chin tuck plus trunk curl until scapulae clear the floor, hold the contraction 5 sec and slowly lower back to the floor, repeated up to 30 times

- ▸ When can comfortably perform 30 repetitions without stopping to rest, increase the resistance for the exercise
- ▸ Cross arms on chest or hold arms behind neck to increase the lever arm resulting in greater demands for the abdominal muscles[57]
- ▸ Perform series of exercises using a trunk curl plus rotation for the oblique abdominal muscles
- ▸ In supine, with one leg flexed 90 degrees at the hip and knee, perform a heel slide of other leg (holding strong abdominal and PFM contractions) to increase the tonic strength of the abdominals[58] and PFM

FUNCTIONAL TRAINING IN SELF-CARE AND HOME MANAGEMENT

- ♦ Self-care and home management
  - • Review all actions, tasks, and activities and postural alignment and PFM contraction for self-care and home management
  - • Injury prevention or reduction
    - ▪ Injury prevention education during self-care and home management
    - ▪ Injury prevention or reduction with lifting and caring for her children
    - ▪ Safety awareness training during self-care and home management

FUNCTIONAL TRAINING IN WORK, COMMUNITY, AND LEISURE INTEGRATION OR REINTEGRATION

- ♦ Work
  - • Review all actions, tasks, and activities and postural alignment and PFM contraction for work
  - • Injury prevention or reduction on the job
  - • Safety awareness while working and at home including body mechanics for lifting and carrying
  - • Increase amount of walking and stair climbing during the day
- ♦ Leisure
  - • Be active and have fun at the same time without concern for SUI
  - • Plan family outings and vacations to include physical activity

ELECTROTHERAPEUTIC MODALITIES

- ♦ Neuromuscular electrical stimulation (NMES) for the PFM
  - • Vary the parameters according to patient comfort and goals

- • Bø, Talseth, and Holme[117] protocol
  - ▪ Biphasic intermittent current at a frequency of 50 Hz with a pulse width of 0.2 milliseconds applied with vaginal electrodes
  - ▪ Patient-selected current intensity may achieve 120 mA
  - ▪ Duty cycles may vary with ability to hold a contraction with "on" time ranging from 0.5 to 10 seconds and "off" time from 0 to 30 seconds
  - ▪ A daily 30-minute session recommended[117]
- • Biofeedback to alert the patient of the quality of the PFM contraction
  - ▪ Visual or audible biofeedback after a preset threshold contraction
  - ▪ sEMG biofeedback from PFM contractions or vaginal pressure sensors selected according to patient comfort or preference
  - ▪ Daily 30-minute session recommended

ANTICIPATED GOALS AND EXPECTED OUTCOMES

- ♦ Impact on pathology/pathophysiology
  - • Physiological response to increased oxygen demand will be improved.
  - • Tissue perfusion and oxygenation is increased.
- ♦ Impact on impairments
  - • Aerobic capacity is increased, her BP is 120/80 mmHg, and her resting HR is approximately 67 bpm after 8 weeks of aerobic conditioning.
  - • Endurance is improved, and she is able to tolerate a 45-minute workout at the gym within 6 weeks.
  - • Energy expenditure per unit of work is decreased.
  - • Muscle performance as evidenced by the ability to sustain a strong active contraction of PFM especially prior to and during sneezing and coughing is improved. (If electrical stimulation or biofeedback are selected by patient, pelvic floor muscle strength is increased and urine leakage during coughing or sneezing is decreased.)
  - • Muscle performance, as measured by improved strength and endurance of PFM, is increased, and pressure readings from the perineometer are increased 15% from baseline within 8 weeks.
  - • Muscle performance of her abdominal muscles is increased to 5/5 within 4 weeks.
  - • Postural alignment, control, and awareness during actions, tasks, and activities within the home and during work and leisure are improved, and SUI when carrying her children is eliminated within 8 weeks.
  - • Relaxation is increased, and she independently incorporates relaxation into her daily routine within 6 weeks.

- Sensory awareness is increased especially for postural alignment.
♦ Impact on functional limitations
  - Ability to lift her children with correct posture and maintained continence is improved.
  - Ability to perform physical actions, tasks, and activities related to self-care, home management, work, community, and leisure is improved.
  - Tolerance of positions and actions, tasks, and activities required for work and leisure is improved.
♦ Risk reduction/prevention
  - Communication enhances risk reduction and prevention of complications.
  - Risk factors are decreased.
  - Risk of secondary impairment is decreased.
  - Safety is improved.
  - Self-management of symptoms is improved.
♦ Impact on health, wellness, and fitness
  - Behaviors that promote healthy nutrition, physical activity, and wellness are promoted and acquired.
  - Decision making is enhanced regarding her health, wellness, and fitness needs.
  - Fitness and health status is improved.
  - Physical capacity and function is improved.
♦ Impact on societal resources
  - Documentation occurs throughout patient management and across all settings and follows APTA's *Guidelines for Physical Therapy Documentation.*[97]
♦ Patient/client satisfaction
  - Access, availability, and services provided will be acceptable to the patient.
  - Awareness of stressors is achieved and response is decreased.
  - Clinical proficiency of the physical therapist is acceptable to the patient.
  - Coordination of care with gynecologist is acceptable to the patient.
  - Patient and family knowledge and awareness of the diagnosis, prognosis, interventions, and anticipated goals and expected outcomes are increased.
  - Patient knowledge of personal and environmental factors associated with the condition is increased.
  - Sense of well-being and control are improved.
  - Stress level as she resolves the SUI is reduced.

REEXAMINATION

Reexamination is performed throughout the episode of care.

DISCHARGE

Mrs. Kim is discharged from physical therapy after a total of 12 physical therapy sessions over 8 weeks and attainment of her goals and expectations. These sessions have covered her entire episode of care. She is discharged because she has achieved her goals and expected outcomes.

PSYCHOLOGICAL ASPECTS

As with any strength and endurance program, progress may appear slow. Mrs. Kim will need frequent encouragement to continue her home program and follow through with the physical therapist's suggestions. Most successful training regimes reported 1 to 6 months of training with considerable cure rates. She will be offered an audiocassette to guide her exercise at home and have regular monthly sessions (after the initial training) with the physical therapist in order to increase the likelihood of compliance with the long-term training.[141] The long-term cosmetic and health benefits of reversing the stress incontinence will be emphasized. In addition, she may keep a log of her incontinence episodes from the time she initiated intervention. This evidence should motivate her to continue to make progress as the incontinence episodes decrease in severity and frequency.

Case Study #3: Diabetes Mellitus

Mrs. Ruth Joseph is a 52-year-old female, post-menopausal, with Type 2 diabetes mellitus for 15 years with numbness in the anterolateral lower legs into the soles of both feet.

PHYSICAL THERAPIST EXAMINATION

HISTORY

♦ General demographics: Mrs. Joseph is a 52-year-old, English-speaking, white female. She is right-hand dominant. She is a high school graduate.
♦ Social history: Mrs. Joseph lives with her husband and two teenage daughters.
♦ Employment/work: Mrs. Joseph works as a supermarket cashier.
♦ Living environment: She lives in a private home with five steps to enter the building and 12 steps to the upper level.
♦ General health status
  - General health perception: Mrs. Joseph reports that

she has controlled the diabetes well over the past 15 years but has noticed general malaise and numbness in the lower legs over the past 3 weeks.

- Physical function: She works 5 days/week, volunteers once a week for a soup kitchen, and walks about 1 to 2 miles, two to three times per week.
- Psychological function: She reports that the change in her condition "has me worried." She denies depression or anxiety.
- Role function: Mother, wife, community volunteer, cashier.
- Social function: She follows the sporting and school activities of her daughters, volunteers weekly, and maintains a moderately active social life.

♦ Social/health habits: She denies smoking and consumes alcohol only on special occasions.

♦ Family history: Her mother had diabetes that caused blindness and polyneuropathy of the hands and feet.

♦ Medical/surgical history: Mrs. Joseph is post-menopausal (x1 year). Diabetes was diagnosed 15 years ago and was managed without injections for 12 years. Her only surgery was a caesarean section for the birth of her second daughter 14 years ago.

♦ Prior hospitalizations: She was hospitalized for the birth of each child.

♦ Preexisting medical and other health-related conditions: She is moderately overweight, but notes that she recently lost 10 pounds following a more stringent diet.

♦ Current condition(s)/chief complaint(s): Mrs. Joseph notes a vague "numbness" along the anterolateral aspects of both lower legs and "tingling" on the soles of both feet.

♦ Functional status and activity level: She is independent in all ADL and IADL. She walks about 1 to 2 miles, two to three times per week.

♦ Medications: Regular insulin twice daily, as indicated with self-monitoring of blood glucose.

♦ Other clinical tests
- Recent blood tests revealed good glucose control: hemoglobin A1C was 6%; fasting blood glucose level was 100 mg/dL.
- Recent urinanalysis showed no glucose present in urine; no hematuria; no proteinuria.
- Bone density studies were WNL at age 51.

SYSTEMS REVIEW

♦ Cardiovascular/pulmonary
- BP: 130/85 mmHg
- Edema: None, however, Mrs. Joseph noted that she has mild bipedal edema after being on her feet for more than 6 hours a day
- HR: 74 bpm
- RR: 13 bpm

♦ Integumentary
- Presence of scar formation: None
- Skin color: WNL
- Skin integrity
  - UE: WNL
  - LE: WNL except for a small area of redness and edema of the medial aspect of the right great toe, adjacent to the nail
  - Integrity of UE and LE nail beds unremarkable

♦ Musculoskeletal
- Gross range of motion: WNL throughout UEs, LEs, and spine
- Gross strength for major muscle groups of the UEs and the hip flexors are WNL. Gross strength limited to the LE muscles
- Gross symmetry
  - Posture appears symmetrical while the patient is standing, slightly protracted shoulders and a slight FHP
  - Gross symmetry of musculature is intact with no areas of obvious hypertrophy or atrophy
- Height: 5'7" (1.702 m)
- Weight: 180 lbs (81.648 kg)

♦ Neuromuscular
- Balance: No unsteadiness based on observation
- Locomotion, transfers, and transitions: WNL, patient notes a tendency to trip when she is fatigued

♦ Communication, affect, cognition, language, and learning style: WNL
- Communication and cognition: Alert and able to communicate needs
- Learning preferences: Active learning style

TESTS AND MEASURES

♦ Aerobic capacity/endurance
- 12-minute distance run/talk test revealed fitness category of fair (walked 0.95 miles in 12 minutes)[142]

♦ Anthropometric characteristics
- BMI: 28.2[103] indicating that she is overweight
- Waist circumference: 30 inches

♦ Circulation
- Pedal pulses examined to assess for arterial problems; bilateral dorsalis pedis (DP) and posterior tibial (PT) artery pulses slightly diminished (1+)
- LE filling time observed
  - In supine, both legs (knees straight) passively elevated to about 45 degrees
  - Nail beds and skin observed for blanching or bluish coloration while both legs are passively elevated for approximately 1 minute
  - If arterial flow is good, very slight blanching or skin color

- Any bluish coloration or leg pain may indicate ischemia
- Assist to seated position with legs dangling over the edge of the table
  ▸ Observe the nail beds and skin for how quickly skin returns to its normal color
  ▸ Delayed refill suggests arterial disease
- Mrs. Joseph was asymptomatic for both legs
- Capillary refill of both great toes appears slightly delayed after nail bed pressure with the patient supine

♦ Cranial and peripheral nerve integrity
  - Cranial nerves: WNL
    - UE sensory: WNL
    - LE
      ▸ Sensory tests: Decreased sensation to light touch over anterolateral aspect of both lower legs (superficial peroneal distribution) and soles of both feet (medial and lateral plantar nerve distributions)
      ▸ Pain (pin prick): WNL
      ▸ Vibration sense around the first MTP joint and both malleoli: WNL
      ▸ Ankle and toe joint proprioception: WNL

♦ Ergonomics and body mechanics
  - Standing posture and the physical demands of her job assessed and she appears to be using appropriate body mechanics

♦ Gait, locomotion, and balance
  - Berg Balance scale: 52/56 indicating minimal risk of fall
  - Gait pattern WNL except a slight tendency toward an increased toe clearance during fast walking for longer than 5 minutes
  - One leg stand for 1 minute without any loss of balance
  - Tandem standing longer than one minute (Resnick and associates observed that women with diabetic neuropathy who could not maintain tandem standing for more than 30 sec were at the greatest risk for falling)[143]
  - Denies a history of falling, dizziness, vertigo, or lightheadedness

♦ Integumentary integrity
  - Bilateral calluses medial to the first and lateral to the fifth MTP
  - Redness on medial aspect of right great toe

♦ Motor function
  - Dexterity and coordination: WNL
  - Nerve conduction velocity (NCV) (Table 3-3): Revealed abnormal sensory nerve action potentials

(SNAP) and motor conduction velocities (MCV) of the superficial and deep peroneal nerves, saphenous, sural, and tibial nerves of both LEs
- EMG conduction studies (Table 3-4) revealed partial denervation of multiple muscles of both LEs; findings suggestive of peripheral polyneuropathy affecting both LEs; UEs not affected at this time

♦ Muscle performance
  - Grip strength with dynamometer was 64 lbs right and 60 lbs left; mean and standard deviation for grip strength for women between 50 and 54 years old are: Right=65.8 ($\pm$ 11.6) lbs; left=57.3 ($\pm$10.7) lbs)[144]
  - MMT
    - UE and trunk: WNL
    - LE: WNL except 4+/5 for quadriceps and ankle plantar bilaterally, and 4/5 for peroneus longus, tibialis anterior and posterior, toe extensors, and flexor and abductor hallucis bilaterally
  - Isokinetic tests for knee flexion and extension and ankle plantarflexion and dorsiflexion: WNL at slow speeds but poor to fair power production at fast speeds
  - Trendelenburg sign: Negative bilaterally
  - Thompson test: Negative bilaterally

♦ Pain
  - No pain in LEs even during brisk walking
  - No reports of "day-after" soreness

♦ Posture
  - Observational assessment revealed:
    - Slight thoracic kyphosis
    - Protracted scapulae
    - FHP

♦ Range of motion
  - Spine: WNL
  - All extremities: WNL except bilateral ankle tightness (dorsiflexion 0 to 5 degrees with knees flexed)
  - Flexibility (muscle length)
    - Tightness of the following muscle groups bilaterally: Hip flexors (iliopsoas and rectus femoris), hip adductors, hamstrings (SLR 0 to 55 degrees bilaterally), ankle plantarflexors (dorsiflexion with knee straight to neutral bilaterally)[145]

♦ Reflex integrity
  - DTR quadriceps, hamstrings, adductors and plantarflexors are 1+ bilaterally

♦ Self-care and home management
  - Interview concerning self-care and home management revealed that they could be performed without difficulty
  - She is fatigued after busy days

♦ Sensory integrity

Peripheral Nerve	SNAP Latency	SNAP Amplitude	MCV
	Table 3-3		
	CASE STUDY #3: TYPE 2 DIABETES MELLITUS PERIPHERAL NERVES TESTED WITH NERVE CONDUCTION VELOCITY RESULTS AND MOTOR CONDUCTION VELOCITY AS APPROPRIATE		
Median nerve, bilateral	WNL	WNL	WNL
Ulnar nerve, bilateral	WNL	WNL	WNL
Superficial peroneal nerve, bilateral	Borderline distal latencies	Low amplitude responses	N/T
Deep peroneal nerve, bilateral	N/T	N/T	Ankle latency is borderline with slow conduction velocity from knee to ankle
Sural nerve, bilateral	Borderline distal latencies	Low amplitude responses	N/A
Saphenous nerve, bilateral	WNL	WNL	N/A
Tibial nerve, bilateral	Prolonged	Low amplitude responses	Ankle latency was prolonged with slow conduction velocity from knee to ankle

MCV=motor conduction velocity, N/A=not applicable, N/T=not tested, SNAP=sensory nerve action potential, WNL=within normal limits

- Proprioception of both hips, knees, ankles, and toes: WNL
- LE vibration sense: WNL bilaterally
♦ Work, community, and leisure integration or reintegration
  - Interview concerning ability to safely manage work, community, and leisure actions, tasks, and activities revealed that they could be done
  - She is fatigued after busy days

EVALUATION

Mrs. Joseph has a long history of Type 2 DM that has required twice daily regular insulin injections over the past 3 years. She reports an insidious onset of "numbness" on the anterolateral aspects of both lower legs along the superficial peroneal nerve distribution. She also notes "tingling" along the soles of both feet consistent with the medial and lateral plantar nerve distributions. Sensory tests show decreased sensation to light touch but not pin prick along those same distributions as well as deep peroneal, sural, and saphenous nerve distributions bilaterally. LE proprioception and vibration sense appear intact. She has quadriceps, ankle, and toe muscle weakness bilaterally. This weakness affects her fast walking when she fatigues and develops a slight high-steppage gait for toe clearance. LE reflexes are present but diminished bilaterally. Integument appears intact with the exception of bilateral calluses medial to the first and lateral to the fifth MTP and redness on the medial aspect of the right great toe. Some LE muscle groups lack flexibility.

DIAGNOSIS

Mrs. Joseph has Type 2 DM complicated by bilateral peripheral neuropathies of the femoral nerve (including the saphenous cutaneous nerve), the sural nerve, the superficial and deep peroneal nerves, and the medial and lateral plantar branches of the tibial nerve. The symptoms are both sensory and motor. Distal symmetric polyneuropathy is the most common form of diabetic neuropathy.[146] Mrs. Joseph has impaired: anthropometric characteristics; circulation; peripheral nerve integrity; gait, locomotion, and balance; integumentary integrity; motor function; muscle performance; posture; and range of motion. She is functionally limited in self-care and home management and in work, community, and leisure actions, tasks, and activities. In addition, Mrs. Joseph is at risk for complications associated with Syndrome X (obesity, HTN, hyperlipidemia, and diabetes).[56] These findings are consistent with placement in Pattern C: Impaired Muscle Performance and Neuromuscular Pattern G: Impaired Motor Function and Sensory Integrity Associated With Acute or Chronic Polyneuropathies. The identified impairments will be addressed in determining the prognosis and the plan of care.

PROGNOSIS AND PLAN OF CARE

Over the course of the visits, the following mutually established outcomes have been determined:
♦ BP is lowered
♦ Cardiovascular fitness is improved

			Table 3-4	

CASE STUDY #3: TYPE 2 DIABETES MELLITUS ELECTROMYOGRAPHY RESULTS SHOWING MUSCLE TESTED, ELECTRICAL ACTIVITY AT REST AND DURING ACTIVE CONTRACTION, AND TYPES OF MOTOR UNITS OBSERVED DURING VOLITIONAL EFFORT

Muscle	Insertional Activity	At Rest	Interference Pattern	Motor Unit Types on Volition
Left deltoid	Normal	Silent	Complete on strong effort	Normal MUs
Left first dorsal interosseous	Normal	Silent	Complete on strong effort	Normal MUs
Rectus femoris, bilateral	Increased	Fibrillation potentials and positive sharp waves	Incomplete on strong effort	Normal MUs and long duration polyphasic MUs
Peroneus longus, bilateral	Increased	Fibrillation potentials and positive sharp waves	Complete on strong effort	Normal MUs and long duration polyphasic MUs
Medial gastronemius, bilateral	Increased	Fibrillation potentials and positive sharp waves	Complete on strong effort	Normal MUs and long duration polyphasic MUs
Tibialis posterior, bilateral	Increased	Fibrillation potentials and positive sharp waves	Complete on strong effort	Normal MUs and long duration polyphasic MUs
Abductor hallucis, bilateral	Increased	Fibrillation potentials and positive sharp waves	Incomplete on strong effort	Normal MUs, long duration polphasic MUs, and large amplitude MUs
Tibialis anterior, bilateral	Increased	Many fibrillation potentials and positive sharp waves	Incomplete on strong effort	Few normal MUs and many long duration polyphasic MUs
Extensor digitorum brevis, bilateral	Increased	Fibrillation potentials and positive sharp waves	Single unit interference pattern on strong effort	Few normal MUs and many long duration polyphasic MUs

- Flexibility of LE muscle groups is improved
- Independence in appropriate skin care is achieved
- Risk factors are reduced
- Strength of quadriceps, ankle, and toe musculature is increased
- Stress is reduced
- Weight loss is achieved

To achieve these outcomes, the appropriate interventions for this patient are determined. These will include: coordination, communication, and documentation; patient/client-related instruction; therapeutic exercise; functional training in self-care and home management; functional training in work, community, and leisure integration or reintegration; and manual therapy techniques.

Based on the diagnosis and prognosis, Mrs. Joseph is expected to require between 9 to 14 visits.[21] Mrs. Joseph has good social support, is motivated, and follows through with her home exercise program. She is not severely impaired and is generally healthy.

INTERVENTIONS

RATIONALE FOR SELECTED INTERVENTIONS

A team approach, with the patient and the primary care physician or endocrinologist in the lead, is vital for proper execution of the multifaceted management of individuals with diabetes. In general, appropriate medication and dietary and exercise prescriptions must be formulated to meet the unique needs of the patient. Physicians, dietitians, physical and occupational therapists, and podiatrists may help the patient manage current problems and prevent future problems. In addition, Mrs. Joseph must make a true commitment to changing certain aspects of her lifestyle.[56,147]

Therapeutic Exercise

Exercise is the choice of physical therapist intervention for individuals with impaired muscle performance. For Mrs. Joseph, restoration of strength and power of muscles affected by the neuropathy will occur through resisted, isokinetic, aerobic, and weightbearing exercises to incorporate the total needs of her system.

Clinicians prescribing exercise for individuals with diabetes must balance the needs of the patient with the systemic issues associated with the disease. Exercise, like diabetes, affects all systems of the body. Therefore, the clinician must make appropriate decisions about the proper level of exercise-induced stress that can be reasonably tolerated by each patient. Exercise prescription will differ for individuals with Type 1 and Type 2 diabetes. Age, duration of symptoms, level of glucose control, presence of co-morbidities, and motivation of the patient must be considered when selecting the appropriate exercises.

The American Diabetes Association offered a position statement about physical activity and exercise for individuals with DM.[44] The benefits and risks of exercise with each type of diabetes are enumerated in the report and are summarized here. The reader is encouraged to access the original article. First, general concepts will be discussed and then specific recommendations for each type of diabetes.

Recommended exercise duration is 30 minutes with a sustained HR less than 60% to 70% of MHR[56] and light to moderate perceived exertion. Three days per week for exercise are recommended but 5 to 7 days may be more effective.[148] Resistive exercises are needed to strengthen the affected muscles, but they also have the benefit of enhancing glucose removal from muscle tissue in postmenopausal women with Type 2 diabetes.[149] In addition, aerobic exercise combined with resistance training helped reduce subcutaneous and visceral adipose tissue. Such reduction was related to improving insulin sensitivity in this sample.[149]

The benefits of regular exercise for individuals with Types 1 and 2 diabetes outweigh the risks for most individuals. Long-term training (three to four times per week, 30 to 60 minutes per session at 50% to 80% VO2max) will assist insulin sensitivity and carbohydrate metabolism in cells of individuals with Type 2.[38,44,49,56] Some serum lipid levels may be improved with regular exercise. Reducing insulin resistance has been shown to have an effect on reducing HTN. In addition, weight loss and maintenance through regular exercise may reduce risks associated with obesity, which is common among diabetics. Controlling lipid levels, weight, and BP are desirable for the prevention of the cardiovascular problems associated with diabetes.[38,44,49,56]

Patients embarking on a new exercise program should have a thorough medical examination with a focus on macro- or microvascular problems associated with the disease that may place the patient at risk during exercise.[44] When indicated and when a patient wishes to embark on a moderate or high intensity aerobic exercise program, a formal graded exercise test is recommended.[44,49] Cardiovascular compromise, such as coronary artery disease (CAD) or PVD, will change the patient's ability to respond to the stress of exercise. In addition, autonomic neuropathy will have a major impact on exercise response. If the patient can tolerate exercise, careful monitoring, a slow progression from lower level to moderate level exercise, and an emphasis of warm-up and cool-down exercise should be incorporated.[38,44,49]

Type 1 diabetes presents a particular challenge when exercise becomes a regular part of the lifestyle of a person with this disease. Good blood glucose control is essential. Self-monitoring and diligent adjustment of insulin and energy intake from food will ensure that someone with Type 1 diabetes can have good physical conditioning without complications.[44,49]

Exercise Precautions

The presence and degree of retinopathy, nephropathy, and neuropathy must all be taken into consideration when prescribing exercise. According to the American Diabetes Association's Clinical Practice Recommendations, patients with proliferative and moderate to severe non-proliferative diabetic retinopathy must avoid activities that could cause a retinal detachment or a vitreous hemorrhage. Anaerobic exercise, Valsalva maneuvers, jarring repetitive movement, and straining must be avoided for these patients. Low impact aerobic exercise, swimming, stationary bicycling, or walking should be selected for cardiovascular training. More frequent assessment of the visual status is also recommended.[44,49]

Renal dysfunction that causes albuminuria will warrant limitation of exercise to low or moderate level activities. Careful monitoring of blood pressure is also indicated.[44,49]

Diabetic autonomic neuropathy (DAN) may cause disturbances in HR and BP regulation, orthostasis, or gastrointestinal and genitourinary problems.[150] Blood pressure responses and thermoregulation during and after exercise may not be normal.[44,151] Adequate hydration and avoiding exercise outdoors in extreme temperatures should be recommended.[44] Disruption of microvascular skin blood flow and sudomotor responses with DAN warrants frequent skin inspection to prevent ulceration or skin fissures.[151] DAN is a significant risk factor for stroke in patients with Type 2 diabetes.[152] The incidence of silent cardiac ischemia and infarction (without symptoms of angina) is greater than with typical individuals with diabetes and coronary artery disease.[153] These people will require formalized testing for exercise tolerance and coronary artery disease including exercise thallium scintigraphy[154] before an exercise regimen is prescribed. A screening tool for cardiac autonomic neuropathy (CAN) includes three ECG tests: HR response to deep breathing (also known as beat-to-beat HR variation or R-R variation), HR response to standing, and the Valsalva maneuver.[150] When DAN is suspected, this screening is an important baseline measure. Prevention of DAN through good glycemic control, MNT, and exercise is essential. When DAN and/or CAN are diagnosed, all factors mentioned above must be considered in determining and monitoring an appropriate, closely supervised, exercise regimen.[151] Rate of perceived exertion should replace MHR as an indicator of exercise intensity.[150]

Peripheral neuropathies may progress to a point where a patient's feet are not sensitive to touch or pressure or stress. In addition, the presence of LE Charcot joints secondary to the diabetes will limit weightbearing exercise. The American Diabetes Association[155] recommends that loss of touch sensation showing an inability to detect a 10 g (5.07) monofilament in the feet would be a cut-off point for allowing strenuous weightbearing exercise. This level of hypoaesthesia indicates a loss of protective sensation. Weightbearing exercise, including prolonged walking, should be avoided in these patients. UE exercise, seated exercise, swimming, and bicycling may be used as substitutes for walking, but the patients must be diligent with monitoring their skin.[155]

Poor peripheral circulation is a common complication of diabetes. Skin care and the prevention of wounds are paramount to maintain the health of the feet and hands.[44]

This topic will be addressed in more detail in Practice Pattern J: Impaired Motor Function, Muscle Performance, Range of Motion, Gait, Locomotion, and Balance Associated With Amputation.

Exercise Safety Issues

Exercise should be avoided or postponed on days when blood glucose levels are less than 100 mg/dL or greater than 250 mg/dL. Individuals experiencing DKA should delay exercising until the hyperglycemia has abated.[38,44] In autonomic neuropathy and Type 1 diabetes, the limit for blood glucose level is reduced to 240 mg/dL, after that, exercise should be postponed until insulin can be administered and control restored.[151]

For individuals following an insulin regimen, exercise should be avoided during the peak hours. Also, late night exercising should not begin suddenly but should be gradually worked into the lifestyle of the patient. In addition to proper hydration 1 to 2 hours before, adequate intake of juices, fruits, and carbohydrate snacks should be used to regulate blood glucose levels during and after exercise.[38,44] Physical therapists should have a supply of fruit juice, honey, water, and easily digested carbohydrate and protein snacks available in case an exercising patient has a hypoglycemic episode.[38]

Manual Therapy Techniques

Improving general LE flexibility and eliminating ROM deficits will reduce stresses placed on LE structures. Strengthening of LE muscle groups will improve function, endurance, and lead to greater cardiovascular fitness. PNF is an excellent hands-on skill that can be individualized to each patient in a safe and effective manner without risk of injury to these patients.

COORDINATION, COMMUNICATION, AND DOCUMENTATION

Communication will occur with family members to engender support for dietary modifications and more frequent and intense exercise. Communication will also occur with her primary care physician to coordinate the exercise and MNT. Regular consultations with her podiatrist and registered dietitian will be encouraged. Because depression and anxiety are common with chronic disease, professional psychological support is suggested.[40] All elements of the patient's management will be documented.

PATIENT/CLIENT-RELATED INSTRUCTION

The patient will be instructed in the varied aspects of MNT, exercise, and appropriate medication for blood glucose control for Type 2 diabetes.[40]

Prevention of obesity through exercise and MNT will be discussed. Prevention or remediation of obesity has significant effects on glucose control.[40,56] In addition to careful nutritional and pharmacological management of blood glucose levels, control of circulating blood lipid levels and HTN are essential in preventing complications associated with Syndrome X (metabolic syndrome).[38,56] Syndrome X is a form of ischemic heart disease characterized by "microvascular angina, exertional angina, or angina without obvious coronary atherosclerosis."[156] Syndrome X includes several conditions associated with CAD: obesity, dyslipidemia, HTN (with elevated systolic BP), and hyperinsulinemia.[38] The latter condition is prevalent with insulin resistance of the tissues (including muscle and adipose) as is found in Type 2 diabetes.[38,56] Mrs. Joseph is not obese, but her BMI is in the overweight category. She notes a recent 10-lb weight loss through dieting. Her BP is 135/80 mmHg indicative of prehypertension.

MNT of individuals with DM must include a basic food plan and strategies to manage appropriate food intake before, during, and after exercise. In addition, MNT is important to manage complications associated with obesity, such as HTN, hyperlipidemia, and nephropathy. A technical review by Franz and associates[43] provides evidence-based, comprehensive recommendations for diabetes treatment and prevention. Only general guidelines will be mentioned here but the reader is encouraged to access the technical review. Franz and associates[43] stated the "goal of nutrition intervention is to assist and facilitate individual lifestyle and behavioral changes that will lead to improved metabolic control."[43] They also acknowledge that MNT must address glycemic, lipid, and weight control, as well as HTN. MNT must consider "the personal and cultural preferences and lifestyle while respecting the individual's wishes and willingness" to change.[43] The registered dietitian provides the best resource for MNT.[43]

Individualized energy intake must balance energy output for weight maintenance. The recommended guidelines for energy intake include 60% to 70% of total daily energy from carbohydrates and monounsaturated fats, 10% to 20% from protein, and less than 10% from saturated fats. Fiber and calcium should also be included. Sucrose and fructose do not need to be avoided, simply balanced within the carbohydrate recommendations. Sodium intake should be monitored to prevent and treat HTN. The registered dietitian can balance these percentages based on the overall health of the individual, need for weight loss, exercise demands on the system, and personal or cultural preferences.[43,49] Support groups with regular weight follow-up are helpful in maintaining motivation for weight loss and maintenance.

Self-management interventions and psychological support (if needed) have been shown to be effective adjuncts to glucose management.[147] Exercise consultations were more effective than exercise instruction manuals for long-term promotion of exercise in a pilot study involving previously sedentary adults with Type 2 diabetes.[157]

Working with the podiatrist, Mrs. Joseph will learn proper foot care and learn about the warning signs of inflammation and integument breakdown. She will receive instruction about selecting proper footwear for her aerobic training.[144,146,155] Mrs. Joseph has normal proprioception and vibration sense in her ankles and toes. If these sensory modalities become diminished secondary to the neuropathy, she will be at increased risk for falling.[144] She needs to understand the implications of joint sensitivity changes and Charcot arthropathy should her condition progress.[143,158]

In addition to the above, the following information and/or instructions will be given to Mrs. Joseph:

♦ A progressive plan of home exercises to increase strength, improve flexibility, improve endurance, and decrease weight

♦ How to monitor blood glucose levels before exercise so that appropriate precautions may be taken

♦ Nutrition supplementation or administration of medication will be adjusted according to her physician's recommendations and to her pre-exercise needs[44,49]

♦ Identification of community resources, including support groups for weight loss, yoga or other relaxation, and stress management

♦ Knowledge of proper foot care and means to monitor integumentary and joint sensory status (see functional training below)

♦ Understanding and reinforcement of the benefit of regular aerobic exercise and weight loss and maintenance of an ideal body weight as a means of preventing Syndrome X[56,156,159] and other complications associated with diabetes (See Pathophysiology of Diabetes for further rationale of benefit of exercise)

♦ The following American Diabetes Association recommendations[44] for patients who exercise regularly will be presented:

● Maintain fluid balance by beginning adequate hydration 2 hours prior to exercise and continuing to drink water during exercise

● Avoid exercising in extreme temperatures

● Monitor skin before and after exercise especially in cases of neuropathy

● Select light weights with more repetitions for weight training; younger individuals may attempt a more intensive program with higher weights, but blood glucose levels should be monitored to set limitations

● Begin an exercise program with early supervision, maintain it through an informal home program, and sustain it with regular follow-up

● Ingest carbohydrates before, during, and after exercise to keep glucose levels stable, which is particularly important with patients with Type 1 diabetes

THERAPEUTIC EXERCISE

♦ Aerobic capacity/endurance conditioning[2]
  ● Mode
    ■ Stationary bicycle and treadmill for aerobic conditioning
  ● Duration
    ■ 20 minutes initially, progressing to 30 or 45 minutes
  ● Intensity
    ■ Moderate: Raising HR to 60% of maximum $(0.60 \times [220-age]=100$ beats per minute$)$[2]
  ● Frequency
    ■ Initially three times a week, alternating with existing walking program

♦ Balance, coordination, and agility training
  ● Weightbearing drills for balance and coordination, such as dance steps, braiding, practice on a balance beam or a strip on the floor
  ● Balance board training progressively increasing the level of difficulty

♦ Body mechanics and postural stabilization
  ● Postural awareness retraining and postural stabilization exercises
    ■ Standing alignment instruction using a full-length mirror for feedback
    ■ Practice lifting and carrying objects of varying sizes and weights while maintaining a neutral lumbar spine
    ■ Quadruped, kneeling, sitting, and standing exercises that incorporate postural stabilization during extremity movements

♦ Flexibility exercises

- Stretching exercises should be done after warming up, using a slow and steady stretch accompanied by deep breathing, and building hold up to 30 to 60 seconds
- Heel cord stretching
  - PNF principles including contract-relax and hold-relax within LE patterns
  - Runner's stretch in weightbearing
  - Towel stretch while seated with knee extended
- Hip flexors, adductors, and plantarflexors
  - Prolonged (1 to 2 minute) stretch focusing on posture and contracting stabilizing muscles
  - Yoga stretching
  - Incorporate as part of warm-up and cool-down for aerobic training
♦ Strength, power, and endurance training
  - Vary program to maintain patient motivation throughout course of treatment
  - Light resistance to extremity movements: free weights, therapeutic band or tubing, or manual resistance
  - PRE (one to three sets of 10 repetitions for each exercise) for the following muscles:
    - Quadriceps: Starting with 10 repetition maximum (RM) weight for SLR, isotonic knee extension in sitting (90 degrees flexion to full extension, concentric and eccentric), and terminal knee extension in supine with thigh support (30 degrees flexion to full extension, concentric and eccentric) and progressing ankle cuff weights as indicated over time
    - Hip flexors: Starting with 90% of 10 RM weight for hip flexion (in sitting with good posture) from 90 degrees flexion to 120 degrees flexion and progressing ankle cuff weights as indicated over time
  - Closed chain exercises
    - Use of therapeutic balls for sitting and standing exercises
    - Dance steps (avoiding sudden, jarring movements)
    - Heel and toe raises in standing
    - LE eccentric exercise, such as partial squat
    - Kinetron
  - Resistive elastic bands or tubing
    - Ankle dorsiflexion, plantarflexion, inversion, and eversion progressing as tolerated (Remind patient to examine her skin before and after using the resistive bands or tubing)
  - Manual resistive exercise
    - LE muscles including PNF techniques with pelvic and extremity patterns in functional positions

FUNCTIONAL TRAINING IN SELF-CARE AND HOME MANAGEMENT

♦ Self-care and home management
  - Bathing
    - Check temperature of the water with hand prior to stepping into a warm or hot bathtub
    - Dry skin of the LEs thoroughly prior to donning socks or shoes
  - Grooming
    - Allow podiatrist to trim toenails to avoid injury
    - Inspect skin of feet in the morning and night and take corrective measures if pressure areas, blisters, or ulcers occur
  - Home activities
    - Practice using vacuum or broom, making beds, and other household activities while maintaining appropriate postural alignment
  - Injury prevention or reduction
    - Injury prevention education during self-care and home management
    - Injury prevention or reduction with use of devices and equipment
    - Safety awareness training during self-care and home management

FUNCTIONAL TRAINING IN WORK, COMMUNITY, AND LEISURE INTEGRATION OR REINTEGRATION

♦ Work
  - Injury prevention or reduction with use of devices and equipment on the job
  - Safety awareness while working including body mechanics for lifting and carrying
  - Increase amount of walking and stair-climbing during the day
  - Inspect feet if pain or tenderness occurs while standing on the job
  - Wear well-fitting, comfortable, and supportive shoes
  - Sit and rest at frequent intervals during work day
♦ Leisure
  - Be active and have fun at the same time
  - Plan family outings and vacations to include physical activity

MANUAL THERAPY TECHNIQUES

♦ Soft tissue mobilization, if needed, to help elongate hip flexors and adductors, hamstrings, and plantarflexors
♦ Myofascial release to improve muscle play

ANTICIPATED GOALS AND EXPECTED OUTCOMES

♦ Impact on pathology/pathophysiology
- Nutrient delivery to tissues will be increased.
- Osteogenic effects of exercise will be improved.
- Physiological response to increased oxygen demand is improved.
- Tissue perfusion and oxygenation is increased.

♦ Impact on impairments
- Aerobic capacity is increased, and her 12-minute walk/run test is improved to 1.12 miles (to put her in the good fitness category) after 6 to 8 weeks.[142]
- Endurance is improved, and she is less fatigued at the end of the day and tolerates longer exercise sessions within 8 weeks.
- Energy expenditure per unit of work is decreased.
- Gait and locomotion are improved, and her Berg Balance scale score is 56/56 at the completion of the 6-week program.
- Gait is improved so her toe clearance during gait at fast speeds is efficient without any tripping as she ambulates.
- Muscle strength and power is increased and quality and quantity of movement between and across body segments is improved. Muscle strength is improved so that her hand grip strength is improved to 65 lbs on the right and 61 lbs on the left, LE MMT scores are 5/5, and power in the quadriceps and hamstrings is improved by 10% during isokinetic testing.
- Postural awareness, alignment, and control during actions, tasks, and activities within the home and during work and leisure are improved, and she will be able to maintain comfortable standing without an excessive thoracic kyphosis or forward head position for 5 minutes within 4 weeks.
- Relaxation is improved, and she independently incorporates relaxation into her daily routine.
- ROM and associated soft tissue restrictions are normalized to eliminate the potential for future injury, and flexibility of hip flexors, hip adductors, and hamstrings is WNL after 6 weeks.
- Sensory awareness is increased, and episodes of "tingling" in the soles of her feet are less frequent after 6 weeks of care.

♦ Impact on functional limitations
- Ability to retain, improve, and perform physical actions, tasks, and activities related to self-care, home management, work, community, or leisure is improved.
- Functional independence in ADL and IADL is increased.
- Level of supervision required for task performance is decreased, and she is independent with her home exercise program.
- Tolerance of positions and actions, tasks, and activities required for work and leisure is improved.

♦ Risk reduction/prevention
- All risk factors, including complications associated with diabetes are decreased.
- Communication enhances risk reduction and prevention of further sequelae of the diabetes or the neuropathy.
- Disability associated with acute or chronic illnesses is reduced.
- Risk of secondary impairment (cardiovascular and integumentary) is reduced.
- Safety of patient, family, significant others, and caregivers is improved.
- Self-management of symptoms is improved.

♦ Impact on health, wellness, and fitness
- Behaviors that promote healthy nutrition, physical activity, and wellness are promoted and acquired.
- Decision making is enhanced regarding her health, wellness, and fitness needs.
- Fitness and health status are improved.
- Physical capacity and function are improved.

♦ Impact on societal resources
- Decision making is enhanced regarding patient health and the use of health care resources by patient, family, significant others, and caregivers.
- Documentation occurs throughout patient management and across all settings and follows APTA's *Guidelines for Physical Therapy Documentation*.[97]
- Utilization of physical therapy services will be optimized.
- Utilization of physical therapy services will result in efficient use of health care dollars.

♦ Patient/client satisfaction
- Access, availability, and services provided are acceptable to the patient.
- Awareness and use of community resources are improved.
- Awareness of stressors is achieved, and response is decreased.
- Care is coordinated with the primary care physician, podiatrist, dietitian, therapists, and family members.
- Clinical proficiency of the physical therapist is acceptable to the patient.
- Coordination of care is acceptable to the patient.
- Patient, family, significant other, and caregiver knowledge, awareness, and understanding of the diagnosis, prognosis, interventions, and anticipated goals and expected outcomes are increased.

- Patient knowledge of personal and environmental factors associated with the condition is increased.
- Sense of well-being and control are improved.

REEXAMINATION

Reexamination is performed throughout the episode of care.

DISCHARGE

Mrs. Joseph is discharged from physical therapy after a total of 12 physical therapy sessions over 8 weeks and attainment of her goals and expectations. These sessions have covered her entire episode of care. She is discharged because she has achieved her goals and expected outcomes.

PSYCHOLOGICAL ASPECTS

In order to monitor her perception of the impact of diabetes and the new program of management on her life, Mrs. Joseph will complete the Diabetes Quality of Life Scale (DQoLS)[160] and the Diabetes Impact Measurement Scale (DIMS)[161] at the initial visit, upon discharge, and at 2-month intervals. The DQoLS measures worries about the future effects of diabetes, social and vocational issues, and impact of and satisfaction with treatment.[162] The DIMS measures well-being, social role fulfillment, morale, and specific and non-specific symptoms.[161] Any negative changes on the scales will be reported to Mrs. Joseph and her physician.

REFERENCES

1. Oatis CA. *Kinesiology: The Mechanics and Pathomechanics of Human Movement.* Philadelphia, Pa: Lippincott Williams & Wilkins; 2004.
2. McArdle WD, Katch FI, Katch VL, eds. *Exercise Physiology.* 4th ed. Baltimore, Md: Williams & Wilkins; 1996.
3. Lieber R. *Skeletal Muscle Structure, Function, and Plasticity.* 2nd ed. Baltimore, Md: Lippincott Williams & Wilkins; 2002.
4. Iyer MB, Mitz AR, Winstein C. Motor 1: lower centers. In: Cohen H, ed. *Neuroscience for Rehabilitation.* 2nd ed. Philadelphia, Pa: Lippincott Williams & Wilkins; 1999:209-242.
5. Guyton AC. Basic neuroscience. *Anatomy and Physiology.* 5th ed. Philadelphia, Pa: WB Saunders; 1991.
6. Lundy-Ekman L. *Neuroscience. Fundamentals for Rehabilitation.* Philadelphia, Pa: WB Saunders; 1998.
7. Kimura J. *Electrodiagnosis in Diseases of Nerve and Muscle: Principles and Practice.* 3rd ed. New York, NY: Oxford Press; 2001.
8. Tanzi MG, Gabay MP. Association between honey consumption and infant botulism. *Pharmacotherapy.* 2002;22(11):1479-1483.
9. Williams PL, Warwick R. *Gray's Anatomy.* 36th ed. Philadelphia, Pa: WB Saunders; 1980.
10. Netter FH. *Atlas of Human Anatomy.* Summit, NJ: Ciba-Geigy Corp; 1989.
11. Moore K. *Clinically Oriented Anatomy.* 3rd ed. Baltimore, Md: Williams & Wilkins; 1992.
12. Hall C, Brody LT. *Therapeutic Exercise Moving Toward Function.* Philadelphia, Pa: Lippincott Williams & Wilkins; 1999.
13. Albert M. *Eccentric Muscle Training in Sports and Orthopaedics.* New York, NY: Churchill Livingstone; 1991.
14. Erim Z, De Luca CJ, Mimeo K, Aoki T. Rank-ordered regulation of motor units. *Muscle Nerve.* 1996;19:563-573.
15. Klass M, Guissard N, Duchateau J. Limiting mechanisms of force production after repetitive dynamic contractions in human triceps surae. *J Appl Physiol.* 2003;96:1516-1521.
16. MacIntosh BR, Rassier DE. What is fatigue? *Can J Appl Physiol.* 2002;27(1):42-55.
17. Rothwell JC. *Control of Human Voluntary Movement.* Rockville, Md: Aspen; 1987.
18. Sahlin K, Tonkonogi M, Sunderland K. Energy supply and muscle fatigue in humans. *Acta Physiol Scand.* 1998;162:261-266.
19. Merton, PA. Voluntary strength and fatigue. *J Physiol.* 1954;123:553-564.
20. Adam A, DeLuca CJ. Recruitment order of motor units in human vastus lateralis muscle is maintained during fatiguing contractions. *J Neurophysiol.* 2003;90:2919-2927.
21. American Physical Therapy Association. Guide to physical therapist practice. 2nd ed. *Phys Ther.* 2001;81:9-744.
22. Tsao CY, Mendell JR. The childhood muscular dystrophies: making order out of chaos. *Semin Neurol.* 1999;19(1):9-23.
23. Beers MH, Berkow R, eds. Muscular disorders. *The Merck Manual of Diagnosis and Therapy.* 17th ed. Whitehouse Station, NJ. Available at http://www.merck.com. Accessed June 17, 2004.
24. Beers MH, Berkow R, eds. Normal laboratory values. *The Merck Manual of Diagnosis and Therapy.* 17th ed. Whitehouse Station, NJ. Available at http://www.merck.com. Accessed June 17, 2004.
25. Brooke M. *A Clinician's View of Neuromuscular Diseases.* 2nd ed. Baltimore, Md: Williams & Wilkins; 1986.
26. National Center on Birth Defects and Developmental Disabilities. Duchenne/Becker Muscular Dystrophy. Available at: http://www.cdc.gov/ncbddd/duchenne/default.htm. Accessed June 17, 2004.
27. Boissonnault WG, Goodman CC. The renal and urologic systems. In: Goodman CC, Boissonnault WG, Fuller KS, eds. *Pathology: Implications for the Physical Therapist.* 2nd ed. Philadelphia, Pa: Saunders; 2003:722-728.
28. National Association for Continence. Media Backgrounder: Stress Urinary Incontinence: Tackling the Last Medical Taboo. Available at: http://www.nafc.org/site2/you/stress/SUIfacts.htm. Accessed November 14, 2003.
29. Abrams P, Blaivas JG, Stanton SL, et al. The standardisation of terminology of the lower urinary tract function. *Scand J Urol Nephrol Suppl.* 1988;114:5-19.
30. Sand PK. In focus: urinary incontinence in post-menopausal women. *Quality Care.* 2003;21(3):1-2.
31. Bø K. Pelvic floor muscle exercises for the treatment of stress

urinary incontinence: an exercise physiology perspective. *Int Urogynecol J Pelvic Floor Dysfunct*. 1995;6:282-291.

32. Kegel AH. Progressive resistance exercise in the functional restoration of the perineal muscles. *Am J Obstet Gynecol*. 1948;56:238-248.

33. Fantl JA, Newman DK, Colling J, et al. *Urinary Continence in Adults: Acute and Chronic Management. Clinical Practice Guideline Update*. Rockville, Md: Agency for Health Care Policy and Research; Publication No. 96-0682, March 1996.

34. Weinberger MW. Conservative treatment of urinary incontinence. *Clin Obstet Gynecol*. 1995;38:175-188.

35. Burgio KL, Matthews KA, Engel BT. Prevalence, incidence and correlates of urinary incontinence in healthy, middle-aged women. *J Urol*. 1991;146:1255-1259.

36. Nygaard IE, Thompson FL, Svengalis SL, et al. Urinary incontinence in elite nulliparous athletes. *Obstet Gynecol*. 1994;84:183-187.

37. Hansen M. *Pathophysiology: Foundations of Disease and Clinical Intervention*. Philadelphia, Pa: WB Saunders; 1998.

38. Goodman CC, Kelly Snyder TE. The endocrine and metabolic systems. In: Goodman CC, Boissonnault WG, Fuller KS, eds. *Pathology: Implications for the Physical Therapist*. 2nd ed. Philadelphia, Pa: Saunders; 2003.

39. DeFronzo RA. The triumvirate: beta-cell, muscle, liver. *Diabetes*. 1988;37:667-687.

40. American Diabetes Association. Standards of medical care for patients with diabetes mellitus. *Diabetes Care*. 2003;26(Suppl 1):S33-S50.

41. Shulman GI. Cellular mechanisms of insulin resistance in humans. *Am J Cardiol*. 1999;84(Suppl 1):3-10.

42. American Diabetes Association. What is type 2 diabetes? Available at: http://www.diabetes.org/type2/type2.jsp. Accessed August 28, 2003.

43. Franz MJ, Bantle JP, Beebe CA, et al. Evidence-based nutrition principles and recommendations for the treatment and prevention of diabetes and related complications. *Diabetes Care*. 2002;25(1):148-198.

44. American Diabetes Association. Physical activity/exercise and diabetes mellitus. *Diabetes Care*. 2003;26(Suppl 1):S73-S77.

45. Mensing C, Boucher J, Cypress M, et al. National standards for diabetes self-management education. *Diabetes Care*. 2003;26(Suppl 1):S149-S156.

46. American Diabetes Association. Gestational diabetes: what it is, and how to treat it. Available at: http://www.diabetes.org/main/info/affected/women/gestation_diab.jsp. Accessed August 28, 2003.

47. The Expert Committee on the Diagnosis and Classification of Diabetes Mellitus. Report of the Expert Committee on the Diagnosis and Classification of Diabetes Mellitus. *Diabetes Care*. 2003;26(Suppl 1):S5-S20.

48. American Diabetes Association. Implications of the diabetes-control and complications trial. *Diabetes Care*. 2003;26(Suppl 1):S25-S27.

49. Diabetes Medical Guidelines Task Force. The American Association of Clinical Endocrinologists medical guidelines for the management of diabetes mellitus: the AACE system of intensive diabetes self-management: 2002 update. *Endocr Pract*. 2002;8(Suppl 1):41-82.

50. American Diabetes Association. Hypoglycemia and employment/licensure. *Diabetes Care*. 2003;26(Suppl 1):S141.

51. National Institute of Diabetes and Digestive and Kidney Diseases. *Hypoglycemia*. Bethesda, Md: National Institutes of Health; 1995: Publication No. 95-3926.

52. American Diabetes Association. Hyperglycemic crises in patients with diabetes mellitus. *Diabetes Care*. 2003;26(Suppl 1):S109-S117.

53. Fenichel GM, Florence JM, Pestronk A, et al. Long-term benefit from prednisone therapy in Duchenne muscular dystrophy. *Neurology*. 1991;41:1874-1877.

54. Carter GT, McDonald CM. Preserving function in Duchenne dystrophy with long-term pulse prednisone therapy. *Am J Phys Med Rehabil*. 2000;79:455-458.

55. American Diabetes Association. Insulin administration. *Diabetes Care*. 2003;26(Suppl 1):S121-S124.

56. Scheen AJ. Current management strategies for coexisting diabetes mellitus and obesity. *Drugs*. 2003;63:1165-1184.

57. Kendall FP, McCreary EK, Provance PG. *Muscles: Testing and Function*. 4th ed. Philadelphia, Pa: Williams & Wilkins; 1993:178-189.

58. Sahrmann SA. *Diagnosis and Treatment of Movement Impairment Syndromes*. St. Louis, Mo: Mosby; 2002.

59. McGee D. *Orthopedic Physical Assessment*. 4th ed. Philadelphia, Pa: WB Saunders; 2002.

60. Hislop HJ, Montgomery J. *Daniels and Worthingham's Muscle Testing*. 6th ed. Philadelphia, Pa: WB Saunders; 1995.

61. Florence JM, Pandya S, King WM, et al. Intrarater reliability of manual muscle test (Medical Research Council Scale) grades in Duchenne's muscular dystrophy. *Phys Ther*. 1992;72:115-122.

62. Barr AE, Diamond BE, Wade CE, et al. Reliability of testing measures in Duchenne or Becker muscular dystrophy. *Arch Phys Med Rehabil*. 1991;72:315-319.

63. Brinkmann JR. Comparison of a hand-held and fixed dynamometer in measuring strength of patients with neuromuscular disease. *J Orthop Sports Phys Ther*. 1994;19:100-104.

64. Bohannon RW. Test-retest reliability of hand-held dynamometry during a single session of strength assessment. *Phys Ther*. 1986;66:206-209.

65. Taylor NF, Dodd KJ, Graham HK. Test-retest reliability of hand-held dynamometric strength testing in young people with cerebral palsy. *Arch Phys Med Rehabil*. 2004;85:77-80.

66. Merlini L, Mazzone ES, Solari A, Morandi L. Reliability of hand-held dynamometry in spinal muscular atrophy. *Muscle Nerve*. 2002;26:64-70.

67. Bohannon RW. Internal consistency of dynamometer measurements in healthy subjects and stroke patients. *Percept Mot Skills*. 1995;81:1113-1114.

68. May LA, Burnham RS, Steadward RD. Assessment of isokinetic and hand-held dynamometer measures of shoulder rotator strength among individuals with spinal cord injury. *Arch Phys Med Rehabil*. 1997;78:251-255.

69. Bohannon RW. Measuring knee extensor muscle strength. *Am J Phys Med Rehabil*. 2001;80:13-18.

70. Smidt GL. *Muscle Strength Testing: A System Based on Mechanics*. Coralville, Iowa: Spark Instruments and Academics Inc; 1984:1-19.

71. Agre JC, Magness JL, Hull SZ, et al. Strength testing with a portable dynamometer: reliability for upper and lower extremities. *Arch Phys Med Rehabil*. 1987;68:454-458.

72. Bohannon RW, Smith J, Hull D, et al. Deficits in lower

extremity muscle and gait performance among renal transplant patients. *Arch Phys Med Rehabil.* 1995;76:547-551.

73. Bohannon RW. Hand-grip dynamometry provides a valid indication of upper extremity strength impairment in home care patients. *J Hand Ther.* 1998;11:158-160.

74. Bohannon RW. Dynamometer measurements of hand-grip strength predict multiple outcomes. *Percept Mot Skills.* 1001;93:323-328.

75. Roberson LD, Mullinax CM, Brodowicz GR, et al. The relationship between two power-grip testing devices and their utility in physical capacity evaluations. *J Hand Ther.* 1993;6:194-201.

76. Kues JM, Rothstein JM, Lamb RL. Obtaining reliable measurement of knee extensor torque produced during maximal voluntary contractions: an experimental investigation. *Phys Ther.* 1992;72:492-504.

77. Basmajian MV. *Muscles Alive: Their Function Revealed by Electromyography.* 4th ed. Baltimore, Md: Williams & Wilkins; 1978.

78. Adams RD, Victor M. *Principles of Neurology.* 3rd ed. New York, NY: McGraw Hill Book Co; 1985.

79. Soderberg G, ed. *Selected Topics in Surface Electromyography for Use in the Occupational Setting: Expert Perspectives.* Public Health Service: US Department of Health and Human Services; 1992.

80. Cram JR, Kasman GS. *Introduction to Surface Electromyography.* Gaithersburg, Md: Aspen Publication; 1998.

81. Nereo NE, Hinton VJ. Three wishes and psychological functioning in boys with Duchenne muscular dystrophy. *J Dev Behav Pediatr.* 2003;24(2):96-103.

82. Shim JY, Kim TS. Relationship between utrophin and regenerating muscle fibers in Duchenne muscular dystrophy. *Yonsei Med J.* 2003;44(1):15-23.

83. Baxter PS, Maltby EL, Quarrell O. Xp21 muscular dystrophy due to X chromosome inversion. *Neurology.* 1997;49(1):260.

84. Centers for Disease Control, National Center for Health Statistics. CDC Growth Charts: United States: Stature-for-age percentiles. Available at: http://www.cdc.gov/nchs/about/major/nhanes/growthchart. Accessed May 30, 2000.

85. Centers for Disease Control, National Center for Health Statistics. CDC Growth Charts: United States: Weight-for-age percentiles. Available at: http://www.cdc.gov/nchs/about/major/nhanes/growthchart. Accessed May 30, 2000.

86. Centers for Disease Control, National Center for Health Statistics. CDC Growth Charts: United States: Body mass index-for-age percentiles. Available at: http://www.cdc.gov/nccdphp/dnpa/bmi/bmi-for-age. Accessed May 30, 2000.

87. Zanardi MC, Tagliabue A, Orcesi S, et al. Body composition and energy expenditure in Duchenne muscular dystrophy. *Eur J Clin Nutr.* 2003;57:273-278.

88. Merlini L, Cicognana A, Malaspina E, et al. Early prednisone treatment in Duchenne muscular dystrophy. *Muscle Nerve.* 2003;27:222-227.

89. Haas A, Pineda H, Haas F, Axen K. *Pulmonary Therapy and Rehabilitation.* Baltimore, Md: Williams & Wilkins; 1979.

90. Kisner C, Colby, L. *Therapeutic Exercise.* 4th ed. Philadelphia, Pa: FA Davis Co; 2002.

91. Harris SE, Cherry DB. Childhood progressive muscular dystrophy and the role of physical therapy. *Phys Ther.* 1974;54(1):4-12.

92. Bakker JP, De Groot IJ, Beelen A, Lankhorst GJ. Predictive factors of cessation of ambulation in patients with Duchenne muscular dystrophy. *Am J Phys Med Rehabil.* 2002;81:906-912.

93. McDonald CM. Physical activity, health impairments, and disability in neuromuscular disease. *Am J Phys Med Rehabil.* 2002;81(11 Suppl):S108-S120.

94. Wanke T, Toifl K, Merkle M, Formanek D, Lahrmann H, Zwick H. Inspiratory muscle training in patients with Duchenne muscular dystrophy. *Chest.* 1994;105:475-482.

95. Lord JP, Behrman B, Varzos N, et al. Scoliosis associated with Duchenne muscular dystrophy. *Arch Phys Med Rehabil.* 1990;71:13-17.

96. Wilkins KE, Gibson DA. The patterns of spinal deformity in Duchenne muscular dystrophy. *J Bone Joint Surg.* 1976;58A:24-32.

97. American Physical Therapy Association. Guidelines for physical therapy documentation. *Guide to Physical Therapist Practice.* 2nd ed. Alexandria, Va: American Physical Therapy Association; 2001:703-705.

98. McDonald DG, Kinali M, Gallagher AC, et al. Fracture prevalence in Duchenne muscular dystrophy. *Dev Med Child Neurol.* 2002;44:695-698.

99. Muscular Dystrophy Association. Facts about Duchenne and Becker muscular dystrophies (DMD and BMD). In what other ways do DBD and BMD affect the body? April, 2000. Available at: www.mdausa.org/publications/fa-dmdbmd-other.html. Accessed November 15, 2003.

100. Winkler G, Zifko U, Nader A, Frank W, et al. Dose-dependent effects of inspiratory muscle training in neuromuscular disorders. *Muscle Nerve.* 2000;23:1257-1260.

101. Mørkved S, Bø K, Fjortoft T. Effect of adding biofeedback to pelvic floor muscle training to treat urodynamic stress incontinence. *Obstet Gynecol.* 2002;100:730-739.

102. Bø K. Pelvic floor muscle strength and response to pelvic floor muscle training for stress urinary incontinence. *Neurourol Urodyn.* 2003;22:654-658.

103. Centers for Disease Control, National Center for Chronic Disease Prevention and Health Promotion. BMI for Adults: What does this all mean? 2003. Available at: http://www.cdc.gov/nccdphp/dnpa/bmi/bmi-means.htm. Accessed June 14, 2004.

104. Jeyaseelan SM, Oldham JA. Electrical stimulation as a treatment for stress incontinence. *British Journal of Nursing.* 2000;9:1001-1007.

105. Sampselle CM. Using a stopwatch to assess pelvic muscle strength in the urine stream interruption test. *Nurse Pract.* 1993;18(1):14-16, 18-20.

106. Sampselle CM, DeLancey JOL. The urine stream interruption test and pelvic muscle function. *Nurs Res.* 1992;41(2):73-77.

107. American Physical Therapy Association. *You Can Do Something About Incontinence: A Physical Therapist's Perspective.* Alexandria, Va: American Physical Therapy Association; 1998.

108. Kegel AH. Stress incontinence of urine in women: physiological treatment. *Journal of the International College of Surgeons.* 1956;25:487-499.

109. Bø K, Hagen RH, Kvarstein B, et al. Pelvic floor muscle exercise for the treatment of female stress urinary incontinence. III. Effects of two different degrees of pelvic muscle exercise. *Neurourol Urodyn.* 1990;9:489-502.

110. Bø K, Finckenhagen HB. Vaginal palpation of pelvic floor muscle strength: intertest reproducibility and comparison between palpation and vaginal squeeze pressure. *Acta Obstet Gynecol Scand.* 2001;80: 883-887.

111. Isherwood PJ, Rane A. Comparative assessment of pelvic floor strength using a perineometer and digital examination. *Br J Obstet Gynecol.* 2000;107:1007-1011.

112. Bø K. Reproducibility of instruments designed to measure subjective evaluation of female stress urinary incontinence. *Scand J Urol Nephrol.* 1994;28:97-100.

113. National Association for Continence. Available at: http://www.nafc.org. Accessed October 10, 2003.

114. Sapsford RR, Hodges PW, Richardson CA, et al. Co-activation of the abdominal and pelvic floor muscles during voluntary exercises. *Neurourol Urodyn.* 2001;20:31-42.

115. Wallace K, Frahm J. Pelvic muscle exercise. *Quality Care.* 2003;21(3):11.

116. Berghmans LCM, Bernards ATM, Hendriks HJM, et al. Guidelines for the physiotherapeutic management of genuine stress incontinence. *Physical Therapy Reviews.* 1998;3:133-147.

117. Bø K, Talseth T, Holme I. Single blind, randomised controlled trial of pelvic floor exercises, electrical stimulation, vaginal cones, and no treatment in management of genuine stress incontinence in women. *BMJ.* 1999;318:487-493.

118. Bø K, Talseth T, Vinsnes A. Randomized controlled trial on the effect of pelvic floor muscle training on quality of life and sexual problems in genuine stress incontinent women. *Acta Obstet Gynecol Scand.* 2000;79:598-603.

119. Fonda D, Woodward M, D'Astoli M, Chin WF. Sustained improvement of subjective quality of life in older community-dwelling people after treatment for urinary incontinence. *Age Ageing.* 1995;24:283-286.

120. Janssen CCM, Lagro-Janssen ALM, Felling AJA. The effects of physiotherapy for female urinary incontinence: individual compared with group treatment. *BJU Int.* 2001;87:201-206.

121. Cammu H, Van Nylen M, Amy JJ. A 10-year follow-up after Kegel pelvic floor muscle exercises for genuine stress incontinence. *BJU Int.* 2000;85:655-658.

122. Mørkved S, Bø K, Schei B, et al. Pelvic floor muscle training during pregnancy to prevent urinary incontinence: a single-blind randomized controlled trial. *Obstet Gynecol.* 2003;101:313-319.

123. Mørkved S, Bø K. Effect of postpartum pelvic floor muscle training in prevention and treatment of urinary incontinence: a one-year follow up. *BJOG.* 2000;107:1022-1028.

124. Wells TJ. Pelvic (floor) muscle exercises. *J Am Geriatr Soc.* 1990;38:333-337.

125. Hay-Smith EJC, Bø K, Berghmans LCM, et al. Pelvic floor muscle training for urinary incontinence in women (Cochrane Methodology Review). In: *The Cochrane Library. Issue 4.* Chichester, UK: John Wiley & Sons, Ltd; 2003.

126. Arvonen T, Fianu-Jonasson A, Tyni-Lenné R. Effectiveness of two conservative modes of physical therapy in women with urinary stress incontinence. *Neurourol Urodyn.* 2001;20:591-599.

127. Johnson ST. From incontinence to confidence. *American Journal of Nursing.* 2000;100:69-76.

128. Fischer W, Linde A. Pelvic floor findings in urinary incontinence: results of conditioning using vaginal cones. *Acta Obstet Gynecol Scand.* 1997;76:455-460.

129. Oláh KS, Bridges N, Denning J, et al. The conservative management of patients with symptoms of stress incontinence: a randomized, prospective study comparing weighted vaginal cones and interferential therapy. *Am J Obstet Gynecol.* 1990;162:87-92.

130. Herbison P, Plevnik S, Mantle J. Weighted vaginal cones for urinary incontinence (Cochrane Methodology Review). In: *The Cochrane Library. Issue 4.* Chichester, UK: John Wiley & Sons, Ltd; 2003.

131. McIntosh LJ, Frahm JD, Mallett VT, Richardson DA. Pelvic floor rehabilitation in the treatment of incontinence. *J Reprod Med.* 1993;38:662-666.

132. Boissonnault WG, Goodman CC. The female genital/reproductive system. In: Goodman CC, Boissonnault WG, Fuller KS, eds. *Pathology: Implications for the Physical Therapist.* 2nd ed. Philadelphia, Pa: Saunders; 2003:757-761.

133. Pages I-H, Jahr S, Schaufele MK, et al. Comparative analysis of biofeedback and physical therapy for treatment of urinary stress incontinence in women. *Am J Phys Med Rehabil.* 2001;80:494-502.

134. Aukee P, Immonen P, Penttinen J, et al. Increase in pelvic floor muscle activity after 12 weeks' training: a randomized prospective pilot study. *Urology.* 2002;60:1020-1024.

135. Weatherall M. Biofeedback or pelvic floor muscle exercises for female genuine stress incontinence: a meta-analysis of trials identified in a systematic review. *BJU Int.* 1999;83:1015-1016.

136. Sung MS, Hong JY, Choi YH, et al. FES-biofeedback versus intensive pelvic floor muscle exercise for the prevention and treatment of genuine stress incontinence. *J Korean Med Sci.* 2000;15:303-308.

137. Sung MS, Choi YH, Back SH, et al. The effect of pelvic floor muscle exercise on genuine stress incontinence among Korean women: focusing on its effects on the quality of life. *Yonsei Med J.* 2000;41:237-251.

138. Blowman C, Pickles C, Emery S, et al. Prospective double blind controlled trial of intensive physiotherapy with and without stimulation of the pelvic floor in treatment of genuine stress incontinence. *Physiotherapy.* 1991;77:661-664.

139. Sand PK, Richardson DA, Staskin DR, et al. Pelvic floor electrical stimulation in the treatment of genuine stress incontinence: a multicenter, placebo-controlled trial. *Am J Obstet Gynecol.* 1995;173:72-79.

140. Goode PS, Burgio KL, Locher JL, et al. Effect of behavioral training with or without pelvic floor electrical stimulation on stress incontinence in women: a randomized control trial. *JAMA.* 2003;290:345-352.

141. Alewijnse D, Metsemakers JFM, Mesters IEPE, et al. Effectiveness of pelvic floor muscle exercise therapy supplemented with a health education program to promote long-term adherence among women with urinary incontinence. *Neurourol Urodyn.* 2003;22:284-295.

142. Resnick HE, Vinik AI, Schwartz AV, et al. Independent effects of peripheral nerve dysfunction on lower-extremity physical function in old age. *Diabetes Care.* 2000;23:1642-1647.

143. Cooper KH. *The Aerobics Program for Total Well-Being.* New York, NY: M. Evans and Co, Inc; 1982:139-141.

144. Mathiowetz B, Kashman N, Volland G, et al. Grip and pinch strength: normative values for adults. *Arch Phys Med Rehabil.*

1995;66:71-72.

145. Salsich GB, Mueller MJ, Sahrmann SA. Passive ankle stiffness in subjects with diabetes and peripheral neuropathy versus an age-matched comparison group. *Phys Ther.* 2000;80:352-362.

146. Vinik AI. Management of neuropathy and foot problems in diabetic patients. *Clin Cornerstone.* 2003;5(2):38-55.

147. Steed L, Cooke D, Newman S. A systematic review of psychosocial outcomes following education, self-management and psychological interventions in diabetes mellitus. *Patient Education and Counseling.* 2003;51:5-15.

148. Hamdy O, Goodyear LJ, Horton ES. Diet and exercise in type 2 diabetes mellitus. *Endocrinol Metab Clin North Am.* 2001;30:883-907.

149. Cuff DJ, Meneilly GS, Martin A, et al. Effective exercise modality to reduce insulin resistance in women with type 2 diabetes. *Diabetes Care.* 2003;26:2977-2982.

150. Vinik AI, Maser RE, Mitchell BD, et al. Diabetic autonomic neuropathy. *Diabetes Care.* 2003;26:1553-1579.

151. Albright AL. Exercise precautions and recommendations for patients with autonomic neuropathy. *Diabetes Spectrum.* 1998;11:231-237.

152. Cohen JA, Estacio RO, Lundgren RA, et al. Diabetic autonomic neuropathy is associated with an increased incidence of strokes. *Auton Neurosci.* 2003;108:73-78.

153. Murray DP, O'Brien T, Mulrooney R, et al. Autonomic dysfunction and silent myocardial ischaemia on exercise testing in diabetes mellitus. *Diabet Med.* 1990;7:580-584.

154. Zola B, Kahn JK, Juni J, et al. Abnormal cardiac function in diabetics with autonomic neuropathy in the absence of ischemic heart disease. *J Clin Endocrinol Metab.* 1986;63:208-214.

155. American Diabetes Association. Preventive foot care in people with diabetes. *Diabetes Care.* 2003;26(Suppl 1):S78-S79.

156. Goodman CC. The cardiovascular system. In: Goodman CC, Boissonnault WG, Fuller KS, eds. *Pathology: Implications for the Physical Therapist.* 2nd ed. Philadelphia, Pa: Saunders; 2003:392.

157. Kirk AF, Higgins LA, Hughes AR, et al. A randomized, controlled trial to study the effect of exercise consultation on the promotion of physical activity in people with type 2 diabetes: a pilot study. *Diabet Med.* 2001;18:877-882.

158. Sinacore DR. Severe sensory neuropathy need not precede Charcot arthropathies of the foot or ankle: implications for the rehabilitation specialist. *Physiotherapy Theory and Practice.* 2001;17:39-50.

159. Toobert DJ, Glasgow RE, Strycker LA, et al. Biologic and quality-of-life outcomes from the Mediterranean Lifestyle Program: a randomized clinical trial. *Diabetes Care.* 2003;26:228-2293.

160. Jacobson AM, De Groot M, Samson JA. The evaluation of two measures of quality of life in patients with type I and type II diabetes. *Diabetes Care.* 1994;17:267-274.

161. Hammond GS, Aoki TT. Measurement of health status in diabetic patients. Diabetes impact measurement scales. *Diabetes Care.* 1999;15:469-477.

162. Garratt AM, Schmidt L, Fitzpatrick R. Patient-assessed health outcome measures for diabetes: a structured review. *Diabet Med.* 2002;19:1-11.

CHAPTER FOUR

Impaired Joint Mobility, Motor Function, Muscle Performance, and Range of Motion Associated With Connective Tissue Dysfunction (Pattern D)

Marie Corkery, PT, MHS, FAAOMPT
Mary Ann Wilmarth, PT, DPT, MS, OCS, MTC, Cert. MDT

ANATOMY

Connective tissue is derived from the embryonic mesenchyme and is composed of cells dispersed in an extracellular matrix. Connective tissues are highly specialized and are differentiated and classified based on the composition of the extracellular matrix. They include tissues, such as the dermis, subcutaneous fat, ligaments, tendons, fascia, cartilage, and bone.[1] Blood is also considered a connective tissue.

As the name implies, connective tissue functions to support and connect other tissues and parts of the body. It provides a mechanical framework, supports nerves and blood vessels, fills space, provides fat storage, repairs tissues, protects against infection, and produces blood cells.

COMPOSITION OF CONNECTIVE TISSUE

The extracellular matrix of connective tissue is composed of a fibrous or fibrillar component and a ground substance or interfibrillar component. The two main types of fibers in the fibrous component are collagen and elastin.[2] The ground substance is composed of glycoproteins, including PGs (proteoglycans) and water, and varies in consistency from rigid to gel- or fluid-like. The cellular component of connective tissue includes circulating cells, such as lymphocytes and macrophages; resident cells, such as fibroblasts

(found in ligaments and tendons); chondroblasts (found in cartilage); osteoblasts (found in bone); and tenocytes (found in tendons).[3]

Fibers

The two most important fibrous components are the insoluble proteins: collagen and elastin.[2] Collagen has the ability to resist tensile loads and allows minimal elongation under tension. Nineteen different types of collagen have been identified. The common structure of all these types is a triple helix made up of three polypeptide chains known as the tropocollagen molecule.[2] These molecules associate with each other to form fibrils that in turn form a number of combinations and eventually fibers (Figure 4-1). Collagen fibers can be found in a wavy configuration that can straighten when tension is applied or when collagen is stretched giving the appearance of slight elongation. Fibril-forming collagens are the most common and include Type I collagen which is found in bones, tendons, ligaments, joint capsules, and the annulus fibrosus of the intervertebral disc. Type II collagen is found in articular cartilage and the nucleus pulposus of the intervertebral disc.[2] The ability of fibril-forming collagen to resist tensile forces provides tensile strength to the human body, limits ROM, and transmits forces. The elastic fibers in the extracellular matrix allow tissue, such as the lungs and blood vessels, to deform and return to their preexisting

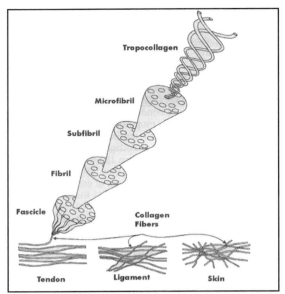

Figure 4-1. Composition of collagen fibers showing the aggregation of tropocollagen crystals as the building blocks of collagen. Organization of the fibers within the connective tissue is related to the function of the tissue. Tissues with parallel fiber orientation, such as tendons, are able to withstand greater tensile loads than tissue such as skin where the fiber orientation appears more random. Reprinted with permission from Kisner C, Colby LA. *Therapeutic Exercise: Foundations and Techniques.* 4th ed. Philadelphia, Pa: FA Davis Co; 2002.

relaxed state. Ligaments, such as the ligamentum flavum, have a large proportion of elastin and therefore allow for more flexibility than tensile strength.

Ground Substance

The PGs function as hydrators, stabilizers, and space fillers of the extracellular matrix.[2] PGs consist of a protein core attached to a glycosaminoglycan (GAG) chain. PG units known as aggregating PGs bind to a hyaluronic acid chain via a link protein. The GAG chains are negatively charged and attract water, thereby helping to hydrate the matrix. The collagen fibers resist the expansion of the PGs resulting in rigidity of the matrix. This aggregating PG forms a high molecular weight structure that has the ability to resist compressive forces. This type of PG is found in the ground substance of articular cartilage. Therefore, tissues subjected to high compressive forces, such as the nucleus pulposus of the intervertebral disc, have a greater proportion of PGs.[2] The other component of the ground substance known as glycoproteins is integral to stabilizing the matrix and linking the matrix to the cell.[2] Ground substance production and viability depends on motion, such as gentle isometric contraction of muscle.[4]

Macroscopic Structure: Types of Connective Tissue

Connective tissue can be divided into connective tissue proper and specialized connective tissue. Connective tissue proper can be subdivided into dense and loose connective tissue. Dense connective tissue is composed primarily of collagen and comprises tendons, ligaments, joint capsules, aponeuroses, and fascia. Loose connective tissue is a looser arrangement of fibers, cells, and ground substance and is found beneath the skin and between muscles and organs.[1] Specialized connective tissues include cartilage, such as hyaline articular cartilage between articulating bones; fibrocartilage found in the intervertebral discs, menisci at the knee, and disc in the TMJ; and elastic cartilage found in the auricle of the ear and the larynx. Adipose tissue is a specialized form of loose connective tissue infiltrated by fat cells. Bone is also a specialized form of connective tissue.[3] Disorders of bone are discussed in Pattern A: Primary Prevention/Risk Reduction for Skeletal Demineralization.

Tendons and ligaments consist of fibroblasts and an extracellular matrix composed of approximately 70% water.[5] There is a varied arrangement of collagen in ligaments due to the need to resist forces in multiple directions. In tendons, there is a parallel arrangement of collagen allowing for resistance of force in one direction and subsequent transmission of force to bone (see Figure 4-1). Tendons and ligaments are surrounded by loose areolar connective tissue. In tendons, this is referred to as a paratenon. In areas of high forces, such as the wrist, there is a parietal synovial layer under the paratenon. It secretes synovial fluid to facilitate tendon gliding. In the area where tendon and ligament attach to bone, there is a gradual alteration in the tendon and ligament structure to become stiffer and more bone like. Forces are transmitted onto a broad area resulting in a stronger attachment.[5]

Fascia, like all connective tissue, is continuous with itself throughout the body. It consists of a thin layer of dense connective tissue without obvious organization of its fibers. The exception to this is superficial fascia or subcutaneous tissue that is not membrane-like but more like packing material.[1] There are two main fascial systems: the internal fascia that lines the thoracic (endothoracic) and the abdominal (endoabdominal) cavities; and the investing fascia that is deep to the superficial fascia and known as deep fascia.[1] The deep fascia envelopes muscles, in some cases blending with the epimysium or providing attachment for muscles. Deep fascia becomes continuous with the periosteum of the bone where muscles attach to bone. Bursae are closed connective tissue sacs lined with a synovial membrane. They are typically flat, but become swollen when infected or injured.[1]

Connective tissue has several mechanical and physical properties including elasticity, which is the ability to return to normal length after elongation, and plasticity, which is the ability to permanently change or deform. As progressive mechanical stress is applied to collagen, the initial response is

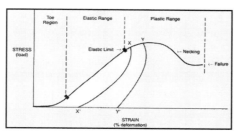

Figure 4-2. Stress-strain curve. When stressed, initially the wavy collagen fibers straighten (toe region). With additional stress, recoverable deformation occurs in the elastic range. Once the elastic limit is reached, sequential failure of the collagen fibers and tissue occurs in the plastic range, resulting in release of heat (hysteresis) and new length when the stress is released. The length from the stress point (X) results in a new length when released (X'); the heat released is represented by the area under the curve between these two points (hysteresis loop). (Y to Y' represents additional length from additional stress with more heat released.) Necking is the region in which there is considerable weakening of the tissue and less force is needed for deformation. Total failure quickly follows even under smaller loads. Reprinted with permission from Kisner C, Colby LA. *Therapeutic Exercise: Foundations and Techniques.* 4th ed. Philadelphia, Pa: FA Davis Co; 2002.

straightening of the crimp in the collagen. The load or stress stays within the physiologic limit of the tissue (toe region) (Figure 4-2). Manual soft tissue mobilization techniques are generally performed in this range, prior to permanent deformation of the collagen (plastic range). As the stress applied increases, there is progressive failure of the collagen, eventually leading to complete rupture at 12% to 15% strain.[4] Viscoelasticity refers to the gradual deformation and recovery that occurs based on the rate of loading and unloading of connective tissues. There is increased tissue resistance to stretch with a fast rate of stretching as compared to a slow rate of stretching. When a high velocity manual therapy technique is applied, there is greater tissue resistance requiring a greater load to elongate the tissues. However, these techniques are generally performed with a small amplitude in order to minimize tissue damage.[4] Connective tissue has the ability to deform over time when a constant load is applied. This is referred to as creep. Stress relaxation is the reduction of stress within a material over time as the material is subject to constant deformation (Figure 4-3). The concepts of stress relaxation and creep are used in the application of splints and static orthoses that are used to reduce contractures or lengthen tissues.[6] Connective tissues have an ability to store some of the mechanical energy applied to them and use it in their movement back to their original status. A loss of energy occurs when tissues are loaded and unloaded as they return

to their original status. This energy loss is known as hysteresis. Heating connective tissues to 37°C to 40°C increases the rate of creep and stress relaxation. This can be used in clinical settings to facilitate the effectiveness of stretching techniques. However, the clinician must be aware that heated connective tissue fails at lower loads than unheated tissue.[6] Thermal energy at 55°C to 65°C produces irreversible shrinkage. This is used in clinical settings, for example, to arthroscopically heat the shoulder capsule to create increased stability.

ANATOMY OF THE TEMPOROMANDIBULAR JOINT

The TMJ, formed by the articulation of the temporal bone and the mandible, allows for mouth opening and closing and jaw movement from side to side. The TMJ is a synovial articulation consisting of two compartments. The superior section is classified as a modified hinge (ginglymoid) and the inferior section is a gliding component (arthrodial). The articular components include the condyle of the mandible, the articular eminence of the temporal bone, the mandibular (glenoid) fossa, and a fibrocartilagenous articular disc. Fibrocartilage lines the articular surfaces, which is advantageous because of its ability to repair itself and because it has less of a propensity to degenerate. The joint is surrounded by a highly innervated and vascular capsule that forms the lateral ligament. There are also two extrinsic ligaments, the stylomandibular and sphenomandibular ligaments, that serve to connect the mandible to the cranium.[7,8]

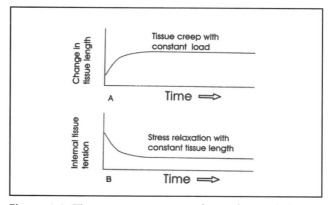

Figure 4-3. Tissue response to prolonged stretch forces as a result of viscoelastic properties. A) Effects of creep. A constant load, applied over time, will result in increased tissue length until equilibrium is reached. B) Effects of stress-relaxation. A load applied with the tissue at a constant length will result in decreased internal tension with the tissue until equilibrium is reached. Reprinted with permission from Kisner C, Colby LA. *Therapeutic Exercise: Foundations and Techniques.* 4th ed. Philadelphia, Pa: FA Davis Co; 2002.

PHYSIOLOGY

Connective tissue is maintained under normal conditions by a delicate balance between synthesis and degradation.[2] This balance may be upset by connective tissue disease, injury, and immobilization. A change in this balance, such as increased or decreased loading, results in a predictable adaptive response.[9]

Tendons and ligaments have limited vascularization that affects their healing process and metabolic activity.[5] They also have a variety of specialized nerve endings including nociceptors for pain and mechanoreceptors that play an important role in proprioception of the joint.[5] The capsule of the knee is innervated with mechanoreceptors as evidenced by the quadriceps inhibition that occurs as a result of capsular distention.[10] Mechanoreceptors in the anterior cruciate ligament (ACL) of the knee have been shown to play a role in knee stability via reflex arcs to the surrounding muscles.[11] Capsuloligamentous structures may play a role in sensory input and act as mechanical stabilizers of the knee joint.[10] Similarly, proprioceptive deficits have been found in patients with capsuloligamentous damage to the shoulder[12,13] and ankle.[14] These deficits are thought to be due to injury of the mechanoreceptors in these structures.

PATHOPHYSIOLOGY

Normal physiology of connective tissue may be altered by disease or injury. Aging also results in a decline in the mechanical properties of connective tissues.[5]

Joint capsules react to abnormal conditions by either elongating, leading to joint hypermobility, or by shortening, leading to joint contractures. Joint capsule contractions can give rise to typical patterns of restriction known as capsular patterns. If only one part of the capsule or additional factors, such as a ligamentous restriction, are responsible for limiting motion, then restrictions may not follow the typical pattern.[15] When assessing passive motion, the examiner can obtain an understanding of the source of the resistance by evaluating the quality of the end feel.[4]

Tendon injuries are described based on the underlying pathology. Tendinosis describes a tendon that has degenerative changes without inflammatory signs. Paratenonitis is inflammation of the outer layer of the tendon known as the paratenon. True tendinitis involves an inflammatory repair response in the tendon and is not as common as previously believed.[16]

Ligament sprains are graded as I, II, or III, based on the severity of damage to the ligament. In a first-degree sprain few fibers are torn, in a second-degree sprain about half the ligament is torn, and in a third-degree sprain all fibers of the ligament are torn.[16]

The synovial membrane reacts to abnormal conditions by producing more fluid effusion, becoming thicker, or forming adhesions with the articular cartilage.[17]

Bursae may become inflamed due to infection, trauma, chronic irritation, or pathological conditions, such as gout.

Degeneration of articular cartilage begins with softening or chondromalacia of the cartilage followed by a fibrillation or splitting of the cartilage surface. If the process continues the cartilage eventually becomes eroded and the underlying bone becomes thick, dense (sclerotic), and eburnated or polished.[17]

Physical examination of connective tissue lesions is based on palpation, assessment of end feel, selective tissue tension tests, joint play assessment, resisted isometric tests, and special tests. Resisted isometric tests primarily test the contractile tissues and may provoke symptoms in the muscle, tendon, or attachment to bone. Some compression of noncontractile tissues may occur with this method (eg, bursa or articular cartilage).[16]

EFFECTS OF IMMOBILIZATION

Physical stress levels of tissues that are below the normal range result in decreased tolerance of the tissues to subsequent stress and changes in their material properties.[9] Studies on the effects of immobilization on connective tissues have primarily been performed on animals. Immobilization of tendons and ligaments has been shown to result in decreased stiffness and weakness at their insertion sites to bone.[18-20] Changes in the organization and content of collagen in intramuscular connective tissue have been found in immobilized skeletal muscle.[21] Immobilization of joints leads to development of fibrofatty connective tissue within the joint space and adherence to cartilage surfaces, adhesions between synovial folds, loss of PG content, decreased ROM, atrophy, and softening of articular cartilage.[18,20,22] Disuse osteoporosis has been found in the immobilized limb.[18,23] The overall effect of these changes is a decreased load bearing capacity of the joint. Of clinical significance to the physical therapist is the fact that many of these changes have been shown to improve with a remobilization program.[19,20] Decreased vascularity of the myotendinous junction that occurred in the gastrocnemius muscle of rats after immobilization has also been shown to be reversed by remobilization.[24] However, results from studies on canines indicate that lengthy immobilization may result in long-term or permanent changes to the biomechanical properties of articular cartilage.[22,25,26] Trauma prior to immobilization accelerates the shortening of dense connective tissue during immobilization. Discussion of impaired joint mobility, motor function, muscle performance, and range of motion associated with localized inflammation falls under Pattern E: Impaired Joint Mobility, Motor Function, Muscle Performance, and Range of Motion Associated With Localized Inflammation. Scar formation is a localized response to trauma and discussion of this mechanism is found in the Integumentary Practice Patterns. The weakening of connective tissue that occurs during immobilization is an important factor to consider to prevent injury by excessive stretching forces during subsequent rehabilitation.[27] Contracted connective tissue may be treated by physically denaturing or rupturing the collagen or by restoring function by stressing collagen within physiologic limits. Stressing collagen within physiologic limits stimulates a biologic process of remodeling.[4,27] The remodeling process involves absorption of the short randomly aligned collagen fibers that limit tissue excursion and replacement by new fibers that are correctly aligned.[27] When essential structures, such as ligaments or tendons, are involved (eg, ACL repairs), excessive stretching may weaken the tissues and provoke an unwanted traumatic inflammatory reaction. In these situations the recommended approach is remodeling. In some cases where there are excessive adhesions causing contractions, such as the palmar fascia in Dupuytren's contracture or early burn scars, weakening or destruction of the scar tissue may be advisable.[27] The application of safe loading to dense connective tissues during immobilization has been advocated to prevent many of the adverse affects of immobilization. This safe loading may be achieved by having patients perform isometric exercises or joint ROM exercises.[6,28]

EFFECTS OF OVERUSE

Physical stress levels that exceed the maintenance range result in increased tolerance of tissue to stress. Tendons and ligaments have shown an ability to adapt to overstressing within a certain range. However, excessively high levels of stress result in tissue injury.[9,29] Overloading of cartilage may result in permanent deformation.[3] Tissue damage to tendons and ligaments from overuse may result in fibroblast proliferation, collagen thickening, and fibrosis.[30] Examination of tissue from patients with chronic overuse tendinopathies has shown a loss of collagen continuity, an increase in ground substance and fibroblasts, and vascular compromise. The lack of inflammatory cells would seem to indicate that chronic overuse tendon injuries involve a degenerative process rather than an inflammatory process.[31] The clinical implication is that physical therapy management of patients with these injuries should focus on load reduction and strengthening rather than anti-inflammatory measures.[32]

EFFECTS OF HORMONES

Hormones may affect the properties of dense connective tissues. For example, the hormone relaxin produced during pregnancy leads to increased extensibility of the pelvic ligaments. Research is being done to examine the role of estrogen in the high incidence of ACL injuries in female athletes.

EFFECTS OF DISEASE

Diabetes Mellitus

Many of the complications of DM involve the connec-

tive tissues resulting in poor wound healing and diminished bone formation. Musculoskeletal complications include Dupuytren's contracture, adhesive capsulitis, and joint contractures in the hand. Patients with diabetes who also have adhesive capsulitis have significant global tightness, as opposed to the typical capsular pattern. When the dominant shoulder is affected, ER and IR are most limited and ER and hyperextension are most limited in the nondominant shoulder.[33] The pathogenesis of the condition is unclear. An analysis of UE ROM in patients with DM found them to be less flexible than controls, particularly in the shoulder and fingers.[34] Decreased collagen production has been found in diabetic rats early after induction of diabetes.[35] Diabetes has also been shown to affect the integrity of articular cartilage in human ankles.[36]

Connective Tissue Diseases

Disease processes cause an alteration in the normal balance between synthesis and degradation of the extracellular matrix in connective tissue.[2]

Ehlers Danlos syndrome is a group of genetically inherited connective tissue disorders characterized by defects in collagen cross-linking.[37] Patients with this disorder suffer from joint hypermobility, subluxations, and dislocations as a result of weak connective tissue.[38] Other diseases that affect dense connective tissues include RA, Sjögrens syndrome, psoriatic arthritis, reactive arthritis, Reiters syndrome, polymyositis and dermatomyositis, systemic lupus erythematosis (SLE), fibromyalgia, reflex sympathetic dystrophy (RSD, also known as complex regional pain syndrome, CRPS), and TMJ disorders. The conditions listed above may also support classification in additional practice patterns.[39]

PATHOPHYSIOLOGY OF COMPLEX REGIONAL PAIN SYNDROME

CRPS, formerly known as RSD, is a disorder that usually develops after an initiating noxious event. The signs and symptoms that follow are out of proportion to the precipitating event. The preferred terminology for this condition, adapted by the International Association for the Study of Pain, is complex regional pain syndrome. The terminology was developed in order to avoid confusion between the diagnostic criteria for RSD and causalgia. CRPS is divided into either Type I or Type II based on the original precipitating injury. Type I (RSD) follows a soft tissue injury and Type II (causalgia) follows a nerve injury.[40,41] Diagnosis is made based on the clinical presentation and the exclusion of conditions that would otherwise account for the signs and symptoms.[42,43] Sympathetic nerve blocks and three phase bone scans are no longer required to confirm the diagnosis.[40]

Clinical criteria include the following: disproportionate pain; altered skin color/temperature (vasomotor); edema; abnormal perspiration at the site (sudomotor); changes in skin texture, hair, or nail at the site (trophic); decreased ROM; and weakness.[43] Thermography can be used to measure temperature asymmetries.[44] The Quantitative Sudomotor Axonal Reflex test assesses sudomotor responses in CRPS. However these tests are not necessary for diagnosis.[40] The exact pathophysiology of CRPS is unknown. It is thought to be due to abnormalities in the peripheral, central, and autonomic nervous systems compounded by psychological and disuse factors as the disease progresses.[40] In some patients a "regional myofascial dysfunction" may play a role in the disease process and active myofascial trigger points may be found in the area.[40,45] CRPS is described as progressing through three stages with the third stage characterized by decreased pain and sometimes irreversible changes including marked trophic changes of the skin and subcutaneous tissues, muscle atrophy, weakness, joint stiffness, and osteoporosis. However, not all patients will progress through these stages or exhibit all signs and symptoms of each stage.[40,41,46] CRPS usually occurs in a distal limb but has been reported in other body regions. It can spread proximally to other areas of the body or recur in the same or other areas.

PATHOPHYSIOLOGY OF TEMPOROMANDIBULAR JOINT DYSFUNCTION

The TMJ and its surrounding structures optimally function within the range of applied forces.[47-49] The TMJ is considered to be a weightbearing joint. Although there are not very many published studies, normal loading has been noted to be from 2 to 27 N with 0 to 40 mm of normal mouth opening.[49,50] Intercuspation (contact of the maxillary and mandibular teeth) and clenching may create a load that starts at 10 N and may exceed 50 N very rapidly.[51]

During chewing, the mandible translates from side to side. The ipsilateral condyle, also called the working condyle, rotates while the contralateral condyle, also called the balancing condyle, translates in anterior, inferior, and medial directions.[49] Tensile strain has been noted to occur in the TMJ in the following: on the balancing side,[51] in the lateral connective tissue structures, during clenching and the end of maximal closure,[49] and at the articular eminence on the head of the condyle with muscular contraction.[49,50] After 1 month of mandibular loading, white rabbits, who were fitted with axial loading chin cup appliances,[52] demonstrated both compressive and tensile loading to the condylar head.[50,53] A significant portion of parafunctional osseous loading occurs secondary to the shearing forces experienced during intercuspation.[49,54]

Nociceptive input is influenced by excessive load to the neural and contractile components of the TMJ. Information that is carried by the afferent A delta and C fibers influence the functional responses and allow for either an adaptive or maladaptive response.[55]

Dysfunctions in the TMJ may be caused by direct trauma, defective occlusion, muscle imbalances, poor posture, or muscle tension.[50,56-59] Cranial nerve V has recently been implicated in TMJ pathomechanics.[49]

When the articular disc is loaded, it is subject to compressive, tensile, and shear forces.[50,52,53,60] Maladaptive temporal and spatial forces may produce the following disc pathologies: dysmorphic changes of size and shape of the disc[60-64]; dysfunctional positional relationships between the disc, condyle, and eminence[62,64-66]; and adaptive histological changes.[49,58,63,64]

PATHOPHYSIOLOGY OF FIBROMYALGIA

Fibromyalgia is a syndrome in which patients report a pattern of consistent tender points. The occurrence of this pattern has been validated by many sources.[67-69] The American College of Rheumatology sponsored a multi-center trial in 1990. The purpose of the trial was to establish criteria which would enable clinicians to diagnose fibromyalgia syndrome (FS). The data for this study were collected from 293 individuals who had been diagnosed with FS and 265 people served as controls. The researchers noted that patients with the diagnosis of FS often presented with fatigue, sleep disturbances, stiffness, paresthesias, headaches, irritable bowel syndrome, Raynaud-like symptoms, depression, and anxiety.[67,70] The results of this trial generated the American College of Rheumatology Criteria for the Classification of Fibromyalgia[70] and are presented in Table 4-1.

The etiology of fibromylagia remains undetermined even though the disease was originally described in 1904.[71] Goldenberg[72] reports that many, rather than a single, factors precipitate the disease. Some of these factors include flu-like viral illness, trauma which can be physical or emotional, or medications (eg, steroid withdrawal). The majority of patients were unable to identify a single causative factor for their symptoms.[67]

Physical or emotional stress is often the precipitating factor that leads fibromylagia to be considered a "stress-related illness." There is a relationship between the intensity of the symptoms and how the patient discerns the severity of the stress.[73] The hypothalamic-pituitary-adrenal axis and the sympathetic nervous system are responsible for the body's response to stress.[74] Imbalance of the autonomic nervous system (ANS) is suspected to be a primary factor in the onset of the pathology.[67]

Patients who are diagnosed with fibromyalgia commonly complain of "hurting all over" and are not able to specifically identify one specific area of pain. These patients often present with a decreased ability to tolerate pain. The pain is chronic with moderate to severe intensity and is often described as burning, radiating, or gnawing and presents in a typical pattern. The diagnosis cannot be confirmed with laboratory or radiological testing; however the process of ruling out other

---

Table 4-1

CRITERIA FOR THE CLASSIFICATION OF FIBROMYALGIA

1. Widespread pain that has become chronic in nature

Definition: Pain is considered widespread when all of the following are present: Pain in the left side of body, pain in the right side of the body, pain above the waist, and pain below the waist. In addition, axial skeletal pain (cervical spine or anterior chest or thoracic spine) must be present. In this definition, shoulder and buttock pain is considered as pain for each involved side. "Low back" pain is considered lower segment pain.

2. Pain in 11 of 18 tender point sites on digital palpation*

Definition: Pain, on digital palpation, must be present in at least 11 of the following 18 tender point sites:

- ◆ Occiput: Bilateral, at the suboccipital muscle insertions
- ◆ Low cervical: Bilateral, at the anterior aspects of the intertransverse spaces at C5-C7
- ◆ Trapezius: Bilateral, at the midpoint of the upper border
- ◆ Supraspinatus: Bilateral, at origins, above the scapular spine near the medial border
- ◆ Second rib: Bilateral, at the second costochondral junctions, just lateral to the junctions on the upper surfaces
- ◆ Lateral epicondyle: Bilateral, 2 cm distal to the epicondyles
- ◆ Gluteal: Bilateral, in upper outer quadrants of buttocks in anterior fold of the muscle
- ◆ Greater trochanter: Bilateral, posterior to the trochanteric prominence
- ◆ Knee: Bilateral, at the medial fat pad proximal to the joint line

For classification purposes, patients will be said to have fibromyalgia if both criteria are satisfied. Widespread pain may have been present for at least 3 months. The presence of a second clinical disorder does not exclude the diagnosis of fibromyalgia.
*Digital palpation should be performed with an approximate force of 4 kg. For tender point to be considered positive, the subject must state that the palpation was painful. "Tender" is not to be considered "painful."
Reprinted with permission from Wolfe F, Smythe HA, Yunus MB, et al. The American College of Rheumatology 1990 criteria for the classification of fibromyalgia. Report of the multicenter criteria committee. *Arthritis Rheum.* 1990;33:160-172.

---

diagnoses is prudent.[67] Differential diagnosis of fibromyalgia and associated conditions are presented in Table 4-2.

IMAGING

The imaging techniques that may be used to assess connective tissues include plain radiographs, arthrography, radionuclide scanning, computed tomography (CT), MRI, and ultrasonography.

Plain radiographs are usually the initial diagnostic method for evaluation of bone injury and disease. They do not show the soft tissues well. Bone appears relatively white (radiopaque) and the soft tissues appear relatively dark (radiolucent).

Arthrography involves the injection of a radiopaque contrast agent with or without air into the synovial cavity. It is used to detect abnormalities of articular cartilage, fibrocartilaginous menisci, capsule, ligaments, tendons, bursae, and synovium. This technique has been replaced by the use of MRI in recent years (eg, for TMJ pathologies).[17]

Arthrography with gadolinium can be used in conjunction with MRI to evaluate intra-articular pathologies. This technique known as direct MR arthrography can be helpful in evaluating partial rotator cuff tears particularly on the underside; capsule and labral abnormalities in the shoulder joint; partial- and full-thickness tears of the collateral ligament of the elbow; tears of the triangular fibrocartilage complex (TFCC) and ligaments in the wrist; labral tears in the hip; recurrent or residual meniscus tears in patients who have had knee surgery; ligament tears in the ankle; osteochondral lesions of articular surfaces; and loose bodies in joints.[75]

Indirect MR arthrography uses intravenously administered gadolinium as a contrast agent and can help visualize vascularized tissue, such as scar tissue. It may be used to help differentiate scar tissue from recurrent disc herniation in the post operative spine.[76]

Radionuclide scanning is a bone scanning technique that detects physiological changes in bone, such as blood perfusion patterns and metabolic activity. This procedure involves the injection of a radioisotopic tracer, usually a technetium 99 m phosphate complex that is taken up by bone. Increased uptake of the tracer can result from infection, tumor, fracture, or synovitis. It is sensitive but not very specific in detecting abnormalities of bones and joints.[76]

The three-phase bone scan is useful for examining orthopedic injuries and can provide additional diagnostic information. It examines initial blood flow, blood pool images that examine soft tissue uptake, and delayed images 2 to 4 hours

Table 4-2

DIFFERENTIAL DIAGNOSIS OF FIBROMYALGIA AND ASSOCIATED CONDITIONS

Differential Diagnosis	Diagnostic Features
RA*	Synovitis, serologic tests, elevated erythrocyte sedimentation rate (ESR)
SLE*	Dermatitis, serositis (renal, CNS, etc)
Polymyalgia rheumatica*	Elevated ESR, elderly, respond to corticosteroids
Myositis	Increased muscle enzymes, muscle weakness
Hypothyroidism*	Abnormal thyroid function tests
Neuropathies	Clinical and EMG evidence of neuropathy

Comorbid Conditions	Relationship to Fibromyalgia
Depression	Present in 25% to 60% of cases
Irritable bowel syndrome	Present in 50% to 80% of cases
Migraine headaches	Present in 50% of cases
Chronic fatigue syndrome	70% of CFS meet criteria for fibromyalgia
Myofascial pain	May be localized form of fibromyalgia

*Fibromyalgia may coexist with these conditions.
Reprinted from Fibromyalgia, Goldenberg DI. *Rheumatology,* Klippel JH, Dieppe PA, eds. 1994, with permission from Elsevier.

after the injection that examine bone activity.[76] It has been used to evaluate bone changes in CRPS particularly in the delayed phase, however, its usefulness in confirming the diagnosis is questionable.[40]

CT uses ionizing radiation to produce computer-enhanced cross-sectional images or slices of the tissues. It provides good resolution of soft tissue and excellent resolution of bony structures.[17]

MRI uses nonionizing radiofrequency radiation and a strong magnetic field. It provides better quality cross sectional images and better soft tissue differentiation than the CT scan. The most commonly used MRI technique is the spin echo sequence used with T1 and T2 weighted images. Tissues such as fat exhibit a bright signal intensity with T1 weighted images, and cortical bone and fibrous tissue have a dark signal intensity. With T2 weighted images, fluids (edema, synovial fluid, cysts) have a high intensity signal. Normal tendons and ligaments have a dark signal intensity in both weightings. T1 images are used to show anatomic detail and T2 images are used to demonstrate soft tissue pathology.[17] The gradient echo technique provides even better soft tissue contrast and is useful in the evaluation of articular cartilage.[76] Contraindications to MRI include presence of pacemaker and aneurysm clips. Of clinical concern is that ferromagnetic metallic implants cause image artifacts.[76]

Ultrasonography for diagnostic purposes may be used to evaluate soft tissue masses (eg, popliteal cysts). It can be used to detect synovial inflammation, tenosynovitis, effusions, tendon tears, and inflammation that can occur in many connective tissue and rheumatological disorders.

PHARMACOLOGY

The following pharmacological agents are utilized in the management of patients with disorders affecting the connective tissues of the body. The generic name of the medication is listed followed by a brand name. This information is obtained primarily from Paget and associates[77] and Mense and Simons.[45] It is a representative list of the medications used with connective tissue diseases, their mechanism of actions, and common side effects.

♦ Analgesics
  • Examples: Acetaminophen (paracetamol) (Tylenol)
  • Action: Analgesic effect is believed to be comparable with aspirin but there is little or no anti-inflammatory effect
  • Side effects: Chronic ingestion and large doses can cause kidney and liver damage and effect bone marrow production, should not be taken with alcohol
♦ Tramadol hydrochloride (Ultram)
  • Action: A synthetic, centrally acting analgesic
  • Side effects: Similar to opioids including lightheadedness, somnolence, nausea, and constipation
♦ Nonsteroidal anti-inflammatory drugs (NSAIDs)
  • Example: Acetylsalicylic acid (aspirin)
    ▪ Action: Analgesic effect is believed to be from inhibition of prostaglandin synthesis, but there may be direct effects on the CNS and white blood cells
    ▪ Side effects: Dyspepsia, gastric ulceration, and bleeding

- Examples: Ibuprofen (Advil, Motrin, Nuprin), indomethacin (Indocin), and naproxen (Naprosyn, Aleve)
  - Action: All inhibit prostaglandin synthesis
  - Side effects: Gastrointestinal bleeding and dyspepsia
- Examples: Celecoxib (Celebrex)
  - Action: Inhibits prostaglandin synthesis via selective inhibition of COX-2 enzymes and thereby have less potential for GI side effects than older NSAIDs
  - Side effects: Dyspepsia and gastrointestinal intolerance
- Other NSAIDs include diclofenac, diflunisal, ketoprofen, ketorolac, oxaprozin, and piroxicam
- Opiod analgesics
  - Examples: Codeine, hydrocodone, meperidine (Demerol), morphine, and propoxyphene hydrochloride (Darvon)
    - Action: Binds to opioid receptors in the spinal cord and brain so used for treatment of moderately severe pain
    - Side effects: Nausea and constipation and risk of physical dependency with chronic pain
- Anticonvulsants
  - Example: Gabapentin (Neurontin)
    - Action: Exact mechanism of action is unknown, used to treat neuropathic pain syndromes
    - Side effects: Somnolence and dizziness
- Other
  - Example: Amitriptyline (Elavil)
  - Action: A tricyclic antidepressant, which is used to treat neuropathic pain; it is thought to block reuptake of a variety of neurotransmitters, particularly serotonin
  - Side effects: Anticholinergic and CNS effects, such as dry mouth and somnolence
- Corticosteroids
  - Examples: Specifically glucocorticoids (hydrocortisone, cortisone, prednisone)
  - Action: Potent anti-inflammatory agents used in the treatment of collagen disease due to their ability to inhibit collagen synthesis and control pain
  - Side effects: Thinning of the subcutaneous tissue, ecchymosis, and delayed wound healing[8]; HTN, weight gain, Cushing's syndrome, glucose intolerance, osteoporosis, and osteonecrosis
  - With the exception of trigger finger, there is a lack of evidence to support the use of corticosteroid injection to treat tendinopathies.[78,79] Intra-articular injections of cortisone can be used to treat inflammation associated with rheumatological conditions[80]

The following pharmacological agents are utilized in the management of patients with CRPS:

- Calcium channel blockers
  - Example: Nifedipine
  - Action: Believed to inhibit contraction of cardiac and smooth muscle by interfering with the release of calcium from the sarcoplasmic reticulum. May help RSD by improving peripheral circulation[81]
  - Side effects: Gastrointestinal effects and headache
- Alpha adrenergic blocker
  - Example: Phenoxybenzamine
  - Action: Prevents the action of circulating catecholamines
  - Side effects: Postural hypotension, reflex tachycardia, and dizziness
- Clonidine
  - Action: Used transdermally for relief of allodynia, thought to reduce peripheral sympathetic nervous system activity by stimulating alpha II adrenergic receptors in the CNS
  - Side effects: Development of hypersensitivity to clonidine, sedation, dryness of the mouth, constipation, headache, and dizziness

The following pharmacological agents are utilized in the management of patients with connective tissue disorders and RA. In addition to NSAIDs and corticosteroids, disease-modifying antirheumatic drugs (DMARDs) are used to treat rheumatological conditions. These drugs are slow acting, and frequent monitoring of patients for side effects is required in many cases. These drugs are thought to slow the progression of the disease and include the following:

- Methotrexate is effective at controlling the inflammatory process
- Sulfasalazine has both anti inflammatory and immunomodulatory effects
- Leflunomide has both immunosuppressive and anti-inflammatory effects
- Antimalarial drugs (hydroxychloroquine) may inhibit antigen presentation and immune response
- D-Penicillamine has been shown to reduce inflammatory synovitis
- Gold salts (oral and injectable) can prevent disease progression, rarely used today due to its side effects and the superior efficacy of other DMARDs
- Minocycline has antibiotic, immunomodulatory, and anti-inflammatory effects
- Biologic agents and immunotherapy, based on recent research that looks at T and B lymphocytes, macrophages, and fibroblasts among others, as potential sites for therapeutic intervention[77]

Medications should be utilized as directed by the patient's physician and can be valuable for those with FS. Randomized, controlled trials using NSAIDs for pain intervention have revealed that (although utilized by physicians) they are not significantly better than using a placebo medication for treatment of FS.[82-84] However, when combined with CNS active medications,[84] there appears to be a synergistic effect that enhances the efficacy of the CNS medication. The most effective pharmacologic interventions appears to be those that improve sleep disturbances.[82-86] Typically, amytriptyline (Elavil) is given (at a dosage of 25 to 50 mg at bedtime) to manage the sleep disturbance. It has been reported in the literature that amytriptyline is associated with significant improvement in pain, sleep, fatigue, patient and physician global assessment, and manual tender point score when compared with placebo or naproxen.[67,83-85,87]

Case Study #1: Complex Regional Pain Syndrome

Mrs. Mary Murphy is a 45-year-old previously active and healthy female who has complex regional pain syndrome Type I of the right foot and ankle.

PHYSICAL THERAPIST EXAMINATION

HISTORY

- General demographics: Mrs. Murphy is a 45-year-old white female whose primary language is English. She is right-side dominant.
- Social history: She is married and has a 15-year-old daughter and two cats.
- Employment/work: Mrs. Murphy is a bookkeeper for a small business firm.
- Living environment: She lives on the second floor of an apartment building with an elevator.
- General health status
  - General health perception: Mrs. Murphy reports that she was in good health prior to this event.
  - Physical function: She has been significantly limited compared to before the injury.
  - Psychological function: She is anxious and irritable due to current condition.
  - Role function: Wife, mother, employee.
  - Social function: She likes to attend her daughter's basketball games.
- Social/health habits: Mrs. Murphy is a non-smoker.
- Family history: Her father has CAD, and her mother has RA.

- Medical/surgical history: Noncontributory.
- Prior hospitalizations: She was hospitalized for the birth of her daughter 15 years ago and for an appendectomy 30 years ago.
- Preexisting medical and other health-related conditions: None.
- Current condition(s)/chief complaint(s): Mrs. Murphy is 2 months status post a Grade I right anterior talofibular ligament sprain that occurred while playing basketball. She was treated in the emergency room and discharged home with crutches for weightbearing as tolerated, with instructions for home use of ice, elevation, and Motrin and Tylenol. Her ankle was wrapped with an ace bandage that she left on for 1 week. Plain radiographs taken in the emergency room were negative for a fracture. After the injury she continued to have pain and swelling gradually increasing in intensity to an excruciating level. She underwent an MRI that was negative. One week ago, she underwent a lumbar sympathetic block that resulted in decreased pain. She has been diagnosed with CRPS Type I and was referred to physical therapy by her orthopedist. She is now complaining of burning shooting pain in the foot and toes that becomes worse at night and in air conditioned/cold rooms. She has pain and difficulty bearing weight on the right foot. She reports that medications do not seem to be of much help. Her chief complaints are inability to put weight on the ball of her foot or squat and difficulty ascending and descending stairs.
- Functional status and activity level: As of yesterday she was able to wear a sneaker and tie the lacings. She has just resumed driving.
- Medications: Motrin 400 mg tid and Ultram 100 mg tid.
- Other clinical tests: The plain films were negative for fracture; MRI was normal; first sympathetic block decreased pain; and she is scheduled for a second sympathetic block next week.

SYSTEMS REVIEW

- Cardiovascular/pulmonary
  - BP: 120/75 mmHg
  - Edema: Moderate edema right foot and ankle
  - HR: 78 bpm
  - RR: 18 bpm
- Integumentary
  - Presence of scar formation: None noted
  - Skin color: Purple/blue discoloration of right foot and ankle
  - Skin integrity: Intact
- Musculoskeletal

- Gross range of motion
  - Both UEs and LLE: WNL
  - Right hip and knee: WNL
  - Significant restrictions noted in right ankle dorsiflexion, inversion, eversion, and first MTP flexion and extension
  - Mild restriction in plantarflexion
- Gross strength
  - Both UEs and LLE: WNL
  - Weakness noted in RLE hip, knee, ankle, and toes
- Gross symmetry: Slight asymmetry due to fear/avoidance
- Height: 5'4" (1.63 m)
- Weight: 150 lbs (68.04 kg)
- Neuromuscular
  - Balance
    - Unable to assess unilateral standing balance on the right due to pain with weightbearing on RLE
    - Unilateral standing balance on left leg is good
  - Locomotion, transfers, and transitions
    - Ambulating independently with one crutch
    - Gait extremely antalgic with decreased weightbearing and push off on the right
    - Independent with transfers and stairs
  - Exhibiting some fear/avoidance behaviors regarding use of right foot and ankle
- Communication, affect, cognition, language, and learning style
  - Communication and cognition: Alert and able to communicate needs
  - Affect: Becomes emotional when discussing pain and lack of function
  - Learning preferences: Visual learner

TESTS AND MEASURES

- Anthropometric characteristics
  - BMI=705 x (body weight [in pounds] divided by height[2] [in inches])
  - Mrs. Murphy's BMI was 25.7 (WHO standard normal for women=19.1 to 25.8)[88,89]
  - Moderate soft tissue edema noted in right foot and ankle and extending proximally 4 inches up the leg
  - Volumetric measurements revealed 10% difference between right and left foot/ankle (shown to be a reliable method of assessing volume changes in patients with LE CRPS)[90]
- Assistive and adaptive devices
  - Using one crutch or support from furniture for ADL

- Circulation
  - DP and PT artery pulses diminished on right
  - Pulses normal on left
- Cranial and peripheral nerve integrity
  - Allodynia noted along dorsum and lateral aspect of right foot and ankle
  - Hyperalgesia along medial aspect of right foot
  - Sensation otherwise intact to light touch in all four extremities
  - SLR test negative bilaterally
- Environmental, home, and work barriers
  - Able to access home and work environments with use of crutch
- Ergonomics and body mechanics
  - Altered body mechanics during activities due to guarding of right foot and ankle, fear/avoidance behavior, and decreased weightbearing on right
- Gait, locomotion, and balance
  - Ambulates independently on level surfaces and stairs with one crutch
  - Extremely antalgic gait with decreased weightbearing and push off on RLE
  - Decreased walking speed; unable to do 6-Minute Walk test, in 1 minute walked 35.5 m
  - Unilateral stance: Painful and unable to independently maintain unilateral stance on right leg; good balance with crutch
- Integumentary integrity
  - Skin of right ankle and foot is cool, cyanotic, and mottled
  - Increased coarse hair growth on dorsum of right distal foot
  - No nail changes noted
  - Hyperhydrosis of right foot
  - Ankle and vasomotor instability with dependent positioning of RLE
- Joint integrity and mobility[91]
  - Joint play left foot and ankle normal throughout
  - Joint play on right revealed the following:
    - Talocrural joint: Distraction, anterior, and posterior glides minimally restricted
    - Subtalar joint: Distraction, medial glide, and lateral glide minimally restricted
    - Talonavicular and calcaneocuboid joints: Minimally restricted
    - TMT joints: Minimally restricted
    - Intermetatarsal joints: Normal throughout
    - First MTP joint: Distraction, A/P, and P/A glides moderately restricted
    - All IP joints and second to fifth MTP joints: Normal

♦ Motor function
  ● Dexterity, coordination, and agility
    ▪ WNL in both UEs and LLE
    ▪ Diminished on the RLE
♦ Muscle performance[92]
  ● MMT revealed the following deviations from normal
    ▪ Right hip abductors and extensors=4/5
    ▪ Right knee extensors=4/5
    ▪ Right ankle plantarflexion in non-weightbearing=3+/5, dorsiflexion=4/5, inversion=4/5, and eversion=3+/5
    ▪ Big toe extension on right=4/5 and flexion=4/5
♦ Pain
  ● The following pain measurements have been shown to correlate well to bedside evaluation of CRPS I of the UE[43]
    ▪ 10 cm VAS[16]
      ‣ VAS: Current pain=6 cm
      ‣ VAS: Effort, pain from exertion (10 ankle pumps)=8 cm
      ‣ VAS: Min, least pain in preceding week=5 cm
      ‣ VAS: Max, worst pain in preceding week=9 cm (with weightbearing and touch)
    ▪ McGill Pain questionnaire[93] (list of pain descriptors experienced over the past week and not at the present moment): Selected 16 words out of 20 pain descriptor groups
♦ Posture
  ● Observational assessment revealed
    ▪ Stands with minimally increased pronation of the left foot, minimal weightbearing on the right leg with right hip and knee flexed
♦ Range of motion
  ● Unable to fully squat due to decreased ROM and pain
  ● Joint active and passive movements[92]
    ▪ Hip WNL bilaterally
    ▪ Right knee WNL bilaterally
    ▪ Ankle
      ‣ Ankle dorsiflexion: R=0 to 5 degrees and L=0 to 17 degrees
      ‣ Ankle plantarflexion: R=0 to 40 degrees and L=0 to 50 degrees
      ‣ Eversion: R=0 to 10 degrees and L=0 to 20 degrees
      ‣ Inversion: R=0 to 15 degrees and L=0 to 30 degrees
    ▪ Toes
      ‣ First MTP (hyper)extension: R=0 to 45 degrees and L=0 to 80 degrees

‣ First MTP flex: R=0 to 15 degrees and L=0 to 35 degrees
‣ All other toes: WNL
● Muscle length[16]
  ▪ Gastrocnemius (ankle dorsiflexion with knee ext): R=5 degrees and L=10 degrees
  ▪ Hamstrings (knee angle with 90 degree hip flexion): R=40 degrees and L=20 degrees
  ▪ Thomas test: WNL
● Soft tissue extensibility
  ▪ Decreased soft tissue extensibility
  ▪ Increased tone and trigger points of right Achilles tendon, gastrocnemius, and soleus muscle complex
♦ Reflex integrity
  ● Patellar and Achilles DTRs=2+ bilaterally
♦ Self-care and home management
  ● Interview concerning ability to safely perform self-care and home management actions, tasks, and activities revealed that she was independent in all activities, but she had limited sitting tolerance to 1 hour and limited ability to squat
  ● Health Status questionnaire SF-36: Used to assess health status and physical function,[94] is one of the few functional outcome tools used to assess outcome measures for patients with CRPS; aspects of it have been used to assess outcomes in UE CRPS[95]
    ▪ Scores were lower than normal in all domains, particularly physical function, role function, and pain
♦ Work, community, and leisure integration or reintegration
  ● Interview concerning ability to safely manage work, community, and leisure actions, tasks, and activities revealed that she was independent in most activities, except she:
    ▪ Had limited sitting tolerance to 1 hour and limited ability to squat
    ▪ Was unable to participate in community and leisure activities involving prolonged walking or standing, such as going shopping to the mall or playing golf
    ▪ Was concerned about missing time from work to attend medical appointments

EVALUATION

Mrs. Murphy was previously active and is in otherwise good health. She has limited insight into her current condition and currently has decreased weightbearing and touch tolerance in the RLE. Additional RLE changes include pain; decreased ROM, muscle performance, and endurance;

strength, gait, and posture deviations; swelling; vasomotor, sudomotor, and trophic changes; and soft tissue restrictions. Functional limitations include limited sitting tolerance, limited ambulation, inability to squat, limited ability to ascend and descend stairs, and diminished capacity for leisure and community actions, tasks, and activities.

DIAGNOSIS

Mrs. Murphy is a patient who has CRPS Type I of the LE and has pain in her right foot and ankle. She has impaired: circulation; cranial and peripheral nerve integrity; ergonomics and body mechanics; gait, locomotion, and balance; integumentary integrity; joint integrity and mobility; motor function; muscle performance; posture; and range of motion. She is functionally limited in self-care and home management and in work, community, and leisure actions, tasks, and activities. These findings are consistent with placement in Pattern D: Impaired Joint Mobility, Motor Function, Muscle Performance, and Range of Motion Associated With Connective Tissue Dysfunction. A diagnosis of CRPS may also support classification in additional practice patterns. This patient is at risk for skeletal demineralization of the RLE and has impaired sensory integrity and integumentary involvement and therefore may also be classified in Pattern A: Primary Prevention/Risk Reduction for Skeletal Demineralization, Neuromuscular Pattern G: Impaired Motor Function and Sensory Integrity Associated With Acute or Chronic Polyneuropathies, and Integumentary Pattern A: Primary Prevention/Risk Reduction for Integumentary Disorders. The identified impairments and functional limitations will be addressed in determining the prognosis and the plan of care.

PROGNOSIS AND PLAN OF CARE

Over the course of the visits, the following mutually established outcomes have been determined:

♦ Ability to perform self-care, home management, work, community, and leisure actions, tasks, and activities is improved

♦ Activity tolerance is improved to allow return to previous functional and leisure actions, tasks, and activities

♦ Edema is reduced

♦ Gait is improved

♦ Improved soft tissue extensibility and muscle tone in RLE

♦ Independent management of symptoms is increased

♦ LE muscle length is increased

♦ Muscle performance is increased

♦ Risk of spread of CRPS proximally is reduced

♦ RLE balance is improved

♦ RLE proprioception is improved

♦ RLE weightbearing tolerance is improved

♦ ROM is increased

Criteria for discharge from physical therapy have been mutually agreed upon by the therapist and patient. Discharge will occur when Mrs. Murphy reaches established functional outcomes and goals, or if she fails to progress toward goals due to complications, or if she declines further treatment.

To achieve these outcomes the appropriate interventions for this patient are determined. These will include: coordination, communication, and documentation; patient/client-related instruction; therapeutic exercise; functional training in self-care and home management; functional training in work, community, and leisure integration or reintegration; manual therapy techniques; electrotherapeutic modalities; and physical agents and mechanical modalities.

There is little information on long-term functional outcomes of patients with this disease. Prognosis is thought to be better with children than adults. Early diagnosis and treatment is recommended.[41,96,97] Mrs. Murphy is expected to require between 12 and 18 visits over a 2- to 3-month period of time. Mrs. Murphy's prognosis for rehabilitation is good based on early diagnosis, improvement of symptoms with sympathetic block, good family support, and relatively early physical therapy intervention.[98]

INTERVENTIONS

RATIONALE FOR SELECTED INTERVENTIONS

Therapeutic Exercise

As ROM improves, appropriate strengthening exercises will be introduced to address the muscle weakness that occurs secondary to reflex inhibition from both pain and disuse.[40,99]

Establishing a baseline level of activity and a quota-based progression system has been advocated for restoring normal motion and promoting functional tolerance in patients with CRPS. This system has been described by Allen,[40] based on the work of Fordyce. A baseline of repetitions or time is established by having the patient perform each activity or exercise until the patient begins to feel pain, muscle weakness, or fatigue. When subsequently performing this exercise in the clinic or at home, the patient is then instructed to perform 80% of the baseline repetitions or the elapsed time. During each subsequent session, the number of repetitions is increased by one or 5% to 10% of the elapsed time. When the number of repetitions reaches 15 with PREs, the resistance is increased and the number of repetitions is dropped to eight. This system can be used to grade aerobic activities based on time or distance. Likewise a quota-based reduction of use of assistive devices may be used. Progression of activity is therefore independent of symptoms of pain.

Ninety-two percent of children with CRPS responded well to an intense exercise program that included desensitization exercises, aerobic exercise training, weightbearing activities, hydrotherapy, and a home exercise program.[97] The authors speculated that one mechanism for improvement might be related to exercise-induced endorphins or other pain-related mediators working through peripheral or central feedback loops.[97] Favorable results were also found in adults with CRPS of the UE after a physical therapy program that included massage, TENS, and exercise.[100]

To prevent skeletal demineralization associated with immobilization, weightbearing exercises with progression to a full weightbearing walking program on a treadmill or land should be encouraged.[5,40] Early weightbearing in a deloaded environment is facilitated in a warm pool. A female who is immersed in water up to the xiphisternum only bears approximately 35% of her total body weight.[101] Hydrotherapy is also beneficial in facilitating edema management and promoting ROM and strength.[40]

Manual Therapy Techniques

Desensitization techniques have been advocated for reducing allodynia.[40,99,102] The affected area is exposed to a series of controlled previously non-nociceptive stimuli. Materials progressing from soft light textured materials (eg, silk) to potentially more irritating rough textured materials (eg, towel) may be used. As the patient becomes accustomed to the material and the painful response diminishes, the next material or stimulus in the sequence is introduced. The goal of desensitization is to allow the patient to tolerate the texture of clothing and objects on the affected area. This restoration of the normal sensory pathway may occur through mechanisms of central habituation or by peripheral inhibition.[99] Soft tissue and joint mobilization techniques are performed within physiologic range to produce tissue remodeling.[4,27]

Joint mobilization techniques are performed to restore normal joint arthrokinematics, provide normal sensory proprioceptive input, and promote synovial fluid exchange that helps maintain nutrient exchange within the joint.[103] The initial treatment is a Grade II traction technique performed with the joint in a resting position.[91,103] Treatment is progressed based on the patient's response to treatment. Joint mobilization techniques are progressed by adding Grade III traction techniques, pre-positioning the joint at the end of the available range prior to mobilization, and adding joint gliding techniques.[103]

Soft tissue mobilization techniques will start with gentle effleurage with the limb elevated above the level of the heart. This position helps to decrease arterial hydrostatic pressure, promote venous and lymphatic drainage, mobilize edema, and reduce pain by mechanical stimulation of mechanoreceptors.[104] This technique performed from distal to proximal for edema reduction has the added benefit of providing a form of desensitization and the pressure used should be adjusted accordingly. Based on the patient's tolerance, deeper kneading or petrissage techniques will be added to help mobilize the tissues, promote circulation, and eliminate metabolic waste from the region.[104] Sustained compression or trigger point release techniques will be used to treat active trigger points. Pressure will be maintained for up to 60 seconds to help promote muscle relaxation via muscle spindle activation and decreasing pain by stimulating the mechanoreceptors.[105]

Electrotherapeutic Modalities

Electrotherapeutic modalities, such as TENS, have been included as part of a successful intervention strategy that included massage and exercise to treat both children and adults with CRPS.[96,100] Because treatments were individualized and parameters were not given in either study, conclusions cannot be drawn on the outcome of TENS treatment alone in these cases. Other authors state that there is little evidence to support the use of TENS or EMS in relieving pain or promoting function in patients with CRPS.[40] Therefore electrotherapeutic modalities were not selected to be included in the intervention program for Mrs. Murphy.

Physical Agents and Mechanical Modalities

Physical agents, such as whirlpool, paraffin, and fluidotherapy, may be used in the initial stages of CRPS to promote circulation, desensitization, and improve skin tone. However, their efficacy has not been studied. Hooshmand has recommended avoidance of ice and soaking the extremity in Epsom salts and warm water.[106] Mrs. Murphy's pain is exacerbated by cold and therefore the use of ice is not recommended. The additional use of paraffin and fluidotherapy was not selected in this case. Hydrotherapy consisting of a pool walking program and exercise is listed in the therapeutic exercise section.

COORDINATION, COMMUNICATION, AND DOCUMENTATION

A coordinated, multidisciplinary approach is important in the management of the patient with CRPS. This team may include the physician, physical therapist, occupational therapist, psychologist, social worker, case manager, nurse, and vocational rehabilitation counselors. Medical management focuses on coordinating care and providing pain and symptomatic relief via medications and other intervention therapies, such as sympathetic blockades, sympathectomy, and use of implantable devices.

Communication will occur with Mrs. Murphy's family as needed to explain therapeutic interventions. All elements of the patient's management will be documented following APTA[39] and facility guidelines. Regular communication with the referring physician will occur to provide updates on

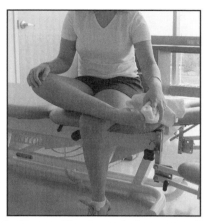

Figure 4-4. Desensitization of the extremity with a towel.

Mrs. Murphy's status.

If Mrs. Murphy's fear/avoidance behaviors and emotional affect are noted to be barriers to treatment, then a referral for psychological intervention will be recommended to her MD. Psychological therapies are useful in identifying psychological co-morbidities that exist, such as anxiety and depression.[40] Cognitive behavioral therapies, such as pain management strategies, biofeedback, relaxation training, and guided imagery, have also been used to treat patients with CRPS.[96]

PATIENT/CLIENT-RELATED INSTRUCTION

The patient will be instructed in the nature and course of her condition, the importance of adherence to a home exercise program, and the potential ramifications of disuse atrophy. Modeling and visual aids will be used to teach the home exercise program to the extent required by the patient. Mrs. Murphy will be encouraged to keep a diary of her home exercise program to record her exercises using the quota-based progression system.

♦ The instructions for her home exercise program will focus on:
 ● Maintenance of weightbearing on the RLE
 ● Use of the RLE as normally as possible, not guarding or splinting the area
 ● Appropriate pacing of physical activity so that a balance between overuse and underuse is maintained
 ● Desensitization of the extremity starting with silk and lightly rubbing the affected area for several minutes twice a day, gradually progressing to more coarse materials, such as cotton and towel (Figure 4-4)
 ● Desensitization with self-massage to the affected foot and ankle
 ● Edema reduction including periodic elevation of the limb throughout the day and use of ankle pumps
 ● Hydrotherapy starting in a warm pool at chest level

with gentle calf and hamstring stretching and a pool-walking program (Figure 4-5)
 ● Improvement of aerobic capacity starting with stationary bicycle and progressing to elliptical machine and treadmill
♦ Self-stretching program for the involved LE
♦ Strengthening exercises of the ankle
 ● Use of correct body mechanics with ADL
♦ Some medical practitioners advocate instruction that addresses dietary factors[106]

THERAPEUTIC EXERCISE

Exercises will be progressed using the quota-based system described earlier, starting each exercise at 80% of baseline and increasing by one repetition or 5% to 10% of time, in subsequent daily sessions.[40]

The key to a successful exercise program is to maintain the delicate balance between an overvigorous approach that will exacerbate symptoms and under-activity of the area that will lead to disuse atrophy and increased symptomatology. Stressing collagen within physiologic limits provides an important stimulus for the remodeling of connective tissue. This stress also influences collagen alignment and formation.[4] Likewise in the rehabilitation of this patient, the optimal stimulus or stress to collagen must be applied in the form of a graded exercise program to stress collagen fibers without overloading them.

♦ Aerobic capacity/endurance conditioning
 ● Exercise progression for these exercises is time based. For example, if the patient tolerates 10 minutes on the stationary bicycle well, she will be started at 8 minutes and then she will increase the time daily by 5% to 10% from this baseline
 ● Mode
  ▪ Bicycle
  ▪ Treadmill

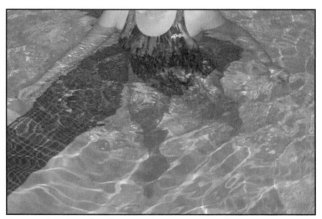

Figure 4-5. Hydrotherapy in warm pool.

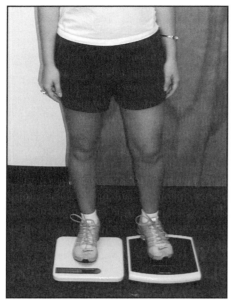

Figure 4-6. Weightbearing status monitored with the use of weighing scales.

- Aquatic program
  - Hydrotherapy starting in a warm pool at chest level with a pool-walking program. Exercise is progressed by time as described above
- Balance, coordination, and agility training
  - Progress from sitting to standing balance
  - Stand on one leg with eyes closed on level ground for proprioceptive retraining
  - Progress to unstable surfaces, such as a balance pad (eg, Airex) or a balance board
- Body mechanics and postural stabilization
  - Verbal cueing and use of a mirror to correct LE postural impairments
- Flexibility exercises
  - Stretching exercises should be done after warming up, using a slow and steady stretch accompanied by deep breathing, and building hold up to 15 to 30 seconds
  - Done two to three times a day, at least two to three repetitions
  - Hamstring stretch: Patient supine, right hip flexed to 90 degrees, hands supporting right posterior thigh and extends right knee to tolerance
  - Gastrocnemius (non-weightbearing): Patient supine with knee extended, towel around foot, and passively dorsiflex ankle
  - Gastrocnemius (progress to weightbearing as tolerated): Standing with a wedge under right foot, right knee extended, and weight shifts forward

- Soleus: Repeat as described above for weightbearing and non weightbearing positions for gastrocnemius with right knee flexed at least 20 degrees
- MTP joint (non-weightbearing): Big toe is manually moved into end range extension, while maintaining IP joint extension
- MTP joint (weightbearing): Big toe is extended upward against a vertical surface, the heel is maintained on the ground, and the ankle dorsiflexed
- Hydrotherapy starting in a warm pool at chest level with gentle calf and hamstring stretching
- Gait and locomotion training
  - Progressive weightbearing encouraged within tolerance
  - Pool walking initiated for early weightbearing in a warm environment. Weightbearing progressed by moving to more shallow water depths
  - Weightbearing status monitored with the use of weighing scales for measurement and to provide visual feedback (Figure 4-6)
  - Use of mirror for visual feedback
- Strength, power, and endurance training
  - A baseline level of activity will first be established for each individual exercise: For example if the patient can tolerate 10 repetitions of an exercise well, then she will begin with eight repetitions of that exercise and increase by one repetition each subsequent session
  - Once she can perform 15 repetitions, resistance will be added and the number of repetitions decreased back to eight and then progressed as before
  - Leg press to facilitate early strengthening and weightbearing
  - Deloaded squats using a deloading bar attached to a lat pulley system, progressing to full weightbearing squats as tolerated; progress exercise by decreasing the amount of deloading, thus increasing the amount of weightbearing
  - Buoyancy resisted exercises performed in the pool for hip and knee strengthening adding resistive equipment to the ankle for increased resistance
  - Hip and knee strengthening exercises using a pulley system or elastic band for resistance
  - Ankle strengthening exercises in all planes using a pulley system or elastic band for resistance
  - Progressive weightbearing within tolerance during exercises
    - Initial weightbearing may occur with exercises, such as bridging
    - A modified plantigrade positioning to promote weightbearing and ankle dorsiflexion
    - The Biomechanical Ankle Platform System

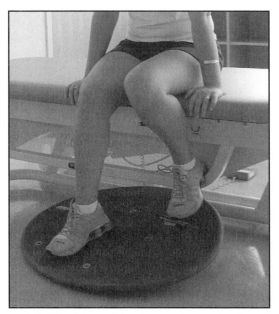

Figure 4-7. BAPS board for increasing weightbearing.

(BAPS board) or other similar device used in a partial-weightbearing position to begin early proprioceptive retraining and ankle ROM exercises

▸ Begin with eight repetitions in a clockwise and counterclockwise direction while seated, and when 15 repetitions can be performed of this exercise, the amount of weightbearing is increased and the number of repetitions decreased back to eight

▸ Weightbearing is progressed incrementally in this way to full weightbearing (Figure 4-7)

Maintenance of a regular exercise program must be instilled in this patient and the outcome depends on adherence to the recommended home exercise program. Achieving an exercise program that the patient will do on a life-long basis is vital to success. Mrs. Murphy will be encouraged to establish a variety of enjoyable activities and alternating activities when possible, to establish a realistic time frame for exercise, and to use entertainment whenever possible (eg, music, TV, books on tape) when performing exercises.

FUNCTIONAL TRAINING IN SELF-CARE AND HOME MANAGEMENT

◆ Self-care and home management
  ● Review and simulation of all actions, tasks, and activities and postural alignment for self-care and home management
  ● Stair climbing (Figure 4-8)
  ● Review of energy conservation techniques

FUNCTIONAL TRAINING IN WORK, COMMUNITY, AND LEISURE INTEGRATION OR REINTEGRATION

◆ Work
  ● Review all actions, tasks, and activities and postural alignment for work
◆ Leisure
  ● Review pool program
  ● Review gym program
  ● Simulated golf activities in clinic with elastic band, plyoball, and golf club

MANUAL THERAPY TECHNIQUES

Manual therapy techniques focus on desensitization, edema, pain control, and increasing ROM with the ultimate goal of restoring function.[40,102]

◆ Massage
  ● Light effleurage to the lower leg and foot, from distal to proximal with limb elevated
◆ Desensitization
  ● Desensitizing starting with silk and lightly rubbing the affected area for several minutes twice a day, gradually progressing to more coarse materials, such as cotton and towel
◆ Mobilization/manipulation
  ● Soft tissue mobilization using light effleurage progressing to deeper muscle kneading and trigger point release techniques as tolerated to the right calf region (Figure 4-9)

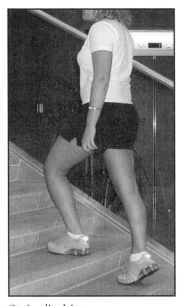

Figure 4-8. Stair climbing.

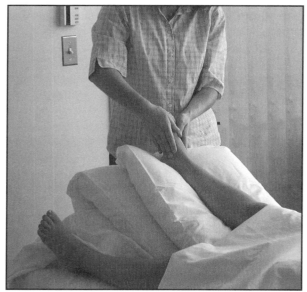

Figure 4-9. Soft tissue mobilization and trigger point releases.

- Edema management and soft tissue mobilization techniques performed in the early stages of treatment and gradually discontinued as the patient progresses to restoring function through activity and exercise
- Joint mobilization techniques
  - Joint gliding oscillation techniques will initially be Grade II and progress to Grades III and IV as tolerated and based on response to treatment[103,107]
  - Grade II traction techniques to the right talocrural, subtalar, and first MTP joints with the joints in the resting position progressing to end range positions and grades as tolerated
  - Anterior and posterior glides to the right talocrural joint at end range
  - Medial and lateral glides to the subtalar joint
  - Anterior and posterior glides to the first MTP joint
  - Talonavicular and calcaneocuboid joint glides
  - TMT joint glides

ANTICIPATED GOALS AND EXPECTED OUTCOMES

- ◆ Impact on pathology/pathophysiology
  - Edema of right foot and ankle is reduced by 50% in 2 to 3 weeks and edema of right foot and ankle is minimal, with <5% difference in volume between both feet, by discharge.
  - RLE allodynia and hyperalgesia are improved.
  - Trigger point irritability is decreased.

- ◆ Impact on impairments
  - Aerobic capacity is increased or maintained.
  - Balance is improved: Right leg standing balance is maintained for at least 60 seconds, in 6 to 8 weeks.
  - Gait and locomotion are improved: Independent ambulation on level surfaces with normal symmetric pattern for up to 15 minutes is achieved initially with straight cane in 2 to 3 weeks and then without assistive device by discharge. Ability to ascend and descend one flight of stairs independently without assistive device and with symmetric step pattern is achieved by discharge.
  - Joint play of the right ankle and foot is increased.
  - Muscle performance is increased: Muscle strength of right ankle plantarflexor and evertor muscles is increased to 4/5 and able to perform a functional squat with minimal complaints of pain in 6 to 8 weeks.
  - Postural control is improved.
  - ROM is increased in 2 to 3 weeks: Right ankle dorsi and plantarflexion is increased by 10 degrees; right inversion and eversion is increased by 10 degrees; right MTP flexion and extension is initially increased by 10 degrees and then increased to 90% of left; right ankle dorsiflexion with knee extended is increased to 10 degrees.
  - Soft tissue extensibility is improved.
  - Weightbearing status is improved: Full weightbearing on RLE is increased to 15 seconds in 2 to 3 weeks and independence in LE weightbearing is achieved by discharge.
- ◆ Impact on functional limitations
  - Ability to perform physical actions, tasks, and activities related to self-care, home management, work, community, and leisure is improved.
- ◆ Risk reduction/prevention
  - Risk factors are reduced.
- ◆ Impact on health, wellness, and fitness
  - Behaviors that promote healthy nutrition, physical activity, and wellness are acquired.
  - Fitness is improved.
  - Health status is improved.
  - Independence in the home exercise and gym programs is achieved.
  - Physical function is improved.
- ◆ Impact on societal resources
  - Documentation occurs throughout patient management and across all settings and follows APTA's *Guidelines for Physical Therapy Documentation.*[39]
- ◆ Patient/client satisfaction
  - Patient and family knowledge and awareness of the diagnosis, prognosis, interventions, and anticipated

goals and expected outcomes are increased.

- Sense of well-being and control is improved.
- Stressors are decreased.

REEXAMINATION

Reexamination is performed throughout the episode of care, particularly as the setting of care changes.

DISCHARGE

Mrs. Murphy is discharged from physical therapy after a total of 18 outpatient physical therapy sessions and attainment of her goals and expectations. These sessions have covered her entire episode of care. She is discharged because she has achieved her goals and expected outcomes.

Case Study #2: Temporomandibular Joint Dysfunction

Dr. Morgan Wright is a 48-year-old female with a diagnosis of temporomandibular joint dysfunction.

PHYSICAL THERAPIST EXAMINATION

HISTORY

- General demographics: Dr. Wright is a 48-year-old black American female. English is her primary language. She is right-hand dominant.
- Social history: She is divorced and lives near family and friends. During this time of her life, they tend to lean on her for support in various ways.
- Employment/work: Dr. Wright is a Departmental Chair at a University. This involves a long commute to and from work each day. She is involved with her community and church and is actively involved in the care of her mother.
- Living environment: Dr. Wright lives alone in her own home with two dogs.
- General health status
  - General health perception: She reports that she was in good health prior to this event.
  - Physical function: Dr. Wright has significantly decreased jaw function compared to the level she had prior to her Colles' fracture. She is not sleeping well due to her stress level and pain. Prior to this episode, she was normally active.
  - Psychological function: She tends to be frustrated

and anxious due to her current condition, bordering on possible depression.

  - Role function: Dr. Wright is both an employee and a caregiver and has focused primarily on these roles. Recently, her typical roles with leisure, community, and social activities have taken a back seat to her work and caregiving, especially since her Colles' fracture.
  - Social function: She likes to run, participate in different sports, walk her dogs, and attend the theater.
- Social/health habits: Dr. Wright was a smoker for 27 years with occasional episodes of non-smoking. She had stopped smoking prior to her wrist injury, but now smokes one to three cigarettes a day.
- Family history: Her father has adult onset DM and her mother has CAD and is status post coronary artery bypass graft (CABG).
- Medical/surgical history: She has been hospitalized for a Colles' fracture, a fibula fracture, and Lyme's disease. She has a history of cervical and lumbar dysfunction.
- Prior hospitalizations: Dr. Wright was hospitalized for the following: open reduction internal fixation (ORIF) s/p Colles' fracture 2 months ago; ORIF s/p right fibula fracture 5 years ago; and Lyme's disease 10 years ago.
- Preexisting medical and other health-related conditions: Dr. Wright has had cervical and lumbar dysfunctions secondary to prior motor vehicle accidents (MVAs). Her neck pain flares up occasionally since her whiplash injury. She uses foot orthotics for walking and running. Dr. Wright has had dental work and TMJ problems intermittently for her entire life. She reports that her dentist has noticed wear patterns on her teeth that suggest bruxism. She feels that she does grind her teeth, sometimes during the day with stress or working at the computer, but more often at night. She states that in the past she has often had pain in her jaw, L>R, upon waking. Her dentist suggested that she try self-help techniques. These have typically helped. Her dentist had recommended an appliance; however, she had never followed up with this due to time constraints and intermittent periods of relief.
- Current condition(s)/chief complaint(s): Dr. Wright experienced a recurrence of left more than right jaw pain and joint noise. Her symptoms were exacerbated over a 2-month period after slipping and falling on an outstretched right wrist and sustaining a Colles' fracture with resulting ORIF. This was due to excessive use of her jaw with chewing because she could not easily cut her food into smaller pieces. While she was in the cast for the Colles' fracture her eating habits changed significantly. Her diet generally consisted of a lot of fruit, including many hard fruits, such as apples. However, this became too painful for her and she discontinued

doing so during that time. In addition, eating fruits like oranges was difficult, if not impossible, because she could not peel the fruit with only her left hand. This also contributed to her eating softer foods, such as yogurt. Dr. Wright is now complaining of left more than right jaw pain that increases with repeated movement of the jaw, such as when talking and/or eating. The pain has been so severe that she has not been able to eat at times. She noted that when her jaw is feeling better, there is no pain at rest. She receives relief with resting in a recumbent position and when refraining from talking or eating.

♦ Functional status and activity level: Talking and eating have become so problematic that Dr. Wright has sought treatment for her jaw pain. She is not exercising (walking and/or running) as she had in the past. She is very busy with her work and caring for her mother. She also finds that she is much slower with her ADL due to the limited use of her right arm secondary to her Colles' fracture and ORIF.

♦ Medications: Motrin 400 mg qd, Tylenol as needed, and calcium 150 mg qd.

♦ Other clinical tests:
  • There has been no recent diagnostic testing for her TMJ.
  • Radiographs taken 10 years previously revealed mild degenerative changes on the left more than right mandibular condyle.

SYSTEMS REVIEW

♦ Cardiovascular/pulmonary
  • BP: 125/85 mmHg
  • Edema: There is minimal edema present in the left TMJ, cheek, and right wrist
  • HR: 75 bpm
  • RR: 22 bpm
♦ Integumentary
  • Presence of scar formation
    ▪ No scars are noted surrounding the TMJ
    ▪ A well-healed scar over palmar aspect of the right wrist is noted
  • Skin color: WNL
  • Skin integrity: Intact
♦ Musculoskeletal[7,49]
  • Gross range of motion
    ▪ Cervical spine is minimally restricted in bilateral rotation and forward flexion and moderately restricted in bilateral sidebending and extension
    ▪ TMJ is significantly restricted with s-curves, joint noise, crepitus, and a click on the L TMJ, more prominent with opening than closing
    ▪ UE ROM is WNL, except for significant restric-

tions noted for the right forearm and wrist
  • Gross strength
    ▪ Cervical spine is WFL
    ▪ Muscle imbalances are noted with FHP and with her breathing pattern
    ▪ TMJ muscle strength is inconsistent due to pain and muscle imbalances not allowing for mandibular opening and closing in midline
    ▪ UE muscle strength is WNL, except for significant weakness noted for the right forearm and wrist
  • Gross symmetry
    ▪ Asymmetry is noted with TMJ mandibular dynamics with all motions: Opening, closing, protrusion, left and right lateral deviation
    ▪ Asymmetry right wrist compared to left
    ▪ Gait asymmetrical with decreased right arm swing
  • Height: 5'10" (1.78 m)
  • Weight: 170 lbs (77.11 kg)
♦ Neuromuscular
  • Balance: Grossly WNL
  • Locomotion, transfers, and transitions
    ▪ She complains of difficulty with static balance when her jaw pain is severe
    ▪ She exhibits some fear/avoidance behaviors regarding use of her jaw and RUE
♦ Communication, affect, cognition, language, and learning style
  • Communication and cognition: Dr. Wright is alert and able to communicate her needs
  • Affect: She becomes emotional when discussing her pain and lack of function
  • Learning preferences
    ▪ She is a visual and auditory learner
    ▪ She is very anxious to learn more about her problems and assist in her recovery to full function

TESTS AND MEASURES

♦ Aerobic capacity/endurance
  • ADL and IADL: She reports being able to complete approximately 70% of her normal activities, but at a very reduced speed
  • Walking
    ▪ She is able to walk approximately 1 mile in 20 minutes
    ▪ Prior to this she was able to walk/jog 5 miles in just under 60 minutes
♦ Anthropometric characteristics
  • BMI=23.18, which is normal
  • Edema

- Moderate soft tissue edema is noted in the area of the left TMJ
- Moderate edema is noted in right wrist compared to left
- Girth right=15 cm, left=13 cm
  - Palpation: There is tenderness in the following areas: L>R masseter, SCM, temporalis, and L>R TMJ
◆ Assistive and adaptive devices
  - None noted for the TMJ
  - A soft splint is used for the right wrist prn
  - She tends to wear the splint most of the day and all night
  - Orthotic for shoes
◆ Cranial and peripheral nerve integrity: Intact for the upper quarter
◆ Environmental, home, and work barriers
  - Dr. Wright is able to access her home and work environments
◆ Ergonomics and body mechanics
  - She exhibits altered body mechanics during activities due to guarding of her head, neck, and RUE with some fear/avoidance behaviors
◆ Gait, locomotion, and balance
  - Dr. Wright ambulates independently on level surfaces and stairs, but with decreased arm swing for the RUE
◆ Integumentary integrity
  - There is increased temperature in the skin over the L>R TMJ and right wrist
  - No nail changes are noted
◆ Joint integrity and mobility[7,49,91]
  - Joint play
    - Left TMJ: Soft end feel limited by pain
    - Right TMJ: Distraction, anterior and posterior glides, and medial and lateral glides are minimally restricted
    - Cervical spine: Moderate P/A restrictions bilaterally and unilaterally in the upper cervical and mid-cervical regions and at the cervico-thoracic (C-T) junction
    - Thoracic spine: Minimal P/A restrictions bilaterally and unilaterally throughout the upper and mid-thoracic regions
    - Right superior and inferior radioulnar joints: Minimally restricted in volar and dorsal glides
    - Right radiocarpal joint: Moderately restricted with dorsal and palmar glides, minimally restricted with medial and lateral glide
    - Right carpometacarpal (CMC) joint: Moderately restricted with dorsal and palmar glides
    - Right intermetacarpal joint: Moderately restricted

with dorsal and palmar glides
    - Interphalangeal joints: WNL
◆ Motor function
  - Dexterity, coordination, and agility are decreased in the RUE
◆ Muscle performance[1,7,92]
  - Strength
    - TMJ: Appears to be decreased, but was not assessed secondary to pain level
    - Cervical and thoracic spines
      ▸ Moderately decreased strength in the deep neck flexors and extensors and general decreased stability
      ▸ Decreased upper back extension and core stabilization
    - Decreased lateral costal and diaphragmatic breathing with excessive upper chest breathing with increased use of the accessory muscles in the neck, especially the scalenes
    - Left wrist: WNL
    - Right wrist
      ▸ Flexion=3-/5
      ▸ Extension=3-/5
      ▸ Radial deviation=2/5
      ▸ Ulnar deviation=2+/5
    - Fingers
      ▸ L=WNL
      ▸ R=3+/5 for all digits.
◆ Pain: The following pain measurements have been shown to correlate well to the evaluation of TMJ dysfunction
  - 10 cm VAS[16]
    - VAS: Current pain 6 cm
    - VAS: Effort, pain from exertion (talking for 5 minutes) 8 cm
    - VAS: Minimum, least pain in preceding week 5 cm
    - VAS: Maximum, worst pain in preceding week 9 cm (chewing)
  - McGill Pain questionnaire[93] (This is a list of pain descriptors experienced over the past week and not at the present moment)
    - Dr. Wright selected 16 words out of 20 pain descriptor groups
◆ Posture
  - FHP
  - Minimal left sidebending and right rotation of head
  - Shoulders protracted
  - Right shoulder low
  - Increased C-T kyphosis, flattened mid-thoracic spine, and minimal increased lordosis[108]

◆ Range of motion
- She is unable to fully open her mouth due to decreased ROM and pain
- ROM[7,16,49,109,110] (Table 4-3)
  - Craniovertebral angle=46 degrees (average range is 42 to 54, placing this individual within the normal range)
  - Cervical ROM measured with the CROM
    - Flexion=0 to 50 degrees
    - Extension=0 to 60 degrees
    - Extension with mouth open=0 to 67 degrees
    - R sidebending=0 to 20 degrees
    - L sidebending=0 to 26 degrees
    - R rotation=0 to 70 degrees
    - L rotation=0 to 65 degrees
  - TMJ: Deviation noted with a right c-curve with slight opening and closing; right s-curve with click with increased opening and closing; right deviation with protrusion; and decreased R lateral deviation
    - Opening=0 to 20 mm, 0 to 34 mm with intermittent clunk
    - Rotation=0 to 24 mm
    - Right lateral deviation=0 to 4 mm
    - Left lateral deviation=0 to 7 mm
    - Protrusion=0 to 2 mm
  - Shoulders and elbows are WNL bilaterally
  - Forearm
    - Forearm pronation: R=0 to 40 degrees, L=0 to 80 degrees
    - Forearm supination: R=0 to 45 degrees, L=0 to 80 degrees
  - Wrist
    - Wrist flexion: R=0 to 5 degrees, L=0 to 17 degrees
    - Wrist extension: R=0 to 40 degrees, L=0 to 50 degrees
    - Ulnar deviation: R=0 to 10 degrees, L=0 to 20 degrees
    - Radial deviation: R=0 to 15 degrees, L=0 to 30 degrees
  - The left hand is WNL, the right hand is WFL
  - Fingers: All finger motions, left=WNL, right=WFL
- Muscle length assessment[7,16,49]
  - Masseter and pterygoids: Decreased right and left
  - Anterior cervical muscles: Decreased right and left
  - Upper trapezius and scalenes: Decreased right and left
  - Suboccipital muscles: Decreased right and left
  - Pectoral muscles: Decreased right and left
  - C-T paraspinals: Increased right and left
  - Decreased soft tissue extensibility, increased tone, and trigger points bilaterally in several areas in the

Table 4-3
TEMPOROMANDIBULAR MOTIONS AND MUSCLES OF MASTICATION[7,16,49,109,110]

Motion	Range of Motion	Predominant Muscle Activity
Mandibular depression (Opening of mouth) Components of opening	35 to 50 mm 60 mm upper limit	Gravity, lateral (external) pterygoid, digastric, mylohyoid, geniohyoid
Rotation	Approximately 25 mm	
Translation	Approximately 10 mm	
Mandibular elevation (Closing of mouth)	From maximal opening to full closure (centric position)	Masseter Temporalis Medial (internal) pterygoid
Mandibular protrusion	2 to 3 mm	Bilateral lateral (external) pterygoid Masseter
Mandibular retrusion	To centric position	Temporalis (posterior fibers) Digastric
Lateral deviation of the mandible	8 to 12 mm 15 mm upper limit Looking for equality side to side	Ipsilateral lateral (external) pterygoid Contralateral medial (internal) pterygoid Masseter Temporalis

jaw, face, neck, and upper back region including the temporalis, masseter, pterygoids, SCM, scalenes, upper trapezius, and C-T paraspinals
- ▶ Exceptions were the muscles of mastication where R>L soft tissue tension
♦ Reflex integrity
- Jaw reflex=2+
- Biceps, triceps, and brachioradialis reflexes=2+ bilaterally
♦ Self-care and home management
- Dr. Wright is independent in self-care and home management actions, tasks, and activities
♦ Sensory integrity: WNL
♦ Ventilation and respiration/gas exchange
- Breathing pattern
  - Decreased lateral costal and diaphragmatic breathing with excessive use of the accessory muscles in the neck
  - She states that she tends to thrust her tongue against her upper teeth especially with swallowing and upon awakening in the morning
♦ Work, community, and leisure integration or reintegration
- She is unable to participate in community and leisure actions, tasks, and activities involving prolonged walking or standing, such as going shopping

EVALUATION

Dr. Wright was previously active and is in otherwise good health. She has moderate insight into her current condition and currently has impaired TMJ function. She has pain, decreased ROM and strength, postural deviations, soft tissue restrictions, and altered mandibular dynamics. Functional limitations include limited endurance for talking and eating and diminished capacity for work, leisure, and community actions, tasks, and activities.

DIAGNOSIS

Dr. Wright has signs and symptoms of both extra-articular TMJ dysfunction and intra-articular TMJ dysfunction with pain. She has impaired: aerobic capacity/endurance; anthropometric characteristics; ergonomics and body mechanics; gait, locomotion, and balance; integumentary integrity; joint integrity and mobility; motor function; muscle performance; posture; range of motion; and ventilation and respiration/gas exchange. She is functionally limited in work, community and leisure actions, tasks, and activities. These findings are consistent with placement in Pattern D: Impaired Joint Mobility, Motor Function, Muscle Performance, and Range of Motion Associated With Connective Tissue Dysfunction.

TMJ disorders may also support classification in additional practice patterns. Since Dr. Wright also has impaired joint mobility, motor performance, and range of motion associated with the fracture of her radius and ulna, she may also be classified in Pattern G: Impaired Joint Mobility, Muscle Performance, and Range of Motion Associated With Fracture. The identified impairments and functional limitations will be addressed in determining the prognosis and the plan of care.

PROGNOSIS AND PLAN OF CARE

Over the course of the visits, the following mutually established outcomes have been determined:
♦ Ability to independently manage symptoms is enhanced
♦ Ability to perform self-care, home management, community, and leisure actions, tasks, and activities is improved
♦ Activity tolerance is improved to allow return to previous functional and leisure actions, tasks, and activities, including talking/eating and walking/jogging
♦ Cervical spine ROM is increased
♦ C-T muscles length-strength relationships are improved
♦ Edema is reduced
♦ Endurance is increased
♦ Patient is independent with home exercise program
♦ RUE ROM is increased
♦ RUE strength is increased
♦ Soft tissue extensibility and muscle tone in upper quarter are improved
♦ Static and dynamic posture is improved
♦ TMJ muscle performance is increased and balanced
♦ TMJ ROM is increased

To achieve these outcomes, the appropriate interventions for this patient are determined. These will include: coordination, communication, and documentation; patient/client-related instruction; therapeutic exercise; functional training in self-care and home management; functional training in work, community, and leisure integration or reintegration; manual therapy techniques; electrotherapeutic modalities; and physical agents and mechanical modalities.

Although there is little information on long-term functional outcomes of patients with this diagnosis, early diagnosis and treatment is recommended.[49] Dr. Wright is expected to require between 8 to 10 visits over a 2- to 3-month period of time. Dr. Wright's prognosis for rehabilitation is good for return to function based on her evaluative findings and her willingness to partake in her rehabilitation and physical therapy interventions.[39,49]

INTERVENTIONS

RATIONALE FOR SELECTED INTERVENTIONS

A multidisciplinary approach is optimal in the management of the patient with TMJ dysfunction. This team may include the physician, physical therapist, dentist, and psychologist. Medical management focuses on coordinating care and providing pain and symptomatic relief via medications if necessary and other intervention therapies.

Psychological therapies are useful in identifying psychological co-morbidities, such as anxiety and depression that may exist.[7,49] Cognitive behavioral therapies, such as pain management strategies, biofeedback, relaxation training, and guided imagery have also been used to treat patients with TMJ dysfunction.[7,49]

Physical self-regulation (Table 4-4) is a useful treatment for patients with TMJ dysfunction since it addresses a wide variety of etiologies except for patients that have experienced external trauma or occlusal dysfunctions. The approach is composed of two sections related to education and additional six sections regarding physiological training activities.[49,103,111]

Therapeutic Exercise

Physical therapist management focuses on promoting occlusal harmony and pain control with the ultimate goal of restoring function.[53] The key to successful treatment is to maintain the delicate balance between an overly vigorous approach that will exacerbate symptoms and underactivity that will lead to disuse atrophy and increased symptoms. Stressing collagen within physiologic limits provides an important stimulus for the remodeling of connective tissue. This also influences collagen alignment and formation.[4] Likewise, the optimal stimulus or stress to collagen must be applied during the rehabilitation process in the form of a graded exercise program designed to stress collagen fibers without overloading them.

As the ROM improves, appropriate strengthening exercises may be introduced to address the muscle weakness that occurs with altered posture, mandibular dynamics, and occlusal deformities.[7,49]

Patients with TMJ dysfunction respond well to a program that includes postural exercises, aerobic exercise training, and a home exercise program.[7,49,108] Postural awareness is a key component of the home exercise program. It is also important for the patient to be cognizant of labor-intensive jaw activities, such as chewing hard foods or gum and excessive talking.

Maintenance of a regular exercise program must be instilled in this patient, and the patient's outcome depends on adherence to the recommended home exercise program.

Achieving an exercise program that the patient will do on a life-long basis is vital to success.

Manual Therapy Techniques

Joint mobilization techniques are performed to restore normal joint arthrokinematics, provide normal sensory proprioceptive input, and promote synovial fluid exchange that helps maintain nutrient exchange within the joint.[103] The initial treatment consists of Grades I and II long axis distraction techniques performed with the joint in a resting position.[49,103] The patient lies supine with the head and trunk supported.[49] Since the patient's pain level is significant and increased soft tissue tension is present, the supine position is the best option to initiate treatment. Treatment is progressed based on the patient's response to treatment. Joint mobilization techniques are progressed by pre-positioning the joint at the end of the available physiological range prior to mobilization and then adding Grade IV long axis distraction techniques.[103]

Soft tissue and joint mobilization techniques are performed within the physiologic range to produce tissue remodeling.[4] Soft tissue mobilization techniques will start with gentle effleurage to the neck, upper back, jaw, and facial regions. These techniques help to mobilize edema and reduce pain by stimulating the mechanoreceptors. Based on the patient's tolerance, deeper kneading or petrissage techniques will be added to help mobilize the tissues, promote circulation, and eliminate metabolic waste from the region, particularly in the neck and upper back regions. Sustained compression or trigger point release techniques may be used to treat active trigger points in the jaw, face, neck, and upper back regions. Pressure should be maintained for up to 60 seconds to help promote muscle relaxation via muscle spindle activation and decreasing pain by stimulation of mechanoreceptors.[104]

Electrotherapeutic Modalities

Supportive treatment in the form of therapeutic modalities is directed toward mediating the symptoms and not the etiology of TMJ dysfunction. This treatment may include the use of electrical stimulation. Such supportive treatment may offer immediate relief of nociception and/or muscle guarding and may be used as an adjunct in preparation for definitive treatment. Supportive therapy is directed towards the symptoms of myalgia, arthralgia, and impaired mobility seen in all types of TMJ dysfunction.[49,112,113]

Physical Agents and Mechanical Modalities

As is the case with electrotherapeutic modalities, so it is with the use of heat, cold, or ultrasound that are directed toward mediating the symptoms and not the etiology of TMJ dysfunction. Such supportive treatment may offer immediate relief of nociception and/or muscle guarding and may be used as an adjunct in preparation for defini-

Table 4-4
PHYSICAL SELF-REGULATION

These exercises work best when you eat the right foods, drink plenty of fluids, and exercise without pain regularly. Practice I, III, IV for 2 minutes six times a day. Practice II and V anytime. Practice VI in bed before sleep.

I. Put self in position of rest: Check clenching and grinding
   1. Practice lips relaxed (usually together), tongue relaxed, teeth slightly apart for 1 minute six times a day.
   2. You are learning the position of rest for the mandible. Do not press your tongue between your teeth. That may induce fatigue.
   3. Teeth should only touch during chewing and swallowing, about 3 minutes/day if you eat for an hour.
II. Practice slow, diaphragmatic breathing
   1. Breathe slowly and regularly from your diaphragm. As you inhale, the stomach should gently rise as the diaphragm contracts. When you exhale, the stomach will move in as the diaphragm relaxes and you slowly let air out.
   2. Slow down your breathing by counting to three or four as you take air in. Then, let used air out for 3 or 4 seconds. Before inhaling again, pause for another 3 to 4 seconds. The pause is when your brain most efficiently uses O_2 and restores proper CO_2 levels to the brain and blood and lets your muscles relax. Proper CO_2 levels let more O_2 and glucose into the brain at each breath.
   3. You are learning diaphragmatic breathing, which restores blood chemistry and relaxes muscles.
   4. If at any time you begin to feel lightheaded or dizzy, you are taking in too much air. Either return to your normal breathing pattern, or better, wait longer between breaths and do not breath deeply.
   5. Remember, slow regular breathing should be very relaxing, but it may take time to relearn.
III. Monitor head position to avoid tilting
   1. Find a comfortable seat, relax your shoulders (slightly sloped but even), place hands in the open position on thighs without crossing legs, and keep head straight up. Eyes should be closed if it feels comfortable.
   2. While practicing lips relaxed, tongue relaxed, teeth slightly apart, exhale while slowly bending head forward without causing pain and then pause with head forward 3 seconds.
   3. Then inhale, taking air into your stomach as you slowly bring your head upright. Pause 1 second before exhaling and bending the head forward again. Do steps 2 and 3 six times per minute.
   4. Do not bend head sideways or bend so far forward that pain is caused. Say my head is supposed to be upright even with relaxed shoulders. When I move my head, I will use both sides of my neck equally.
   5. You are learning neutral shoulder position and improving blood supply to the area.
IV. Ease upper back tightness: Straighten rounded shoulders
   1. Raise hands up as if conducting a choir. Move arms and shoulders backward and forward without causing pain.
   2. Repeat motion slowly six times in 30 seconds.
   3. You are learning neutral shoulder position and improving blood supply to the area.
V. Take brief relaxation breaks
   1. Start with 5 minutes at a time, gradually increase relaxation time by 1 minute each session up to 20 to 25 minutes.
   2. Take at least two relaxation breaks each day during your training.
   3. You are learning to take periods of rest where the mind allows the body to rest.
VI. Begin sleep in relaxed position: Control nighttime grinding
   1. Lie on your back and practice slow breathing for 5 minutes while keeping lips relaxed and teeth slightly apart.
   2. Then say aloud six or seven times "I will not clench my teeth." Picture yourself sleeping with your mouth relaxed.
   3. Start off sleeping on your back. Don't worry if you move.

Reprinted with permission from American Association of Oral and Maxillofacial Surgeons. OMS Knowledge Update. Managing facial pain. *Anesthesia*. Vol 3. Rosemont, Ill: American Association of Oral and Maxillofacial Surgeons; 2001:1992.

tive treatment. Supportive therapies are directed toward the symptoms of myalgia, arthralgia, and impaired mobility seen in all types of TMJ dysfunction.[49,112,113]

Other

For optimal care the patient is referred back to her dentist to assess the possible benefit of occlusal therapy with an occlusal appliance or splint. The purpose of occlusal therapy is to provide a predictable and stable contact for the opposing arch. Occlusal appliances are used to protect the teeth from bruxism, promote an orthopaedically stable occlusal and condylar posture, and provide a neutral occlusal environment that may inhibit neuromuscular hypersensitization.[49,112]

COORDINATION, COMMUNICATION, AND DOCUMENTATION

Communication will occur with Dr. Wright to explain the therapeutic interventions. Documentation occurs throughout patient management and across settings and follows APTA's *Guidelines for Physical Therapy Documentation*[39] and facility guidelines. Regular communication with the referring physician will occur to provide updates on Dr. Wright's status. If Dr. Wright's fear/avoidance behaviors and emotional affect are noted to be barriers to treatment, then a referral for psychological intervention will be recommended to her physician. Dr. Wright will be referred to her dentist for assessment of her need for an occlusal appliance or splint.

PATIENT/CLIENT-RELATED INSTRUCTION

Communication will take place with Dr. Wright to explain the nature and course of her condition, the importance of adherence to a home exercise program, and the potential ramifications of non-compliance with her program.

- ◆ Dr. Wright will be instructed in a home exercise program focusing on:
  - Aerobic conditioning starting with walking on the treadmill and progressing to walking outdoors and then jogging and finally running
  - Appropriately pacing physical activity maintaining a balance between overuse and underuse
  - A self-stretching program
  - Avoiding labor-intensive jaw activities
  - Importance of diaphragmatic breathing and relaxation
  - Importance of maintaining proper posture
  - Importance of using the jaw and RUE as normally as possible and not guarding or splinting the involved area
  - PSR (see Table 4-4)
  - Strengthening exercises
- ◆ Instruction in correct body mechanics with ADL

- ◆ Dr. Wright will be encouraged to establish a variety of enjoyable activities and alternating activities when possible, to establish a realistic time frame for exercise, and to use entertainment whenever possible, such as listening to music when doing weight exercises or while walking outside and watching TV while on the treadmill
- ◆ Modeling and visual aids will be used to teach the home exercise program
  - These will include the use of a mirror for visual feedback for jaw and postural exercises

THERAPEUTIC EXERCISE

- ◆ Aerobic capacity/endurance conditioning
  - Practice jaw relaxation, deep breathing, and maintain appropriate posture when performing aerobic conditioning
  - Start with 5 to 10 minutes and progress to 30 to 45 minutes at 80% of THR for three to five times per week
  - Treadmill walking per American College of Sports Medicine Guidelines
    - Duration may be 5 minutes at first, but gradually increase
    - Exercise 3 to 5 days each week
    - Warm up for 5 to 10 minutes before aerobic activity
    - Maintain exercise intensity for 30 to 45 minutes
    - Gradually decrease the intensity of the workout, then stretch to cool down during the last 5 to 10 minutes
    - Estimate MHR and determine lower and upper limits and exercise at a HR that is between the upper and lower limits[114]
    - The Borg Rating of Perceived Exertion scale may be used once the limits have been determined[115]
  - Walking outdoors
  - Jogging outdoors
- ◆ Body mechanics and postural stabilization
  - Monitor head position
    - Keep head in a neutral position without tilting or excessive forward position to assist the performance of the exercises in the program
    - A conscious awareness of this with self-correction should be performed a minimum of six times per day, hourly, and/or as necessary
  - Shoulder position
    - Keep shoulders neutral and relaxed and perform shoulder shrugs emphasizing the relaxation portion of the exercise
    - Shoulder circles backward-forward-backward should be performed six times per day, hourly and/or as necessary

- Cervical retraction exercises
  - Start in supine with a progression to sitting
  - Perform with relaxed shoulder and jaw positions
  - Hold for 5 seconds each and repeat 5 to 10 times
  - Maintain jaw relaxation throughout exercise
  - Perform 5 to 10 repetitions twice a day, morning and evening
- Verbal cueing and use of a mirror will be incorporated to correct postural impairments
- Mandibular dynamics training
  - Use a mirror for visual feedback for opening and closing in midline
  - First practice tip-to-tip opening for maintenance of protrusion, then opening and closing in neutral
  - Initially, toothpicks can be used for ease of viewing
    - Place a toothpick gently between the center top and another toothpick between the bottom incisors when using the mirror as necessary

♦ Flexibility exercises
- Stretching exercises should be done after warming up, using a slow and steady stretch accompanied by deep breathing, and building hold up to 30 to 60 seconds
- Quadruped with wrists in neutral leaning on the fist if tolerated, or plantigrade leaning on a table or firm surface, performing alternating trunk flexion and extension for general ROM and flexibility
  - Progress to extended wrist as tolerated
- Practice opening and closing doorknobs to increase pronation and supination
- Instruct patient in self stretching for wrist flexion and extension
- Upper trapezius and scalene stretching with and without the use of a towel for stabilization
  - The towel can be draped over one shoulder and pulled with the hands while stretching is performed in the direction opposite to the towel stabilization
- Pectoral stretching
  - Scapula retraction and shoulder horizontal abduction with flexed elbow, unilaterally in a doorway at various levels of shoulder flexion or in a corner of a room with arms resting on the walls for stabilization
  - Maintain jaw relaxation throughout and monitor for anterior shoulder capsule stretch versus pectoral stretch
- Levator scapula stretching

- Sitting patient flexes, sidebends, and rotates head to the side opposite the tight muscle
  - Patient places the ipsilateral UE over the top of the head for stabilization
  - The opposite hand grasps the base of the chair and the patient leans away and slightly forward from the stabilizing hand
- Cervical retraction with minimal forward nodding of the head with jaw relaxation for suboccipital stretching
- TMJ rotation (controlled opening) with the tongue on the roof of the mouth
  - To be done two to three times a day, two to three repetitions, and held for at least 15 to 30 seconds

♦ Relaxation
- Put the jaw in the rest position and maintain throughout the day
  - The resting position of the jaw should be where the teeth are apart allowing for approximately 2 mm of freeway space (space between tips of upper and lower teeth)
  - Practice for 1 minute six times per day
- Perform jaw rotation by opening the jaw while the tip of the tongue is lightly contacting the roof of the mouth
  - Do not push forward on the teeth with the tongue and do not force the rotation motion
  - By allowing primarily rotation, the pressure on the TMJ itself can be reduced and the jaw muscles are more relaxed
- Practice slow diaphragmatic and lateral costal breathing
  - Breathe in slowly through the nose to upper chest and then more deeply to diaphragm and the lateral chest region
  - Maintain jaw relaxation with deep breathing
  - Perform six times per day with other exercises, hourly, and/or as necessary for relaxation
- Take brief relaxation breaks six times per day, hourly, and/or as necessary throughout the day
  - Verbal or audible cues may be helpful as reminders especially when starting the program
- Begin sleep in a restful and relaxed position incorporating deep breathing, proper supportive posture, and relaxed jaw position

♦ Strength, power, and endurance training
- Alternating isometrics for the jaw in neutral initially using a mirror
  - Maintain neutral posture while performing the exercises
  - Hold for 5 seconds for 5 to 10 repetitions two to

three times per day
- Tubing or pulley system exercises for the following
  - Bilateral scapula retraction in various positions
  - Shoulder flexion, abduction, and extension while maintaining axial extension
- Modified prone press-ups
- Patient sitting with forearm supported on table, grasp a hammer for resisted pronation and supination 5 to 10 repetitions two to three times per day
- Patient sitting with forearm in pronation over the end of a table. Starting with a one pound weight extend wrist against gravity 5 to 10 repetitions two to three times per day
  - Modify forearm position to allow for strengthening of wrist flexion, ulnar deviation, and radial deviation

FUNCTIONAL TRAINING IN SELF-CARE AND HOME MANAGEMENT

- ◆ Self-care and home management
  - Assessment of mandibular dynamics with talking, chewing, and posture with ADL and IADL
  - Review of home actions, tasks, and activities including simulation of activities using correct body mechanics and postural alignment
  - Review of techniques of physical self-regulation

FUNCTIONAL TRAINING IN WORK, COMMUNITY, AND LEISURE INTEGRATION OR REINTEGRATION

- ◆ Work
  - Review of work actions, tasks, and activities including simulation of activities using correct body mechanics and postural alignment
- ◆ Leisure
  - Review walking, jogging, and ADL with proper posture and jaw relaxation
  - Review of home and gym program
  - Simulated activities, such as driving and computer work in clinic with Theraband and plyoball

MANUAL THERAPY TECHNIQUES

- ◆ Massage
  - For edema and pain management
  - Light effleurage to the masseters, temporalis, and upper trapezius muscles
- ◆ Mobilization/manipulation
  - Soft tissue
    - Light effleurage and progressing to deeper muscle kneading and trigger point release techniques

as tolerated to the neck, upper back, and facial region
  - Soft tissue mobilization techniques will be performed in the early stages of treatment and gradually discontinued as the patient progresses to restoring function through activity and exercise
- Peripheral joints
  - Grades III and IV volar and dorsal glide of the proximal and distal radius on the ulna
  - Grades III and IV distraction of proximal carpals from the distal radius
  - Grades III and IV anterior, posterior, medial, and lateral glide of the proximal carpals from the distal radius
  - Grades I and II long axis distraction techniques to the TMJ with the joint in the resting position progressing to end range positions and Grades III and IV
  - Mobilization with long axis distraction and protrusion for additional joint distraction and increased protrusion
  - Medial and lateral glides of the TMJ as above to normalize capsular restrictions, TMJ ROM, and mandibular dynamics
  - Joint gliding oscillation techniques initially at Grades I and II and progressing to Grades III and IV as tolerated and based on response to treatment[7,49,91,103]

ANTICIPATED GOALS AND EXPECTED OUTCOMES

- ◆ Impact on pathology/pathophysiology
  - Pain level is decreased by three points on the VAS scale in 2 to 3 weeks and averages 1 to 2 cm by discharge.
  - Soft tissue tension in neck, upper back, and jaw muscles is decreased to WFL.
- ◆ Impact on impairments
  - Aerobic capacity is increased.
  - Endurance is improved.
  - Gait and locomotion are improved: Walking 5 to 10 minutes per day is achieved initially and at end of treatment able to walk for up to 15 minutes (approximately 1 mile) on treadmill, daily.
  - Joint mobility and soft tissue flexibility are increased.
  - Length-tension relationship of neck, upper back, and jaw muscles are such that neutral posture can be maintained during static and dynamic ADL 80% of the time.
  - Motor performance is improved as evidenced by

enhanced quality and quantity of movement between and across body segments.

- Muscle strength is improved with right wrist and fingers increased to 4/5.
- Postural control, both static and dynamic, is improved to WFL in 2 to 3 weeks and WNL by discharge.
- Relaxation is increased.
- ROM and associated soft tissue restrictions will be normalized to decrease the patient's level of pain and to eliminate the potential for future injury.
- ROM of the TMJ is increased in 2 to 3 weeks, as evidenced by opening by 10 mm, R lateral deviation by 4 mm, L lateral deviation by 2 mm, protrusion by 1 mm, and rotation by 2 mm.
- ROM of the right wrist is increased in all directions by 10 degrees in 2 to 3 weeks and will be WNL by discharge.
- ROM of the left TMJ is increased at end of treatment to within 90% of the right TMJ and all TMJ motions are WNL.
- Sensory awareness is increased.

♦ Impact on functional limitations
- Functional talking and chewing of soft foods are increased by 50% initially in 2 to 3 weeks and at end of treatment able to perform functional talking throughout a normal workday and chewing of all but hard foods without any exacerbation of TMJ dysfunction symptoms.

♦ Risk reduction/prevention
- Self-management of symptoms is improved in 2 to 3 weeks, and patient is independent by discharge.

♦ Impact on health, wellness, and fitness
- Behaviors that promote healthy nutrition, physical activity, and wellness are promoted and acquired.
- Fitness is improved.
- Health status is improved to WNL and to previous level of function.
- Independence in the home exercise and gym programs is achieved.
- Physical capacity is improved.
- Physical function is improved.

♦ Impact on societal resources
- Documentation occurs throughout patient management and across all settings and follows APTA's *Guidelines for Physical Therapy Documentation.*[39]

♦ Patient/client satisfaction
- Patient awareness and use of community resources are improved.
- Patient knowledge, awareness, and understanding of the diagnosis, prognosis, interventions, and anticipated goals and expected outcomes are increased.
- Patient knowledge of personal and environmental

factors associated with the condition is increased.
- Sense of well-being and control are improved to WNL and to a level above her previous level of function.

REEXAMINATION

Reexamination is performed throughout the episode of care.

DISCHARGE

Dr. Wright is discharged from physical therapy after a total of eight physical therapy sessions. These sessions have covered her entire episode of care. She is discharged because she has achieved her goals and expected outcomes.

Case Study #3: Fibromyalgia Syndrome

Mrs. Rosa Ruiz is a 43-year-old previously active and healthy female who has fibromyalgia syndrome.

PHYSICAL THERAPIST EXAMINATION

HISTORY

♦ General demographics: Mrs. Ruiz is a 43-year-old Cuban-American female. She is equally fluent in English and Spanish. Ms. Ruiz is right-hand dominant.

♦ Social history: She is married with three children.

♦ Employment/work: Mrs. Ruiz is a stay at home mother of three who is actively volunteering at the children's school. She had worked full-time as a lawyer until 7 years ago when her third child was born.

♦ Living environment: She lives in a home in the suburbs with her husband and three children.

♦ General health status
- General health perception: She reports that she was in good health prior to her initial diagnosis.
- Physical function: Her function is severely limited compared to before the FS.
- Psychological function: Mrs. Ruiz is depressed due to her current condition. This has gradually worsened as her symptoms of FS also worsened.
- Role function: Wife, mother, volunteer.
- Social function: She likes to attend her children's school activities and athletic events. She also loves to cook and entertain. However, at this time if she entertains in her home she will be in bed for 2 to 3 days afterwards. If she goes shopping one day, then she will

most likely have to spend the next day in bed.

♦ Social/health habits: She is a nonsmoker and drinks alcohol on a social basis.

♦ Family history: Her father has had myocardial infarctions, and her mother has HTN, scleroderma, RA, and Raynaud's syndrome.

♦ Medical/surgical history: Mrs. Ruiz had febrile convulsions until she was 5 years of age. Eleven years ago she had sarcoidosis with a left pulmonary sarcoid. She had unexplained infertility and took Pergonal injections for ovarian hyperstimulation. This resulted in three pregnancies, the last one with twins. She was on bedrest for 2 months and miscarried one of the fetuses. Her FS was exacerbated after the birth of her third child. She recently developed irritable bowel syndrome and has occasional migraines.

♦ Prior hospitalizations: Mrs. Ruiz was hospitalized previously due to a tonsillectomy and the births of her children.

♦ Preexisting medical and other health-related conditions: The patient has sarcoidosis, irritable bowel syndrome, and migraine headaches.

♦ Current condition(s)/chief complaint(s): Mrs. Ruiz first started having problems at the age of 23 and was given the diagnosis of multiple sclerosis by two different neurologists at the age of 26. She did not have any specific intervention at that time. Five years later she was referred to a rheumatologist who gave her the diagnosis of FS. She recently experienced a flare-up of her symptoms of FS and was referred to physical therapy by her rheumatologist. She is now complaining of increased pain and fatigue. The pain can be located throughout her body and does not follow any predictable pattern following her activities. She has not been doing any regular exercise and would like to improve her condition and ability to complete her ADL.

♦ Functional status and activity level: Mrs. Ruiz is now barely functioning in order to complete her ADL. She has to take frequent rests and is not even walking for exercise because it feels like it is too much for her.

♦ Medications: For the past 6 weeks Mrs. Ruiz has taken Advil or Aleve as needed.

  • She had been on various other medications in the past, including the following:

    ▪ Elavil 10 to 20 mg qd at night for 5 years, Paxil 10 mg qd for 1 year, and serotonin.

    ▪ The serotonin was discontinued due to an adverse skin reaction.

    ▪ She has also discontinued the other two drugs as well due to increasing side effects of "fog myalgia" and heart palpitations.

♦ Other clinical tests

  • Mrs. Ruiz just completed 2 weeks of wearing a Holter monitor.

• She had experienced tachycardia and vertigo and fainted three times within the past few months.

• It was determined that her heart function was WNL.

SYSTEMS REVIEW

♦ Cardiovascular/pulmonary
  • BP: 130/80 mmHg
  • Edema: None
  • HR: 78 bpm
  • RR: 18 bpm

♦ Integumentary
  • Presence of scar formation: None
  • Skin color: WNL
  • Skin integrity: Intact
  • Mrs. Ruiz reports Raynaud-like symptoms

♦ Musculoskeletal
  • Gross range of motion: BUEs and BLEs on the low end of WFL and limited by pain
  • Gross strength: BUEs and BLEs 4-/5 and limited by pain
  • Gross symmetry: Grossly equal for BUEs and BLEs
  • Height: 5'1" inch (1.55 m)
  • Weight: 115 lbs (52.16 kg)

♦ Neuromuscular
  • She is independent with balance, locomotion, transfers, and transitions, but is slow and performs them with obvious discomfort
  • Her gait appears somewhat slow and laborious, but is WFL

♦ Communication, affect, cognition, language, and learning style
  • Communication and cognition: Mrs. Ruiz is alert and able to communicate her needs
  • Affect: She becomes emotional when discussing her pain and lack of function
  • Learning preferences: She learns best via both verbal and visual means

TESTS AND MEASURES

♦ Aerobic capacity/endurance
  • 6-Minute Timed Walk test: She tolerated 4 minutes and completed almost three laps of 60 meters each, reporting 4 on the Borg scale prior to testing and 6 after testing[116]
  • Timed stair climbing-descent test: She was able to complete one flight of stairs slowly and with increased pain and fatigue[117]

♦ Anthropometric characteristics
  • BMI=21.7 (this is considered to be in the normal range)[118]
  • No edema or nail changes are noted

- The skin of both her hands and feet are noted to be cool
♦ Assistive and adaptive devices
  - No assistive devices are noted at the time of the initial evaluation
♦ Cranial and peripheral nerve integrity
  - Sensation intact to light touch in all four extremities
♦ Environmental, home, and work barriers
  - She is able to access her home, although she has difficulty with stairs and often tries to avoid them when she is in severe pain
♦ Ergonomics and body mechanics
  - Mrs. Ruiz has altered body mechanics during her activities due to her generalized guarding and fear/avoidance behavior
♦ Gait, locomotion, and balance
  - Mrs. Ruiz ambulates independently
  - She is able to stand statically on both feet for 50 seconds with eyes opened
  - She is unable to tolerate unilateral stance
  - Dynamic balance not assessed
♦ Joint integrity and mobility[91]
  - Joint play: Not assessed due to the patient's level of pain
  - The end feels were generally soft and limited by pain
♦ Motor function
  - Dexterity, coordination, and agility WFL in both UEs and LEs
♦ Muscle performance[67,92]
  - Grip strength with a hand-held dynamometer was 22 kg for the left hand and 32 kg for the right hand
    - This is considered poor with the average norm for both hands combined being 59 to 64 kg[119,120]
  - UE MMT revealed 4-/5 strength throughout
  - LE MMT revealed 4/5 strength throughout, except for 4-/5 for bilateral hamstrings
♦ Pain
  - Palpation revealed the following pattern of tenderness and trigger points, bilaterally: Suboccipital region, upper trapezius, scalenes, SCM, supraspinatus, lateral epicondyle more than medial epicondyle region, costochondral junctions, thoracolumbar paraspinal region, gluteals, piriformis, greater trochanter, tensor fascia lata, distal hamstrings, and gastrocsoleus
  - 10 cm VAS[92-94]
    - VAS: Current pain 9 cm
    - VAS: Effort, pain from exertion (ADL) 10 cm
    - VAS: Minimum, least pain in preceding week 4 to 5 cm

  - VAS: Maximum, worst pain in preceding week 10+ cm (with ADL)
- Stanford Health Assessment questionnaire and Fibromyalgia Impact questionnaire[67]
  - Tolerance of disease=3/10 (10=tolerating very well)
  - Assessment of disease activity=severe (scale=none, mild, moderate, severe)
  - Assessment of ability to rest/sleep=3/10 (10=best sleep ever)
  - Fatigue level=8/10 (10=worst fatigue possible)
- McGill Pain questionnaire[93] (list of pain descriptors experienced over the past week and not at the present moment)
  - She selected 14 words out of 20 pain descriptor groups
♦ Posture
  - Mrs. Ruiz has a FHP, rounded shoulders, minimal increased kyphosis, and minimally decreased lordosis in standing
  - In sitting her posture is slouched
  - She is not comfortable standing for very long during the assessment of her posture
♦ Range of motion[16,67]
  - UEs on the low end of WFL and limited by pain
  - LEs on the low end of WFL and limited by pain
  - Muscle length, soft tissue extensibility, and flexibility[16,67]
    - Generalized decreased muscle length, decreased soft tissue extensibility, increased tension and trigger points throughout the body as noted previously and with complaints of pain during assessment[67]
♦ Reflex integrity
  - DTRs WNL bilaterally
♦ Self-care and home management
  - She is independent in self-care and home management actions, tasks, and activities, but at a decreased level from previously
♦ Sensory integrity: WFL bilaterally
♦ Work, community, and leisure integration or reintegration
  - Often unable to participate in community and leisure actions, tasks, and activities for more than a few hours without having to be in bed for 2 to 3 days after the event or activity
  - Health Status questionnaire SF-36 used to assess health status and physical function[94]
    - Mrs. Ruiz's score was 80 which is considered low[121]

EVALUATION

Mrs. Ruiz has had limited activity for an extended period of time and thus her return to function will be gradual. She has moderate insight into her condition and currently has limitations including the following: pain; decreased ROM, strength, and flexibility; soft tissue restrictions; altered posture and gait; and decreased endurance. Mrs. Ruiz's functional limitations include decreased ability to perform IADL and diminished capacity for leisure and community actions, tasks, and activities.

DIAGNOSIS

Mrs. Ruiz is a patient with FS and diffuse pain. She has impaired: aerobic capacity and endurance; ergonomics and body mechanics; gait, locomotion, and balance; joint integrity and mobility; muscle performance; posture; and range of motion. She is functionally limited in self-care and home management and in work, community, and leisure actions, tasks, and activities. These findings are consistent with placement in Pattern D: Impaired Joint Mobility, Motor Function, Muscle Performance, and Range of Motion Associated With Connective Tissue Dysfunction. Fibromyalgia may also support classification in additional practice patterns. The identified impairments and functional limitations will be addressed in determining the prognosis and the plan of care.

PROGNOSIS AND PLAN OF CARE

Over the course of Mrs. Ruiz's visits, the following mutually established outcomes have been determined:
♦ Ability to perform self-care, home management, community, and leisure actions, tasks, and activities is improved
♦ Activity tolerance is improved to allow return to most previous functional and leisure actions, tasks, and activities
♦ Endurance is improved
♦ Gait is improved
♦ Independent management of relaxation, energy conservation, and joint protection are increased
♦ Independent management of symptoms is increased
♦ Muscle length tension relationships are improved
♦ Muscle performance is increased
♦ ROM is increased
♦ Soft tissue extensibility is increased

To achieve these outcomes, the appropriate interventions for this patient are determined. These will include: coordination, communication, and documentation; patient/client-related instruction; therapeutic exercise; functional training in self-care and home management; functional training in work, community, and leisure integration or reintegration; manual therapy techniques; and electrotherapeutic modalities.

There is little information on long-term functional outcomes of patients with FS. The studies that have been completed demonstrate that pain, tender points, and significant functional loss may persist over time.[67,72,122,123] Prognosis is thought to be better with early diagnosis and treatment.[67,123] Mrs. Ruiz is expected to require between 18 and 26 visits over a 3- to 4-month period of time. Mrs. Ruiz's prognosis and rehabilitation are fair to good due to the chronic nature of her problem.

INTERVENTIONS

RATIONALE FOR SELECTED INTERVENTIONS

A multidisciplinary approach is important in the management of the patient with FS. This team may include the physician, physical therapist, occupational therapist, psychologist, social worker, case manager, nurse, or vocational rehabilitation counselors.[67]

Therapeutic measures that could prove useful are biofeedback, meditation, acupuncture, injection of tender points with local anesthetic or corticosteroids, modalities including heat or cold (depending on patient preference), massage, and exercise. These methods of treatment do not have extensive well-controlled trials; however, cardiovascular fitness,[123] EMG biofeedback,[124] cognitive-behavior interventions,[125,126] and hypnosis[127] have been studied.[67] Interestingly, hypnosis was determined to be better than physical therapy in 40 patients with refractory fibromyalgia.[127] The hypnosis group demonstrated better outcomes in pain, fatigue, and patient global assessment of pain. However, this did not prove to be the case in the tender points group.[67]

Psychological therapies are useful in identifying psychological co-morbidities that exist, such as anxiety and depression.[67] Goldenberg recommends referral for psychological or psychiatric work up because 25% of patients with fibromylagia do manifest concurrent psychopathology.[72] Cognitive behavioral therapies, such as pain management strategies, biofeedback, relaxation training, and guided imagery have also been used to treat patients with FS.[67,72]

Physical therapy management for FS focuses on the following: enhancing peripheral and central analgesia, improving sleep disturbances, diminishing mood disturbances, and increasing blood flow to muscle and superficial tissues.[72]

Patient/Client-Related Instruction

Education is of paramount importance in the successful treatment of FS. This includes education of both the patient and the family. Freundlich and Leventhal[128] highly

Table 4-5
APPROACHES TO HELP ACHIEVE SELF-EFFICACY IN FIBROMYALGIA

1. Perform exercises that suit your ability and interest including mild aerobic exercises.
2. Select a healthy balanced diet, no caffeine, no heavy meals within 3 hours of bedtime. Stop smoking and alcohol ingestion.
3. Avoid habits that aggravate and overuse muscles by pacing and prioritizing tasks and activities.
4. Develop consistent sleep habits: Go to bed and arise at the same time every day.
5. When medication for sleep is needed, take it with the evening meal to reduce hangover effect the next morning.
6. Get professional help and develop strategies to live with chronic pain.
7. Use coping strategies to manage stress.
8. Do not expect miracles. Set reachable goals within several months, not days or hours.

Reprinted with permission from Sheon RP, Moskowitz RW, Goldberg VM. *Soft Tissue Rheumatic Pain*. 3rd ed. Baltimore, Md: Williams & Wilkins; 1996:286. Copyright 1996, Williams & Wilkins Publishers.

recommended that the initial approach to treatment should include patient education and reassurance with respect to two important issues. First, the patient needs to be informed that FS is not a psychiatric disturbance and secondly, that it is not a rare disorder. Furthermore, the physical therapist should reassure the patient that it is not deforming or life threatening, although it frequently becomes a chronic condition that requires the patient to become the chief manager of her disease. Measures for helping the patient to improve self-efficacy are presented in Table 4-5.[67,129]

Therapeutic Exercise

The physical therapist utilizes therapeutic exercise to promote the proper amount of activity and pain control with the ultimate goal of restoring function.[67,72] The key to successful treatment is to maintain the delicate balance between an overly vigorous approach that will exacerbate symptoms and underactivity that will lead to disuse atrophy and increased symptoms. Stressing collagen within physiologic limits provides an important stimulus for the remodeling of connective tissue. This also influences collagen alignment and formation.[4] Likewise in the rehabilitation of this patient, the optimal stimulus or stress to collagen must be applied in the form of a graded exercise program to stress collagen fibers without overloading them.

Various investigators have suggested that exercise training is beneficial for the treatment of FS.[67,123,128-137] A therapeutic exercise regimen that is reported to be beneficial by most patients is aquatic therapy. Some authors have described a water therapy protocol for fibromyalgia syndrome that focuses on total body fitness, stretching, and strengthening specific areas of the body.[138] The authors suggested the protocol include deep-water warm-up, deep-water interval training, waterpower exercises, stationary kicking training, stretching, UE exercises, and swimming or assisted swimming. For patients who find that any kind of pounding activity makes their tender points worse, non-weightbearing exercises like swimming or riding a stationary bicycle are ideal.[9]

A stationary bicycle may be used to promote aerobic conditioning and LE ROM and strengthening. Maintenance of a regular exercise program must be instilled in this patient, and the patient's outcome depends on adherence to the recommended appropriate home exercise program. Achieving an exercise program that the patient will do on a life-long basis is vital to success.

The results of studies regarding exercise training for FS indicate that persons who exercise demonstrate improvement in such variables as work capacity, physical endurance, tender point pain threshold, and psychological stress indicators. While these reports are welcomed, there are limitations evident including small sample sizes; questions related to duration, frequency, and intensity of exercise; and lack of longitudinal data of the effects of exercise on FS. It appears that those studies where formal coping skills training in pain management are combined with exercise training can help individuals effectively manage FS.[9,130-139]

Additional types of exercises that may be beneficial for the patient with FS are presented in Table 4-6 and include aerobic exercise, aquatic therapy, and Tai Chi.[67,129]

Manual Therapy Techniques

Soft tissue mobilization techniques are performed within physiologic range to produce tissue remodeling.[4] Manual techniques that might be tried (according to the tolerance of the patient) are massage, myofascial release, and pressure techniques for tender points. The patient should be taught self-management techniques with such aids as a tennis ball or frozen water balloon to help with pressure friction massage techniques.[67]

Electrotherapeutic Modalities

Electrotherapeutic modalities, such as biofeedback, have been included as part of a successful intervention strategy

	Table 4-6
	EXERCISES FOR FIBROMYALGIA

Exercise	Parameters
Stretching	Low intensity; low repetitions, slow duration.
Posture alignment	Breathing exercises, correct body alignment and body mechanics, sleep postures and positioning, movement education such as Feldenkrais or Alexander techniques.
Manual techniques	Myofascial release; pressure point massage; self-treatment techniques with tennis balls, frozen water balloons, or frozen ice cups.
Tai Chi	A form of Eastern exercises that are slow and sequential and allow the person to learn relaxation skills, peace of mind, increase flexibility, improve endurance, and decrease his or her pain.
Aerobic exercise	Encourage a fitness program that can be tolerated by the patient and one he or she will adhere to regularly. Combining the use of the pool, an exercycle at home, walking program, and videotapes with non-impact aerobic exercises to be done from 1 to 10 minutes, each exercise allows a full 30-minute exercise program. The patient should be taught to monitor his or her HR and exertion.
Aquatic therapy	Very good for stretching activities, walking for 20 to 30 minutes, and aerobic conditioning for those persons who do not tolerate land exercises well. Use of flotation devices may be useful.
Adherence	Lifestyle and exercise changes, periodic tune-ups for adherence and outcome assessment, exercise logs, reminder phone calls, regular progress reports, buddy system.

Reprinted with permission from Sheon RP, Moskowitz RW, Goldberg VM. *Soft Tissue Rheumatic Pain.* 3rd ed. Baltimore, Md: Williams & Wilkins; 1996:287. Copyright 1996, Williams & Wilkins Publishers.

for patients with FS. Ferraccioli and associates[124] found that persons who completed an EMG-biofeedback training program (vs those who completed a sham EMG-biofeedback program) improved significantly in decreasing pain, morning stiffness, and tender points.

COORDINATION, COMMUNICATION, AND DOCUMENTATION

A coordinated, multidisciplinary approach is important in the management of the patient with FS. The team may include the physician, physical therapist, occupational therapist, psychologist, social worker, and vocational rehabilitation counselor as appropriate. Medical management focuses on coordinating care and providing pain and symptomatic relief via medications and other intervention therapies.

Communication will occur with Mrs. Ruiz's family as needed to explain therapeutic interventions. All elements of the patient's management will be documented following APTA and facility guidelines. Regular communication with the referring physician and with her psychologist will occur to provide updates on Mrs. Ruiz's status.

PATIENT/CLIENT-RELATED INSTRUCTION

The nature and course of her condition, the importance of adherence to an appropriate home exercise program, and the potential ramifications of not following through with her home program will be provided to Mrs. Ruiz.

Mrs. Ruiz will be instructed in her home exercise program focusing on:

♦ The importance of maintaining aerobic conditioning

♦ A progressive plan of home exercises to increase strength, improve flexibility, and improve endurance

♦ Appropriately pacing physical activity maintaining a balance between overuse and underuse with energy conservation

♦ Importance of protecting her joints, but using her extremities as normally as possible

♦ Identification of community resources, including groups

if appropriate, for stress management, relaxation, Tai Chi, aquatic therapy, and yoga

♦ Importance of maintaining a stretching program

♦ Importance of performing relaxation techniques on a regular basis

♦ Instruction in correct body mechanics with ADL and IADL

Mrs. Ruiz will be encouraged to establish a variety of enjoyable and alternating activities when possible, to establish a realistic time frame for exercise and to use entertainment whenever possible when doing exercises. She can use music when exercising or walking, she can walk outside with friends or family members, and she can watch TV while on the stationary bicycle or treadmill. Modeling and visual aids will be used as necessary to teach the home exercise program.

THERAPEUTIC EXERCISE

♦ Aerobic capacity/endurance conditioning[140]

- Stationary bicycle, walking and/or treadmill for aerobic conditioning

  - Duration: 10 minutes initially, progressing to 30 or 45 minutes with time based exercise progression

  - Intensity: Moderate raising HR to 60% of maximum [0.60 x (220–age)=100 beats per minute][140]

  - Frequency: Initially three times a week and progressing to five times a week

- Aquatic program

  - Mode: Water walking, pool exercises, and/or swimming with time based exercise progression

  - Frequency: Initially can be done in place of one of the above-mentioned aerobic capacity/endurance conditioning exercises and increased in frequency as tolerated by the patient

♦ Body mechanics and postural stabilization

- Postural awareness retraining and postural stabilization exercises

- Standing alignment instruction using a full-length mirror for feedback

- Practice lifting and carrying objects of varying sizes and weights, starting with small, light objects, while maintaining a neutral lumbar spine and neutral wrist position

- Quadruped, kneeling, sitting, and standing exercises that incorporate postural stabilization during extremity movements

♦ Flexibility exercises

- Stretching exercises should be done after warming up, using a slow and steady stretch accompanied by deep breathing, and building hold up to 15 to 30 seconds

- Performed two to three times per day, at least two to three repetitions, rather than performing only once per day for 5 to 10 repetitions

- UE and LE stretches

- PNF principles including contract-relax and hold-relax within UE and LE patterns

- Emphasis on areas that are most involved with tender points and limited mobility

- Performed within patient's tolerance

- Trunk flexibility and mobility

  - Quadruped flexion and extension exercise holding flexion for 5 to 10 seconds, gently moving into extension and holding for 5 to 10 seconds and then repeating the entire sequence three to five times

- Neck and upper back flexibility and mobility

  - Upper trapezius stretch: Tuck chin and gently tip the left ear to the left shoulder while keeping the arms relaxed at the side, holding for 15 to 30 seconds, repeating two to three times on each side

  - Gently perform half circles for the head and neck, letting the chin drop to the left and then bringing to the right and repeating three to five times to each side

  - Keeping head in a neutral and relaxed position, gently rotate both shoulders backward 5 to 10 times

- LE stretching

  - In supine, flex hip to 90 degrees and stabilize behind thigh with both UEs, gently extend LE as far as tolerated 5 to 10 times

  - In standing, heel cord stretch

    ‣ Lunge position with forward LE flexed and back LE extended at the hip and knee and heel on the floor

    ‣ Stabilize trunk with both hands on the wall

    ‣ Lean forward to stretch the back calf

♦ Strength, power, and endurance training

- Vary program to maintain patient motivation throughout course of treatment

- Any combination, as appropriate, of the exercises below can be used in conjunction with an aerobic and flexibility exercise program

  - Light resistance to all extremity movements: free weights, therapeutic band or tubing, or manual resistance

  - Progressive resisted exercises (one to three sets of 10 repetitions for each exercise)

    ‣ Quadriceps: Starting with 10 RM weight for SLR, isotonic knee extension in sitting (90 degrees flexion to full extension, concentric and eccentric), and terminal knee extension in supine with thigh support (30 degrees flexion to full extension, concentric and eccentric) and progressing ankle cuff weights as indicated over time

> ▶ Modify positions to allow for strengthening of all additional LE muscles

- Closed chain exercises
- Use of therapeutic balls for sitting and standing exercises for stabilization, postural awareness, balance, and transfers
- LE eccentric exercise, such as partial squat
- Bilateral scapula retraction in standing with trunk stabilization for 10 repetitions
- PNF techniques and patterns can be used in functional positions

FUNCTIONAL TRAINING IN SELF-CARE AND HOME MANAGEMENT

- ◆ Self-care and home management
  - Review of home and work actions, tasks, and activities, including simulation of activities using correct body mechanics and postural alignment
  - Review of energy conservation techniques

FUNCTIONAL TRAINING IN WORK, COMMUNITY, AND LEISURE INTEGRATION OR REINTEGRATION

- ◆ Leisure
  - Review of leisure actions, tasks, and activities, including simulation of activities using correct body mechanics and postural alignment
  - Review of energy conservation techniques
  - Be active and have fun at the same time
  - Plan family outings and vacations to include physical activity
  - Review of pool and gym program

MANUAL THERAPY TECHNIQUES

- ◆ Soft tissue mobilization
  - Light effleurage and petrissage progressing to deeper muscle kneading and trigger point release techniques as tolerated to the involved areas
  - Soft tissue mobilization techniques will be performed in the early stages of treatment and gradually discontinued as the patient progresses to restoring function through activity and exercise

ELECTROTHERAPEUTIC MODALITIES

- ◆ Biofeedback training to decrease pain, morning stiffness, and tender points

ANTICIPATED GOALS AND EXPECTED OUTCOMES

- ◆ Impact on pathology/pathophysiology
  - Pain level is decreased by 2 cm on the VAS in 2 to 3 weeks and averages 3 to 4 cm by discharge.
- ◆ Impact on impairments
  - Aerobic capacity is increased.
  - Endurance is improved.
  - Energy expenditure per unit of work is decreased.
  - Gait and locomotion is improved as evidenced by walking initially 15 minutes four times per week in 2 to 3 weeks and increasing to walking 30 minutes four to five times per week by discharge.
  - Joint mobility and soft tissue flexibility are increased to WFL by discharge.
  - Muscle performance as measured by improved strength and power is increased and quality and quantity of movement between and across body segments is improved to WFL by discharge.
  - Postural alignment, control, and awareness during actions, tasks, and activities are improved.
  - Relaxation is increased.
  - ROM and associated soft tissue restrictions are normalized to decrease the patient's level of pain and to eliminate the potential for future injury.
  - Sensory awareness is increased.
- ◆ Impact on functional limitations
  - Ability to retain, improve, and perform physical actions, tasks, and activities related to self-care, home management, work, community, or leisure is improved.
  - Functional independence in ADL and IADL is increased.
  - Level of supervision required for task performance is decreased to moderate in 2 to 3 weeks and no supervision is required at discharge.
  - Tolerance of positions and actions, tasks, and activities is improved.
- ◆ Risk reduction/prevention
  - Disability associated with acute or chronic illnesses is reduced.
  - Self-management of symptoms is improved so that patient is independent at discharge.
- ◆ Impact on health, wellness, and fitness
  - Behaviors that promote health, physical activity, and wellness are promoted and acquired.
  - Decision making is enhanced regarding patient health and the use of health care resources by patient, family, significant others, and caregivers.
  - Fitness is improved.
  - Health status is improved.

- Independence in the home exercise and gym programs is achieved.
- Physical capacity is improved.
- Physical function is improved.

♦ Impact on societal resources
  - Documentation occurs throughout patient management and across all settings and follows APTA's *Guidelines for Physical Therapy Documentation.*[39]
  - Utilization of physical therapy services will be optimized.
  - Utilization of physical therapy services will result in efficient use of health care dollars.

♦ Patient/client satisfaction
  - Access, availability, and services provided are acceptable to the patient.
  - Awareness and use of community resources are improved.
  - Clinical proficiency of the physical therapist is acceptable to the patient.
  - Communication will optimize attainment of the goals.
  - Coordination of care is acceptable to the patient.
  - Patient and family knowledge, awareness, and understanding of the diagnosis, prognosis, interventions, and anticipated goals and expected outcomes are increased.
  - Patient knowledge of personal and environmental factors associated with the condition is increased.
  - Sense of well-being and control is improved.
  - Stress level as she resolves the SUI is reduced.
  - Stressors are decreased to WFL.

REEXAMINATION

Reexamination is performed throughout the episode of care.

DISCHARGE

Mrs. Ruiz is discharged from physical therapy after a total of 24 physical therapy sessions over 14 weeks. These sessions have covered her entire episode of care. She is discharged because she has achieved her goals and expected outcomes.

REFERENCES

1. Rosse C, Gaddum-Rosse P. *Hollinshead's Textbook of Anatomy.* 5th ed. Philadelphia, Pa: Lippincott-Raven; 1997.
2. Culav EM, Clark CH, Marilee MJ. Connective tissues: matrix composition and its relevance to physical therapy. *Phys Ther.* 1999;79:308-310.
3. Levangie PK, Norkin CC. *Joint Structure and Function: A Comprehensive Analysis.* 3rd ed. Philadelphia, Pa: FA Davis Co; 2001.
4. Hertling H, Kessler RM. *Management of Common Musculoskeletal Disorders: Physical Therapy Principles and Methods.* 3rd ed. Philadelphia, Pa: Lippincott; 1996.
5. Nordin M, Frankel VH. *Basic Biomechanics of the Musculoskeletal System.* 3rd ed. Philadelphia, Pa: Lippincott Williams & Wilkins; 2001.
6. Oatis CA. *Kinesiology: The Mechanics and Pathomechanics of Human Movement.* Philadelphia, Pa: Lippincott Williams & Wilkins; 2003.
7. Bennett AC. Temporomandibular disorder and orofacial pain. In: HSC 13.3.5 *Physical Therapy for the Cervical Spine and Temporomandibular Joint.* Orthopaedic Section, APTA, Inc, 2003.
8. Gross AR, Aker PD, Goldsmith CH, Peloso P. Physical medicine modalities for mechanical neck disorders. *Cochrane Database Syst Rev.* 2000;2:CD000961.
9. Mueller MJ, Maluf KS. Tissue adaptation to physical stress: a Proposed "physical stress theory" guide to physical therapist practice, education, and research. *Phys Ther.* 2002;82:383-403.
10. Kennedy JC, Alexander AJ, Hayes KC. Nerve supply of the human knee and its functional importance. *Am J Sports Med.* 1982;10:329-335.
11. Solomonow M, Baratta R, Zhou BH, et al. The synergistic action of the anterior cruciate ligament and thigh muscles in maintaining joint stability. *Am J Sports Med.* 1987;15:207-213.
12. Lephart SM, Warner JJP, Borsa PA, Fu FH. Proprioception of the shoulder joint in healthy, unstable, and surgically repaired shoulders. *J Shoulder Elbow Surg.* 1994;3:371-380.
13. Guanche C, Knatt T, Solomonow M, Lu Y, Baratta R. The synergistic action of the capsule and shoulder muscles. *Am J Sports Med.* 1995;23:301-306.
14. Garn SN, Newton RA. Kinesthetic awareness in subjects with multiple ankle sprains. *Phys Ther.* 1988;11:1667-1671.
15. Cyriax JH. *Textbook of Orthopaedic Medicine, Vol 1. Diagnosis of Soft Tissue Lesions.* 8th ed. London, England: Balliere Tindall; 1982.
16. Magee DJ. *Orthopedic Physical Assessment.* 4th ed. Philadelphia, Pa: WB Saunders; 2002.
17. Salter RB. *Textbook of Disorders and Injuries of the Musculoskeletal System.* 3rd ed. Baltimore, Md: Williams & Wilkins; 1999.
18. Akeson WH, Amiel D, Abel MF, Garfin SR, Woo SL. Effects of immobilization on joints. *Clin Orthop.* 1987;219:28-37.
19. Woo SL, Gomez MA, Sites TJ, Newton PO, Orlando CA, Akeson WH. The biomechanical and morphological changes in the medial collateral ligament of the rabbit after immobilization and remobilization. *J Bone Joint Surg (Am).* 1987;69:1200-1211.
20. Schollmeier G, Sarkar K, Fukuhara K, Uhthoff HK. Structural and functional changes in the canine shoulder after cessation of immobilization. *Clin Orthop.* 1996;323:310-315.
21. Jarvinen TA, Jozsa L, Kannus P, Jarvinen TL, Jarvinen M. Organization and distribution of intramuscular connective tissue in normal and immobilized skeletal muscles. An immunohistochemical, polarization and scanning electron miscropic study. *J Muscle Res Cell Motil.* 2002;23:245-254.
22. Haapala J, Arokoski J, Pirttimaki J. Incomplete restoration

of immobilization induced softening of young beagle knee articular cartilage after 50-week remobilization. *Int J Sports Med.* 2000;21:76-81.

23. Matsumato F, Trudel G, Uhthoff HK, Backman D. Mechanical effects of immobilization on the Achilles' tendon. *Arch Phys Med Rehabil.* 2003;84:662-667.

24. Kvist M, Hurme T, Kannus P, et al. Vascular density at the myotendinous junction of the rat gastrocnemius muscle after immobilization and remobilization. *Am J Sports Med.* 1995:23:359-364.

25. Kiviranta I, Tammi M, Jurvelin J, Arokoski J, Saamanen AM, Helminen HJ. Articular cartilage thickness and gly-cosaminoglycan distribution in the young canine knee joint after remobilization of the immobilized limb. *J Orthop Res.* 1994;12:161-167.

26. Haapala J, Arokoski J, Pirttimaki J, et al. Remobilization does not fully restore immobilization induced articular cartilage atrophy. *Clin Orthop.* 1999;362:218-229.

27. Currier DP, Nelson RM. *Dynamics of Human Biologic Tissues.* Philadelphia, Pa: FA Davis Co; 1992.

28. Kanuus P. Immobilization or early mobilization after an acute soft tissue injury? *Physician Sportsmedicine.* 2000;28:55-56,59-60,62-63.

29. Hayashi K. Biomechanical studies of the remodeling of knee joint tendons and ligaments. *J Biomech.* 1996;29:707-716.

30. Barr AE, Barbe MF. Pathophysiological tissue change associated with repetitive movement: a review of the evidence. *Phys Ther.* 2002;82:173-188.

31. Khan KM, Cook JL, Taunton JE, Bonar F. Overuse tendinosis, not tendinitis. Part 1: a new paradigm for a difficult clinical problem. *Physician Sportsmedicine.* 2000;28:38-48.

32. Cook JL, Khan KM, Maffulli N, Purdam C. Overuse tendinosis, not tendinitis. Part 2: applying the new approach to patellar tendinopathy. *Physician Sportsmedicine.* 2000;28:31-32,35-36,39-41.

33. Goodman C, Kelly Snyder TE. The endocrine and metabolic systems. In: Goodman CC, Boissonnault WG, Fuller KS, eds. *Pathology Implications for the Physical Therapist.* 2nd ed. Philadelphia, Pa: WB Saunders; 2003.

34. Schulte L, Roberts MS, Zimmerman C, Ketler J, Simon LS. A quantitative assessment of limited joint mobility in patients with diabetes. Goniometric analysis of upper extremity passive range of motion. *Arthritis Rheum.* 1993;36:1429-1443.

35. Spanheimer RG, Umpierrez GE, Stumpf V. Decreased collagen production in diabetic rats. *Diabetes.* 1988;37:371-376.

36. Athanasiou KA, Fleischli JG, Bosma J, et al. Effects of diabetes mellitus on the biomechanical properties of human ankle cartilage. *Clin Orthop.* 1999;368:182-189.

37. Rote NS. Inflammation. In: McCance KL, Huether SE, eds. *Pathophysiology. The Biologic Basis for Disease in Adults and Children.* 4th ed. St. Louis, Mo: Mosby; 2002.

38. Lehman TJ. Childhood rheumatic diseases. In: Paget SA, Gibofsky A, Beary JF, eds. *Manual of Rheumatology and Outpatient Orthopedic Disorders. Diagnosis and Therapy.* 4th ed. Philadelphia, Pa: Lippincott, Williams &Wilkins; 2000.

39. American Physical Therapy Association. Guide to Physical therapist practice. 2nd ed. *Phys Ther.* 2001;81:9-744.

40. Galer BS, Schwartz L, Allen RJ. Complex regional pain syndromes—type I: reflex sympathetic dystrophy, and type II: causalgia. In: Loeser JD, ed. *Bonica's Management of Pain.* 3rd ed. Philadelphia, Pa: Lippincott Williams & Wilkins; 2000.

41. Gellman H, Markiewitz AD. Reflex sympathetic dystrophy. In: Brotzman SB, Wilk KE, eds. *Clinical Orthopaedic Rehabilitation.* 2nd ed. St. Louis, Mo: Mosby; 2003.

42. Rho RH, Brewer RP, Lamer TJ, Wilson PR. Complex regional pain syndrome. *Mayo Clin Proc.* 2002;77:174-180.

43. Oerlemans HM, Oostendorp RAB, de Boo T, Perez RS, Goris RJ. Signs and symptoms in complex regional pain syndrome type I/reflex sympathetic dystrophy: judgement of the physician versus objective measurement. *Clin J Pain.* 1999;15:224-232.

44. Bruehl S, Lubenow TR, Nath H, Ivankovich O. Validation of thermography in the diagnosis of reflex sympathetic dystrophy. *Clin J Pain.* 1996;12:316-325.

45. Mense S, Simons DG. *Muscle Pain: Understanding Its Nature, Diagnosis and Treatment.* Philadelphia, Pa: Lippincott, Williams & Wilkins; 2001.

46. Strakowski JA, Wiand JW, Johnson EW. Upper limb musculoskeletal pain syndromes. In: Braddom RL, ed. *Physical Medicine and Rehabilitation.* 2nd ed. Philadelphia, Pa: WB Saunders; 2000.

47. Clarke NG, Townsend GC. Distribution of nocturnal bruxing patterns in man. *J Oral Rehabil.* 1984;11:717-721.

48. Trenouth MJ. The relationship between bruxism and temporomandibular joint dysfunction as shown by computer analysis of nocturnal tooth contact patterns. *J Oral Rehabil.* 1979;6:81-87.

49. Mormile CS. Evaluation and treatment of temporomandibular dysfunction from a multidisciplinary perspective. In: HSC 13.3.6 *Physical Therapy for the Cervical Spine and Temporomandibular Joint.* Orthopaedic Section, APTA, Inc, 2003.

50. Rocabado M. Arthrokinematics of the temporomandibular joint. *Dent Clin North Am.* 1983;27:573-594.

51. Helkimo M. Epidemiologica surveys of dysfunction of the masticatory system. *Oral Science Review.* 1976;7:54-69.

52. Turk DC, Rudy TE. A dual-diagnostic approach assess TMD patients. *J Mass Dent Soc.* 1995;44:16-19.

53. Fricton JR, Nelson A, Monsein M. IMPATH: microcomputer assessment of behavioral and psychosocial factors in craniomandibular disorders. *Cranio.* 1987;5:372-381.

54. Levitt SR, Mckinney MW, Lundeen TF. The TMJ scale: cross-validation and reliability studies. *Cranio.* 1988;6:17-25.

55. Macfarlane TV, Gray RJM, Kinsey J, et al. Factors associated with temporomandibular disorder, pain dysfunction syndrome (PDS): Manchester case-control study. *Oral Dis.* 2001;7:321-330.

56. Seligman DA, Pullinger AG. A multiple stepwise logical regression analysis of trauma history and 16 other history and dental cofactors in females with temporomandibular disorders. *Journal of Orofacial Pain.* 1996;10:351-361.

57. Lundh H, Westesson PL. A three-year follow-up of patients with reciprocal temporomandibular clicking. *Oral Surg Oral Med Oral Pathol Oral Radiol Endod.* 1987;63:530-533.

58. Castro L. Importance of occlusal status in the research diagnostic criteria of craniomandibular disorders. *Journal of Orofacial Pain.* 1995;9:98.

59. Katzberg, RW, Westesson PL, Tallents RH, et al. Anatomical disorders of the temporomandibular joint disc in asymptomatic subjects. *J Oral Maxillofac Surg.* 1996;54:147-153.

60. De Laat A, Soontjens N. Association between oral habits and signs/symptoms of temporomandibular disorders in Flemish adolescent girls (in process citation). *J Oral Rehabil.* 2002;29:884.

61. Ciancaglini R, Testa M, Radaelli G. Association of neck pain with symptoms of temporomandibular dysfunction in the general adult population. *Scandinavian Journal of Rehabilitation Medicine.* 1999;31:17-22.

62. Curran SL, Carlson CR, Okeson JP. Emotional and physiological responses to laboratory challenges: patients with temporomandibular disorders versus matched control subjects. *Journal of Orofacial Pain.* 1996;10:141-150.

63. Harper RP, Schneiderman E. Condylar movement and centric relation in patients with internal derangement of the temporomandibular joint. *J Prosthet Dent.* 1996;75:67-71.

64. Elfving L, Helkimo M, Magnusson T. Prevalence of different temporomandibular joint sounds, with emphasis on disc-displacement in patients with temporomandibular disorders and controls. *Swed Dent J.* 2002;26:9-19.

65. Leader JK, Boston JR, Rudy TE, et al. The influence of mandibular movements on joint sounds in patients with temporomandibular disorders. *J Prosthet Dent.* 1999;81:186-195.

66. John MT, Zwijnenberg AJ. Interobserver variability in assessment of signs of TMD. *International Journal of Prosthodontics.* 2001;14:265-270.

67. Moncur C. Fibromyalgia syndrome. In: HSC 12.2.1 *Orthopaedic Interventions for Selected Disorders.* Orthopaedic Section, APTA, Inc, 2002.

68. Yunus MB, Masi AT, Calabro JJ, Miller KA, Feigenbaum SL. Primary fibromyalgia (fibrositis): clinical study of 50 patients with matched normal controls. *Semin Arthritis Rheum.* 1981;11:151-157.

69. Campbell SM, Clark S, Tindall EA, Forehand ME, Bennett RM. Clinical characteristics of fibrositis. I. A "blinded," controlled study of symptoms and tender points. *Arthritis Rheum.* 1983;26:817-824.

70. Wolfe F, Smythe HA, Yunus MB, et al. The American College of Rheumatology 1990 criteria for the classification of fibromyalgia. Report of the multicenter criteria committee. *Arthritis Rheum.* 1990;33:160-172.

71. Gowers WR. A lecture on lumbago. Its lessons and analogues. *BMJ.* 1904;1:117-121.

72. Goldenberg DL. Fibromyalgia. In: Klippel JH, Dieppe PA, eds. *Rheumatology.* London, England: Mosby-Year Book Ltd; 1994.

73. Crofford L, Demitrack M. Evidence that abnormalities of central neurohormonal systems are key to understanding fibromyalgia and chronic fatigue syndrome. *Rheum Dis Clin North Am.* 1996;22:267-284.

74. Martínez-Lavín M, Hermosillo A, Rosas M, et al. Circadian studies of autonomic nervous balance in patients with fibromyalgia. *Arthritis Rheum.* 1998;41:1966-1971.

75. Steinbach LS, Palmer WE, Schweitzer ME. MR Arthrography. *Radiographics.* 2002;22:1223-1246.

76. Schneider R. Diagnostic imaging techniques. In: Paget SA, Gibofsky A, Beary JF, eds. *Manual of Rheumatology and Outpatient Orthopedic Disorders. Diagnosis and Therapy.* 4th ed. Philadelphia, Pa: Lippincott, Williams & Wilkins; 2000.

77. Paget SA, Gibofsky A, Beary JF, eds. *Manual of Rheumatology and Outpatient Orthopedic Disorders. Diagnosis and Therapy.*

78. Speed CA. Corticosteroid injections in tendon lesions. *BMJ.* 2001;18:382-386.

79. Paavola M, Kannus P, Jarvinen TA, Jarvinen TL, Jozsa L, Jarvinen M. Treatment of tendon disorders. Is there a role for corticosteroid injection? *Foot Ankle Clin.* 2002;7:501-513.

80. Boissonnault WG, Goodman C. Bone, joint and soft tissue disorders. In: Goodman CC, Boissonnault WG, Fuller KS, eds. *Pathology Implications for the Physical Therapist.* 2nd ed. Philadelphia, Pa: Saunders; 2003.

81. Smith MB. The peripheral nervous system. In: Goodman CC, Boissonnault WG, Fuller KS, eds. *Pathology Implications for the Physical Therapist.* 2nd ed. Philadelphia, Pa: Saunders; 2003.

82. Goldenberg DL. Treatment of fibromyalgia syndrome. *Rheum Dis Clin North Am.* 1989;15:91-104.

83. Goldenberg DL, Felson DT, Dinerman H. A randomized controlled trial of amitryptaline and naproxen in the treatment of patients with fibromyalgia. *Arthritis Rheum.* 1986;29:1371-1377.

84. Russell IJ, Fletcher EM, Michalek JE, et al. Treatment of primary fibrositis/fibromyalgia syndrome with ibuprofen and alprazolam. A double-blind placebo-controlled study. *Arthritis Rheum.* 1991;35:552-560.

85. Carrette S, Bell MJ, Reynolds WJ, et al. Comparison of amitryptaline, cyclobenzaprine and placebo in the treatment of fibromyalgia: a randomized, double-blind clinical trial. *Arthritis Rheum.* 1994:37;32-40.

86. Bennett RM, Gatter RA, Campbell SM, et al. A comparison of cyclobenzaprine and placebo in the management of fibrositis: a double-blind controlled study. *Arthritis Rheum.* 1988;31:1535-1542.

87. Freundlich B, Leventhal L. Diffuse pain syndromes: the fibromyalgia syndrome. In: Klippel JH, ed. *Primer on the Rheumatic Diseases.* Atlanta, Ga: Arthritis Foundation; 1997:123-127.

88. World Health Organization. *Preventing and Managing the Global Epidemic of Obesity: Report of the World Health Organization Consultation of Obesity.* Geneva, Switzerland: WHO; 1997.

89. USDA Center for Nutrition Policy and Promotion. Body mass index and health. *Nutrition Insights.* 2000;March.

90. Perez RS, Oerlemans HM, Zuurmond WW, De Lange JJ. Impairment level sumscore for lower extremity complex regional pain syndrome type I. *Disabil Rehabil.* 2003;25:984-991.

91. Kaltenborn FM. *Manual Mobilization of the Joints. Volume I: The Extremities.* 5th ed. Oslo, Norway: Olaf Norlis Bokhandel; 1999.

92. Palmer ML, Epler ME. *Fundamentals of Musculoskeletal Assessment Techniques.* 2nd ed. Philadelphia, Pa: Lippincott, Williams & Wilkins; 1998.

93. Melzak R. The McGill pain questionnaire: major properties and scoring methods. *Pain.* 1975;1:277-299.

94. Guccione A. Functional assessment. In: O'Sullivan SB, Schmitz TJ, eds. *Physical Rehabilitation Assessment and Treatment.* 4th ed. Philadelphia, Pa: FA Davis Co; 2001.

95. Schasfoort FC, Bussmann JB, Stam HJ. Outcome measures for complex regional pain syndrome type I: an overview in the context of the international classification of impairments,

disabilities and handicaps. *Disabil Rehabil.* 2000;22:387-398.

96. Lee BH, Scharff L, Sethna NF et al. Physical therapy and cognitive–behavioral treatment for complex regional pain syndromes. *J Pediar.* 2002;141:135-140.

97. Sherry DD, Wallace CA, Kelley C, Kidder M, Sapp L. Short- and long-term outcomes of children with complex regional pain syndrome type I treated with exercise therapy. *Clin J Pain.* 1999;15:218-223.

98. Kemler MA, Rijks CP, de Vit HC. Which patients with chronic reflex sympathetic dystrophy are most likely to benefit from physical therapy? *Journal of Manipulative and Physiological Therapeutics.* 2001;24:272-278.

99. Berger P. The role of the physiotherapist in the treatment of complex peripheral pain syndromes. *Pain Reviews.* 1999;6:211-232.

100. Oerlemans HM, Oostendorp RA, de Boo T, van der Laan L, Severens JL, Goris JA. Adjuvant physical therapy versus occupational therapy in patients with reflex sympathetic dystrophy/complex regional pain syndrome type I. *Arch Phys Med Rehabil.* 2000;81:49-56.

101. Martin G. Aquatic therapy in rehabilitation. In: Prentice WE, Voight MI, eds. *Techniques in Musculoskeletal Rehabilitation.* New York, NY: McGraw-Hill; 2001.

102. Stanton-Hicks M, Baron R, Boas R, et al. Complex regional pain syndromes: guidelines for therapy. *Clin J Pain.* 1998;14:155-166.

103. Kisner C, Colby LA. *Therapeutic Exercise. Foundations and Techniques.* 4th ed. Philadelphia, Pa: FA Davis Co; 2002.

104. Domenico G, Wood EC. *Beard's Massage.* 4th ed. Philadelphia, Pa: WB Saunders; 1997.

105. Travel JG, Simons DG. *Myofascial Pain and Dysfunction. The Trigger Point Manual.* Baltimore, Md: Williams & Wilkins; 1983.

106. Hooshmand H. *Chronic Pain Reflex Sympathetic Dystrophy Prevention and Management.* Boca Raton, Fla: CRC Press; 1992.

107. Maitland GD. *Peripheral Manipulation.* 3rd ed. Boston, Mass: Butterworth-Heinemann; 1991.

108. Kraus SL, ed. *Temporomandibular Disorders.* New York, NY: Churchill Livingstone; 1994.

109. Norkin CC, White DJ. *Measurement of Joint Motion: A Guide to Goniometry.* 2nd ed. Philadelphia, Pa: FA Davis Co; 1995.

110. Richardson JK, Iglarsh ZA. *Clinical Orthopaedic Physical Therapy.* 2nd ed. Philadelphia, Pa: WB Saunders; 2006.

111. American Association of Oral and Maxillofacial Surgeons. Anesthesia, "Managing Facial Pain." *OMS Knowledge Update.* 2001;3:92.

112. Okeson JP. *Management of Temporomandibular Disorders and Occlusion.* 5th ed. St. Louis, Mo: Mosby; 2003.

113. Dawson PE. *Evaluation, Diagnosis, and Treatment of Occlusal Problems.* 2nd ed. St. Louis, Mo: Mosby; 1989.

114. American College of Sports Medicine Guidelines. Available at: http://www.acsm.org/index.asp. Accessed September 21, 2004.

115. Borg GAV. Psycho-physical bases of perceived exertion. *Med Sci Sports Exerc.* 1982;14:377-381.

116. American Thoracic Society. ATS statement: guidelines for the Six-Minute Walk test. *Am J Respir Crit Care Med.* 2002;166:111-117.

117. Hunt S, McEwen S. Measuring health status: a new tool for clinicians and epidemiologists. *JR Coll Gen Pract.* 1985;35:185-188.

118. Body mass index. Available at: http://www.nhlbi.nih.gov/about/oei/index.htm. Accessed December 10, 2004.

119. Grip strength. Available at: http://faculty.camdencc.edu/pdilorenzo/102home_files/GRIPSTRENGTHTESTNORMS.doc. Accessed December 10, 2004.

120. Hanten WP, Chen WY, Austin AA, et al. Maximum grip strength in normal subjects from 20 to 64 years of age. *J Hand Ther.* 1999;12(3):193-200.

121. Ware JE Jr, Snow KK, Kosinski M, Gandek B. *SF-36 Health Survey Manual and Interpretation Guide.* Boston, Mass: The Health Institute, NEMC; 1993.

122. Felson DT, Goldenberg DL. The natural history of fibromyalgia. *Arthritis Rheum.* 1986;20:1522-1526.

123. Hawley DJ, Wolfe F, Cathey MA. Pain, functional disability and psychological status: a 12-month study of severity in fibromyalgia. *J Rheumatol.* 1988;15:1551-1556.

124. Ferraccioli G, Ghiereli L, Scita F. EMG-biofeedback training in fibromyalgia syndrome. *J Rheumatol.* 1987;14:820-825.

125. Nielson WR, Walker C, McCain GA. Cognitive behavioral treatment of fibromyalgia syndrome: preliminary findings. *J Rheumatol.* 1992;19(1):99-103.

126. Bradley LA. Cognitive behavioral therapy for primary fibromyalgia. *J Rheumatol.* 1989;19:131-136.

127. Haanen HCB, Hoenderdos HTW, van Romunde LKJ, et al. Controlled trial of hypnotherapy in the treatment of refractory fibromyalgia. *J Rheumatol.* 1991;18:2-75.

128. Freundlich B, Leventhal L. Diffuse pain syndromes: the fibromyalgia syndrome. In: Klippel JH, ed. *Primer on the Rheumatic Diseases.* Atlanta, Ga: Arthritis Foundation; 1997:123-127.

129. Sheon RP, Moskowitz RW, Goldberg VM. *Soft Tissue Rheumatic Pain.* 3rd ed. Baltimore, Md: Williams & Wilkins; 1996:287.

130. Bennett RM, Clark SR, Goldberg L, et al. Aerobic fitness in patients with fibrositis. *Arthritis Rheum.* 1989;32:454-460.

131. Mannerkorpi K, Burckhardt CS, Bjelle A. Physical performance characteristics of women with fibromyalgia. *Arthritis Care Research.* 1994;7:123-129.

132. Jacobsen S, Holm B. Muscle strength and endurance compared to aerobic capacity in primary fibromyalgia syndrome. *Clin Exp Rheumatol.* 1992;10:419-420.

133. Jacobsen S, Danneskiold-Samsoe B. Dynamic muscular endurance in primary fibromyalgia compared with chronic myofascial pain syndrome. *Arch Phys Med Rehabil.* 1992;72:170-173.

134. Jacobsen S, Danneskiold-Samsoe B. Isometric and isokinetic muscle strength in patients with fibrositis syndrome. *Scand J Rheumatol.* 1987;16:61-65.

135. Mengshoel AM, Forre O, Komnaes HB. Muscle strength and aerobic capacity in primary fibromyalgia. *Clin Exp Rheumatol.* 1990;8:475-479.

136. Mengshoel AM, Komnaes HB, Forre O. The effects of 20 weeks of physical fitness training in female patients with fibromyalgia. *Clin Exp Rheumatol.* 1992;10:345-349.

137. Clark SR. Prescribing exercise for fibromyalgia patients. *Arthritis Care Research.* 1994;7:221-225.

138. Nichols DS, Glenn TM. Effects of aerobic exercise on pain perception, affect, and level of disability in individuals with fibromyalgia. *Phys Ther.* 1994;74:327-332.

139. Martin L, Nutting A, MacIntosh BR, Edworthy SM, Butterwick D, Cook J. An exercise program in the treatment of fibromyalgia. *J Rheumatol.* 1996;23:1051-1053.

140. McArdle WD, Katch FI, Katch VL, eds. *Exercise Physiology.* 4th ed. Baltimore, Md: Williams & Wilkins; 1996.

CHAPTER FIVE

Impaired Joint Mobility, Motor Function, Muscle Performance, and Range of Motion Associated With Localized Inflammation (Pattern E)

Roslyn Sofer, MA, PT, OCS

ANATOMY

The tissues involved with this practice pattern include muscle, tendon, fascia, joint capsule, synovial membrane, and bursa. The anatomy and physiology of skeletal muscle are discussed in Pattern C: Impaired Muscle Performance and Pattern I: Impaired Joint Mobility, Motor Function, Muscle Performance, and Range of Motion Associated With Bony or Soft Tissue Surgery. The anatomy and physiology of the connective tissues of the musculoskeletal system are found in Pattern D: Impaired Joint Mobility, Motor Function, Muscle Performance, and Range of Motion Associated With Connective Tissue Dysfunction.

PHYSIOLOGY

PHASES OF HEALING

The healing process begins immediately post trauma and is divided into three phases: inflammatory response, fibroblastic repair, and maturation/remodeling. The time frames for these phases overlap one another and therefore cannot be thought of as having definitive beginnings or endings.

Decisions on how and when to treat, treatment alterations, and treatment progression must be based not only on the time frames of the phases of healing but also on the patient's signs and symptoms[1] (Figure 5-1).

Inflammatory Response Phase: 2 to 4 Days Post Initial Injury

The signs and symptoms of this phase are redness, swelling, tenderness, and increased temperature around the injured area. The original injury damages individual cells causing a release of chemicals. This chemical release initiates the inflammatory response. In order to localize and/or dispose of injury byproducts and exudates (ie, blood and damaged cells), leukocytes and other phagocytic cells are brought to the injured tissue. This process is called phagocytosis and sets the stage for the repair process. The inflammatory response phase may be divided into local vascular effects, fluid exchange, and alterations and migration of leukocytes from blood to the tissues.[1]

Local Vascular Effects

The immediate vascular response is vasoconstriction that lasts for 5 to 10 minutes. Spasm of the local blood vessels presses the endothelial linings of each side together, producing a localized decrease in blood flow. This is followed by vasodilation that creates a transitory increase in blood flow. The vasodilation then slows the blood flow in the area. This slower blood flow eventually progresses to stagnation and

TISSUE HEALING PROCESS

Inflammatory Response Phase
Local Vascular Effects
Fluid Exchange Effects
Leukocyte Migration

Fibroblastic Repair Phase
Scar Formation

Maturation-Remodeling Phase
Collagen Fiber Realignment

Figure 5-1. Stages of the healing process of musculoskeletal tissues.

stasis of blood and plasma. This initial effusion lasts for approximately 24 to 36 hours.

The next part of the vascular response is clot formation. When the blood vessel is injured, the collagen fibers are exposed and the platelets and leukocytes adhere to them, eventually forming clots. These clots obstruct the lymphatic fluid drainage and localize the injury response. The release of a protein molecule called thromboplastin from the damaged cell begins the process of clot formation. This molecule changes prothrombin to thrombin, which converts fibrinogen into a sticky fibrin clot that closes down the blood supply to the injured area. Clot formation occurs approximately 12 hours after injury and is completed within about 48 hours.

Fluid Exchange

As the vascular response is occurring, there is a release of chemicals that helps to limit the amount of exudates and swelling post injury. Vasodilation and increased cell permeability occur as a result of the release of histamine and leukotaxin from the injured mast cells. The chemical necrosin is responsible for phagocytic activity. The amount of post-injury edema is directly dependent on the number of blood vessels that are injured.

Leukocyte Migration

The result of the above processes is the walling off of the injured area during the inflammatory stage of healing. The fibroblastic stage begins when the leukocytes migrate into the area and phagocytize most of the foreign debris.

Fibroblastic Repair Phase

This phase begins within the first few hours post injury and may last as long as 4 to 6 weeks. Scar formation occurs during this phase. The lack of oxygen getting to the tissue causes endothelial capillary buds to start to grow into the wound. These buds bring oxygen and nutrients to the area

so that the wound may heal aerobically and regenerate tissue. As the fibrin clot breaks down, a delicate network of connective tissue called granulation tissue forms. Granulation tissue consists of fibroblasts, collagen, and capillaries. It is usually a reddish mass of granular connective tissue that fills in the gaps during the healing process.

As capillaries continue to grow into the area, fibroblasts accumulate at the wound site, arranging themselves parallel to the capillaries. They synthesize an extracellular matrix consisting of protein fibers, collagen fibers, and elastin. At about the sixth or seventh day, the fibroblasts also begin producing collagen fibers that are deposited in a random fashion throughout the forming scar. As the collagen proliferates, the tensile strength of the wound increases. The wound strength is proportional to the rate of collagen synthesis. As the tensile strength increases, the number of fibroblasts decreases. At this point, minimal scar tissue has been formed and the maturation phase begins.

There is a gradual decrease in the signs and symptoms of inflammation although tenderness to palpation and pain with movements that stress the area of injury may continue. With continued scar formation, this tenderness and pain gradually lessen and then disappear.[1]

Maturation-Remodeling Phase

This phase may take up to several years to complete. During this stage, the collagen fibers that make up the scar tissue are remodeled according to the tensile forces that are applied. Breakdown and synthesis of collagen is ongoing, with a steady increase in the tensile strength of the scar matrix. The principle of specific adaptation to imposed demand (SAID) states that the body remodels soft tissue, such as ligament and tendon, as a response to alterations in external loading. As the tissue is subjected to specific stresses and strains, the collagen fibers are realigned parallel to the lines of tension for maximum strength and efficiency.[2] By the end of the third week, the scar is fairly strong and the tissue gradually assumes normal appearance and function, although the scar is rarely as strong as the normal tissue.[1]

Chronic Inflammation

Inflammation is considered to be chronic when the acute inflammatory response is not successful at eliminating the cause of the inflammation and restoring the tissue to its normal physiological equilibrium. When inflammation becomes chronic, the leukocytes are replaced with macrophages, lymphocytes, and plasma cells that accumulate in the loose connective tissue matrix in the area of the injury. This accumulation causes chronic edema. Presently there is no explanation for why acute inflammation converts to chronic inflammation. It may be due to continued microtrauma secondary to overuse or overload of a particular structure. There is no specific time frame in which acute inflammation converts to the chronic classification. Chronic inflammation is usually resistant to both physical and pharmacological treatments.

When the inflammatory response is persistent, there is continued release of inflammatory products that creates extended fibroplasias and excessive fibrogenesis. These may lead to irreversible tissue damage. If fibrosis occurs in synovial structures, conditions such as adhesive capsulitis of the shoulder may develop. If fibrosis occurs in extra-articular tissues such as tendons, ligaments, bursa, and muscles, lack of flexibility and/or decreased strength may occur.[1]

General Factors that May Delay Healing

The following factors may all delay the healing process:
- ♦ Age: With increased age, cellular regeneration requires more time.
- ♦ General health: As the number of health issues with which the body has to deal increases, the less effectively it can cope with the additional stress of a musculoskeletal injury.
- ♦ Inadequate protein, vitamins, and excessive heavy metals in the system: This will affect the body's ability to synthesize new tissue.
- ♦ Local infection: This will not allow the inflammatory process to resolve.
- ♦ Presence of co-morbidities, such as diabetes and peripheral vascular disease: Effective vascularization is of prime importance to tissue healing. If these are compromised, healing will be compromised.
- ♦ Tobacco and/or alcohol use: Use of these substances creates vascular compromise.
- ♦ Type of tissue: Each tissue type has its own healing time.[3]

PATHOPHYSIOLOGY

For the pathophysiology related to the joint capsule and the synovial membrane, see Pattern D: Impaired Joint Mobility, Motor Function, Muscle Performance, and Range of Motion Associated With Connective Tissue Dysfunction.

Disease, injuries, and the normal aging processes have an effect on each of the tissues of the musculoskeletal system. Primary injury to these tissues may be either acute or chronic. They may occur as a result of macro- or microtrauma. Macrotrauma is defined as an acute trauma with immediate pain and disability. Examples of macrotrauma include fractures, dislocations, sprains, strains, and contusions. Microtrauma is defined as overuse injuries due to repetitive overloading of a tissue or repetitive use of a tissue with incorrect mechanics. Examples of microtrauma include myositis, tendinitis, tenosynovitis, fasciitis, synovitis, bursitis, or neuritis. Regardless of the cause of the trauma (micro or macro), once an injury has occurred, all of these tissues follow a similar pattern of healing.[1]

INJURIES TO MUSCLES

Muscle injuries involve contusions, lacerations, strains, compartment syndromes, and denervation. The most common muscle injury is a strain. Strains occur when the musculotendinous unit is either overstretched or forced to contract against excessive resistance. If the muscle's extensibility or tensile capabilities are exceeded, there may be damage to the muscle fibers, the musculotendinous junction (most common), the tendon, or the tendinous attachment to bone. Strains are classified into first, second, or third degree.[1] Table 5-1 delineates the classification of strains.

Characteristics of Muscle Strain

Muscle strain has a history of acute onset. The mechanism of injury may be due to overstretch or excessive loading. Pain is localized to the area of injury that is often in the vicinity of the musculotendinous junction. In severe cases, there may be discoloration due to pooling of blood distal to the site of injury. Muscle weakness may be present if the strain is second or third degree.

The hallmark symptom is pain with muscle contraction.

		Table 5-1	
SIGNS AND SYMPTOMS OF FIRST-, SECOND-, AND THIRD-DEGREE MUSCLE STRAINS			
Signs or Symptoms	*First Degree*	*Second Degree*	*Third Degree*
Muscle fiber injury	A few muscle fibers are torn	Almost half of muscle fibers are torn	Complete tear of all muscle fibers (rupture)
Weakness	Mild	Moderate to severe	Severe
Muscle spasm	Mild	Moderate to severe	Severe
Loss of function	Mild	Moderate to severe	Severe
Swelling	Mild	Moderate to severe	Moderate to severe
Palpable defect	No	No	Yes
Pain with contraction	Mild	Moderate to severe	None to mild
Pain with stretching	Yes	Yes	No
PROM	Limited	Limited	May be limited due to edema

	Table 5-2		
SIGNS AND SYMPTOMS OF FIRST-, SECOND-, AND THIRD-DEGREE MUSCLE CONTUSIONS			
Signs or Symptoms	First Degree	Second Degree	Third Degree
Tissue damage	More superficial tissues are crushed	Superficial and some deeper tissues are crushed	Deeper tissues are crushed; fascia surrounding muscle may rupture, allowing swollen muscle tissue to protrude
Weakness	None	Mild to moderate	Moderate to severe
Muscle spasm	None	None	Sometimes
Loss of function	Mild	Moderate	Severe
Ecchymosis	Mild	Moderate	Severe
Swelling	Mild	Moderate	Severe
PROM	Unaffected	Mild limitation	Moderate to severe limitation due to swelling

Depending on the degree of the strain, there also may be pain when the muscle is stretched and pain with palpation of the muscle belly.

Characteristics of Muscle Contusion

Muscles may also be subject to contusions as a result of a direct blow. Contusions are classified into first-, second-, and third-degree injuries. Table 5-2 delineates the classification of contusions.

Muscle contusions are characterized by the presence of edema and discoloration. Pain is found with palpation of the injured area, with muscle contraction, and with stretch of the muscle belly. The pain is often local to the area of injury.[4]

Muscle Healing

The healing process of muscles is similar to that of other tissues. Initially, hemorrhage and edema are followed almost immediately by phagocytosis to clear debris. Within a few days, there is proliferation of ground substance and fibroblasts begin producing a gel-type matrix that surrounds the connective tissue, leading to fibrosis and scarring. Simultaneously, myoblastic cells form in the area of injury that eventually leads to regeneration of new myofibrils. This begins regeneration of both connective and muscle tissue.

Regardless of the severity of the strain, the time required for rehabilitation is lengthy, usually longer than for ligament sprains. These debilitating strains often occur in larger muscle groups such as the hamstrings and the quadriceps. Treatment may take 6 to 8 weeks. Return to full activity too soon often causes reinjury.

Healing after a muscle contusion follows the general inflammatory healing process as previously described. One complication that may occur after a muscle contusion is myositis ossificans (also referred to as heterotopic ossification or HO). Small pieces of calcium are deposited in the injured area. These deposits may significantly impair active and passive mobility.[1]

INJURIES TO TENDONS

Tendons may be injured at the musculotendinous junction, in the body of the tendon itself, or at the bony insertion site. A tendon may be completely or partially torn, inflamed, or strained. When tension is generated in a tendon at a slow rate, injury is more likely to occur at the tendon-bone junction than at other regions. At a faster rate of tension development, the actual tendon is the more common site of failure. For the total muscle tendon unit, the most likely site of injury is either the muscle belly or the myotendinous junction.[5]

Tendinitis is a general term that has been used to describe many different pathologic conditions of a tendon. Tendinitis, according to the American Academy of Orthopedic Surgeons, replaces the old terminology of tendon strain or tear. It is defined as a symptomatic degeneration of the tendon with vascular disruption and an inflammatory response.[6]

Almekinders and colleagues[7] did a systematic review of etiology, diagnosis, and treatment of tendinitis. The authors noted that the diagnosis of tendinitis, that is, actual inflammation of tendon tissue, is not seen clearly in patho-anatomic studies. The authors further stated that conclusive evidence was not found to confirm repetitive mechanical load as a major factor in the etiology of tendinitis.

Paratenonitis is a term used to replace tenosynovitis, tenovaginitis, and peritendinitis. It is an inflammation of the paratenon only, regardless of the presence or absence of a synovial lining.[7] These conditions may occur when the tendon rubs over a bony prominence or is subjected to friction forces as it travels through tight spaces. In these areas of high friction, the tendons are usually surrounded by synovial sheaths that decrease the friction of movement. If the tendon that is gliding through a synovial sheath is subject to overuse, inflammation may occur. Inflammation most commonly occurs but is not limited to the flexor digitorum superficialis at the wrist or hand, flexor digitorum profundus at the wrist or hand, and the biceps tendon at the shoulder. The inflammatory process produces byproducts that are sticky and tend to cause the sliding tendon to adhere to the synovial sheath surrounding it.[1] The histological findings in paratenonitis are inflammatory cells in the paratenon or peritendinous areolar tissue.

If the tendinitis is chronic there will be evidence of tendon degeneration, loss of normal collagen structure, and loss of cellularity in the area, but absolutely no signs of an inflammatory response in the tendon. The cellular response involves replacement of leukocytes with macrophages and plasma cells.[1]

Symptoms depend on the severity of the dysfunction of the tendon. The hallmark symptom is pain with muscle contraction that causes a pull on the tendon. The amount of resistance necessary to elicit pain decreases as the amount of inflammation increases. Additional symptoms that may occur include pain when the tendon is stretched, pain with palpation of the tendon, edema in the area around the tendon, and crepitus. Crepitus is a crackling sound usually caused if the paratenon adheres to the surrounding structures when the tendon is moving. The chemical products of inflammation that accumulate in the irritated tendon may cause adhesions that will limit the extensibility of the tendon.[1]

There is no exact method of distinguishing between a muscle and tendon dysfunction except by areas of tenderness; that is, a tendon dysfunction may be tender over the tendon itself or the musculotendinous junction, but not over the muscle belly.

Tendinosis is a condition in which the tendon shows significant degenerative changes, possibly due to aging, microtrauma, or vascular compromise. There are no clinical or histological signs of inflammation.[1]

Although tendon dysfunctions may occur in any tendon, there are areas of the body that are particularly susceptible. In the UE, the most common areas of tendinous lesions are the supraspinatus and long head of biceps brachii (which are often involved in impingement syndromes); pronator teres and flexor carpi radialis (also known as medial epicondylitis, golfer's elbow, racquetball elbow, swimmer's elbow, and Little League elbow); extensor carpi radialis brevis (also known as lateral epicondylitis or tennis elbow); and abductor pollicus longus and extensor pollicus brevis (also known as de Quervain's tenosynovitis).[1] In the LE, the most common areas of tendinous lesions are the rectus femoris, iliopsoas, hamstrings near their distal attachments, patellar tendon (also known as jumper's knee), popliteus tendon, peroneal tendon, anterior tibial tendon, flexor hallucis longus tendon, posterior tibialis tendon, and Achilles tendon.[8]

Tendons may be partially or completely torn. Tears may occur due to macro- or microtrauma. The most frequently torn tendons are supraspinatus, biceps, patella, Achilles, posterior tibial, and peroneal. Spontaneous rupture of tendons may occur in individuals who receive local corticosteroid injections or who are diagnosed with RA or SLE.[9]

Tendon Healing

In order for an injured tendon to heal well, the site of injury must be both strong and flexible. There must be enough deposition of collagen to achieve good tensile strength. However, if collagen synthesis becomes excessive, fibrosis and adhesions may form in the surrounding tissue and interfere with tendon function. Over time, and with the appropriate application of stretching and strengthening forces, the collagen cross-links in the scar remodel to allow efficient tendon function. If the injury has occurred in a tendon that is surrounded by a synovial sheath, there is a significant risk that scar formation will severely limit tendon gliding.[1]

Time Frame for Healing

Healing tendons must be protected from excessive forces of overstretch or contraction. It is not until the fourth or fifth week that the tensile strength has improved enough to tolerate a strong pull.[1] The tissue continues to heal for several months but never achieves its pre-injury levels of strength and extensibility.[8]

INJURIES TO LIGAMENTS

An injury to a ligament is called a sprain. The most common classification of ligamentous injury is first, second, and third degree. Table 5-3 delineates the classification of sprains. Sprains are characterized by a history of acute onset. The mechanism of injury may be either overstretch or excessive force. Pain is localized over the area of injury. If examination occurred prior to onset of effusion, joint instability may be detected. If the injury is severe, there may be joint subluxation or dislocation.[4]

Ligaments are highly resistant to tensile forces. Frequently a third-degree sprain will result in an avulsion fracture at the bony insertion of the ligament rather than a substance tear of the ligament.

Ligament Healing

Ligaments heal using the same basic processes as noted for the previous tissues. Ligament sprains can be intra-articular (within the confines of the joint capsule) or extra-articular (outside of the joint capsule).

If the injury is extra-articular, bleeding occurs in the subcutaneous space. Vascular proliferation, new capillary growth, and fibroblastic activity take place during the next 6 weeks. All of this activity creates a fibrin clot that eventually is mixed with collagen and ground substance. This forms the scar that acts as a bridge between the torn ends of the ligament. Initially, collagen fibers are arranged in a random woven pattern with little organization and the scar is soft and viscous.[1] Over the next few months, the collagen fibers

		Table 5-3	
Signs and Symptoms of First-, Second-, and Third-Degree Ligamentous Sprains			
Signs or Symptoms	*First Degree*	*Second Degree*	*Third Degree*
Ligament fiber injury	A few ligamentous fibers are torn	Almost half of ligamentous fibers are torn	Complete tear of all ligamentous fibers (rupture)
Results of stress tests	<5 mm distraction	5 to 10 mm distraction	>10 mm distraction
Muscle weakness	Mild	Mild to moderate	Mild to moderate
Loss of function	Mild	Moderate to severe	Severe (instability)
Swelling	Mild	Moderate	Moderate to severe
Pain with stretching	Yes	Yes	No
PROM	Limited	Limited	May increase mobility due to instability or decrease mobility due to edema

realign themselves in response to progressive stresses and strains to which they are subjected. Full scar maturation may take as long as 12 months.[8] The length of time for full scar maturation depends on mechanical factors, such as length of time of immobilization, how well the torn ends were apposed, and the patient's age and health status. Ligament failure may be due to the body's failure to produce enough scar tissue, the surgeon's failure to reconnect the ligament to the appropriate location on the bone, or excessive mechanical forces being applied too early by the patient or the physical therapist.

If an intra-articular ligament is sprained, bleeding occurs inside the joint capsule until either clotting occurs or the increasing pressure stops the bleeding. An intra-articular ligament tear will usually require surgical repair because the synovial fluid dilutes the hematoma therefore preventing formation of a fibrin clot and spontaneous healing.

When a ligament is completely torn, the full stability of the joint will probably not be completely restored. Whether or not a surgical repair is performed, it is necessary to increase the muscle/tendon strength around the joint to reinforce the ligament.

A ligament's tensile strength decreases with immobilization. Therefore, it is necessary to minimize periods of immobilization and progressively stress the injured ligament, bearing in mind the stage of healing and the tensile strength.[1]

INJURIES TO JOINT CAPSULES

The joint capsule may develop inflammation (capsulitis) either spontaneously or as a result of trauma. The most common capsulitis occurs at the shoulder joint and is known as adhesive capsulitis. It is also often referred to as frozen shoulder. The term adhesive capsulitis was first noted by Neviaser. He described a clinical condition of decreased shoulder movement that appeared to result from an inflammatory process that changed the compliance of the joint capsule connective tissues and resulted in fibrosis and thickening of the capsule and ligaments. Nevasier described four stages of adhesive capsulitis. In Stage 1, there are complaints of ache at rest and pain at ends of ranges. This stage lasts about 3 months and ends with decreased shoulder mobility, mostly due to pain. In Stage II, there is progressive loss of shoulder mobility due to capsular fibrosis. Stage III is characterized by progressive loss of ROM and impaired scapulohumeral rhythm, with fewer complaints of pain. At this stage, symptoms may have been present for 9 to 14 months. In Stage IV, which Nevasier called the "thawing stage," there is a slow improvement in shoulder ROM.[10] These stages were previously referred to as freezing (Stage II), frozen (Stage III), and thawing (Stage IV).

According to Hannafin and associates,[11] the pathogenesis of adhesive capsulitis is probably a cascade of cellular events that begins with an inflammatory reaction. There is an increase in vascularity and presence of inflammatory cells in the synovium. The synovitis results in a fibroblastic response within the adjacent capsule. The etiology is typically unknown. It is possibly the result of microtrauma, macrotrauma, or an autoimmune response. The result of the chronic inflammatory response may be fibrosis that results in thickening of the normally thin and redundant capsule with associated contracture of the collagen fibers.

Adhesive capsulitis is a dysfunction that is most often seen in women between the ages of 40 and 60 years. Fifteen percent of patients develop the disorder bilaterally.[12] The condition may be associated with DM, hyperthyroidism, ischemic heart disease, and lung diseases, such as tuberculosis, emphysema, and chronic bronchitis. It may also develop 6 to 9 months after a CABG procedure.[3]

INJURIES TO BURSAE

Bursae are segments of synovial membrane that contain small amounts of synovial fluid that permit friction-free motion of surrounding structures. If excessive movement or trauma occurs, the bursa can become irritated and inflamed. It reacts by producing large amounts of synovial fluid. As the fluid accumulates in the bursa, pressure increases and causes irritation of the pain receptors in the area. Common areas of bursal inflammation are the inferior/medial scapula border, subacromial/subdeltoid area, olecranon, greater trochanter, ischial tuberosity, iliopectineal area, and the retrocalcaneal area.[1]

If a bursa is chronically irritated its walls become thickened and tough. Pain occurs when nearby joints are moved and compress the bursa. This may create a noncapsular pattern of restriction of motion. Pain at rest may occur if there is a significant amount of synovial fluid in the bursa and nociceptive receptors are stimulated.[8] The subacromial, olecranon, and prepatella bursae are most commonly irritated.[1]

EFFECTS OF IMMOBILIZATION

The effects of immobilization on connective tissue are discussed in the chapter on Pattern D: Impaired Joint Mobility, Motor Function, Muscle Performance, and Range of Motion Associated With Connective Tissue Dysfunction.

Whether muscle is immobilized or subjected to disuse, there is a loss of both strength and endurance. A decrease in both the size and the number of muscle fibers occurs. The exact effects depend on the fiber type of the muscle and the position that the muscle was in during the period of immobilization. Type I muscle fibers are the most likely to atrophy during immobilization. If the muscle is immobilized in a lengthened position, the negative effects of the immobilization are somewhat diminished. Many animal model studies have shown that early mobilization may prevent muscle atrophy after injury or surgery.[13]

EFFECTS OF OVERUSE

The effects of overuse on the various connective tissues are discussed in the chapter on Pattern D: Impaired Joint Mobility, Motor Function, Muscle Performance, and Range of Motion Associated With Connective Tissue Dysfunction.

When a muscle is overused, two types of soreness can occur. The first type is acute and occurs with muscle fatigue during or immediately after exercise. The second type is called delayed onset muscle soreness (DOMS) that begins about 12 hours post activity, increasing in intensity for 24 to 48 hours, then gradually subsiding within 3 to 4 days. The mechanism of DOMS is not clear. Historically, there have been theories that the cause of DOMS was lactic acid build-up or localized spasm of MUs. These theories have been disproved. Presently, it is thought that DOMS may be caused by small tears in muscle tissue (most likely due to eccentric or isometric exercise) or by connective tissue damage at the musculotendinous junction.[1]

EFFECTS OF DISEASE

Many disease processes may create localized inflammation within the musculoskeletal system. People who have DM tend to have higher rates of tendon contractures, tenosynovitis, joint stiffness, capsulitis, and osteoporosis. People with chronic renal failure tend to have increased incidence of tendon failure due to dialysis treatments.[12] Systemic diseases such as diabetes, hyperthyroidism, and RA are associated with secondary adhesive capsulitis. In addition, patients with a history of myocardial infarction, cerebrovascular accidents, tuberculosis, chronic lung disease, pulmonary cancer, scleroderma, and postmastectomy are also predisposed to secondary adhesive capsulitis.[3]

IMAGING

Plain radiographs are often the first imaging techniques performed. However, the information gleaned from this source is limited. MRI or CT will provide more relevant information for patients with localized inflammation. For detailed information about these imaging techniques refer to Pattern D: Impaired Joint Mobility, Motor Function, Muscle Performance, and Range of Motion Associated With Connective Tissue Dysfunction and Pattern F: Impaired Joint Mobility, Motor Function, Muscle Performance, Range of Motion, and Reflex Integrity Associated With Spinal Disorders.

PHARMACOLOGY

When a person initially becomes aware of pain, self-treatment may begin with OTC medications for pain relief or anti-inflammation. Some common OTC medications that are often used include Tylenol, Advil, Aleve, Motrin, or generic variations. If these offer minimal to no relief, the physician will often prescribe medications that are either analgesic, anti-inflammatory, or a combination of both (depending on the severity of the patient's symptoms). Analgesics such as Ultracet, Darvocet, or Percocet or anti-inflammatory medications may be prescribed. Analgesics and anti-inflammatory drugs have been described in detail in Pattern D: Impaired Joint Mobility, Motor Function, Muscle Performance, and Range of Motion Associated With Connective Tissue Dysfunction.

Case Study #1: Plantar Fasciitis

Jared St. Clair is a 22-year-old healthy male who developed pain in his right heel while training for a half marathon and was diagnosed with plantar fasciitis.

PHYSICAL THERAPIST EXAMINATION

HISTORY

♦ General demographics: Mr. St. Clair is a 22-year-old black American male whose primary language is English. He is left-hand dominant.

♦ Social history: Mr. St. Clair is single and lives alone.

♦ Employment/work: He is a full-time law student. He has a part-time job as a bicycle messenger.

♦ Living environment: He lives alone in a one-bedroom apartment on the fifth floor of an elevator building.

♦ General health status
  • General health perception: Mr. St. Clair considers himself to be in excellent health.
  • Physical function: He perceives his physical function as normal.
  • Psychological function: Normal.
  • Role function: Full-time student, bicycle messenger.
  • Social function: Mr. St. Clair is very involved in athletic activities. He participates in his college basketball and swimming clubs. He also is a recreational runner and is presently training for his first half marathon.

♦ Social/health habits: He is a non-smoker and a social drinker.

♦ Family history: His parents are alive and in good health.

♦ Medical/surgical history: Mr. St. Clair had a left ACL reconstruction after a basketball injury 3 years ago.

♦ Preexisting medical and other health-related conditions: None.

♦ Current condition(s)/chief complaint(s): He has pain localized in his right heel. The pain occurs with any weightbearing activity and is worse in the morning.

♦ Functional status and activity level: Mr. St. Clair has refrained from playing basketball and running since pain began 3 weeks ago. He has continued with all other activities.

♦ Medications: None.

♦ Other clinical tests: Plain radiographs of his right foot were normal.

SYSTEMS REVIEW

♦ Cardiovascular/pulmonary
  • BP: 110/70 mmHg
  • Edema: Slight edema on plantar surface of right calcaneous as compared to left
  • HR: 65 bpm
  • RR: 10 bpm

♦ Integumentary
  • Presence of scar formation: A well-healed and non-adherent scar is noted on anterior left knee secondary to ACL reconstruction 3 years ago
  • Skin color: WNL
  • Skin integrity: WNL

♦ Musculoskeletal
  • Gross range of motion
    ▪ WNL for LLE and right hip and knee
    ▪ Right foot and ankle were moderately limited in dorsiflexion and inversion and WNL in plantarflexion and eversion
  • Gross strength: WNL for LLE, 4/5 to 5/5 for RLE
  • Gross symmetry
    ▪ Cervical, thoracic, and lumbar curves: WNL
    ▪ Right ilium anteriorly rotated as compared to left
    ▪ Right knee valgus as compared to left
    ▪ Right foot pronated as compared to left
  • Height: 6'1" (1.85 m)
  • Weight: 182 lbs (82.55 kg)

♦ Neuromuscular: WNL

♦ Communication, affect, cognition, language, and learning style
  • Communication, affect, and cognition: WNL
  • Learning preferences: Visual learner

TESTS AND MEASURES

♦ Aerobic capacity/endurance
  • Patient ordinarily runs 5 miles in 30 minutes three times weekly

♦ Anthropometric characteristics
  • BMI=705 x (body weight [in pounds] divided by height^2 [in inches])
  • Mr. St. Clair's BMI=24.07
  • BMI values between 18.5 and 24.9 are considered normal[14]
  • Observation reveals slight edema over the plantar surface of the calcaneous

♦ Assistive and adaptive devices
  • Patient has a dorsiflexion night splint

♦ Cranial and peripheral nerve integrity: WNL

♦ Ergonomics and body mechanics

- When patient is in school or on the bicycle during his job as a messenger, he displays appropriate ergonomics and body mechanics
- If he attempts his normal impact recreational activities, he minimizes heel contact on his right foot

◆ Gait, locomotion, and balance
- Observational gait analysis on level surfaces at preferred cadence walking revealed symmetrical step size and cadence with no hint of attempts to favor RLE
- Observational gait analysis of uphill walking (on treadmill) at speed of 3.0 mph revealed an antalgic gait with minimization of weightbearing on RLE from initial contact through push-off phases of gait
- Patient was unable to run on level surface due to pain in right heel
- Single leg stance balance was unimpaired
  - Patient could balance for greater than 3 minutes on either LE with eyes open or closed on both stable and unstable surfaces

◆ Integumentary integrity
- Examination of the soles of the feet revealed excessive callus on medial plantar surface of calcaneous of right foot

◆ Joint integrity and mobility
- Right foot: Spread of the distal tibia/fibular joint, superior fibular glide, posterior glide of talus on distal tibia/fibular joint, talar tilt into supination and dorsal glide of the first MTP joint were moderately hypomobile
- Right foot: Talar tilt into pronation was minimally hypermobile
- All other joints: WNL

◆ Motor function
- Dexterity, coordination, and agility: WNL

◆ Muscle performance
- MMT of LLE was WNL
- MMT of RLE
  - 4/5 gluteus maximus, piriformis, gluteus medius, posterior tibialis, flexor hallucis longus and brevis, flexor digitorum longus and brevis
  - 5/5 strength in all other muscles

◆ Orthotic, protective, and supportive devices
- Patient states that he has tried OTC inserts in his shoes with no change in symptoms

◆ Pain
- Mr. St. Clair was asked to rate his pain using the NPS
- The NPS is a simple self-reported 11-point pain scale (0 to 10, with 0 being "no pain" and 10 being pain "as bad as it can be")
- The patient rates his pain intensity over the past 24 hours

- Stratford and Spadoni[15] have found that the 90% confidence interval (CI) was ± 2 points on the scale and the true change estimates are ±3 points that means that a change of three points is necessary in order to be confident that a true change in pain has occurred
- Mr. St. Clair reports that pain is 0/10 when nonweightbearing, 8/10 at initial weightbearing in the morning, and 3/10 when walking during an average day

◆ Posture
- Cervical, thoracic, and lumbar curves were WNL
- Right ilium was anteriorly rotated as compared to left
- Right knee was positioned in slight valgus as compared to the left
- Right foot posture showed calcaneal valgus and forefoot pronation as compared to the left

◆ Range of motion
- Joint PROM was WNL throughout except right dorsiflexion 0 to 5 degrees and inversion 0 to 7 degrees
- SLR test: right=60 degrees, left=60 degrees and mobility was limited by hamstring tightness
- Muscle length
  - Three muscle Thomas test
    ▸ Tightness right rectus femoris and iliopsoas
    ▸ Right TFL was WNL
    ▸ LLE muscle groups were WNL

◆ Reflex integrity: WNL

◆ Self-care and home management
- Patient is independent in all self-care and home management actions, tasks, and activities

◆ Sensory integrity: WNL

◆ Work, community, and leisure integration or reintegration
- Mr. St. Clair is able to continue his work and student responsibilities, but has refrained from his leisure actions, tasks, and activities at this time

EVALUATION

Mr. St. Clair's history and risk factors previously outlined indicate that he is a healthy 22-year old black American male who developed plantar fasciitis while training for a half marathon. He has a gait deviation, muscle tightness, right knee joint malalignment, decreased joint ROM, and decreased muscle strength. At present, the patient has symptoms of pain and inability to tolerate impact on the right foot.

Examination results may lead one to believe that the fasciitis may be caused from a more proximal dysfunction. Postural examination revealed that the right ilium was anteriorly rotated. When the ilium is anteriorly rotated, the acetabulum takes a more downward facing position creating a relatively longer femur on that side. This will create a functionally long LE. The body has several ways in which it may compensate for a functionally long LE. Unilateral foot pronation and genu valgus each contribute to making a LE functionally shorter compared to the opposite side.[8] The source of the leg length discrepancy may be originating from the muscle length asymmetry in the rectus femoris and iliopsoas. When one or both of these muscles are tight, they create a constant pull on the anterior ilium. The muscle weakness of the gluteus maximus, piriformis, gluteus medius, posterior tibialis, flexor hallucis longus and brevis, and flexor digitorum longus and brevis is a result of the excessive strain on these muscles to control the deceleration of the limb as the foot is going into early and rapid pronation.

DIAGNOSIS

Mr. St. Clair has been diagnosed with plantar fasciitis of the right foot. In addition, he has impaired: anthropometric characteristics; gait, locomotion, and balance; integumentary integrity; joint integrity and mobility; muscle performance; posture; and range of motion. He is functionally limited in work, community, and leisure actions, tasks, and activities. These findings are consistent with placement in Pattern E: Impaired Joint Mobility, Motor Function, Muscle Performance, and Range of Motion Associated With Localized Inflammation. These impairments and functional limitations will be addressed in determining the prognosis and the plan of care.

PROGNOSIS AND PLAN OF CARE

Over the course of the visits, the following mutually established outcomes have been determined:

♦ Gait is normalized initially during walking and then progressing to running via conscious effort at appropriate weight distribution
♦ Integumentary integrity is improved
♦ Joint integrity and mobility are improved so that normal joint mobility in the right ankle and foot is achieved
♦ Knowledge is obtained of the importance of a regular appropriate stretching and strengthening program
♦ Muscle performance is increased
♦ Normal muscle length in RLE is achieved
♦ Normal muscle strength in RLE is achieved
♦ Pain is eliminated during weightbearing
♦ Patient is educated in appropriate distribution pattern of body weight on foot during gait
♦ Physical function is improved
♦ Postural control is improved
♦ Return to his previous running regime is achieved so that

he may achieve his goal of running in a half marathon
♦ ROM is improved
♦ Self-awareness of weight distribution over the right foot during gait is achieved

To achieve these outcomes, the appropriate interventions for this patient are determined. These will include: coordination, communication, and documentation; patient/client-related instruction; therapeutic exercise; functional training in work, community, and leisure integration or reintegration; manual therapy techniques; prescription, application, and, as appropriate, fabrication of devices and equipment; electrotherapeutic modalities; and physical agents and mechanical modalities.

Based on the diagnosis and prognosis, Mr. St. Clair is expected to require between 10 and 16 visits over an 8-week time period. Mr. St. Clair has good social support, is motivated, and will follow through with his home exercise program. He is not severely impaired and is very healthy.

INTERVENTIONS

RATIONALE FOR SELECTED INTERVENTIONS

Therapeutic Exercise

It is important that Mr. St. Clair maintains or increases his fitness level until he can resume his normal training program. This will be accomplished via non-weightbearing aerobic activities. When weightbearing is not painful, Mr. St. Clair will gradually add running to his fitness activities. Simultaneously, it is necessary to restore strength, power, flexibility, and endurance to all RLE musculature so that Mr. St. Clair will not have difficulty resuming his running program when pain is alleviated. When Mr. St. Clair walks uphill or runs he reports pain in his right heel. Without interventions, Mr. St. Clair may develop excessive stress in other body areas, eventually leading to repetitive stress injuries in knee, hip, or back. Closed chain exercises that strengthen muscles functionally combined with education encouraging awareness of normal weight distribution patterns on the foot during regular and uphill walking and running will contribute to avoiding future injuries.[16,17]

Flexibility of the right rectus femoris, iliopsoas, and hamstrings must be improved bilaterally, in order to regain pelvic symmetry. Normal flexibility also reestablishes the length-tension relationship of these muscles to allow for optimum function.[18] Adaptive shortening of the calf muscles and Achilles tendon may put a person at risk for plantar fasciitis.[8] Stretching and flexibility exercises of the Achilles tendon are important to allow normal range of dorsiflexion to occur.

Manual Therapy Techniques

Mr. St. Clair demonstrates pelvic asymmetry and decreased joint capsule flexibility of the talocrural, subtalar, and hallux MTP joints. Greenman defines a muscle energy technique as a "manual medicine treatment procedure that involves the voluntary contraction of the patient's muscle, in precisely controlled direction, at varying levels of intensity, against a distinctly executed counterforce applied by the operator."[19] Isometric and concentric types of muscle contraction are most commonly used in muscle energy techniques. The isometric technique is primarily used to inhibit the antagonistic muscle via the law of reciprocal innervation. Following relaxation of the hypertonic agonist, inhibition of the antagonist muscles is decreased and a more equal balance of muscle tone occurs. Concentric muscle contraction may then be used to strengthen or reeducate those antagonist muscles.[19] Examination revealed that Mr. St. Clair's right ilium was anteriorly rotated. This is often due to tight and hypertonic hip flexors (agonist) that may be released using a muscle energy technique involving an isometric contraction. This is followed by concentric contraction of the antagonist (hip extensors) for strengthening and muscle reeducation.[20]

According to Maitland,[21] mobilizations are passive movements that can be performed either as oscillations of small or large amplitudes anywhere within the ROM or sustained stretch with or without small oscillations at the end of the ROM. The oscillatory movements may be done using the joint's accessory movement or physiological movement. Maitland states that mobilization may be used to restore structures within a joint to their normal positions and to stretch stiff joint structures in order to restore normal ROM. Mobilization techniques will be used to mobilize Mr. St. Clair's foot, ilium, and ankle.[8]

Prescription, Application, and, as Appropriate, Fabrication of Devices and Equipment

It is suggested that Mr. St. Clair use a silicone heel pad in his walking and running shoes. By raising the heel slightly, some tension is taken off the plantar fascia and the silicone material creates a cushioning effect that does not bottom out. Pfeffer and associates[22] found that Achilles tendon and plantar fascia stretches plus silicone heel inserts produced significantly better results than stretching and rubber inserts, felt inserts, custom orthoses, or stretching alone.

It is also suggested that Mr. St. Clair use a dorsiflexion night splint to maintain a prolonged stretch on the plantar fascia and the Achilles tendon. Since the fascia will be more flexible, initial weightbearing in the morning will be less painful. Powell and colleagues[23] found that splinting alone, without stretching or exercise, produced significant improvement in symptoms. Batt and associates[24] found that

patients treated with anti-inflammatory medication, stretching, silicone heel pad, and a custom-made night splint had a significantly greater decrease in their symptoms as compared to those patients who did not have a night splint as part of their treatment.

Electrotherapeutic Modalities/Physical Agents and Mechanical Modalities

Several possible modalities may be used for this patient. However, there is minimal evidence as to the effectiveness of most modalities. The most commonly used modalities for plantar fasciitis are ultrasound, phonophoresis, and iontophoresis. Atkins and Crawford[25] did a systematic review of treatments for the painful heel in which eleven randomized, controlled trials were reviewed. Although many more studies have been done, they have not met rigorous standards. The authors stated that even the more rigorous studies done used a small sample size and therefore did not provide true evidence of treatment efficacy. The findings of this review were based on six trials that evaluated the efficacy of lasers, ultrasound, and steroid injections versus heel pads, insoles with and without magnetic foil, and the Bioelectron MKII. The Bioelectron MKII is an experimental device that produces a beam of electrons delivered to the skin surface via a probe that is reported to decrease tissue acidity thereby restoring normal pH to the inflamed tissues. The authors found no differences between the various treatments.

Iontophoresis with dexamethasone, steroid injections, extracorporeal shock wave therapy (ECST), and night splints were interventions that did show statistically significant differences in pain.[25] Gudeman and colleagues[26] found that iontophoresis in conjunction with traditional modalities provided the most immediate results while at 1-month follow-up there was no difference between iontophoresis and traditional modalities. Crawford and associates[27] found that ultrasound at a dosage of 0.5 w/cm^2, 3 MHz, pulsed 1:4, for 8 minutes was no more effective than placebo in the treatment of heel pain.

ECST is a relatively new procedure that delivers shock waves to specific body areas. The technique was initially used to break up kidney stones. The exact mechanism of action is not well understood. The shock waves generated by the machine may disrupt calcium deposits, increase diffusion of cytokines across blood vessel walls, and/or promote new bone formation. The most common chronic musculoskeletal conditions that have been treated with ECST are heel spurs, plantar fasciitis, lateral or medial epicondylitis, and calcific tendinitis in the shoulder. The literature reports conflicting results when reporting the clinical efficacy of ECST for any of the body areas mentioned.[28-31]

COORDINATION, COMMUNICATION, AND DOCUMENTATION

Communication will occur with Mr. St. Clair only, since his family is not involved with any of his care. All elements of Mr. St. Clair's management will be documented.

PATIENT/CLIENT-RELATED INSTRUCTION

The patient will be instructed about his current condition and impairments. Mr. St. Clair will receive an explanation of how his pelvic dysfunction relates to his foot pain. He will be given ample opportunity to ask questions. The patient will understand the importance of his home exercise program and the outcomes that can be expected, and he will receive a written home exercise program with pictures. This exercise program will change appropriately, as his needs change. Exercises will be taught and then reviewed in the same session and again at future encounters as many times as needed to ensure that they are done correctly.

THERAPEUTIC EXERCISE

- ◆ Aerobic capacity/endurance conditioning
  - Mr. St. Clair will work to maintain/increase his fitness level without significant weightbearing on his LEs
  - He may use combinations of bicycle, upper body ergometer, rowing machine, or swimming to maintain or improve his fitness level until he can safely and comfortably resume weightbearing exercises
  - For healthy individuals, THR for exercise is 65% to 90% of age-adjusted maximum heart rate (AAMHR) for 15 to 60 minutes per session at least 3 days per week
  - The THR range calculation is between 0.65 (220-age) and 0.90 (220-age)[32]
- ◆ Flexibility exercises
  - Stretching exercises should be done after warming up, using a slow and steady stretch accompanied by deep breathing, and building hold up to 30 to 60 seconds
  - Muscle lengthening of the rectus femoris and iliopsoas using PNF contract-relax method[33]
  - Self-stretching will be taught of the gastrocnemius/soleus muscle group (runner's stretch), lunges with a neutral spine to stretch anterior hip muscles, and manual self-stretch of the plantar fascia by passively moving toes into extension while ankle is kept in maximum dorsiflexion
  - Stretch of the posterior LE muscles using a slant board or Prostretch
- ◆ Gait and locomotion training
  - Instruct patient to have lateral calcaneal pressures at initial contact phase of gait followed by weight shift-ing medially so that the pressure is on the first MT at push-off
  - Initially practice on level surfaces and progress to inclines using preferred speed
  - Practice on treadmill beginning at slower speeds such as 1 mph and progress to higher speeds according to patient's tolerance and ability
- ◆ Strength, power, and endurance training
  - Open chain exercises:
    - PNF LE diagonals #1 and #2 (D1 and D2) for RLE using manual resistance and combination of isotonics[33]
    - Free weights using the DeLorme method (10 RM) to strengthen LE musculature with emphasis on hip external rotators and gluteus medius and posterior tibialis and ankle/foot invertors to control pronation[7]
    - Elastic bands/tubing with use of progressively thicker bands to increase resistance as patient's strength improves
    - Strengthen toe flexors/foot intrinsics
      - ► While resting foot on towel, use toe flexors to bunch towel, moving the towel from toes toward heel
      - ► Pick up marbles or other objects with toes
  - CKC exercises to strengthen the same muscles must be incorporated in order to transition the previous exercises into function
    - Parameters for CKC must take into consideration the variables of force, speed, complexity, and control of movement
    - Exercise should start in gravity eliminated or reduced positions and progress by increasing the weightbearing forces
    - CKC exercises should begin in a single plane and progress to include multiple planes
    - Exercises may also begin by allowing UE support for balance and then removal of that support[7]
      - ► Wall squats
      - ► Lunges
      - ► Heel raises
      - ► Toe walking
      - ► Walking on outside borders of feet
      - ► Use exercise equipment including stairclimber, leg press, total gym, shuttle

FUNCTIONAL TRAINING IN WORK, COMMUNITY, AND LEISURE INTEGRATION OR REINTEGRATION

- ◆ Leisure
  - Mr. St. Clair will be encouraged to return to a run-

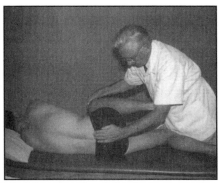

Figure 5-2. Muscle energy technique used to posteriorly rotate the right ilium. Initiate by positioning the patient with the right ilium in maximum posterior rotation. The practitioner's hand monitors motion at the right SI join. Reprinted with permission from Greenman P. *Principles of Manual Medicine.* 2nd ed. Baltimore, Md: Williams & Wilkins; 1996:353.

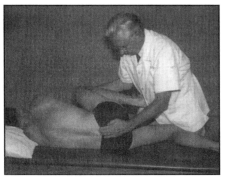

Figure 5-3. Muscle energy technique used to posteriorly rotate the right ilium. The patient attempts to straighten the right leg by pushing against the practitioner's hip. The ilium is then moved further into posterior rotation and the procedure is repeated. Reprinted with permission from Greenman P. *Principles of Manual Medicine.* 2nd ed. Baltimore, Md: Williams & Wilkins; 1996:353.

ning program starting with minimal distances, such as a half mile three times weekly, with a very gradual increase in distance by adding a half mile per week
- He will use his pain as a monitor during and after his training sessions
- He will also be educated as to the necessity of checking his running shoes and changing them when they are worn

MANUAL THERAPY TECHNIQUES

♦ Mobilization/manipulation
  - To correct the right anteriorly rotated ilium
    - Use a muscle energy technique that engages the right hamstrings and gluteus maximus to posteriorly rotate the ilium
      ▸ Patient is lying on left side, with left hip and knee flexed and RLE extended
      ▸ Therapist uses one finger over the right sacroiliac joint to monitor motion and then introduces hip flexion, abduction, and ER of the right hip until the barrier of ilial posterior rotation is reached
      ▸ Patient exerts three to five isometric muscle contractions against the therapist's resistance and holds for 3 to 7 seconds
      ▸ The isometric force activates the hamstrings and gluteal muscles that pull the ilium into posterior rotation[19] (Figures 5-2 and 5-3)
  - Mobilize the right ilium posteriorly: this can be done in addition to muscle energy techniques if necessary
    - Patient is lying on left side with right hip and

knee flexed so that the iliosacral joint is at the end of its range of posterior rotation
    - The patient's upper trunk is rotated to the right as far as possible in order to limit vertebral motion in the thoracic and lumbar spines
    - The therapist stands facing the patient and contacts the right ASIS with the right hand and the right ischial tuberosity with the left hand
    - The therapist rotates the ilium posteriorly by simultaneously pushing in a posterior/inferior direction with the right hand and in an anterior/superior direction with the left hand[34] (Figure 5-4)
  - To improve right talocrural joint dorsiflexion[21]
    - Perform posterior glide of talus on the distal tibia/fibular joint with the ankle at or close to maximum dorsiflexion, Grade III or IV
    - Perform anterior glide of the distal tibia/fibular joint with the ankle at or close to maximum dorsiflexion, Grade III or IV

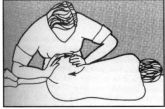

Figure 5-4. Posterior rotation mobilization of left ilium. Reprinted from *Practical Orthopedic Medicine.* Corrigan B, Maitland GD. Page 331, 1983, with permission from Elsevier.

- Perform anterior/posterior glides of the tibia with the fibula stabilized to enhance the spread of the distal tibia/fibular joint, Grade IV
- Perform anterior/posterior glides of the fibula with the tibia stabilized to enhance the spread of the distal tibia/fibular joint, Grade IV
- To increase right hallux MTP extension[21]
  - Perform distraction of the MTP joint
  - Perform dorsal glide (anterior glide) of the proximal phalanx on the first MT, Grade III or IV
  - Perform medial/lateral glides of the proximal phalanx on the first MT, Grade III or IV
- To lengthen plantar fascia
  - Place the fascia in lengthened position and apply soft tissue mobilization (STM) techniques such as cross friction, strumming, deep effleurage, etc
  - Passively elongate the plantar fascia by maximally dorsiflexing the ankle and extending the toes[35]

PRESCRIPTION, APPLICATION, AND, AS APPROPRIATE, FABRICATION OF DEVICES AND EQUIPMENT

- ◆ Orthotic devices
  - The patient will use a dorsiflexion night splint to maintain a prolonged stretch on the plantar fascia
  - Mr. St. Clair may try custom foot orthotics if the splint and silicone pad do not achieve total relief of symptoms
- ◆ Protective devices
  - It is suggested that Mr. St. Clair use a silicone heel pad in his walking and running shoes to absorb shock and raise the heel slightly thereby taking some tension off the plantar fascia

ELECTROTHERAPEUTIC MODALITIES

- ◆ Electrotherapeutic delivery of medications
  - Iontophoresis with dexamethasone will be used to decrease pain and inflammation

PHYSICAL AGENTS AND MECHANICAL MODALITIES

- ◆ Thermotherapy
  - Hydrocollator packs will be used to apply moist heat to the plantar fascia to increase tissue extensibility[8]

ANTICIPATED GOALS AND EXPECTED OUTCOMES

- ◆ Impact on pathology/pathophysiology
  - Pain is decreased to 0/10 while walking.

- Soft tissue inflammation, edema, and restriction are reduced.
- ◆ Impact on impairments
  - Endurance is increased.
  - Energy expenditure per unit of work is decreased.
  - Flexibility of rectus femoris, iliopsoas, and TFL are improved.
  - Gait is improved to normal cadence with full weight-bearing on the RLE. Patient is able to run pain-free on level surfaces.
  - Joint mobility in all joints of the right foot is normal.
  - Muscle performance (strength, power, and endurance) is increased.
  - Muscle strength is increased to 5/5 in gluteus maximus, piriformis, gluteus medius, posterior tibialis, flexor hallucis longus and brevis, flexor digitorum longus and brevis.
  - Pain on weightbearing in the morning is 0/10.
  - Plantar fascia flexibility is improved.
  - Postural control is improved. Bony alignment of the pelvis, knee, and foot are WNL.
  - ROM is improved in right dorsiflexion to 10 degrees and inversion to 15 degrees.
  - Walking speed is increased.
- ◆ Impact on functional limitations
  - Ability to assume or resume required work, community, and leisure roles is achieved.
  - Ability to independently perform physical actions, tasks, and activities related to ADL/IADL in self-care, home management, work, community, and leisure with or without assistive devices and equipment is improved.
- ◆ Risk reduction/prevention
  - Risk factors are reduced.
  - Risk of secondary impairments is reduced.
- ◆ Impact on health, wellness, and fitness
  - Behaviors that foster healthy habits, wellness, and prevention are acquired.
  - Decision making is enhanced regarding health, wellness, and fitness needs.
  - Fitness, health status, physical capacity, and physical function are improved.
- ◆ Impact on societal resources
  - Available resources are maximally utilized.
  - Documentation occurs throughout patient management and follows APTA's *Guidelines for Physical Therapy Documentation.*[36]
- ◆ Patient/client satisfaction
  - Clinical proficiency and interpersonal skills of the physical therapist are acceptable to patient/client.

- Patient's knowledge and awareness of the diagnosis, prognosis, interventions, and understanding of anticipated goals and expected outcomes are increased.
- Sense of well-being is improved.

REEXAMINATION

Reexamination is performed throughout the episode of care.

DISCHARGE

Mr. St. Clair was discharged after 11 visits. Anticipated goals for elimination of pain, return to full mobility and strength, and ability to resume a full running training schedule were achieved. He was discharged because he achieved his goals and expected outcomes.

Case Study #2: Adhesive Capsulitis

Mrs. Barbara Brooks is a 58-year-old female who developed an insidious onset of right shoulder pain 2 months ago.

PHYSICAL THERAPIST EXAMINATION

HISTORY

- General demographics: Mrs. Brooks is a 58-year-old white female whose primary language is English. Her highest educational level is high school. She is right-hand dominant.
- Social history: She is married with three grown children, all of whom live out of the home. She lives with her husband in a co-operative high-rise apartment building.
- Employment/work: She works as a bookkeeper and general clerical person for a real estate company.
- General health status
  - General health perception: Mrs. Brooks perceives herself as healthy.
  - Physical function: She has moderate limitation in ADL and IADL due to pain and inability to raise her RUE overhead or behind back.
  - Psychological function: Mrs. Brooks is angry and frustrated due to pain and limitations in function.
  - Role function: Wife, mother, full-time bookkeeper.
  - Social function: She participates in frequent social functions, and her leisure activities include reading and bicycle riding.

- Social/health habits: Mrs. Brooks smokes one pack per week and is a social drinker (wine with dinner about once per month).
- Family history: Her mother died of breast cancer 10 years ago. Her father is alive, but in failing health due to diabetes, heart disease, and HTN.
- Medical/surgical history: She has had a history of Type 2 diabetes that was diagnosed when she was 54 years old.
- Current condition(s)/chief complaint(s): Mrs. Brooks had an insidious onset of right shoulder pain, starting about 2 months ago. The pain became most severe 1 month ago and has now started to subside. Her symptoms were unchanged after 2 weeks of self-treatment. The physician gave her Celebrex, with minimal change. After 1 month, the physician injected the shoulder. The injection decreased the pain, although she still cannot sleep on her right side. She continues to complain of severely decreased mobility and severe functional limitations in her right shoulder.
- Functional status and activity level: Prior to this episode she was exercising at least 2 hours 1 day per week. Now she is unable to do any functional activities that require reaching above 80 degrees or behind her back with her RUE. However, she accomplishes all of her ADL activities with adaptations and modifications, and she is able to perform all work activities.
- Medications: She is taking Glucophage for the diabetes and took an anti-inflammatory medication for 1 month only. Currently she is taking Advil prn.
- Other clinical tests: The plain radiographs showed mild arthritis in her right shoulder. An MRI was not done at this time.

SYSTEMS REVIEW

- Cardiovascular/pulmonary
  - BP: 135/85 mmHg
  - Edema: No edema noted in extremities
  - HR: 80 bpm
  - RR: 12 bpm
- Integumentary
  - Presence of scar formation: None
  - Skin color: WNL
  - Skin integrity: Intact
- Musculoskeletal
  - Gross range of motion
    - Cervical ROM
      - Flexion WNL
      - Moderate decreases in extension, rotation, and lateral bending to each side
    - Thoracic ROM
      - Upper thoracic spine WNL except for moderate decrease in extension

- ▸ Mid and lower thoracic spine WNL
  - Gross ROM in LUE: WNL
  - Gross ROM of right shoulder moderately limited
  - Gross ROM of right elbow, forearm, wrist, and hand: WNL
  - Gross strength
    - Gross strength for cervical, LUE, and right elbow, wrist and hand: WNL
    - Gross strength of right shoulder: 4-/5
  - Gross symmetry: Kyphoscoliosis
  - Height: 5'4" (1.62 m)
  - Weight: 150 lbs (68.04 kg)
- ◆ Neuromuscular: WNL
- ◆ Communication, affect, cognition, language, and learning style
  - Communication, affect, and cognition: WNL
  - No apparent learning barriers
  - Learns well via written and auditory methods

TESTS AND MEASURES

- ◆ Aerobic capacity/endurance
  - Patient leads a moderately sedentary lifestyle
  - Her maximum physical exertion is bicycling outdoors for 2 miles 1 day per week
- ◆ Anthropometric characteristics
  - BMI=705 x (body weight [in pounds] divided by height^2 [in inches])
  - Mrs. Brooks' BMI=25.8
  - BMI values between 25 and 29.9 are considered overweight[14]
  - No edema noted in RUE
- ◆ Assistive and adaptive devices: None
- ◆ Cranial and peripheral nerve integrity: WNL
- ◆ Environmental, home, and work barriers: None
- ◆ Ergonomics and body mechanics
  - She tends to lift and carry using her back rather than the UE and LE musculature
  - When working at a desk or keyboard, she tends to maintain her trunk in a forward flexed posture
- ◆ Gait, locomotion, and balance: WNL
- ◆ Integumentary integrity: WNL
- ◆ Joint integrity and mobility
  - Right GH joint: All accessory and joint play movements were moderately hypomobile
  - Right AC and SC joints: Accessory and joint play movements were mildly hypomobile
  - Right ST joint
    - Mildly hypomobile in upward and downward rotation and adduction

- Scapular movements of elevation and abduction were WNL
- ● Cervical spine mobility testing using PPIVM testing[34]
  - Flexion: WNL
  - Extension: Moderately restricted from C5 to C7 with hard end feel
  - Rotation: Moderately restricted from C5 to C7 with hard end feel bilaterally
- ● Thoracic spine mobility testing using PPIVMs[34]
  - Flexion: WNL
  - Extension: Moderately restricted from T1 to T5 with hard end feel
  - Rotation: Moderately restricted from T1 to T5 with hard end feel bilaterally
- ◆ Motor function
  - Dexterity, coordination, and agility: WNL
- ◆ Muscle performance
  - MMT revealed the following:
    - Right shoulder flexion=4-/5
    - Right shoulder extension=4+/5
    - Right shoulder abduction=4-/5
    - Right shoulder ER=4-/5
    - Right shoulder IR=4/5
    - Right shoulder horizontal adduction=5/5
    - Right scapula upward rotators=4-/5
    - Right scapula adductors=4-/5
  - MMT below right shoulder and all of LUE were WNL
  - SH rhythm was impaired with excessive scapula elevation during attempted shoulder flexion and abduction
  - Grip strength dynamometry
    - Right=50 lbs
    - Left=45 lbs
    - According to Mathiowetz, the mean grip strength in the 55 to 59-year-old age group was 57.3 lbs for the right hand and 47.3 lbs for the left hand[37]
- ◆ Orthotic, protective, and supportive devices: None
- ◆ Pain
  - On the NPS (0=no pain and 10=worst possible pain), pain in the right shoulder was rated as 3/10 at rest and 6/10 with activity[15]
- ◆ Posture
  - FHP
  - Mild kyphoscoliosis, right thoracic, left lumbar
  - Right shoulder girdle elevated with right scapula winged and anteriorly tilted
  - Scapulae abducted bilaterally
- ◆ Range of motion

- Cervical spine measured with a CROM
  - Flexion=0 to 65 degrees
  - Extension=0 to 20 degrees
  - Rotation right=0 to 45 degrees
  - Rotation left=0 to 45 degrees
  - Sidebend right=0 to 20 degrees
  - Sidebend left=0 to 10 degrees
- Right shoulder AROM (goniometry)
  - Flexion=0 to 85 degrees
  - Abduction=0 to 65 degrees
  - ER=0 to 20 degrees
  - IR=0 to 60 degrees
- Behind back: Patient was able to reach her wrist only to the level of the buttocks
- Pain noted when approaching the end ranges of active movement
- Right shoulder PROM
  - Passive motion 3 degrees greater than AROM in all directions with pain at end ranges
- Left shoulder: AROM and PROM were WFL
- ROM of all joints below shoulders: WNL bilaterally
- Muscle length and soft tissue extensibility and flexibility
  - There was decreased flexibility of right pectoralis major, pectoralis minor, latissimus dorsi, subscapularis, and upper trapezius
- Muscle tension (palpation)
  - Palpation revealed mild tenderness over anterior and medial GH joint line, supraspinatus, and long head of biceps tendons
  - Spasm of right pectoralis major, pectoralis minor, and subscapularis
- Reflex integrity
  - DTRs: WNL in all four extremities
- Self-care and home management
  - She has difficulty with all grooming and reaching activities that require moving shoulder above 80 degrees
  - She is unable to tuck shirt into back of pants and unable to take off or put on bra in a traditional fashion
  - She has been able to maintain independence in all actions, tasks, and activities with modifications and adaptations
- Sensory integrity: WNL in both UEs
- Work, community, and leisure integration or reintegration
  - She is able to continue with her pasttimes of reading and bicycle riding
  - She reports no difficulty with social functions that do not require overuse of her UE

EVALUATION

Mrs. Brooks's examination indicated that she is a 58-year-old female patient with Type 2 diabetes who developed insidious onset of right shoulder pain, stiffness, and weakness. Although she has not curtailed any of her ADL or IADL activities, she is performing them with difficulty due to the pain and limited ROM of her right shoulder.

Mrs. Brooks's shoulder mobility findings fall into a capsular pattern, and her examination results were compatible with a diagnosis of adhesive capsulitis. The term capsular pattern was first described by Cyriax.[38] He defined a capsular pattern as a specific ratio of limitations of passive ROM that implies that the entire joint capsule is involved. The capsular pattern of the shoulder is accepted as having the most limitation, proportionately, in ER. This is followed by limitation in abduction and then IR. The concept of a capsular pattern is based on empirical findings and tradition rather than scientific research.[8]

DIAGNOSIS

Mrs. Brooks is an individual with DM and adhesive capsulitis with pain in her right shoulder. She has impaired: aerobic capacity/endurance; ergonomics and body mechanics; joint integrity and mobility; muscle performance; posture; and range of motion. She is functionally limited in self-care and home management and in work, community and leisure actions, tasks, and activities. These findings are consistent with placement in Pattern E: Impaired Joint Mobility, Motor Function, Muscle Performance, and Range of Motion Associated With Localized Inflammation. These impairments and functional limitations will be addressed in determining the prognosis and the plan of care.

PROGNOSIS AND PLAN OF CARE

Over the course of the visits, the following mutually established outcomes have been determined:
- Ability to perform self-care, home management, work, community, and leisure actions, tasks, and activities with a minimum of compensatory movement patterns is increased
- Joint mobility in the right shoulder girdle is improved
- Muscle spasm of the pectoral and subscapularis muscles is decreased
- Muscle strength of the right shoulder girdle is improved
- Normal SH rhythm is achieved
- Pain at rest and with activity is eliminated
- Posture is improved

To achieve these outcomes, the appropriate interventions are determined. These will include: coordination, communication, and documentation; patient/client-related instruction; therapeutic exercise; functional training in self-care and home management; functional training in work, community, and leisure integration or reintegration; manual therapy techniques; electrotherapeutic modalities; and physical agents and mechanical modalities.

Based on the diagnosis and prognosis, Mrs. Brooks is expected to require between 16 to 24 visits over a period of 12 weeks. Mrs. Brooks is angry and has a history of diabetes, but she has good social support and is relatively healthy.

INTERVENTIONS

RATIONALE FOR SELECTED INTERVENTIONS

There have been few, well-controlled studies on the treatment of adhesive capsulitis. Existing studies have not established a superior method of treatment. Physical therapy may include manual techniques, such as soft tissue and joint mobilization, muscle and/or fascial stretching, and muscle strengthening. Modalities such as electrical stimulation, ultrasound, iontophoresis, heat, or cold may also be included. Interventions by physicians may include local steroid injection, intra-articular injection of sodium hyaluronate,[39] capsular distension,[40] or arthroscopic surgery.[41] No one technique or set of treatments has been proven to be most effective.

Therapeutic Exercise

Since Mrs. Brooks has not been using her right shoulder girdle, it is expected that she will have weakness secondary to disuse and muscle inhibition caused by pain.[8] Weakness may be a result of poor timing of shoulder girdle musculature, especially impairment in scapulohumeral rhythm. Improvement in muscle strength, power, and endurance may be achieved by doing resistive exercises using any external force including gravity, cuff weights, dumbbells, or elastic resistance. It is also necessary to do functional exercises so that there is carryover into daily activities.[17]

To address these issues, interventions must include postural awareness, strengthening of the deep cervical musculature, thoracic extensors, scapula musculature, and the rotator cuff.

Manual Therapy Techniques

Although passive joint mobilization has been an accepted physical therapy intervention, the exact arthrokinematic movement at the GH joint is becoming controversial as biomechanical studies have become more sophisticated. Several studies[42,43] have now shown that there is very little inferior glide of the humeral head in the glenoid fossa during shoulder elevation. These studies have shown that inferior glide does not occur with active or passive shoulder elevation. They demonstrate that when the arm begins to elevate, the humeral head first translates superiorly approximately 1 to 3 mm, then remains relatively centered within the glenoid fossa. It is the function of the rotator cuff muscles to maintain the humerus centered in the glenoid. In spite of the latest information regarding kinematics of the GH joint, there have been studies that demonstrate significant changes in the GH joint after intervention using mobilization.

Tovin and Greenfield[44] noted that if the patient has low irritability and capsular restriction, he or she may require aggressive joint and STM. Vermeulen and associates[45] in a multiple subject case report found that after 3 months of treatment with end-range mobilization techniques for adhesive capsulitis of the shoulder, there were significant improvements in active and passive abduction, flexion, and ER. There was also an increase in the mean fluid capacity of the GH joint by the end of the study.

Physical Agents and Mechanical Modalities

There have been no studies to document the effectiveness of any modality as a stand-alone treatment for adhesive capsulitis of the shoulder. Since Mrs. Brooks states that her pain is 3/10 at rest and 6/10 with activity, moist heat or ultrasound may be useful to decrease inflammation and decrease muscle spasm and tightness. Funk and colleagues[46] found that 20 minutes of moist heat application to the hamstrings resulted in increased flexibility when compared to three sets of 30 seconds of static stretching alone. This may be extrapolated to the usefulness of moist heat application prior to stretching at the shoulder. Klaiman and associates[47] found that ultrasound was effective at decreasing pain and pressure sensitivity in a variety of tendinitis and fasciitis conditions. In this study, there was no significant difference between ultrasound and phonophoresis. Esenyel and colleagues[48] studied the effectiveness of ultrasound treatment and trigger point injection in combination with stretching exercises on myofascial trigger points in the upper trapezius muscle. The results showed a statistically significant decrease in pain intensity and increase in pressure pain threshold for both treatment groups compared to the control group. Ebenbichler and associates[49] found that ultrasound produced significant short-term improvement in strength, electroneurography, and subjective complaints for at least 6 months in patients with mild to moderate idiopathic carpal tunnel syndrome. On the negative side, Oztas and colleagues[50] demonstrated a statistically significant improvement in both therapeutic and placebo ultrasound groups in patients with carpal tunnel syndrome. Gursel and associates[51] did a randomized controlled trial on patients with soft tissue disorders of the shoulder (supraspinatus and biceps tendinosis, partial rotator cuff tear). The patients all received physical therapy modalities and exercise. One group also received ultrasound. There was no significant difference between the outcomes of the treatment and the control group.

Like all physical therapy modalities, the effectiveness of TENS has not been consistently documented. However, many studies indicate that TENS does have an analgesic effect. Resende and colleagues[52] induced hyperalgesia in rats' paws by injection of carrageenan. They found a 100% inhibition of the hyperalgesia after a 20-minute application of either high (130 Hz) or low (10 Hz) frequency TENS. The low frequency TENS had a longer lasting effect. Chesterton and associates[53] in a double blind study used a pressure algometer to measure the effects of TENS parameters of frequency, intensity, and stimulation site on pressure pain thresholds at the first dorsal interosseous muscle of healthy volunteers. The high frequency, high intensity segmental and combined stimulation groups showed rapid onset and significant hypoalgesic effects that were sustained for 20 minutes in the high frequency segmental group.

The purpose of any of the above modalities is to decrease pain and increase soft tissue extensibility so that it will be easier to elongate those tissues with mobilization and stretching.[1] Modalities may be eliminated as they reach their maximum usefulness.

COORDINATION, COMMUNICATION, AND DOCUMENTATION

The findings of the examination are discussed with Mrs. Brooks. A plan of care is formulated and discussed with her. Importance of compliance with her home exercise program for postural reeducation, stretching, and strengthening will be emphasized. All elements of the patient's management will be documented.

PATIENT/CLIENT-RELATED INSTRUCTION

She will be informed that although the exact etiology of adhesive capsulitis is unknown, people with Type 2 diabetes are at greater risk. Her chronic poor posture at her desk and keyboard may be a contributing factor to her shoulder problem. Mrs. Brooks will be given a written home exercise program with pictures and explanations of the exercises. This program will be upgraded as her status changes. Mrs. Brooks will be educated about the use of self-administered thermal agents and/or modalities for carryover of interventions to the home.

THERAPEUTIC EXERCISE

- ◆ Aerobic capacity/endurance conditioning
  - Patient will use the upper body ergometer for 10 minutes three times per week
  - She will bicycle for 20 minutes five times per week, exercising at a HR of between 130 and 146 that is at 80% to 90% of her AAMHR[32]

- ◆ Body mechanics and postural stabilization
  - Chin tucks
    - Start from the supine position, with the minimal number of pillows under the patient's head as is necessary for comfort
    - Teach the patient to tuck her chin and be aware of the lengthening of the neck so that the back of the skull moves away from the bottom of the neck
    - Progress quickly to doing these same exercises in seated and standing positions
    - Progress to adding scapula retraction and depression
    - Be certain that when seating or standing, the patient is not substituting with lumbar extension
  - Lumbar spine alignment
    - Teach patient the relationship between lumbar spine position and its effect on cervical/thoracic position
    - Teach patient to maintain a lumbar neutral position while seated
      - ▹ This may include education about proper type of furniture and its effect on posture and use of a lumbar support pillow for the lumbar spine

- ◆ Flexibility exercises
  - Stretching exercises should be done after warming up, using a slow and steady stretch accompanied by deep breathing, and building hold up to 30 to 60 seconds
  - Cervical AROM
  - Corner stretch for anterior chest muscles and fascia
  - PNF contract/relax techniques to increase:
    - Stretch of cervical muscles, including upper trapezii, scalenes, and SCMs
    - Stretch of shoulder muscles including internal and external rotators, pectoralis major, latissimus dorsi, and levator scapulae
  - Wand exercises in supine
    - Patient holds any straight, light object, such as a cane, long umbrella, or mop stick, with one hand close to each end
    - Raise both arms overhead as far as possible holding the stretch for 30 seconds while trying to breathe and relax
    - From the overhead position, keep elbows straight and move wand from side to side (adduction and abduction)
    - Do same as above, but start with elbows in 90 degrees of flexion and shoulder in about 45 degrees of abduction using the wand to stretch into ER
  - Wand exercises in standing
    - Hold wand behind the back with one hand hold-

ing each end, stretch back (into extension) as far as possible
- Slide wand up back as far as possible
- Towel exercise in standing to stretch into flexion and behind back
  - Hold towel end with right hand and reach overhead so towel dangles behind the back
  - Grasp other end of towel with left hand and pull the towel down with the left hand to stretch the right shoulder into flexion
  - Reverse hand position so the left hand pulls the right shoulder higher behind the back
- Wall walk
  - Slide hand or walk fingers up wall as high as possible
- Strength, power, and endurance training
  - Manual scapula strengthening exercises using PNF techniques of anterior elevation/posterior depression and posterior elevation/anterior depression[33]
  - Lying prone retract scapula down and back to activate lower trapezius and lift arms up as high as possible
    - Do this at first with arms at sides, progressing to arms at 90 degrees abduction and then with arms overhead (if possible) in the scaption position
  - Manual shoulder strengthening exercises using D1 and D2 PNF patterns[33]
  - Strengthening of all rotator cuff muscles using elastic bands, dumbbells, and/or Velcro cuff weights
  - Closed chain exercises for the shoulder girdle
    - Quadruped position
      ‣ Rock forward and backward straight and diagonally
      ‣ Lift left arm and right leg simultaneously
      ‣ Do push-ups maintaining weight equally on right and left arms
      ‣ Do push-up with a plus
        ○ A push-up with an additional scapula protraction to activate the serratus anterior
    - Wall push-ups and wall push-ups with a plus
  - Physioball exercises
    - Patient is prone on Physioball and walks forward with ball under abdomen until most of the body weight is on both hands
    - From this position, the patient can:
      ‣ Push the ball away from her hands and then pull the ball toward her hands
      ‣ Do push-ups
      ‣ Lift the left arm up and balance on the ball using the RUE
    - While standing, bounce the Physioball rhythmically first using each hand alternately, and then

using the right hand only
- Using an overhand technique, throw the physioball against a wall and catch it
  ‣ If this is too difficult, substitute a lighter ball. Progress this exercise by throwing higher and/or a longer distance each time
- If there is access to aquatic therapy, either formal or informal, Mrs. Brooks will be encouraged to participate
  ‣ Initially activity in water should be geared to buoyancy-supported exercises to achieve relaxed, pain-free movement
  ‣ Exercises may then be progressed (as the patient's comfort level allows) to water resisted exercises and swimming
  ‣ Swimming should begin with strokes that do not challenge end ranges (eg, elementary back stroke, dog paddle, or side stroke on uninjured side) and progress to crawl, regular backstroke, and breaststroke

FUNCTIONAL TRAINING IN SELF-CARE AND HOME MANAGEMENT

- Self-care
  - Mrs. Brooks will be given suggestions for compensatory accomplishment of ADL tasks until her impairments decrease
    - Turn bra to front for closure or purchase front-closing bras
    - Dress upper body by inserting affected arm first
    - Obtain long-handled comb/brush to groom hair
    - Obtain long-handled sponge to wash mid/low back
- Home management
  - Mrs. Brooks will be given suggestions for compensatory accomplishment of IADL actions, tasks, and activities until her impairments decrease

FUNCTIONAL TRAINING IN WORK, COMMUNITY, AND LEISURE INTEGRATION OR REINTEGRATION

- Work, community, and leisure
  - Mrs. Brooks will be given suggestions for compensatory accomplishment of these tasks until her impairments decrease
- Devices and equipment use and training
  - Mrs. Brooks will be advised to use a "reacher" in order to remove objects from high shelves until her mobility and strength improve
  - As an alternative, she can either move frequently

used objects to lower shelves or use a step stool to reach higher areas

MANUAL THERAPY TECHNIQUES

- ◆ Mobilization/manipulation
  - STM
    - Any form of STM that would elongate muscles/tissues that are tight or in spasm may be utilized
    - Muscles that are most commonly tight and must be addressed include the pectoralis major and minor, intercostals of ribs 1 through 7 or 8, subscapularis, latissimus dorsi, and teres major[31]
  - Joint mobilization: All glides should be done in Grades III and IV in order to stretch the joint capsule[21]
    - ST joint
      - ▸ Since there is no capsule at this joint, the following movements stretch primarily muscles and soft tissue
        - ○ Distraction to increase all physiological movements
        - ○ Upward rotation and adduction to increase physiological movement of shoulder flexion
        - ○ Depression and downward rotation to increase physiological movement of IR
    - GH joint
      - ▸ Lateral distraction to increase all physiological movements
      - ▸ Posterior glide to increase physiological movement of flexion and IR
      - ▸ Inferior glide to increase physiological movement of abduction
      - ▸ Anterior glide to increase physiological movement of extension and ER
    - SC joint
      - ▸ Inferior glide to increase physiological movement of scapula elevation
      - ▸ Superior glide to increase physiological movement of scapula depression
      - ▸ Posterior glide to increase physiological movement of scapula adduction
    - AC joint
      - ▸ Posterior, anterior, superior, and inferior glides to increase joint play and improve physiological movements in all directions
    - Low cervical/upper thoracic spines
      - ▸ The last 20 degrees of shoulder flexion and abduction are actually spinal movements
      - ▸ If the right shoulder is brought into full range of abduction or flexion, the upper thoracic spine moves into sidebend left

- ▸ If both UEs are moved into 180 degrees flexion, the last 20 degrees comes from upper thoracic extension
- ▸ As Mrs. Brooks gets closer to about 160 degrees of flexion or abduction, it is important to add mobilization of the low cervical/upper thoracic spines to allow the last degrees of motion to occur[54,55]
- ▸ Manual cervical distraction to improve general intervertebral mobility[34]
- ▸ Anterior glide of the SPs of low cervical and upper thoracic areas to improve mobility into extension[34]

ELECTROTHERAPEUTIC MODALITIES

- ◆ Electrical stimulation
  - TENS or high voltage stimulation to modulate pain[1]

PHYSICAL AGENTS AND MECHANICAL MODALITIES

- ◆ Sound agents
  - Continuous ultrasound to the shoulder for thermal effect[1]
- ◆ Thermotherapy
  - Hydrocollator packs for 20 minutes to the cervical spine and right shoulder girdle to increase tissue extensibility[8]

ANTICIPATED GOALS AND EXPECTED OUTCOMES

- ◆ Impact on pathology/pathophysiology
  - Pain is decreased to 1/10 with activity and 0/10 with rest.
  - Soft tissue inflammation, edema, and restriction are reduced.
- ◆ Impact on impairments
  - Endurance is increased.
  - Flexibility of right pectoralis major, pectoralis minor, latissimus dorsi, subscapularis, and upper trapezius is improved.
  - Mobility of right shoulder girdle and cervical and thoracic spines is improved in all directions.
  - Muscle spasms are eliminated.
  - Muscle strength of right shoulder girdle is improved to 4+/5 with normal SH rhythm. Grip strength is increased to 57 lbs in the right hand.
  - Muscle tension (palpation) is no longer tender over anterior and medial GH joint line, supraspinatus, and long head of biceps tendons.

- Posture is improved. Forward head is improved. Posture while working at the computer is improved.
- ROM is improved in cervical, thoracic, and right shoulder girdle joints to 85% to 95% of normal.
- Spasm of right pectoralis major, pectoralis minor, and subscapularis is decreased.

♦ Impact on functional limitations
  - Ability to assume or resume required self-care, home management, work, community, and leisure roles is improved.
  - Ability to independently perform physical actions, tasks, and activities related to ADL/IADL in self-care, home management, work, community, and leisure with or without assistive devices and equipment is increased.
  - Ability to raise RUE overhead and behind back for dressing is improved.
  - Ability to return to previous exercise level is achieved.

♦ Risk reduction/prevention
  - Risk factors are reduced.
  - Risk of secondary impairments is reduced.

♦ Impact on health, wellness, and fitness
  - Behaviors that foster healthy habits, wellness, and prevention are acquired.
  - Decision making is enhanced regarding health, wellness, and fitness needs.
  - Physical function is improved.

♦ Impact on societal resources
  - Available resources are maximally utilized.
  - Documentation occurs throughout patient management and follows APTA's *Guidelines for Physical Therapy Documentation.*[36]

♦ Patient/client satisfaction
  - Case is managed throughout the episode of care.
  - Clinical proficiency and interpersonal skills of the physical therapist are acceptable to the patient/client.
  - Patient's knowledge and awareness of the diagnosis, prognosis, interventions, and understanding of anticipated goals and expected outcomes are increased.

REEXAMINATION

Reexamination is performed throughout the episode of care.

DISCHARGE

Mrs. Brooks is discharged from physical therapy after a total of 20 physical therapy sessions over 12 weeks. These sessions have covered her entire episode of care. She is dis-

charged because she has achieved her goals and expected outcomes.

Case Study #3: Lateral Epicondylitis

Charles Kang is a 45-year-old male computer programmer who has been renovating his house for the past 3 months and has been diagnosed with right lateral epicondylitis.

PHYSICAL THERAPIST EXAMINATION

HISTORY

♦ General demographics: Mr. Kang is a 45-year-old male of Asian-American descent whose native language is English. He is a college graduate with a master's degree in computer programming. Mr. Kang is right-hand dominant.

♦ Social history: Mr. Kang grew up in an immigrant household. His parents came from Hong Kong. He is married with a 5-year-old daughter and an 8 year-old son.

♦ Employment/work: Mr. Kang works as a computer programmer. His job responsibilities include the use of a keyboard 5 out of 8 hours per day.

♦ Living environment: He lives in a private ranch-style house in the suburbs.

♦ General health status
  - General health perception: Mr. Kang considers himself to be in excellent health, in spite of having borderline HTN.
  - Physical function: He perceives his physical function as normal.
  - Psychological function: Normal.
  - Role function: Father, husband, computer programmer.
  - Social function: Mr. Kang is very involved in family activities, such as hiking and camping. He coaches his son's baseball team and his daughter's soccer team.

♦ Social/health habits: He is a non-smoker and a social drinker (two to three drinks and three glasses of wine per month).

♦ Family history: Mr. Kang's mother has Type 2 diabetes. His father died 3 years ago secondary to a MVA.

♦ Medical/surgical history: He sustained a left distal fibula fracture secondary to a skiing accident 6 years ago. He has no residual deficits in the LLE. All other systems are noncontributory.

♦ Preexisting medical and other health-related conditions: Mr. Kang has borderline HTN controlled with diet and exercise.

♦ Current condition(s)/chief complaint(s): Mr. Kang reports an insidious onset of right forearm pain starting about 8 weeks ago. He was building shelving systems and cabinets for his den. He states that the condition has been worsening in the past 4 weeks. He complains that he is limited in his ability to work at the keyboard.

♦ Functional status and activity level: Mr. Kang has deferred further renovation of his den secondary to increased pain. He purchased and is using a "tennis elbow brace" upon advice of a friend but has had only minimal relief.

♦ Medications: He has treated himself with Aleve once daily for 4 weeks with minimal relief.

♦ Other clinical tests: None.

SYSTEMS REVIEW

♦ Cardiovascular/pulmonary
  ● BP: 140/85 mmHg
  ● Edema: None noted
  ● HR: 80 bpm
  ● RR: 10 bpm

♦ Integumentary
  ● Presence of scar formation: None
  ● Skin color: WNL
  ● Skin integrity: WNL

♦ Musculoskeletal
  ● Gross range of motion
    ■ LUE, right elbow, forearm, and fingers were WNL
    ■ There were mild decreases in ROM in right shoulder flexion, ER, IR, and wrist extension
  ● Gross strength
    ■ LUE WNL
    ■ Right shoulder girdle, shoulder, and hand demonstrated mild to moderate weakness
  ● Gross symmetry: Upper quarter is grossly symmetrical
  ● Height: 5'11" (1.80 m)
  ● Weight: 170 lbs. (77.11 kg)

♦ Neuromuscular: WNL

♦ Communication, affect, cognition, language, and learning style
  ● Communication, affect, and cognition: WNL
  ● No apparent learning barriers
  ● Learns well via written and auditory methods

TESTS AND MEASURES

♦ Aerobic capacity/endurance

● Mr. Kang exercises three times weekly for 30 minutes each on a treadmill and bicycle ergometer
● He exercises at a HR of between 140 and 157, which is at 80% to 90% of his AAMHR[32]

♦ Anthropometric characteristics
  ● BMI=705 x (body weight [in pounds] divided by height[2] [in inches])
  ● Mr. Kang's BMI=23.7
  ● BMI values between 18.5 and 24.9 are considered normal[14]
  ● Edema: Circumferential measurements of forearms 1 inch distal to humeral epicondyles were equal

♦ Cranial and peripheral nerve integrity: Intact

♦ Ergonomics and body mechanics
  ● Patient does not have adequate lumbar support while sitting at his work station
  ● His keyboard is higher than it should be
  ● The monitor is too high for appropriate eye gaze

♦ Joint integrity and mobility
  ● Right shoulder anterior and posterior glides moderately hypomobile
  ● Right humero/ulna joint: WNL
  ● Right humero/radial joint: WNL
  ● Right proximal radio/ulna joint: WNL
  ● Right wrist anterior glide of radiocarpal and midcarpal joints moderately hypomobile
  ● Cervical spine mobility testing using PPIVM testing[34]
    ■ Flexion: WNL
    ■ Extension: Moderately restricted from C5 to C7 with hard end feel
    ■ Rotation: Moderately restricted from C5 to C7 with hard end feel, bilaterally
  ● Thoracic spine mobility testing using PPIVMs
    ■ Flexion: WNL
    ■ Extension: Moderately restricted from T1 to T5 with hard end feel

♦ Motor function
  ● Finger manipulative and dexterity skills were WNL

♦ Muscle performance
  ● MMT of LUE: WNL
  ● MMT right shoulder WNL except:
    ■ Lower trapezius=4-/5
    ■ Infraspinatus=4-/5
    ■ Teres minor=4/5
    ■ Subscapularis=4/5
  ● MMT right elbow and forearm: WNL
  ● MMT right hand WNL except:
    ■ Flexor pollicus longus=3+/5
    ■ Flexor digitorum profundus of second and third digits=3+/5

- Grip strength testing with hand dynamometer:
  - Right: 80 lbs with reports of pain in lateral epicondyle area
  - Left: 100 lbs and pain free
  - The mean grip strength for males in the 45- to 49-year-old age group is 109.9 with a SD of 23.0 for the right hand and 100.8 with a SD of 22.8 for the left[37]
- Pinch grip testing
  - WNL for left hand
  - When testing the right hand, the patient could only perform pulp-to-pulp pinch and not tip-to-tip pinch
  - This is a positive Pinch Grip test that indicates anterior interosseus nerve entrapment[56]
  - The anterior interosseus nerve (a motor branch of the median nerve) may become entrapped as it passes between the two heads of the pronator teres muscle
  - The nerve innervates the flexor pollicis longus, lateral half of the flexor digitorum profundus, and the pronator quadratus muscles
  - Distal interphalangeal (DIP) flexion of the thumb, index, and middle fingers are weak or paralyzed therefore impairing tip-to-tip pinch
- ◆ Orthotic, protective, and supportive devices
  - Patient is using a tennis elbow splint
  - Patient is using a tennis elbow counterforce brace in order to distribute the tension of the muscle pull over a larger area so that the force per unit area is decreased
- ◆ Pain
  - On the NPS, Mr. Kang reported pain intensity to be 0/10 at rest and 8/10 with activities that require sustained stress or strength of right elbow/wrist/hand complex[15]
- ◆ Posture
  - Mild FHP
  - Right shoulder higher than left
  - Both scapulae are abducted, right greater than left
- ◆ Range of motion
  - Cervical spine AROM, measured using a CROM
    - Flexion: WNL
    - Extension=20 degrees with motion occurring mostly at upper cervical spine
    - Rotation=40 degrees left and 40 degrees right
    - Sidebending=15 degrees left and 15 degrees right
  - Right shoulder PROM measured using a standard goniometer
    - ER=0 to 45 degrees
    - IR=0 to 50 degrees

- Flexion=0 to 170 degrees
- Abduction=0 to 170 degrees
- Right elbow PROM: WNL
- Right forearm PROM: WNL
- Right wrist PROM
  - Extension=0 to 15 degrees
  - Flexion=WNL
  - Radial and ulnar deviation=WNL
- Muscle tightness
  - Suboccipital muscles
  - Pectoral muscles, bilaterally
  - SCM muscles, bilaterally
  - Right extensor carpi radialis brevis
- Special tests
  - Cozen's test was positive for lateral epicondylitis[52]
  - Pinch grip test was positive for anterior interosseus nerve entrapment[56]
- Muscle tension (palpation)
  - Tenderness noted over the right lateral epicondyle, common extensor tendon insertion and pronator teres muscle
- ◆ Reflex integrity
  - UE DTRs were WNL, bilaterally
- ◆ Self-care and home management
  - Independent in all areas
- ◆ Work, community, and leisure integration or reintegration
  - He is having difficulty with posture and keyboard placement during work activities
  - He is able to continue to participate in family activities
  - He is able to continue coaching

EVALUATION

Mr. Kang's examination indicated that he is a fairly healthy 45-year-old male who developed gradual onset of right elbow and forearm pain and weakness due to repetitive strain injury of the wrist extensors. He has weakness and decreased ROM in his right wrist. He reports pain that increases with activity. His posture is altered, especially during his work actions, tasks, and activities. He is able to carry out all ADL, IADL, and work activities with discomfort and some compensatory strategies.

DIAGNOSIS

Mr. Kang has right lateral epicondylitis with pain. In addition he has impaired: ergonomics and body mechanics; joint integrity and mobility; muscle performance; posture; and range of motion. He in functionally limited in work, community, and leisure actions, tasks, and activities. These findings are consistent with placement in Pattern E: Impaired Joint Mobility, Motor Function, Muscle Performance, and Range of Motion Associated With Localized Inflammation. These impairments and functional limitations will be addressed in determining the prognosis and the plan of care.

PROGNOSIS AND PLAN OF CARE

Over the course of the visits, the following mutually established outcomes have been determined:

♦ Ability to perform work actions, tasks, and activities is improved

♦ Joint integrity and mobility are improved

♦ Muscle performance is increased

♦ Pain is decreased

♦ Physical function is improved

♦ Postural control is improved

♦ ROM is improved

To achieve these outcomes, the appropriate interventions are determined. The plan of care will include: coordination, communication, and documentation; patient/client-related instruction; therapeutic exercise; functional training in work, community, and leisure integration or reintegration; manual therapy techniques; prescription, application, and, as appropriate, fabrication of devices and equipment; electrotherapeutic modalities; and physical agents and mechanical modalities.

Based on the diagnosis and prognosis, Mr. Kang is expected to require between 8 and 16 visits over a period of 8 weeks. Mr. Kang has good social support, is motivated, and will follow through with his home exercise program. He is not severely impaired and is healthy.

INTERVENTIONS

RATIONALE FOR SELECTED INTERVENTIONS

Therapeutic Exercise

Mr. Kang demonstrates extreme stress applied to the right elbow and wrist musculature due to excessive use of carpentry tools such as screwdrivers, hammers, and saws. Proximal muscular stabilization is decreased due to weakness of the right shoulder rotators that fatigue easily. This shifts even more stress to the elbow, wrist, and hand. His poor posture (forward head and increased thoracic kyphosis) places the scapula in an abnormal resting position on the thorax. This leads to abnormal SH rhythm and decreased efficiency of the shoulder girdle muscles and places more stress on the elbow, wrist, and hand.[57] Restoring muscle flexibility, power, and

endurance to the shoulder girdle, forearm, wrist, and hand will allow each area to adequately cope with the added work stresses.[58]

Manual Therapy Techniques

Restoring muscle function and balance without addressing posture and joint mobility will not be effective. Strengthening muscles with the proximal and distal segments in poor alignment may result in injury to those muscles. When thoracic spine mobility is limited in extension, the scapula develops an abnormal position on the thoracic spine, and the scapula musculature develop altered recruitment patterns due to overstretch weakness. Joint and STM of the cervical and thoracic spines will allow the scapula to rest in an appropriate position on the thoracic spine. This will restore normal length-tension relationships of the scapula musculature and allow the muscles of the shoulder girdle to function in a balanced fashion.[18,59]

Shoulder mobility was impaired in IR and ER. Both of these directions must be addressed with joint mobilization so that joint capsule tightness does not interfere with the ability of the rotator cuff musculature maintaining the humeral head centered in the glenoid fossa.

Muscle flexibility impairments in the cervical spine may be addressed with soft tissue and myofascial release techniques to allow the head to achieve a balanced position on the cervical spine.[35]

Flexibility impairment of the extensor carpi radialis brevis may be addressed by use of cross friction massage,[1] myofascial release, and stretching.[35]

Electrotherapeutic Agents

Electrotherapy, such as high voltage current or TENS, may be used for pain modulation.[52,53,60]

Iontophoresis is the process of transferring ions from an electrolytic solution through the skin by means of an electric current. Dexamethasone sodium phosphate is one commonly used anti-inflammatory agent. Applying iontophoresis with dexamethasone to the lateral epicondyle may help to decrease the inflammation during the acute and subacute phase.[60]

Physical Agents and Mechanical Modalities

Cold packs may be used to create pain inhibition and reduce inflammation and reduce muscle guarding and spasm.[8]

COORDINATION, COMMUNICATION, AND DOCUMENTATION

The findings of the examination are discussed with the patient. All elements of Mr. Kang's management will be documented.

PATIENT/CLIENT-RELATED INSTRUCTION

The patient will be instructed about his current condition and impairments. It will be explained to Mr. Kang that the most probable etiology of his pain is a repetitive strain injury of the right forearm that occurred as a result of excessive and repeated muscle overuse when working on the reconstruction project at home. This extra work combined with his continuous work at the keyboard created severe stress on specific muscles that resulted in his painful condition.

A plan of care is formulated and discussed with the patient. Mr. Kang will be given a program of self-care at home. This will consist of application of cold, self-massage to decrease pain and edema, exercises to elongate the wrist extensor muscles, and progressive stretching and strengthening of the scapula, shoulder, and hand muscles that were found to be weak. He will also be instructed in workplace ergonomics to prevent future reinjury.

THERAPEUTIC EXERCISE

- ◆ Body mechanics and postural stabilization
  - Patient is taught that posture starts with a balanced pelvis
  - Patient will learn pelvic rocking in order to move into and out of a neutral spine or use a support for the lumbar spine when sitting
  - The concept that the low back and pelvic position affect thoracic and cervical spine position will be reinforced
  - The concept that the head should be balanced on the neck will also be reinforced
  - Exercises for cervical axial extension starting in supine and progressing to sitting and standing will be performed
- ◆ Flexibility exercises
  - Cervical and thoracic AROM
  - Corner stretch to open anterior chest
  - "L" bar exercises to stretch IR and ER of the shoulder[1]
  - Progressive stretching of right dorsal forearm
    - Start with passive stretch into wrist flexion with the elbow flexed
    - Progress to same stretch with fingers flexed
    - Progress to same stretch with elbow straight
    - Add shoulder IR to stretch
    - Full stretch will include finger flexion, wrist flexion, ulnar deviation, elbow extension, shoulder IR, and shoulder extension
- ◆ Strength, power, and endurance training
  - Strengthening of the deep cervical flexors
  - Manual resistive exercises (MREs)
    - Scapula PNF patterns anterior elevation/posterior depression with emphasis on posterior depression, bilaterally
    - Manual resistance may be done using isotonic, eccentric, and/or combination of isotonic techniques[33]
    - Progress to PNF D2 RUE pattern using isotonic, eccentric, and combination of isotonic contractions with emphasis on forearm, wrist, and hand[33]
  - Strengthening of flexor pollicus longus and flexor profundus of index and middle fingers
  - Strengthening of flexor pollicus longus and flexor profundus of the index and middle fingers using therapeutic putty exercises and a Power Web elastic hand exerciser
  - PRE using the DeLorme method (10 RM) to strengthen the right shoulder and wrist musculature[7]

FUNCTIONAL TRAINING IN WORK, COMMUNITY, AND LEISURE INTEGRATION OR REINTEGRATION

- ◆ Mr. Kang will be taught appropriate ergonomics in the workplace in order to avoid increasing stress on the forearm while at work
  - He will be taught that his chair should provide adequate lumbar support, with his thighs approximately parallel to the floor and his feet resting comfortably on the floor
  - His keyboard height should allow his elbows to rest at 90 degrees with his wrists in neutral or slight flexion
  - The monitor should be positioned so that the eyes gaze downward at about a 10- to 15-degree slope[8]
  - He will be instructed to take frequent breaks from the keyboard in order to stretch his upper quarter
- ◆ He will be taught to perform a stretching program at specific time intervals during the workday. This program will include stretching of the cervical spine, shoulder, elbow, forearm, wrist, and fingers

MANUAL THERAPY TECHNIQUES

- ◆ Mobilization/manipulation
  - Soft tissue techniques[35]
    - To the muscle bellies of the dorsal right forearm
    - Cross friction massage to common extensor tendon of the right forearm
    - STM of suboccipital muscles
    - STM and myofascial release to the pronator teres in order to free the anterior interosseus nerve
  - Mobilization techniques[21,34]
    - Manual cervical distraction

- Anterior glide on the SPs of the low cervical spine (Grades III and IV)
- Anterior glide on the SPs of mid and upper thoracic spine (Grades III and IV)
- Anterior glide of the GH joint to increase physiological movement of ER (Grades III and IV)
- Posterior glide of the GH joint to increase physiological movement of IR (Grades III and IV)
- Neural gliding techniques to free the anterior interosseus nerve[61]
  - Since the anterior interosseous nerve is a branch of the median nerve, the median nerve dominant upper limb tension test 1 (ULTT 1) will be used
    - Patient is supine
    - The physical therapist depresses the scapula, abducts the humerus to 110 degrees, supinates the forearm, extends the wrist and fingers, laterally rotates the shoulder, and extends the elbow
  - The use of neural gliding techniques have general guidelines, but leave specific progressions up to the clinical judgment of the physical therapist and the patient's response
  - The initial technique must move into ranges in which the therapist senses resistance and tension or pain is felt by the patient
  - This would be the equivalent of a Grade III joint mobilization
  - Oscillations are performed for about 20 seconds
  - The techniques may be repeated several times, based on the patient's response
  - Key symptoms should be reassessed immediately after treatment
  - The therapist should always begin treatment with neural glides conservatively and progress slowly, since excessively aggressive treatment may irritate the patient's symptoms
- PROM
  - Passive range of the cervical spine to improve upper cervical flexion, rotation, and sidebending to each side
  - Passive range of the right shoulder to improve IR and ER
  - Passive range of the right wrist to improve extension

PRESCRIPTION, APPLICATION, AND, AS APPROPRIATE, FABRICATION OF DEVICES AND EQUIPMENT

- ♦ Orthotic devices
  - Use of a lateral epicondylitis brace may be effective in helping to distribute forces away from the lateral epicondyle
  - Be sure that the patient is using it correctly
  - The patient must be educated as to appropriate placement, tightness, and frequency of use during the day—the pad must be over the extensor muscle belly and secured tightly enough to keep the brace in place, but not to create edema in the forearm below the brace

ELECTROTHERAPEUTIC MODALITIES

- ♦ Electrotherapeutic delivery of medications
  - Iontophoresis with dexamethasone to relieve inflammation[60]
  - Electrical stimulation
  - TENS for pain relief[52,53,60]
- ♦ These modalities should be discontinued when it is determined that they have reached their maximum therapeutic benefit

PHYSICAL AGENTS AND MECHANICAL MODALITIES

- ♦ Cryotherapy
  - Cold packs will be applied to decrease edema
- ♦ Sound agents
  - Ultrasound to decrease inflammation[60]

ANTICIPATED GOALS AND EXPECTED OUTCOMES

- ♦ Impact on pathology/pathophysiology
  - Pain is decreased to 0/10 with activity.
  - Soft tissue inflammation, edema, and restriction are reduced.
- ♦ Impact on impairments
  - Endurance is increased.
  - Mobility in cervical and thoracic spines, right shoulder, and right wrist is improved.
  - Muscle flexibility of suboccipitals, right extensor carpi radialis brevis, and bilateral SCMs and pectorals are improved.
  - Muscle performance (strength, power, and endurance) is increased to 4+/5 in the deep cervical flexors, scapula adductors, and upward rotators, right shoulder, elbow, wrist, and hand. Grip strength is increased to 100 lbs in the right hand.
  - Postural control of head, neck, right shoulder, and scapula is improved.
  - ROM of the cervical spine is WFL, right shoulder ER is increased to 60 degrees, right IR is increased to 65, and right wrist extension is increased to 40 degrees.

♦ Impact on functional limitations
  • Ability to assume or resume required self-care, home management, work, community, and leisure roles is improved.
  • Ability to independently perform physical actions, tasks, and activities related to ADL/IADL in self-care, home management, work, community, and leisure with or without assistive devices and equipment is increased.
  • Ability to integrate appropriate posture while using the computer is achieved.
♦ Risk reduction/prevention
  • Risk factors are reduced.
  • Risk of secondary impairments is reduced.
  • Self-management of symptoms is improved.
♦ Impact on health, wellness, and fitness
  • Behaviors that foster healthy habits, wellness, and prevention are acquired.
  • Decision making is enhanced regarding health, wellness, and fitness needs.
  • Fitness, health status, physical capacity, and physical function are improved.
♦ Impact on societal resources
  • Available resources are maximally utilized.
  • Documentation occurs throughout patient management and follows APTA's *Guidelines for Physical Therapy Documentation.*[36]
♦ Patient/client satisfaction
  • Clinical proficiency and interpersonal skills of the physical therapist are acceptable to patient/client.
  • Patient's knowledge and awareness of the diagnosis, prognosis, interventions, and understanding of anticipated goals and expected outcomes are increased.
  • Sense of well-being is improved.

REEXAMINATION

Reexamination is performed throughout the episode of care.

DISCHARGE

Mr. Kang is discharged from physical therapy after a total of 13 visits over 8 weeks. These sessions have covered his entire episode of care. He is discharged because he has achieved his goals and expected outcomes.

REFERENCES

1. Prentice WE, Voight MI. *Techniques in Musculoskeletal Rehabilitation.* New York, NY: The McGraw-Hill Companies; 2001.
2. Oatis C. *Kinesiology: The Mechanics and Pathomechanics of Human Movement.* Philadelphia, Pa: Lippincott Williams & Wilkins; 2004.
3. Goodman CC, Boissonnault, WG. *Pathology: Implications for the Physical Therapist.* Philadelphia, Pa: WB Saunders; 1998.
4. Hamill J, Knutzen K. *Biomechanical Basis of Human Movement.* 2nd ed. Philadelphia, Pa: Lippincott Williams & Wilkins; 2003.
5. Cotran RS, Kumar V, Collins T. *Pathologic Basis of Disease.* 6th ed. Philadelphia, Pa: WB Saunders; 1999.
6. Hall CM, Brody LT. *Therapeutic Exercise Moving Toward Function.* Philadelphia, Pa: Lippincott Williams & Wilkins; 1999.
7. Almekinders LC, Temple JD. Etiology, diagnosis and treatment of tendonitis: an analysis of the literature. *Med Sci Sports Exerc.* 1998;30(8):1183-1190.
8. Dutton M. *Manual Therapy of the Spine.* New York, NY: McGraw-Hill; 2002.
9. Arnoczky SP. Physiologic principles of ligamentous injuries and healing. In: Scott WN, ed. *Ligament and Extensor Injury Mechanisms of the Knee.* St. Louis, Mo: Mosby; 1991.
10. Neviaser JS. Adhesive capsulitis of the shoulder. *J Bone Joint Surg.* 1945;27:211.
11. Hannafin JA, DiCarlo ED. Wickiewicz TL. Adhesive capsulitis: capsular fibroplasias of the glenohumeral joint. *J Shoulder Elbow Surg.* 1994;38(5).
12. Siegel LB, Cohen NJ, Gali EP. Adhesive capsulitis: a sticky issue. American Family Physician. April 1999. http://www.aafp.org/afp/990401ap/1843.html. Accessed June 16, 2004.
13. Nordin M, Frankel VH. *Basic Biomechanics of the Musculoskeletal System.* 3rd ed. Baltimore, Md: Lippincott Williams & Wilkins; 2001.
14. USDA Center for Nutrition Policy and Promotion. Body mass index and health. *Nutrition Insight.* 2000;March.
15. Stratford PW, Spadoni G. The reliability, consistency, and clinical application of a numeric pain rating scale. *Physiotherapy Canada.* 2001;53:88-91,114.
16. Carroll TJ, Riek S, Carson RG. Neural adaptations to resistance training. *Sports Med.* 2001;31(12):829-840.
17. Behm DG, St-Pierre DMM. The effects of strength training and disuse on the mechanisms of fatigue. *Sports Med.* 1998;25(3):173-189.
18. Sahrmann SA. *Diagnosis and Treatment of Movement Impairment Syndromes.* St. Louis, Mo: Mosby; 2002.
19. Greenman P. *Principles of Manual Medicine.* 2nd ed. Baltimore, Md: Williams & Wilkins; 1996.
20. Chaitow L. *Muscle Energy Techniques.* New York, NY: Churchill Livingstone; 1997.
21. Maitland G. *Peripheral Manipulation.* 2nd ed. London, England: Butterworth-Heinemann; 1991.
22. Pfeffer G, Bacchetti P, Deland J, et al. Comparison of custom and prefabricated orthoses in the initial treatment of proximal plantar fasciitis. *Foot Ankle Int.* 1999;20(4):214-221.
23. Powell M, Post WR, Keener J, Weardon S. Effective treatment of chronic plantar fasciitis with night splints: a crossover prospective randomized outcome study. *Foot Ankle Int.* 1998;19(1):8-10.
24. Batt ME, Tanjii JL, Skattum N. Plantar fasciitis: a prospective randomized clinical trial of the tension night splint. *Clin J Sport Med.* 1996;6(3):158-162.

25. Atkins D, Crawford F, Edwards J, et al. A systematic review of treatments for the painful heel. *Rheumatology.* 1999;38:968-973.

26. Gudeman SD, Eisele SA, Heidt RS Jr, et al. Treatment of plantar fasciitis by iontophoresis of 0.4% dexamethasone: a randomized double-blind, placebo controlled study. *Am J Sports Med.* 1997;25(3):312-316.

27. Crawford F, Snaith M. How effective is therapeutic ultrasound in the treatment of heel pain? *Ann Rheum Dis.* 1996;55(4):265-267.

28. Buchbinder R, Ptasznik R, Gordon J, et al. Ultrasound-guided extracorporeal shock wave therapy for plantar fasciitis: a randomized control study. *JAMA.* 2002;288(11):1364-1372.

29. Haake M, Konig R, Decker T, et al. Extracorporeal shock wave therapy for lateral epicondylitis: a randomized multicentered trial. *J Bone Joint Surg (Am).* 2002;84(11):1982-1991.

30. Seed CA, Richards C, Nichols D, et al. Extracorporeal shock wave therapy for tendonitis of the rotator cuff: a double blind randomized controlled trial. *J Bone Joint Surg (Br).* 2002;84(4):509-513.

31. Melikyan EY, Shahin E, Miles J, et al. Extracorporeal shock wave treatment for tennis elbow: a randomized double blind study. *J Bone Joint Surg (Br).* 2003;85(6):852-858.

32. Rothstein JM, Roy SH, Wolf SL. *Rehabilitation Specialist's Handbook.* Philadelphia, Pa: FA Davis Co; 1998.

33. Adler SS, Beckers D, Buck M. *PNF in Practice.* 2nd ed. New York, NY: Springer-Verlag; 2000.

34. Maitland G. *Vertebral Manipulation.* Boston, Mass: Butterworth-Heinemann; 2002.

35. Cantu RI, Grodin AJ. *Myofascial Manipulation: Theory and Clinical Application.* 2nd ed. Baltimore, Md: Aspen Publishers; 2001.

36. American Physical Therapy Association. Guide to physical therapist practice. 2nd ed. *Phys Ther.* 2001;81:9-744.

37. Mathiowetz V, Kashman N, Volland G, Weber K, Dowe M, Rogers S. Grip and pinch strength: normative data for adults. *Arch Phys Med Rehabil.* 1985;66:69-72.

38. Cyriax J. *Textbook of Orthopedic Medicine, Diagnosis of Soft Tissue Lesions.* 8th ed. London, England: Bailliere Tindall; 1982.

39. Itokazu M, Matsunaga T. Clinical evaluation of high-molecular-weight sodium hyaluronate for the treatment of patients with periarthitis of the shoulder. *Clin Ther.* 1995;17:946-955.

40. Rizk TE, Gavant AL, Finals RS. Treatment of adhesive capsulitis with arthrographic capsular distention and rupture. *Arch Phys Med Rehabil.* 1994;75:803-807.

41. Pollack RG, Duralde XA, Flatow EL, Bigliani LU. The use of arthroscopy in the treatment of resistant frozen shoulder. *Clin Orthop.* 1994;July(304):30-36.

42. Graichen H, Stammberger T, Bonel H, et al. Glenohumeral translation during active and passive elevation of the shoulder girdle: a 3D open MRI study. *J Biomech.* 2000;33:609.

43. Kelker, Flatow E, Bigliani L. A stereophotogrammetric method to determine the kinematics of the glenohumeral joint. *Advance Bioengineering.* 1992;(49):143.

44. Tovin BJ, Greenfield BH. Impairment-based diagnosis for the shoulder girdle. In: Tovin BJ, Greenfield BH, eds. *Evaluation and Treatment of the Shoulder: An Integration of the Guide to Physical Therapist Practice.* Philadelphia, Pa: FA Davis Co; 2001.

45. Vermeulen HM, Obermann WR, Burger BJ, Kok GJ, Rozing PM, Van den Ende CHM. End-range mobilization techniques in adhesive capsulitis of the shoulder joint: a multiple subject case report. *Phys Ther.* 2000;80:1204-1213.

46. Funk D, Swank AM, Adams KJ, Treolo D. Efficacy of moist heat pack application over static stretching on hamstring flexibility. *J Strength Cond Res.* 2001;15(1)123-126.

47. Klaiman MD, Shrader JA, Danoff JV, Hicks JE, Pesce WJ, Farland J. Phonophoresis versus ultrasound in the treatment of common musculoskeletal disorders. *Med Sci Sports Exerc.* 1998;30(9):1349-1355.

48. Esenyel M, Caglar N, Aldemir T. Treatment of myofascial pain. *Am J Phys Med Rehabil.* 2000;79(1):48-52.

49. Ebenbichler GR, Resch KL, Nicolakis P, Uhl F, Ghanem AH, Flalka V. Ultrasound treatment for treating the carpal tunnel syndrome: randomized "sham" controlled. *BMJ.* 1998;316(7133):731-737.

50. Oztas O, Turan B, Bora I, Karaskaya MK. Ultrasound therapy effect in carpal tunnel syndrome. *Arch Phys Med Rehabil.* 1998;79(12):1540-1544.

51. Gursel YK, Ulus Y, Bilgic A, Dincer G, van der Heijden G. Adding ultrasound in the management of soft tissue disorders of the shoulder: a randomized placebo-controlled trial. *Phys Ther.* 2004;84(4):336-343.

52. Resende MA, Sabino GG, Candido CR, Pereira LS, Francischi JN. Local transcutaneous electrical stimulation (TENS) effects in experimental inflammatory edema and pain. *Eur J Pharmacol.* 2004;504(3):217-222.

53. Chesterton LS, Foster NE, Wright CC, Baxter GD, Barlas P. Effects of TENS frequency, intensity and stimulation site parameter manipulation on pressure pain thresholds in healthy human subjects. *Pain.* 2003;106(1-2):73-80.

54. Porterfield JA, DeRosa C. *Mechanical Shoulder Disorders.* St. Louis, Mo: Saunders; 2004.

55. Bang MD, Deyle GD. Comparison of supervised exercise with and without manual physical therapy for patients with shoulder impingement syndrome. *J Orthop Sports Phys Ther.* 2000;30(3):126-137.

56. Konin JG, Wiksten DL, Isear JA, Brader H. *Special Tests for Orthopedic Examination.* Thorofare, NJ: SLACK Incorporated; 2002.

57. Ellenbecker T. *Clinical Examination of the Shoulder.* St. Louis, Mo: Elsevier Saunders; 2004.

58. Kisner C, Colby LA. *Therapeutic Exercise Foundations and Techniques.* Philadelphia, Pa: FA Davis Co; 2002.

59. Basmajian JV, Nyberg R. *Rational Manual Therapies.* Baltimore, Md: Williams & Wilkins; 1993.

60. Michlovitz S. *Thermal Agents in Rehabilitation.* 3rd ed. Philadelphia, Pa: FA Davis Co; 1996.

61. Butler DS. *Mobilization of the Nervous System.* New York, NY: Churchill Livingstone; 1992.

CHAPTER SIX

Impaired Joint Mobility, Motor Function, Muscle Performance, Range of Motion, and Reflex Integrity Associated With Spinal Disorders (Pattern F)

Lorna King, MSc, PT, MTC
Elaine Rosen, PT, DHSc, OCS, FAAOMPT
Sandra Rusnak-Smith, PT, DHSc, OCS

ANATOMY

Only pertinent basic anatomy for this pattern is detailed below. For a more in-depth understanding of the anatomy of the spine, the reader is encouraged to refer to *Gray's Anatomy*[1] and Bogduk and Twomey's *Clinical Anatomy of the Lumbar Spine*.[2]

The spinal column is made up of 33 vertebral segments which allow both stability and flexibility to the axial skeleton (Figure 6-1). The spinal column protects the spinal cord and spinal nerves, supports the trunk, transmits forces from the LEs and UEs, and provides attachments for connective tissue, muscles, and ribs. The spinal column is divided into cervical, thoracic, lumbar, and sacral regions. These regions curve in the sagittal plane with the cervical and lumbar regions having lordotic curves and the thoracic and sacral regions having kyphotic curves.

ANATOMY OF THE SPINE

Bony Elements

A typical vertebra is made up of a body anteriorly and an arch posteriorly, which together form the neural arch containing the spinal cord (Figure 6-2). At the junction of the vertebral body and the neural arch is the intervertebral foramen, which contains the spinal nerves, blood, and lym-

phatic vessels. An intervertebral disc connects each body. The vertebral body varies in size, shape, and proportions in different regions of the spine. The vertebral body gives rise to two short, thick, rounded pedicles posteriorly. The pedicles give rise to the superior and inferior articular processes that form the synovial zygapophyseal (facet) joints. The shapes of the facets of the zygapophyseal joints contribute to the available motion at the different levels of the spine. The laminae continue from the pedicles and curve posteromedially to complete the vertebral foramen and give rise to the SP. Transverse processes project laterally from the junction between the pedicle and the lamina and in the thoracic spine provide attachments for the ribs.[1]

Regional Variations

The different regions of the spinal column have variations in the bony elements of the typical vertebra that specifically relate to the function of that particular region. Following is a brief synopsis of the regional variations.

Cervical Spine

There are seven cervical vertebrae. Each has a foramen in the transverse process called the foramen transversarium for passage of the vertebral artery. Other features specific to the cervical vertebrae (C3-C6) include a small, relatively broad body with raised lateral lips called uncinate processes, a short bifid SP, and the formation of an articular pillar on each

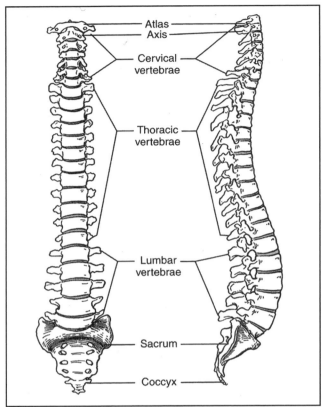

Figure 6-1. The spinal column. Reprinted from *Hollinshead's Functional Anatomy of the Limbs and Back*. 7th ed. Jenkins DB. Page 200, 1998, with permission from Elsevier.

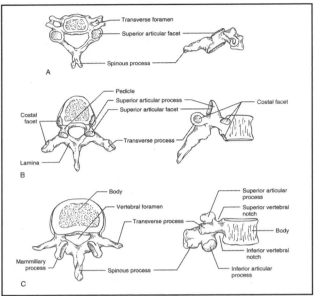

Figure 6-2. Typical cervical, thoracic, and lumbar vertebra. Reprinted from *Hollinshead's Functional Anatomy of the Limbs and Back*. 7th ed. Jenkins DB. Page 201, 1998, with permission from Elsevier.

side by the articulation of the superior and inferior articular processes. The joint plane of the cervical facet joints is generally described as approximately 45 degrees to the vertical.[1] There are three cervical vertebrae that need to be considered separately: C1 (the atlas), C2 (the axis), and C7 (vertebra prominens). C1 supports the head. It has no vertebral body and instead surrounds and articulates with the dens of C2 thus providing an axis for rotation of the atlas and the head. C7 has a long SP and is easy to palpate, although differentiation between C6, C7, and T1 is required.

Thoracic Spine

There are 12 thoracic vertebrae. Thoracic vertebrae increase in size caudally due to increased loading from above.[2] A unique feature of the thoracic vertebrae is the presence of facets for articulation with the ribs. A typical thoracic vertebra has lateral costal facets on the thoracic vertebral bodies that are for articulations with the head of the ribs. There are also facets on the transverse processes of the thoracic vertebrae T1-10 for articulation with the costal tubercle of ribs 1-10. Other features specific to the thoracic vertebrae include a gradual change in the size of the vertebral

bodies from a more cervical dimension in the upper thoracic vertebrae, uniquely thoracic in the mid thoracic area, and then to more lumbar characteristics in the lower thoracic area. The joint plane of the thoracic facet joints is described as approximately 15 to 20 degrees to the vertical plane.[2] There is a change in the orientation of the thoracic facet joints usually around T10, 11, or 12 whereby the superior articular processes are thoracic, that is, they face posterolaterally and the inferior articular processes are similar to those of the lumbar vertebrae, that is, they face anterolaterally and are transversely convex. This transitional vertebra marks the site of a sudden change in degree from rotational to nonrotational function.[1]

Lumbar Spine

There are five lumbar vertebrae. The main difference in the lumbar vertebrae is their large size in comparison to the cervical and thoracic vertebrae. The kidney-shaped bodies of the lumbar vertebrae are wider transversely and deeper anteriorly. The vertebral foramen is triangular, larger than the thoracic but smaller than the cervical levels.[1] The superior articular processes have facets that are vertical and concave and face posteromedially. The inferior articular processes have vertical, convex facets that face anterolaterally. The fifth lumbar vertebra that has the largest vertebral body is significantly deeper in the front, contributing to the lumbosacral angle.[1] In contrast, the SP of the fifth lumbar vertebra is relatively small and blunt.[3]

Sacrum and Coccyx

The sacrum is a large triangular fusion of five vertebrae forming the posterior wall of the pelvic cavity.[1] The sacrum is wedged between the two innominate bones.[1] The sacrum articulates superiorly with the L5-S1 intervertebral disc and the L5 vertebra and inferiorly with the coccyx. The sacrum is curved longitudinally and is convex on the posterior surface and concave on the anterior surface.[1] The base of the sacrum is the upper surface of the first sacral vertebra. The superior articular facets of the first sacral vertebra articulate with the inferior articular facets of the L5 vertebra. The anterior edge of the first sacral vertebra is known as the sacral promontory. The vertebral foramen is triangular, and the transverse processes are very different from those of the lumbar vertebrae. They are fused together to give rise to two important structures, the superior part of the sacral lateral mass or ala and the lateral auricular surface that articulates with the ilium forming the sacroiliac joint. The sacral canal is formed by the sacral vertebral foramina and contains the cauda equina. Inferiorly is the sacral apex that has a facet for articulation with the coccyx. The coccyx is a small triangular bone consisting of four rudimentary vertebrae.[1]

LIGAMENTS OF THE SPINE

Atlanto-Occipital Joints

Ligaments of the atlanto-occipital joints consist of the articular capsules and the anterior and posterior atlanto-occipital membranes.

Atlanto-Axial Joints

The cruciform ligament is composed of the transverse ligament, which is a broad, strong band arching across the atlantal ring behind the dens. It is attached laterally to a small tubercle on the medial side of each atlantal lateral mass. From the upper margin of the transverse component, a strong median longitudinal band (superior longitudinal band of the cruciform ligament) arises and inserts into the basilar part of the occipital bone between the apical ligament of the dens and the tectorial membrane. The inferior longitudinal band, when present, is the downward longitudinal projection that attaches to the posterior surface of the axis.

Each of the lateral atlanto-axial joints includes an accessory ligament posteromedially that attaches below to the axial body and above to the lateral atlantal mass near the transverse ligament.[1]

Ligaments Connecting the Axis and the Occipital Bone

These include the alar ligaments that are thick cords about 11 mm long that extend from the longitudinally ovoid flattenings on the posterolateral aspect of the apex of the dens horizontally and laterally to the roughened areas on the medial side of the occipital condyles. The apical liga-ment of the dens fans out from the apex of the dens into the anterior margin of the foramen magnum between the alar ligaments.[1]

Ligaments of the Spine (Figure 6-3)

The Anterior Longitudinal Ligament

The anterior longitudinal ligament (ALL) is a strong band extending along the anterior surfaces of the vertebral bodies and intervertebral discs.[1] It is attached to the occipital bone superiorly and to all vertebrae continuing caudally until it reaches the upper surface of the sacrum.[1] The ALL is several layers deep.[1] The structure of the ALL allows it to resist vertical separation of the anterior ends of the vertebral bodies, thereby limiting anterior bowing of the spine during extension movements.[2]

The Posterior Longitudinal Ligament

The posterior longitudinal ligament (PLL) is found on the posterior surface of the vertebral bodies and lies in the vertebral canal. It is attached to the body of C2 and the sacrum. The structure of the PLL is different from the ALL as it is separated from its attachments by the basivertebral veins.[1] In addition, at the cervical and upper thoracic areas, the PLL is broad and of uniform width, whereas at the lower thoracic and lumbar areas, it narrows over the vertebral bodies and is broader over the discs.[1] The structure of the PLL allows it to resist separation of the posterior ends of the vertebral bodies.[2]

Ligaments of the Posterior Elements

The supraspinous ligament (SSL) lies in the midline and attaches to the posterior edges of the SPs. *Gray's Anatomy* describes this ligament as "a strong fibrous cord connecting the tips of the SP from C7 to the sacrum."[1] Bogduk and Twomey, however, question whether the supraspinous ligament is truly a ligament due to the presence of intertwining tendinous fibers of the dorsal layer of the thoracolumbar fascia and the aponeurosis of the longissimus thoracis.[2] The functions of the thoracolumbar fascia and longissimus thoracis, via their tendinous fibers within the supraspinous ligament, include maintenance of posture, stability of the lumbar spine in the flexed position, and flexion and extension of the spine.

The ligamentum nuchae is the continuation of the supraspinous and interspinous ligaments in the neck.[2] However, the ligamentum nuchae differs structurally from the inter- and supraspinous ligaments as it consists of fibro-elastic fibers.[2] The function of the ligamentum nuchae is to limit flexion of the cervical spine.

The ligamentum flavum (LF) is a short, thick ligament that joins the laminae of each consecutive vertebra. The lateral portion of the ligamentum flavum attaches to the anterior aspect of the zygapophyseal joints and forms the anterior capsule.[2] The ligamentum flavum is unique in its histological

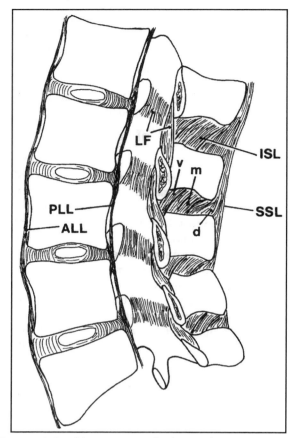

Figure 6-3. Ligaments of the spine (v=ventral, m=medial, d=dorsal). Reprinted from *Clinical Anatomy of the Lumbar Spine.* 2nd ed. Bogduk N, Twomey LT. Page 45, 1991, with permission from Elsevier.

thicknesses of the intervertebral discs vary within the different regions of the spine and within the disc themselves.[1] In the cervical and lumbar areas the discs are thicker anteriorly, which contributes to the lordotic curve in the sagittal plane. In the thoracic region the discs are of uniform thickness, and the kyphotic curve is mainly due to the shape of the thoracic vertebral bodies. Discs are avascular except for their peripheries, which are supplied by adjacent blood vessels.[1] Each disc consists of an outer annulus fibrosus and an inner nucleus pulposus.

The microstructures of the annulus fibrosus and the nucleus pulposus are both composed of water, PGs, and collagen. Collagen offers flexibility and high tensile strength. More than a dozen different types of collagen exist in the body. Type I collagen is tensile in nature and found in tissues routinely subjected to tension and compression.[1] Type II collagen is more elastic and found in tissues habitually exposed to pressure.[1]

Both Types I and II collagen fibers are found in the annulus fibrosus. These fibers are arranged in a highly ordered pattern in sheets called lamellae. The lamellae in turn are arranged in concentric rings around the nucleus pulposus. Each lamella overlaps in alternately oblique directions.[3] In the lumbar spine the lamellae are thick in the anterior and lateral portions of the annulus but are finer and more tightly packed in the posterior portion.[2] It has been suggested that the posterior fibers run more vertically predisposing to herniation.[2] Vascularity and neural ingrowth are present in the peripheral one-third of the annulus.

The nucleus pulposus is a semi-fluid mass of mucoid material. It is nearer the disc's posterior surface in the cervical and lumbar regions of the spine. The fluid nature of the nucleus pulposus allows it to be deformed under pressure. If it is subjected to pressure from any direction it will attempt to deform, thereby transmitting the pressure in all directions.[2] The PG molecules have the property of attracting and retaining water. The difference in composition between the annulus and the nucleus is in their relative concentrations of materials. The nucleus pulposus consists predominantly of PGs and water and some Type II collagen. The annulus fibrosus consists of water, PGs, and a higher concentration of Type I collagen fibers.[2] PGs inflate the disc due to their high osmotic pressure and close-packed nature and are able to maintain disc hydration even when high external loads are applied making it harder for water to escape. Collagen is responsible for providing a structural network to allow the disc to act as a joint and shock absorber. The individual fibers entangle the PG chains keeping them in the tissue. Water inflates the disc and provides 70% to 80% of its volume.[3] Thus, the principle functions of the disc are to allow movement between the vertebral bodies and to transmit loads from one vertebral body to the next. Variations in posture will alter the amount of pressure and the degree of annular tension being sustained by the disc. Nachemson[4] has found that there is greater pressure

composition, being composed of 80% yellow elastin fibers and 20% collagen fibers.[2] Thus, the ligamentum flavum is essentially an elastic ligament that may assist the flexed spine to return to the erect position, prevent nipping of the capsule of the zygapophyseal joints, and may reduce the risk of nerve root compromise.[2]

The interspinous ligament (ISL) connects adjacent SPs. This ligament is thin and almost membranous.[1] The direction of the fibers of the interspinous ligament resists separation of the SPs thereby limiting forward bending of the intervertebral joint.[2]

JOINTS OF THE SPINE

Joints of the Vertebral Bodies

All vertebrae, from the second cervical to the first sacral, are united by fibrocartilaginous intervertebral discs between their bodies and by the ALL and PLL. The intervertebral discs unite the adjacent surfaces of the vertebral bodies. The

exerted on the disc in the sitting position than in the standing position.

JOINTS OF THE VERTEBRAL ARCHES

The zygapophyseal joints, located between the superior articular facet of one vertebra and the inferior articular facet of the subadjacent vertebra, are synovial and vary in shape. These joints are contained within a thin, loose articular capsule, which attaches peripherally.[1] The zygapophyseal joints also contain small meniscoid structures.[1] In the cervical spine the joint planes are approximately 45 degrees to the vertical allowing for flexion, extension, lateral flexion, and rotation of the cervical spine.[3] In the thoracic spine the joint planes are approximately 60 degrees to the vertical allowing for flexion, lateral bending, and rotation which is limited by the ribs. In the lumbar spine, the facet planes may vary in orientation and shape. However, the primary motions are flexion and extension with limited sidebending and rotation. The zygapophyseal joints are innervated by the adjoining spinal nerves.

THE VERTEBRAL CANAL AND THE INTERVERTEBRAL FORAMINA

The alignment of successive vertebral foramina forms the vertebral canal. The shape of the vertebral canal varies throughout the length of the spine. The spinal cord runs the length of the vertebral canal ending approximately at the level of the L1-2 intervertebral disc. The cauda equina is formed by the lumbar, sacral, and coccygeal nerve roots.

The intervertebral foramina are the main routes of entry and exit to the vertebral canal.[1] The intervertebral foramina contain a segmental mixed spinal nerve and its sheaths, two to four recurrent meningeal (sinuvertebral) nerves, spinal arteries, and venous plexuses.[1] The boundaries of a typical intervertebral foramina are as follows: superiorly, the inferior aspect of the pedicle of the vertebra above; inferiorly the superior border of the pedicle of the vertebra below; anteriorly the dorsal aspect of the disc; and posteriorly the facet joint and the ligamentum flavum. These are important clinically because of the susceptibilities of their contents to multiple disorders.[1]

SPINAL NERVES

The spinal nerves lie in the intervertebral foramina and are connected to the spinal cord by the ventral and dorsal spinal roots. Of importance clinically are where the spinal nerves exit and their relationship to the intervertebral disc. In the cervical region the nerve root exits above the correspondingly numbered vertebra, so that the C5 root would be affected by prolapse of the C4/5 disc.[1] However, since there are eight cervical nerve roots and only seven cervical vertebrae, this relationship changes at the cervico-thoracic junction, so that below this level the nerve root emerges below the corresponding numbered vertebra.[1]

In the lumbar spine, the nerve root leaves the vertebral column laterally above the disc and is affected by a prolapsed disc at one level above its exit.[1] For example, the L5 root that emerges between L5 and S1 is usually affected by disc prolapse between L4 and L5.[1]

The spinal nerves divide into small dorsal rami and larger ventral rami after they exit the intervertebral foramina. The dorsal rami in turn divide into medial and lateral branches to supply the muscles and skin of the posterior regions of the neck and trunk.[1] The ventral rami of the spinal nerves supply the limbs and anterolateral aspects of the trunk. The cervical, lumbar, and sacral ventral rami connect near their origins to form plexuses.

Each typical spinal nerve contains somatic and visceral fibers. The somatic fibers are efferent and afferent. The efferent fibers innervate skeletal muscles. The afferent fibers carry information from receptors in the skin, subcutaneous tissue, muscles, fascia, and joints.[1] The visceral fibers are also efferent and afferent and belong to the ANS.

The sinuvertebral nerves are recurrent branches of the ventral rami that reenter the intervertebral foramina to be distributed within the spinal canal.[2] Here these mixed sensory and sympathetic nerves divide into transverse, ascending, and descending branches distributed to the dura mater, walls of blood vessels, periosteum, ligaments, and intervertebral discs.[2]

MUSCULATURE OF THE SPINE

A description of the actions and clinical relevance of the muscles of the spine is found in Table 6-1, and Figure 6-4 is intended primarily as a review of the muscles evaluated during examination of a patient.

KINESIOLOGY

BIOMECHANICS

The pertinent biomechanics of the spine for this pattern relate to the function of the intervertebral disc and movements of the different regions of the spine. This information provides the framework upon which a thorough examination, diagnosis, and rationale for intervention selection is made. For more detailed information on biomechanics of the spine it is suggested that the reader review White and Panjabi's *Clinical Biomechanics of the Spine*.[11]

The limited deformation of the intervertebral discs, the shape of the zygapophyseal joints, and the ligaments of the spinal column restrict movement between the vertebrae. Although movements between individual vertebrae are small, their summation gives a larger range to the vertebral column in flexion, extension, lateral flexion, and rotation.[1]

Table 6-1
MUSCLES OF THE SPINE

Muscles	Actions	Clinical Relevance
Suboccipital Muscles Recti capitis posteriors major and minor Obliqui capitis superior and inferior	Suboccipital muscles are extensors of the head at the atlanto-axial joints and rotators of the head and atlas on the axis.	The suboccipital muscles are a common trigger point source of post-traumatic headache.
Cervico-Thoracic Muscles		
Longus capitis	Flexes the head.	Same as for longus colli.
Longus colli	Forward flexes the neck. The superior oblique part creates lateral flexion. The inferior oblique part creates contralateral rotation.	Contraction of these deep neck flexors may be difficult after whiplash. Longus colli atrophy may affect the alignment of the head on neck.
Scaleni	Acting from below, the scalenus anterior flexes and sidebends the cervical spine and rotates it contralaterally. Acting from above, it helps to elevate the first rib. Acting from below, scalenus medius sidebends the cervical spine ipsilaterally. Acting from above, it helps to raise the first rib. The scalene muscles, particularly scalenus medius, are active during inspiration, even during quiet breathing in the erect posture. When the second rib is fixed, the scalenus posterior creates ipsilateral sidebending of the lower part of the cervical spine. When its upper attachment is fixed, it helps to elevate the second rib.	Tightness or spasm of these muscles can elevate the first and second ribs. The proximity of the scaleni muscles to the lower brachial plexus and subclavian artery and vein can give rise to compression syndromes, such as thoracic outlet syndrome.
Splenius capitis and splenius cervicis	Simultaneous contraction of the splenii pull the head directly in a posterior direction. Unilateral contraction pulls the head into slight rotation ipsilaterally.	Injury to these muscles may occur during any accident causing whiplash. It has been suggested that postural stresses that overload extension or rotation of the head and neck are likely to initiate and perpetuate splenius cervicis trigger points. It is important during examination of the patient to measure pectoralis major and minor tightness and the overall effect on posture and motion.
Sternocleidomastoid (SCM)	Acting alone, one SCM will tilt the head toward the ipsilateral shoulder, simultaneously rotating the head so as to turn the face to the other side. When acting together from below, the SCM also causes level rotation from side to side and the muscles draw the head forward. The two muscles are also used to raise the head when the body is supine and can assist in forced inspiration.	Torticollis, a postural deformity is due to a contracture of the SCM. This muscle can be injured in MVAs and should be evaluated for bruising and muscle spasm.

continued

	Table 6-1 (continued)	
	MUSCLES OF THE SPINE	
Muscles	*Actions*	*Clinical Relevance*
Trapezius	The trapezius assists in stabilizing the scapula during movements of the arm. With the levator scapulae, the upper fibers of the trapezius elevate the scapulae. With the serratus anterior, the trapezius rotates the scapula forward so that the arm can be raised above the head. With the rhomboids, the trapezius retracts the scapula. With the shoulder fixed, the trapezius may bend the head and neck backward and laterally.	It has been suggested that the trapezius is the muscle most affected by trigger points.[5]
Trunk Muscles		

Abdominal muscles:
  Rectus abdominis
  Obliquus externus
  Obliquus internus
  Transversus
  abdominis
	The abdominal muscles provide a firm but elastic wall that retains the abdominal viscera in position. When the thorax and the pelvis are fixed, the active contraction of these muscles creates a compressive force on the abdominal viscera.
	When the pelvis is fixed, the recti from both sides aided by the oblique abdominal muscles flex the lumbar spine; when the thorax is fixed they draw the front of the pelvis upward.
	If the muscles are active only on one side, the trunk is side bent to that side.
	The external oblique turns the front of the abdomen contralaterally, and the internal oblique ipsilaterally.
		Studies of motor control of the internal oblique and transversus abdominis have resulted in increased attention to instructing patients in exercises to increase the strength and endurance of these specific abdominal muscles for lumbar stabilization.[56,57]

Erector spinae	As a group these muscles function together to extend the cervical, thoracic, and lumbar spines. Asymmetrically they can cause ipsilateral side-bending and rotation. The erector spinae muscle complex lies in a groove on the side of the vertebral column covered in the lumbar and thoracic regions by the thoracolumbar fascia, serratus posterior inferior below, and rhomboids and splenii above.	These muscles play an important role in lumbar stabilization.
Multifidus Lumbar components of longissimus and iliocostalis	These muscles, in conjunction with the erector spinae muscles, are extensors of the spine.[6] They also contribute to lateral flexion and rotation of the spine. The multifidus also acts as a prime stabilizer of the lumbar spine and reinforces the articular capsule of the zygapophyseal joints.[7]	Clinically, it is important to note that wasting and local inhibition of the lumbar multifidus have been reported in a group of patients with a first episode of acute/sub-acute low back pain.[8] In a follow-up study it was also reported that without therapeutic intervention, the multifidus did not regain its original size or function, and the recurrence rate of low back pain in this group of patients was high. However, it was reported that the deficit could be reversed with an appropriate exercise program.[8]

continued

Table 6-1 (continued)
MUSCLES OF THE SPINE

Muscles	Actions	Clinical Relevance
Quadratus lumborum	The quadratus lumborum fixes the last rib and acts as a muscle of inspiration by helping to stabilize the lower attachments of the diaphragm. With the pelvis fixed, the quadratus acts upon the vertebral column, flexing it to the same side.	Tightness and spasm of this muscle is a common finding on examination of patients with low back pain.
Psoas	The psoas acts together with iliacus, the combination being referred to as the iliopsoas. These muscles thus flex the thigh on the pelvis and bend the trunk and pelvis forward against resistance. The psoas muscles are continuously active in erect posture.[9]	The roots of the lumbar plexus enter the muscle directly, and the plexus is lodged within it.
Iliacus	See above.	If the iliacus is shortened or in spasm, it may cause the pelvis to anteriorly rotate and increase the lumbar lordosis.
Thoracolumbar Fascia		It has been suggested that this fascial complex is important to the dynamic stability of the lumbar spine. It also serves as an attachment site for several key muscles of the trunk: latissimus dorsi, internal oblique, and transversus abdominis.[10]

The Intervertebral Disc

The main functions of the disc are to allow movements between the vertebral bodies and to transmit loads from one vertebral body to the next.[2] Both the nucleus pulposus and annulus fibrosus are involved in weightbearing. Compression of the intervertebral disc causes increased pressure in the nucleus pulposus. This increased pressure of the nucleus results in increased tension in the annulus. Tension on the annulus prevents the nucleus from expanding radially, and thus the pressure on the nucleus is exerted vertically on the vertebral end plates. The load is then passed from vertebra to vertebra via the vertebral end plate.[2] Another important role of the disc is that of a shock absorber of the spine. This same mechanism causes the speed of the force applied to the disc to attenuate, slowing the rate at which the applied force is transmitted to the vertebra.[2] It is important to understand that injury to any of these structures will affect the transmission of forces through the disc.

Biochemical changes, such as drying out of the disc, an increase in collagen, and a decrease in elastin, make the disc more fibrous. Fissures may occur in the annulus fibrosus.[12] As the outer layers of the annulus are innervated, these changes may lead to discogenic back pain.

BIOMECHANICS

Cervical Spine

Occipito-Atlanto Joints

White and Panjabi have suggested that the occipito-axial joints are relatively unstable. Their limited stability comes from the cup-shaped configuration of the occipito-axial joint surfaces, their capsules, and the anterior and posterior atlanto-occipital membranes.[12] Further stability is provided by the ligaments between the occiput and axis and the alar and apical ligaments. These joints allow for 3 degrees of freedom: axial rotation, flexion and extension, and lateral flexion.

The relative instability of the occipito-axial joints and the atlanto-axial joints are of particular relevance to physical therapists who treat patients with neck pain following trauma and/or patients with RA. There are a variety of possible traumatic upper cervical spine injuries, including fracture of the posterior arch of C1, fracture of the dens, and compression fractures. It is therefore very important to ensure that patients with neck pain secondary to a traumatic event have had radiographs to rule out cervical spine fractures. Radiographic studies should include an open-mouth view of the dens.

Atlanto-Axial Joints

Articulation of the atlas to the axis is at three mechanically linked synovial joints: two between the lateral masses; and one median articulation between the dens of the axis, the anterior arch, and the transverse ligament of the atlas. Movement of the atlanto-axial joint consists almost exclusively of rotation of the axis. Rotation takes place in the trochoid joint between the odontoid and the posterior aspect of the anterior arch of C1 and the lateral masses. The odontoid stays in place and the osteoligamentous ring turns around it. The alar ligaments limit rotation with a minor contribution from the accessory atlanto-axial ligament. There is no evidence of opening between the atlanto-odontoid and atlanto-axial joints noted on x-ray during flexion and extension.[13] The odontoid is held in place by the transverse ligament. Upper cervical sidebending and rotation are always coupled to the opposite side.[14]

Mid-Cervical Spine

In the cervical spine the upward inclination of the superior articular facets allows for flexion and extension. Flexion of the cervical spine occurs in the sagittal plane with a ROM of 80 to 90 degrees. In flexion, the upper vertebral body tilts and slides anteriorly. During flexion the facets barely engage, and it is therefore an unstable position. The nuclear material is displaced posteriorly. Flexion is limited by the tension developed in the PLL, the ligamentum nuchae, and the ligamentum flavum and by the apposition of the projecting lower lips of vertebral bodies on the sub-adjacent bodies.

Extension also occurs in the sagittal plane with a total ROM of 70 degrees, 15 degrees occurring at the occipito-axial joints. In extension, the overlying vertebral body tilts and slides posteriorly. The intervertebral space narrows posteriorly and the anterior fibers of the annulus widen. Extension is limited by the ALL and is limited cephalically by locking of the posterior edges of the superior facets of C1 in the occipital condylar fossae and caudally by the slipping of the inferior processes of C7 into grooves inferoposterior to the first thoracic superior articular process. This is the close packed position and is therefore maximally congruent with maximal stability.

Lateral flexion occurs in the frontal plane with a ROM of 20 to 45 degrees in each direction of which the majority of the movement takes place in the suboccipital joints. In lateral flexion, the facets slide upward (open) on the contralateral side, while on the ipsilateral side the facets slide downwards (close). Lateral flexion is limited by the ipsilateral uncinate process and the contralateral capsule.[13] Lateral flexion is usually coupled with rotation below C2.[2]

Rotation occurs in the transverse plane with a ROM of 70 to 90 degrees in each direction of which half of the range occurs at occipito-axial and atlanto-axial joints.[3] During rotation, an inferior glide of the facet occurs on the ipsilateral side. The amount of rotation that occurs with

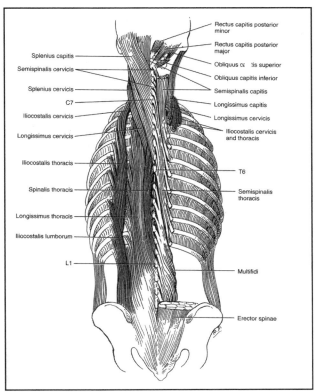

Figure 6-4. Muscles of the spine. Reprinted from *Hollinshead's Functional Anatomy of the Limbs and Back.* 7th ed. Jenkins DB. Page 215, 1998, with permission from Elsevier.

sidebending decreases from C2-7. The greatest amount of rotation occurs at C1-C2. Cervical sidebending and rotation are coupled movements to the same side.[14]

Thoracic Spine

Flexion of the thoracic spine occurs in the sagittal plane with a ROM of 20 to 45 degrees. In flexion, the inferior articular processes of the uppermost (superior) vertebra glide anteriorly and upwardly over the superior facets of the vertebrae below (inferior) allowing both facets to open. The interspaces between the vertebrae open, and the nuclear material is displaced posteriorly. Flexion is limited by the tension developed in the interspinous ligament, the ligamentum flavum, the supraspinous ligament, the capsular ligaments of the joints between the articular processes, and the PLL.

Extension also occurs in the sagittal plane with a ROM of 25 to 45 degrees. In extension, the inferior articular processes of the uppermost (superior) vertebrae glide posteriorly and downward over the superior facets of the vertebrae (inferior) below causing both facets to close. The thoracic vertebrae approximate posteriorly, and the nucleus is displaced anteriorly. Extension is limited by both the articular processes and SPs. The ALL is taut while the PLL, the ligamentum flavum, and the interspinous and supraspinous ligaments are relaxed. Extension of the thoracic vertebra also occurs during bilateral elevation of the arms.[15]

Lateral flexion occurs in the frontal plane with a ROM of 20 to 40 degrees in each direction. In lateral flexion, the facets slide upward (open) on the contralateral side, while on the ipsilateral side the facets slide downward (close). The interspaces on the ipsilateral side approximate, and the nuclear material is displaced towards the contralateral side. Lateral flexion is limited by the approximation of the articular processes on the side of the movement and by the contralateral ligamentum flavum and intertransverse ligaments. Sidebending is usually coupled with rotation.

Rotation occurs in the transverse plane with a ROM of 35 to 50 degrees in each direction. The degree of rotation of a vertebra is limited because of its connection to the bony thorax. During rotation, the articular facets slide relative to each other, which creates rotation of the vertebral body above in relation to the one below. The inferior facets of the superior vertebra slide on the superior facet of the inferior vertebra. Rotation and twisting of the intervertebral disc then occurs.

In the thoracic spine, sidebending and rotation are believed to occur to the opposite side (ie, sidebending to the right will be coupled with rotation to the left) when the individual is in neutral alignment in an erect posture. However, it appears that the direction of the rotation may vary and is dependent upon whether the motion occurs above or below the apex of the curve. In the frontal plane, rotation appears to be coupled in the opposite direction to normal physiological sidebending when the motion occurs below the apex of the sidebending curve. When the movement occurs above the apex, rotation appears to be coupled in the same direction as the sidebending.[13,14,16]

If the individual is in a forward bend position, the sidebending and rotation will occur to the same side (ie, sidebending to the right will be coupled with rotation to the right). The direction of coupling that occurs in backward bending remains controversial. Many sources[13,14,16] agree that if the individual is in a backward bend position and then sidebends, rotation will occur to the opposite side (ie, sidebending to the right will be coupled with rotation to the left). Greenman[14] postulated that the type of coupling may be related to whether the movement occurs above or below the apex of the thoracic spine or to which movement (sidebending vs rotation) occurs first. He reported that if sidebending is introduced first, rotation will occur to the opposite side, and if rotation is introduced first, sidebending will occur to the same side.

Lumbar Spine

During flexion there is a reversal of the lumbar lordosis that occurs mainly at the upper lumbar levels.[2] Forward flexion is achieved by each lumbar vertebra rotating from its posteriorly tilted position in the upright lordotic position to the neutral position that relieves the posterior compression of the intervertebral discs and zygapophyseal joints.[2]

Flexion of the lumbar spine occurs in the sagittal plane with a ROM of 40 to 60 degrees. In flexion, the inferior facets of the superior vertebra glide anteriorly and superiorly over the superior facets of the inferior vertebrae allowing both facets to open. During flexion the interspaces between the vertebrae open, and the nuclear material is displaced posteriorly. Flexion is limited by the tension developed in the PLL, supraspinous and interspinous ligaments, and the ligamenum flavum while the ALL is relaxed.

Extension also occurs in the sagittal plane with a ROM of 20 to 35 degrees. In extension, the inferior articular processes of the superior vertebrae glide posteriorly and downward over the superior facets of the inferior vertebrae below causing both facets to close. During extension the lumbar vertebrae approximate posteriorly, and the nucleus is displaced anteriorly. Extension is limited by the articular processes and SPs and by the tension developed in the ALL. The PLL, supraspinous and interspinous ligaments, and the ligamentum flavum are relaxed.

Lateral flexion occurs in the frontal plane with a ROM of 15 to 20 degrees in each direction. In lateral flexion, the facets slide upward (open) on the contralateral side, while on the ipsilateral side the facets slide downward (close). During lateral flexion the interspaces on the ipsilateral side approximate, and the nuclear material is displaced towards the contralateral side. Lateral flexion is limited by the approximation of the articular processes on the side of the movement and by the contralateral ligamentum flavum and intertransverse ligaments. Sidebending is usually coupled with rotation.

Rotation occurs in the transverse plane with a ROM of 3 to 18 degrees in each direction. During rotation, the articular facets slide relative to each other, which creates rotation of the vertebral body above in relation to the one below. Thus, the inferior facets of the superior vertebra slide on the superior facet of the inferior vertebra. Rotation and twisting of the intervertebral disc then occurs.

In the lumbar spine, when an individual is standing erect in neutral alignment, sidebending and rotation are coupled to opposite sides (ie, sidebending to the right will be coupled with rotation to the left).

If the individual is in a forward bent position, the sidebending and rotation appear to be coupled to the same side (ie, sidebending to the right will be coupled with rotation to the right). If the individual is in a backward bent position, then sidebending and rotation appear to be coupled to opposite sides.[14]

It has been speculated that the high incidence of clinically evident disc disease at L4-5 and L5-S1 may be related to the mechanics.[11]

PATHOPHYSIOLOGY

A wide variety of pathological conditions are associated with the spine. It is not the intention of this section to review an exhaustive list of pathologies. In addition, lumbar spine pain may be due to visceral or vascular disease.[17] The following pathological conditions represent the most common conditions referred to outpatient physical therapy. It is important to realize that unlike the extremities, it is much more difficult to pinpoint the precise structure or structures responsible for pain in the spine. This difficulty has resulted in a number of classification systems for categorization of disorders of the spine, particularly the lumbar spine.[11] Herein lies the necessity of making a diagnosis based on the examination of the patient.

MUSCLE STRAINS/SPRAINS

Muscle strains or sprains may be caused by injury to a number of structures including muscle, ligament, and fascia.[11] In a systematic discussion of the structures most likely to be injured in a traumatic flexion injury of the lumbar spine, Bogduk and Twomey suggested that muscle is the most likely structure and is commonly strained as a result of a flexion injury of the lumbar spine.[2] Under strain, muscles characteristically fail near their musculotendinous junction.[18] The muscles of the spine are polysegmental, myotendinous junctions occurring throughout the back.[18] This results in the potential for muscle sprains occurring both in the deep and superficial muscles of the spine. Trigger points often occur concurrently with back pain and may produce point tenderness and muscle spasm. The etiology of trigger points is still not understood.[19] It has been suggested that they represent acute or recurrent sprain of individual strands of the back muscles.[18]

DISC PROTRUSION AND HERNIATION

This clinical diagnosis is probably the most discussed pathology of the spine. The terms disc bulge, disc herniation, and disc prolapse are often used indiscriminately. Disruption of the annular fibers allows for prolapse, and therefore a portion of the annulus is displaced. This then allows the nucleus to follow the displaced segment of the annulus. Originally described by Mixter and Barr, disc herniation is very common, particularly at the lumbar level.[20] The most referenced classification system is described by Macnab[21] (Table 6-2). Disc herniations may produce central or peripheral pain, muscle weakness, muscle spasm, sensory loss, or reflex changes.

SPONDYLOLISTHESIS

Herbinaux, a Belgian obstetrician, first described spondylolisthesis in 1782.[3] Spondylolisthesis (from the Greek spondylo meaning spine and listhesis meaning slide) is a condition where one spinal vertebrae slips, usually forward, on the one below it.[22] This condition may be caused by trauma that creates a fracture in the posterior portion of the vertebrae; degeneration of the joints between the vertebrae; structural weakness resulting from bone disease; fatigue fractures; anatomical anomalies or variations that cause a disruption of the posterior part of the vertebrae (spondylolysis); or congenital malformation of the sacrum.

Wiltse and associates[23] categorized spondylolisthesis into five groups (Table 6-3). All of these groups ultimately allow

Table 6-2	
MACNAB'S CLASSIFICATION OF DISC HERNIATION	
Classification Name	*Definition*
Type I peripheral annular bulge	The annulus protrudes circumferentially beyond the peripheral rims of the vertebral bodies.
Type II localized annular bulge	A discrete eminence; when producing signs to warrant operation, the myelographic defect is unilateral. The annular fibers themselves remain intact, and on incision the nucleus does not extrude.
Type I prolapsed intervertebral disc	Displaced nuclear material is confined solely by a few strands of annulus, and on incision of these, the nucleus spontaneously extrudes.
Type II extruded intervertebral disc	The nuclear material displaced has already burst through the restraining annulus and lies under cover of the PLL.
Type III sequestered intervertebral disc	Extruded nuclear material lies free in the spinal canal. It may remain trapped between the nerve root and disc, or may migrate to lie behind the vertebral body in the nerve root "axilla," in the intervertebral foramen or in the mid-line just anterior to the dural sac.

Reprinted with permission from Macnab I. *Backache*. 2nd ed. Baltimore, Md: Williams & Wilkins; 1977.

Table 6-3
CLASSIFICATION AND ETIOLOGY OF SPONDYLOLISTHESIS

Type of Spondylolisthesis	Description
I	Dysplastic (congenital)
II	Isthmic (spondylolytic)
III	Degenerative
IV	Traumatic
V	Pathological

Reprinted with permission from Wiltse LL, Newman PH, Macnab I. Classification of spondylolysis and spondylolisthesis. *Clin Orthop.* 1976;117(June):23-29.

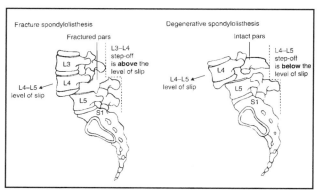

Figure 6-5. Spondylolisthesis. From McKinnis LN: *Fundamentals of Musculoskeletal Imaging.* 2nd ed. FA Davis Co, Philadelphia, 2005, p. 272, with permission. Adapted from Greenspan, pp. 10-42.

for the development of instability due to failure of the locking mechanism between the two vertebrae. The two types more likely to be seen by a physical therapist are Type II, isthmic (spondylolytic) spondylolisthesis, and Type III, degenerative spondylolisthesis.

Isthmic spondylolisthesis results from a defect in the pars interarticularis (Figure 6-5). The defect separates the vertebra in two, allowing for the anterior portion to slip forward while the posterior portion remains fixed. Isthmic spondylolisthesis is found two times more frequently in men, and white men and women have the diagnosis more commonly than black American men and women.[22]

Degenerative spondylolisthesis occurs secondary to osteoarthritic changes in the facet joints that may result in abnormal alignment. Degenerative spondylolisthesis is five times more common in women and usually occurs after the age of 40. Black American women are three times more likely to develop degenerative spondylolisthesis than white women. L4-L5 is the most common area (6 to 10 times greater than any other level) and the amount of slippage is proportional to the amount of disc degeneration. The slip rarely exceeds 33% of the length of the adjacent vertebral body.[3,22]

The most commonly used grading system for spondylolisthesis is the one proposed by Meyerding[24] in 1947. The degree of slippage is measured as the percentage of distance the translated superior vertebral body has moved relative to the superior end plate of the inferior vertebra. Classifications use the following grading system:
♦ Grade 1: 1% to 25% slippage
♦ Grade 2: 26% to 50% slippage
♦ Grade 3: 51% to 75% slippage
♦ Grade 4: 76% to 100% slippage
♦ Grade 5: Greater than 100%

Lumbar spine lateral and bilateral oblique plain radiographs are used to diagnose and grade the amount of slippage. The pars interarticularis defect, commonly described as a "Scotty dog with a collar," is most readily visible on bilateral oblique views.[22] Patients with Grades III and IV displacements may develop instability in their spine because of the greater degree of slippage present.

Symptoms may include low back pain that may radiate to the buttocks and legs. The pain may not follow a particular pattern. Stiffness or loss of flexibility may also be present. An actual "step" or ledge may be felt in the spine in the area above the spondylolisthesis.

DEGENERATIVE DISC DISEASE

Degenerative disc disease (DDD) is also referred to as degenerative arthritis, OA, osteoarthrosis, degenerative facet disease, and spondylosis. The majority of individuals have degenerative changes after the age of 60 years. In those patients with DDD, males are more commonly affected in the younger-than-45-years-old group and females in the older-than-55-years-old group. This condition may occur earlier in some individuals based on genetic factors, work, or lifestyle differences.

DDD involves disruption of the normal annular fibers of the disc to such an extent that the disc is no longer able to maintain adequate mechanical function. This may be associated with the degenerative arthritic process of the vertebral bodies and/or intervertebral joints.[11] DDD is a non-inflammatory degeneration of the disc with simultaneous reactive change in the neighboring structures leading to osteophytic outgrowths. The clinical syndrome involving the cervical spine is more common and severe than that of the lumbar spine.[25]

DDD may produce symptoms that may include pain in the back or pain radiating into one or both legs, paresthesia, anesthesia, weakness of the muscles in the legs, or loss of reflexes (eg, knee jerk). The pain is most commonly felt with movement or activity and may be relieved by rest.

STENOSIS

Spinal stenosis is a condition that may be congenital or may develop later in life. The most common cause is degenerative joint disease. Spinal stenosis may also occur as a result of previous spinal surgery (eg, spinal fusion) or as a result of some systemic diseases (eg, Paget's disease).

Spinal stenosis is the abnormal narrowing of the neural canal and/or intervertebral foramina. The narrowing is responsible for compression of the spinal cord and/or the nerve roots. Signs and symptoms are due to vascular compromise of the venous plexus related to the cauda equina and the nerve roots and may include anesthesia, paresthesia, weakness, loss of reflexes, and pain. Patients typically have pain and sensory changes in their back or in one or both legs. The symptoms are exacerbated by walking and eased with a stooping posture or sitting.

SCOLIOSIS

Scoliosis is a descriptive term to depict abnormal lateral curves in the spinal column. It is a condition that can affect the spine throughout the life spectrum. Either an "S" or "C" shaped curve is present when the spine is viewed from the back. These curves are named by the directions of their convexity. The degree of the curve(s) is measured on an x-ray. Scoliosis may be structural when actual bony changes exist or functional where the curve is reversible. There are many causes of scoliosis including congenital spine deformity, genetic conditions, neuromuscular disorders, and limb length inequality. Idiopathic scoliosis of the structural type comprises 85% of all types of scoliosis.[26] Four categories of idiopathic scoliosis exist based on age: 1) infantile, children ages 3 years and under; 2) juvenile, ages 3 to 9 years; 3) adolescent, ages 10 to 18 years; and 4) adult, after skeletal maturity. The most common form of idiopathic scoliosis is adolescent idiopathic scoliosis representing about 80% of idiopathic cases.[26] Symptoms are dependent on the degree of the curve and may include loss of flexibility and function, spasm, pain, and fatigue. In severe, longstanding cases, individuals may experience respiratory compromise, difficulty breathing, and shortness of breath.

IMAGING

A number of modalities are available for imaging of the spine (Table 6-4). X-ray or radiography is the oldest and most widely available modality for imaging of the spine.[27] The four other imaging tests commonly used in assessing the anatomy of the spine are myelography, CT scan, MRI scan, and CT myelography.[28] X-rays tend to be the first imaging technique of choice. However, not all patients with back or neck pain will have x-rays prior to seeing a physical therapist. For example, it has been recommended that patients with acute low back pain (ie, back pain for less than 3 months) do not have x-rays taken as part of a routine evaluation by a physician within the first month of symptoms.[29] This is due to the poor correlation between x-ray findings and low back problems.[28] However, x-rays are recommended when red flags are present.[29] These include recent significant trauma, history of prolonged steroid use, osteoporosis, a patient that is over 70 years old, prior diagnosis of cancer, recent infection, fever over 100 degrees, intravenous (IV) drug abuse, back pain that is worse at rest, or unexplained weight loss. Posing questions to rule out red flags must be mandatory for every physical therapist seeing patients with spinal pain. MRI, CT, CT myelography, and myelography are tests that are used to define remediable anatomic pathologic conditions.[2] Again recommendations exist for the use of all four tests.[22] MRI is the most frequently used test.[29] MRI is non-invasive, and because it does not require the use of ionizing radiation, it is therefore safer than plain x-ray, CT scan, and myelography.[29] In studies of subjects without low back pain, disc herniations and disc degeneration have been found.[30] Furthermore, some authors have cautioned against the use of MRI to replace x-rays as there is no long term difference in disability, pain, or general health status, and there may be a higher surgical rate among patients undergoing MRI scan. For example, incidental anatomic findings may confuse the exact source of the patient's symptoms.[31]

PHARMACOLOGY

Common pharmacological agents used in treating these diagnoses may be found in Table 6-5.

Case Study #1: Disc Herniation

Ms. Debra Smith is a 37-year-old healthy female with a diagnosis of multi-level disc herniations.

PHYSICAL THERAPIST EXAMINATION

HISTORY

♦ General demographics: Ms. Smith is a 37-year-old English-speaking white female. She has a diploma from a business school. She is right-hand dominant.

♦ Social history: She is married and has no children.

♦ Employment/work: She is a computer trainer.

♦ Living environment: Ms. Smith lives with her husband in a two-story house with stairs.

♦ General health status

Table 6-4

RADIOGRAPHIC AND IMAGING TECHNIQUES FOR THE SPINE[28,29]

Imaging Technique	Information Provided	Advantages	Disadvantages
X-ray	Bony and structural abnormalities detected	Assesses alignment of the spine Comparison of vertebral body and disc space size Assessment of bone density and architecture Detection of unilateral or bilateral spondylolisthesis Evaluate possible ankylosing spondylitis Effective at ruling out fractures, tumor, or infection in patients with "red flags" Comparative value	Gross evaluation of soft tissues only Increased radiation exposure Not effective for diagnosing lumbar nerve root impingement, herniated disc, spinal stenosis, or for ruling out early stage cancer or infection[29]
MRI	MRI has emerged as the procedure of choice for diagnostic imaging of the lumbar spine[23] MRI uses magnetic fields to produce computer-generated axial and sagittal cross-sectional images of the body[28]	Noninvasive Lack of ionizing radiation Multiplanar capabilities Usually does not require contrast High-contrast resolution Direct visualization of the spinal cord and disc and pathology Visualizes an entire region	Contraindicated in certain patients (eg, pacemaker, vascular clips)
CT	CT scans use multiple x-ray beams projected at different angles and levels to produce computer-generated axial cross-sectional images of the body[28]	Minimal irradiation No need for contrast Visualizes disc herniation-location, size, migration, disc sequestration Evaluates the status of spinal canal and epidural space Good tissue contrast Measurements (canal, dural sac) 3-D reconstruction	Limited exam to two to three levels Contents of thecal sac are not well seen Difficult if scoliosis or postural changes are present
Myelogram	Plain myelography uses plain x-ray, taken after a nonionic water-soluble contrast media is injected into the spinal canal via a lumbar puncture needle, to produce images of the borders and contents of the dural sac[28]	Visualizes the entire subarachnoid space, spinal cord, and nerve roots Better visualization of disc herniation and nerve root abnormalities Allows dynamic studies (flexion and extension) Useful in patients with severe scoliosis or spinal stenosis	Invasive Potential side effects from intrathecal subarachnoid contrast (headaches, nausea, seizures) Poor visualization of spinal cord or nerve roots above a block Does not visualize the extradural segment of the nerve roots and epidural space
CT myelogram	CT-myelography uses a CT scan, done after a contrast media injected into the dural sac in the same manner as for plain myelography, to produce axial cross-sectional images of the spine that enhance distinction between the dural sac and its surrounding structures	Combines the advantages of CT and the opacification of the subarachnoid space Better visualization of neural foramen, spinal cord, and nerve roots	Intrathecal contrast Requires a clinical and/or myelographical lesion level

	Table 6-5			
PHARMACOLOGICAL AGENTS USED FOR PATIENTS WITH SPINAL DISORDERS				
Medication	*Examples*	*Primary Effects*	*Mechanism of Action*	*Adverse Effects/ Rehabilitation Concerns*
Opioid analgesics	Hydrocodone, Vicodin, fentanyl, Durgesic patch	Analgesic	Synthetic narcotic that interacts with opioid receptors in CNS	Hepatic, renal toxicity Lightheadedness, dizziness Sedation Nausea, vomiting Drug dependence
Nonopioid analgesics	NSAIDs (eg, OTC ibuprofen, aspirin, others; prescription fenoprofen; prescription COX-2 inhibitors [Celebrex])	Analgesic Anti-inflammatory Antipyretic	Inhibit synthesis of PGs by inhibiting cyclooxygenase	Gastric irritation Headache Hepatic, renal toxicity Overdose: Aspirin intoxication
	Acetaminophen	Analgesic Antipyretic No anti-inflammatory effect	Selective inhibition of PG biosynthesis in the CNS	Liver toxicity with high doses
Glucocorticoids	Prednisone, cortisone	Anti-inflammatory	Inhibit function of inflammatory cells	Breakdown effect on bone, ligament, tendon, skin Salt/water retention Increased rate of infection Gastric ulcers Glaucoma Adrenal suppression
Muscle relaxants	Valium	Selective decrease of skeletal muscle excitability	Increases inhibitory effects of gamma-amino-buteric-acid (GABA)	Generalized weakness Drowsiness
	Soma		Decreases excitatory input onto alpha motor neuron by acting on the polysynaptic reflex arc	
	Neurontin		Enhances GABA effects in cord	
Psychotropics	Antidepressants	Decrease depression Decrease chronic low back pain	Increase stimulation of postsynaptic receptors by prolonging the effects of neurotransmitters	Time lag before beneficial effects Chance of increased depression during initial treatment

Adapted with permission from course notes of "Pharmacology in Rehabilitation." Instructor Charles C. Ciccone, PT, PhD.

- General health perception: Ms. Smith reported that she is in good health.
- Physical function: Normal.
- Psychological function: Normal.
- Role function: Wife, computer instructor.
- Social function: She enjoys exercising and travels frequently.
♦ Social/health habits: She reports that she is a non-smoker. She had been able to walk daily on a treadmill for 1 hour prior to this episode.
♦ Family history: Ms. Smith's maternal grandmother had a heart attack in her 50s.
♦ Medical/surgical history: She has hypothyroidism, which is well controlled with medication.
♦ Prior hospitalizations: None.
♦ Preexisting and other health related conditions: She has hypothyroidism.
♦ Current condition(s)/chief complaint(s): Ms. Smith reports initially feeling weakness in her right foot about 6 weeks ago. She felt sharp pain from her low back area radiating down her right posterior thigh into the lateral leg and dorsum of the foot as she was getting out of her car while on a business trip 3 weeks ago. The pain in her back has improved but she continues to have pain and weakness in her right leg.
♦ Functional status and activity level: She reports difficulty with all ADL. She is unable to work and unable to exercise.
♦ Medications: Ms. Smith is taking synthetic thyroid hormone replacement (Synthroid), aspirin, and vitamin E.
♦ Other clinical tests: Plain radiographs showed narrowing of the disc space at L3-4, L4-5, and L5-S1. MRI of the lumbar spine showed a L4-5 herniated nucleus pulposus, with freely extruded disc fragment impinging on the right L5 nerve root sleeve origin in the lateral recess and degenerative changes and disc bulging/protrusions at T11-12, L1-2, L2-3, and L4-5.

SYSTEMS REVIEW

♦ Cardiovascular/pulmonary
- BP: 130/75 mmHg
- Edema: None
- HR: 72 bpm
- RR: 12 bpm
♦ Integumentary
- Presence of scar formation: None
- Skin color: WNL
- Skin integrity: WNL
♦ Musculoskeletal
- Gross range of motion as ascertained from the lower quarter examination

- Moderately restricted in lumbar extension, bilateral sidebending, and rotation
- Severely restricted in flexion
- All motions limited by pain
- Gross strength: Decreased strength of the trunk and right lower leg
- Gross symmetry: Right lateral lumbar shift, atrophy noted in the right leg
- Height: 5'0" (1.52 m)
- Weight: 100 lbs (37.32 kg)
♦ Neuromuscular
- Balance: WNL
- Locomotion: Difficulty maintaining ankle dorsiflexion during heel strike on the right
- Transfers: Independent
- Transitions: Independent
♦ Communication, affect, cognition, language, and learning style
- Communication, affect, cognition: WNL
- Learning preferences: Visual learner

TESTS AND MEASURES

♦ Aerobic capacity/endurance
- Unable to be assessed at this time secondary to pain
- Was ambulating 1 mile a day on the treadmill prior to this episode
♦ Anthropometric characteristics
- BMI=705 x (body weight [in pounds] divided by height^2 [in inches])
- Ms. Smith's BMI=19.58, this is considered to be normal[32]
♦ Assistive and adaptive devices
- None used
♦ Cranial and peripheral nerve integrity
- Cranial nerves were intact
- Motor distribution of L4 and L5 nerve root was decreased
- Sensation was decreased to light touch and pin prick on the right medial and lateral aspect of the leg and lateral border of the right foot
♦ Environmental, home, and work barriers
- Ms. Smith is unable to work at this time
- She has difficulty negotiating the flight of stairs at home and demonstrates a nonreciprocal pattern
♦ Ergonomics and body mechanics
- Analysis of body mechanics during self-care, home management, work, community, and leisure actions, tasks, and activities revealed that Ms. Smith was limited in these activities due to pain and altered posture
- The score on the ODQ, a self-reporting patient

questionnaire, was 34%, indicating low disability[33]

◆ Gait, locomotion, and balance
- Analysis of walking on even surfaces showed an increased time from heel strike to foot flat on the right side compared to the left

◆ Joint integrity and mobility
- Joint integrity and mobility assessment entails not only the osteokinematic and arthrokinematic analysis, but also the structural integrity of the joint and includes special tests designed to assess ligamentous stability, compression, distraction tests, impingement tests, and joint play[34]
  - Lumbar spine
    - Lumbar flexion: PPIVM testing was moderately restricted, and end feel was muscular at all levels of the lumbar spine
    - Lumbar extension: PPIVM was mildly restricted, and end feel was empty at all levels of the lumbar spine
    - Lumbar sidebending: PPIVM was mildly restricted on the left, and moderately restricted on the right
    - Lumbar rotation: PPIVM was mildly restricted to the right and moderately restricted to the left, and end feel was muscular at all levels of the lumbar spine
    - PAIVM performed using P/A glides on the lumbar SPs: Moderately restricted
  - Pelvis
    - Provocation tests of the sacro-iliac joints included compression, distraction, and Gaenslen's test
    - None of these passive motion tests reproduced the patient's pain
  - Hip joints
    - Hip flexion and extension were limited bilaterally at end ranges
    - SLR was mildly restricted bilaterally by tight hamstrings
    - All other motions were WNL

◆ Motor function
- Dexterity and coordination: Intact
- Agility: Mildly impaired secondary to pain and weakness

◆ Muscle performance
- MMT revealed the following deviations from normal
  - Abdominals: 4/5
  - Back extensors: 4/5
  - LE
    - Hip flexors: Left=4/5, Right=4/5
    - Hip extensors: Left=4/5, Right=4/5
    - Hip abductors: Left=4/5, Right=4/5
    - Ankle dorsiflexors: Left=5/5, Right=3/5
    - Extensor hallucis longus: Left=5/5, Right=3/5
- Muscle tension (palpation)
  - Spasm
    - Thoracic and lumbar paraspinals R > L
    - Bilateral gluteus medius

◆ Orthotic, protective, and supportive devices
- None used

◆ Pain
- NPS revealed pain of 8/10 (0=no pain and 10=worst possible pain) located in the lumbar spine and radiating into the right leg when bending forward[35]
- Pain is eased with left sidelying

◆ Posture
- Observational assessment done from all perspectives
  - Lateral view: Decreased lumbar lordosis
  - Anterior view: Right lumbar lateral shift, decreased weightbearing through the right leg and foot
  - Posterior view: Right lumbar lateral shift, decreased weightbearing through the right leg and foot

◆ Range of motion
- Functional range of motion
  - Decreased ability to bend forward for dressing and tying shoe laces
  - Decreased ability to look over or behind either shoulder
- Joint active and passive movement
  - Lumbar spine motion was measured using an inclinometer
  - Intratester reliability was found to be high (ICC>0.9) and intertester reliability was found to be high (ICC=0.9)[36]
    - Flexion=25 degrees
    - Extension=5 degrees
    - Lateral flexion R=20 degrees
    - Lateral flexion L=40 degrees
    - Rotation R=20 degrees
    - Rotation L=20 degrees
- Muscle length
  - Hamstring tightness bilaterally
  - Rectus femoris tightness bilaterally

◆ Reflex integrity
- Testing of DTRs or myotatic reflexes revealed bilateral quadriceps reflex=2+ and bilateral ankle (Achilles) reflex=2+

◆ Self-care and home management
- Interview concerning ability to safely perform self-care and home management actions, tasks, and activities found that the patient could manage to

shower and dress but required help for shopping, laundry, and housework
♦ Work, community, and leisure integration or reintegration
  • The patient is unable to work at this time
  • Interview concerning ability to safely manage community and leisure actions, tasks, and activities revealed that the patient had difficulty driving for longer than 15 minutes due to increase in low back and right leg pain
  • The patient is unable to exercise at this time

EVALUATION

Ms. Smith's history as outlined is significant for right foot weakness followed by an exacerbation of back and right leg pain. She reports significant pain aggravated by sitting and eased with left sidelying. This has resulted in Ms. Smith's inability to work. She has a right lumbar lateral shift, limited ROM of the lumbar spine, weakness in the right dorsiflexors and extensor hallucis longus, impaired posture, and difficulties with all ADL. Her medical history is significant for HTN, hypothyroidism, and high cholesterol. Ms. Smith previously exercised daily by walking on the treadmill to maintain cardiovascular endurance. She is currently unable to do this.

DIAGNOSIS

Ms. Smith is a patient who has multi-level herniated discs with pain in her back and right leg. In addition, she has impaired: aerobic capacity; peripheral nerve integrity; ergonomics and body mechanics; gait, locomotion, and balance; joint integrity and mobility; motor function; muscle performance; posture; range of motion; and reflex integrity. She is functionally limited in self-care and home management and in work, community, and leisure actions, tasks, and activities. She also has home barriers. These findings are consistent with placement in Pattern F: Impaired Joint Mobility, Motor Function, Muscle Performance, Range of Motion, and Reflex Integrity Associated With Spinal Disorders. The identified impairments and functional limitations will be addressed in determining the prognosis and the plan of care.

PROGNOSIS AND PLAN OF CARE

Over the course of the visits, the following mutually established outcomes have been determined:
♦ Ability to perform physical actions, tasks, and activities related to self-care, home management, work, community, and leisure is improved
♦ Body mechanics during self-care, home management, work, community, and leisure actions, tasks, and activities is improved

♦ Daily exercise program is re-established
♦ Gait is improved
♦ Muscle performance is increased
♦ Pain is reduced
♦ Posture is improved
♦ Return to work is achieved
♦ Risk of secondary impairment is reduced
♦ Risk factors are reduced
♦ ROM is increased

To achieve these outcomes the appropriate interventions for this client are determined. These will include: coordination, communication, and documentation; patient/client-related instruction; therapeutic exercise; functional training in self-care and home management; functional training in work, community, and leisure integration or reintegration; manual therapy techniques; electrotherapeutic modalities; and physical agents and mechanical modalities.

Based on the diagnosis and prognosis, Ms. Smith is expected to require between 8 to 10 visits over a 6-week period of time. Mrs. Smith is not severely impaired, is generally healthy, and follows through with her home exercise program.

INTERVENTIONS

RATIONALE FOR SELECTED INTERVENTIONS

Therapeutic Exercise

Sackett defined evidence-based practice as "the conscientious, explicit and judicious use of current best evidence in making decisions about the care of individual patients."[37] There is persistent controversy about the best exercise program for patients with low back pain. Although there is little agreement on specific regimes, there is a consensus that exercise plays a major role in the treatment of mechanical low back pain.[38]

Patients with low back pain may have decreased ROM[39] and decreased trunk strength.[40,41] Physical therapists use pain levels and the impairment measures of ROM and trunk strength to assist in forming a rationale to treat the patient. However, it is important to realize that the correlation between impairment measures and disability scores is generally low.[42]

Exercises for this patient may include repeated movements, postural exercise, stretching, strengthening, and aerobic conditioning. Various types of exercise programs have been advocated for patients with low back pain. These include extension exercises, flexion exercises, generalized strengthening, aerobic exercise, stretching, or any combination of these exercise types. There are a number of factors to be considered when reviewing the pertinent literature relating to therapeutic exercise. A major problem when investigating patients with low back pain is that the precise medical diagnosis is unknown in 80% to 90% of the cases.[43] One explanation for the lack of positive research findings from randomized trials is that patients with non-specific low back pain are regarded as a homogenous group with all patients equally likely to succeed or fail with any particular treatment.[44] Most studies divide patients into groups with acute low back pain (ie, less than 3 months' duration of pain) and chronic low back pain (ie, greater than 3 months' duration). It may be that patients with low back pain do not neatly fall into these two groups; hence there is a need for valid and reliable classification systems for patients with low back pain.[44] It therefore may be difficult to determine which treatment approach should be applied and how it will directly affect the specific pathological condition responsible for the back pain.[45]

The difficulty in formulating a diagnosis has led to the creation of a number of classification systems from both the medical[46] and physical therapy[47] professions. McKenzie[12] proposed a classification system in which patients undergo an examination including assessing the available motion of the trunk, noting how it influences their pain, and then classifying them as having a postural, dysfunctional, or derangement syndrome.[12] In 1995, another classification system was developed by Delitto and associates.[44,46,48] They established seven groups that were based on information provided by the patient and gathered by the physical therapist during their examination. The groups include immobilization, lumbar mobilization, sacroiliac mobilization, extension syndrome, flexion syndrome, lateral shift, and traction. They suggested that treatment interventions should be based on the classification of the patient.

Another problem is the complexity of the mixture of physical and psychosocial factors that occur in patients with low back pain.[49] No one single measure of severity of low back pain or predictor for outcome of treatment is considered to be the gold standard.[50] Therefore, a variety of measures are used to examine the impairment and functional disabilities caused by low back pain.

The use of therapeutic exercise as an approach to patient care in physical therapy may be traced back to the 1920s.[51] In the 1930s and 1940s, Williams combined an understanding of the mechanics of the spine, especially the region of the intervertebral foramina, with the concept of the trunk as a closed cylinder pressurized by the abdominal muscles.[52] This gave rise to William's flexion exercise program (posterior pelvic tilt in three positions, abdominal strengthening, and low back stretching exercises). The intent of these exercises was to increase the height of the intervertebral foramina and strengthen the abdominal wall.[52] At the same time, Cyriax[53] described the difference between referred and radicular pain. He recognized that any low back structure, if injured, could refer pain into the LE and was not necessarily due to nerve root irritation. He advocated extension-hyperextension exer-

cises to compress the posterior part of the disc and "push" the nuclear contents anteriorly. McKenzie[12] began to review Cyriax,[53] Kapandji,[13] and his own clinical results and subsequently developed the McKenzie system of treatment. The McKenzie method is a mechanical diagnosis and therapy program based on the centralization of symptoms. This phenomenon occurs when LE pain associated with low back pain begins to diminish and centralize with repeated movements. Centralization is one of the most important contributions made by McKenzie and allows the physical therapist and the patient to monitor the effect of treatment.[12] Patients are examined to determine which spinal movements cause changes in their symptoms. The symptoms may either centralize or peripheralize.[12] Centralization is the most important clinical guide and helps to establish the direction of movement that will reduce the mechanical deformation. McKenzie stated that an increase or peripheralization is just as reliable in indicating which movements should be avoided because they exaggerate the mechanical deformation. It has been suggested that the mechanism of centralization may be due to reduction of intradiscal pressure and decreased pressure on the nerve root.[12]

In the 1980s and 1990s, the functional restoration programs of Mayer and Hazard became popular.[50,51] These programs were an attempt to treat the multifaceted problem of low back pain with attention to pain control, strengthening and conditioning exercises, and also address the psychological aspects of chronic low back pain. Yet another treatment philosophy is that proposed by Sahrmann[54] who suggested that the majority of spinal dysfunctions were the result of microtrauma associated with faulty alignment, stabilization, and movement patterns.[54] She stresses the importance of exercises that stabilize the spine.

Stabilization training was introduced as a multi-faceted program of education, flexibility, strength, coordination, and endurance training to prevent repetitive micro trauma to the spinal structures responsible for pain and degeneration. This concept of exercise for the spine was a combination of approaches.[55] More recently there has been interest in very specific retraining of a precise co-contraction pattern of the deep trunk muscles, transversus abdominis, and the multifidus.[56] The rationale for the use of this type of exercise is to provide pain relief in patients with low back pain by retraining dysfunctional muscles, thereby enhancing stability of the lumbar spine segments.[57]

Manual Therapy Techniques

Manual therapy techniques include the use of skilled hands to enhance tissue extensibility, joint mobility, modulate pain, decrease spasm, and reduce soft tissue swelling.[58] Improvements in ROM, pain, and function have been demonstrated with manual physical therapy interventions for painful, stiff spines and extremity joints.[16,34,59]

Muscle tightness leading to shortened positions and soft

tissue restrictions requires the use of soft tissue massage and myofascial release.[60]

Prolonged shortening of the soft tissues ultimately leads to joint hypomobility. Mobilization techniques that are directed towards the restricted motion may be applied to the lumbar spine and LEs using Grades III and IV mobilizations.[34] In addition, Grades I and II oscillation techniques[34] may be applied to the same joints for pain relief.[16] Wyke[61] noted that pain relief may be produced through stimulation of the Types I and II joint receptors located in the ligaments and joint capsule.

Patients receiving spinal manipulation as part of their care required less anti-inflammatory and analgesic medications.[62] Patients who received manual therapy as part of their treatment protocol demonstrated more rapid and greater improvement in their physical performance.[63] Although a systematic review of 36 randomized controlled studies did not support the efficacy of manipulation,[63] indications were noted that manipulation might be effective for certain types of patients.[64]

Electrotherapeutic Modalities

This patient may benefit from the use of TENS. The major physiological and therapeutic effect of TENS is the reduction of pain. This is thought to occur by triggering and modulating the PNS and CNS through a series of neurohormonal, neurophysiological, and cognitive systems.[65] With appropriate application of the TENS unit, the patient's treatment may be augmented and facilitated yielding reduced pain.

Treatment for this patient may also be augmented with the use of EMS. EMS may be used to reduce soft tissue edema by creating a pumping effect through repeated muscle contraction. Muscle spasm may be reduced using the tetanizing effect of EMS on the muscle. Studies demonstrating this effect have only been performed in the levator ani muscle. Some evidence indicates that EMS may increase blood flow in the muscles following repetitions of muscle contraction.[65]

Physical Agents and Mechanical Modalities

Ultrasound may be incorporated as an adjunct in the treatment of this patient to introduce a thermal effect, decrease the inflammatory response, decrease pain, and enhance tissue healing. The thermal effect may be produced when the sound wave passes through the involved tissue, since vibration is initiated by cycles of high pressure. A simultaneous mechanical effect occurs secondary to cavitation in the tissues that disrupts the cell membrane, thus enhancing skin permeability and decreasing the inflammatory response and concurrent pain.[65]

Hot packs may also be incorporated into this patient's treatment to promote tissue healing, decrease joint stiffness, and ultimately create relaxation of the tissues with a subsequent reduction of pain.[65]

COORDINATION, COMMUNICATION, AND DOCUMENTATION

Communication will occur with Ms. Smith regarding all components of her care. Documentation following APTA's *Guidelines for Physical Therapy Documentation*[58] will occur including changes in impairments and functional limitations and changes in interventions. All elements of patient/client management and outcomes of interventions will be documented.

PATIENT/CLIENT-RELATED INSTRUCTION

Ms. Smith will be instructed in the expectations for rapid recovery and possibility of recurrence of symptoms based on the natural history of low back symptoms.[66] Providing the client with the relevant education regarding her impairments, disability, and diagnosis gives her an understanding of her problem and the role of movement in her rehabilitation.[12] It has been shown that there is value to providing information on self-management for patients with low back pain and that this may lead to improved function, less doctor visits, less sick time from work, and less anxiety for the patient.[67-69]

Ms. Smith will understand the basic anatomy and biomechanics of the lumbar spine as it relates to her diagnosis. She will be informed on how different positions and movements effect lumbar intervertebral discs and surrounding structures.[70] Based on this understanding, she will be advised on resting positions and also activity to maintain aerobic capacity, such as walking. Activity modification will include advice on bending, lifting, sitting, and prolonged postures.[71] She will be instructed on the importance of frequently changing positions, and this will be underlined with the instructions on therapeutic exercise.

THERAPEUTIC EXERCISE

♦ Aerobic capacity/endurance conditioning
  ● Exercise progression for these exercises is time based
  ● For example, if the patient tolerates 10 minutes at 3.5 mph on the treadmill well, she will be started at 8 minutes at 2.5 mph and will increase the time daily by 5% to 10% from this baseline
  ● Frequency: Daily
♦ Balance, coordination, and agility training
  ● Tandem walking
  ● Braiding
  ● Obstacle courses of increasing difficulty
♦ Body mechanics and postural stabilization
  ● Body mechanics training
    ■ Appropriate sitting posture for work and leisure activities—in this case the patient should maintain the lumbar lordosis
    ■ Appropriate use of body mechanics while sitting

at the computer and performing housework
- ■ Appropriate lifting and carrying instructions, including maintaining the lordosis, flexing at the hips, and using a flat back lift
- ■ Appropriate bending instructions
- ● Postural awareness training
  - ■ Verbal cueing and use of a mirror to correct spinal shift and maintain lordosis
  - ■ Proper alignment of head, cervical, thoracic, and lumbar spines
  - ■ Axial extension to achieve position of no more than 2 inches from the deepest portion of the cervical lordosis to the apex of the thoracic kyphosis[72]
  - ■ Scapula retraction and depression
  - ■ Elevation of the sternum
  - ■ Proper postural position during transitions
    - ‣ From supine to sitting, standing, and walking
    - ‣ From sit to kneel
    - ‣ From 1/2 kneel to stand
    - ‣ To functional activities at work
    - ‣ To functional activities at leisure
  - ■ Reminder notes all around home, car, office
- ● Postural control training
  - ■ Postural alignment and repositioning
  - ■ Shoulder rolls
  - ■ Scapula squeezes
  - ■ Exercises for centralization of pain
    - ‣ Correction of shift in standing: Physical therapist stands to the right side of the patient's trunk and pulls the pelvis toward that side
    - ‣ Extension in standing: Patient places hands behind pelvis and extends backward
    - ‣ Self-correction of shift in standing against the wall
    - ‣ Self-correction of shift in prone
    - ‣ Repeated extension exercises in prone lying with shift correction
      - ◆ The patient starts by lying prone for 5 minutes and then lying prone in extension for another 5 minutes
      - ◆ Progress to modified press-ups in groups of 10 repetitions up to a total of 30 to 40 press-ups while symptoms are monitored[12]
      - ◆ If extension in lying causes reduction of pain and/or centralization of pain then the patient is instructed on how to maintain the lumbar lordosis at all times, for example, sitting with a lumbar roll
      - ◆ Home exercise program at this time includes shift correction, repetition of extension exercise every waking hour for the next 24

hours, and maintenance of lumbar lordosis in all positions
- ◆ As the patient improves, she can discontinue lying prone and lying prone in extension and gradually reduce repeated extension in lying to two to three times a day
- ◆ Once the shift is corrected and the pain has centralized, flexion is introduced
- ● Postural stabilization activities[73]
  - ■ Pelvic neutral by finding mid range between anterior and posterior pelvic tilt in supine in hooklying
  - ■ Maintain pelvic neutral and isolate UE and LE movement
    - ‣ Hip abduction
    - ‣ Heel slides
    - ‣ Knee extension
    - ‣ Unilateral SLR
    - ‣ Bilateral SLR
    - ‣ March in place
    - ‣ Add repetitions as appropriate, for example starting with one set of 10, increase by sets of 10
    - ‣ Start without weights and add weights as appropriate, for example, add 1 lb weights to each extremity after patient is able to perform 30 reps
  - ■ Glut sets
  - ■ Bridging
  - ■ Unilateral bridging
  - ■ Maintain bridge and add hip flexion right and then left
  - ■ Maintain bridge and add knee extension right and then left
  - ■ Decrease base of support
  - ■ Utilize ball for supine exercises
  - ■ Prone glut sets
  - ■ Utilize exercise ball for prone exercises
    - ‣ Arm raises unilateral and then bilateral in prone, progressing to quadruped
    - ‣ Leg raises unilateral prone, progressing to quadruped
    - ‣ Bilateral leg raises
    - ‣ Alternate opposite arm and leg
  - ■ Bilateral standing on a stable surface with perturbations
  - ■ Unilateral stance on stable surfaces
  - ■ Unilateral stance on stable surface with perturbations
  - ■ Incorporate the use of the foam roller and unstable surfaces like wobble board or foam rubber

cushion in sitting and standing
- ‣ Bilateral standing on foam rubber cushion
- ‣ Unilateral standing on foam rubber cushion
  - ■ Challenge patient out of center of gravity/base of support
  - ■ Utilize balance beam
- ◆ Flexibility exercises
  - ● Stretching exercises should be done after warming up, using a slow and steady stretch accompanied by deep breathing, and building hold up to 30 to 60 seconds
  - ● Lumbar ROM in all directions
  - ● Hamstring stretching in supine with affected LE placed on the wall while stabilizing pelvis
  - ● Rectus femoris stretch while in Thomas test position on the mat
- ◆ Strength, power, and endurance training
  - ● LE weight training for hip flexion, extension, abduction, and ankle dorsiflexion starting, for example, with a low weight for 8 to 12 reps and progressing according to patient's tolerance
  - ● Total gym closed chain squats
  - ● Cable column for hip strengthening in all directions
  - ● BAPS board for ankle movements
  - ● Trampoline including jogging in place

FUNCTIONAL TRAINING IN SELF-CARE AND HOME MANAGEMENT

- ◆ Self-care and home management
  - ● Review resting positions in bed and chair
  - ● Review precautions of exercises including the importance of stabilizing the pelvis, not twisting the trunk, and holding objects close to the body
  - ● Review how to manage leg pain that is exacerbated by following the extension exercise protocol
  - ● Review standing and sitting postures with tips on stabilizing the trunk, maintaining correct head and neck alignment, and maintaining the lumbar lordosis
  - ● Restart walking program on home treadmill

FUNCTIONAL TRAINING IN WORK, COMMUNITY, AND LEISURE INTEGRATION OR REINTEGRATION

- ◆ Work
  - ● Review driving position: Keep lumbar lordosis while sitting in driver's seat, make sure that seat is properly placed from the steering wheel to allow for hands to be at 4 o'clock and 8 o'clock on the steering wheel, adjust seat height, adjust rearview and side mirrors to limit neck and trunk rotation

- ● Review use of carrying equipment: Make sure to use a flat back bend to reach for equipment, lift with legs not back, make sure that object is straight ahead, carry close to trunk, limit carrying load to tolerance
- ● Review ways to prevent prolonged, static postures
  - ■ Make sure to change positions often, for example, every 15 to 20 minutes
  - ■ Get up from sitting position and extend and walk for a few minutes before returning to sitting position
- ● Practice lifting from different heights and different weights

MANUAL THERAPY TECHNIQUES

- ◆ Massage
  - ● Connective tissue massage/myofascial release[60]
    - ■ Hamstrings, hip flexors, paraspinal muscles
- ◆ Mobilization/manipulation
  - ● Soft tissue
    - ■ Lumbar paraspinal muscles
    - ■ Hip flexors
    - ■ Hamstrings
  - ● Spinal and peripheral joints[16,34]
    - ■ Manual distraction to lumbar spine to increase intervertebral space and improve intervertebral mobility
    - ■ Grades III and IV mobilizations performed in the resting position, progressing the physiological position of the joint to follow the pathological end range until patient reaches the anatomical limit
      - ‣ PAIVM to increase lumbar flexion and extension
      - ‣ P/A glide of SPs or bilateral transverse processes of lumbar spine to increase mobility
      - ‣ Transverse glide of SPs to the right to increase left rotation and to the left to increase right rotation
      - ‣ Unilateral P/A on right and left transverse processes to increase rotation in both directions

ELECTROTHERAPEUTIC MODALITIES

- ◆ EMS or TENS to decrease pain and spasm

PHYSICAL AGENTS AND MECHANICAL MODALITIES

- ◆ Sound agents
  - ● Ultrasound to decrease the pain and enhance tissue perfusion and oxygenation
- ◆ Thermotherapy

- Hot packs to increase muscle extensibility and decrease spasm in lumbar spine muscles

ANTICIPATED GOALS AND EXPECTED OUTCOMES

♦ Impact on pathology/pathophysiology
  - Joint restriction is reduced by 25%.
  - Muscle spasm is decreased from moderate to minimal.
  - Neural compression is decreased.
  - Nutrient delivery to tissue is increased.
  - Pain is decreased from 8/10 to 3/10 on the NPS and from 34% to 15% on the Oswestry scale.
  - Soft tissue inflammation, edema, and restriction are reduced.
  - Tissue perfusion and oxygenation are increased.

♦ Impact on impairments
  - Aerobic capacity is increased so that patient is able to ambulate one mile each day.
  - Endurance is increased with return to treadmill walking at prior level of function.
  - Joint integrity and mobility of hips and lumbar spine are improved by 25%.
  - Motor function is improved so that agility is WNL.
  - Muscle length is improved to WNL.
  - Muscle strength of hip flexors, extensors, and abductors are 5/5, and right anterior tibialis and extensor hallucis longus are 4/5.
  - Postural control is improved. Lateral shift is corrected and normal lordosis is regained.
  - Quality of movement is improved.
  - Relaxation is increased.
  - ROM of lumbar spine and hip joint is improved to WFL.

♦ Impact on functional limitations
  - Ability to assume or resume required self-care, home management, work, community, and leisure roles is improved.
  - Ability to independently perform physical actions, tasks, and activities related to ADL/IADL in self-care, home management, work, community, and leisure with or without assistive devices and equipment is increased.
  - Able to drive for 30 to 45 minutes in proper position without pain.
  - Able to reciprocally climb one flight of stairs.
  - Able to resume previous exercise program.
  - Able to tie shoes independently without pain.
  - Tolerance of positions and actions, tasks, and activities is increased.

♦ Risk reduction/prevention
  - Awareness of precautions and correct resting positions is achieved.
  - Risk factors are reduced.
  - Risk of secondary impairments is reduced.
  - Self-management of symptoms is improved.

♦ Impact on health, wellness, and fitness
  - Behaviors that foster healthy habits, wellness, and prevention are acquired.
  - Decision making is enhanced regarding health, wellness, and fitness needs.
  - Fitness, health status, physical capacity, and physical function are improved.

♦ Impact on societal resources
  - Available resources are maximally utilized.
  - Documentation occurs throughout patient management and across all settings and follows APTA's *Guidelines for Physical Therapy Documentation.*[58]

♦ Patient/client satisfaction
  - Case is managed throughout the episode of care, including initial, interim, and discharge letters to any referring physician and documentation to the payer group if required.
  - Clinical proficiency and interpersonal skills of the physical therapist are acceptable to patient.
  - Coordination of care is acceptable to patient.
  - Patient's knowledge and awareness of the diagnosis, prognosis, interventions, and understanding of anticipated goals and expected outcomes are increased.
  - Sense of well-being is improved.

REEXAMINATION

Reexamination is performed throughout the episode of care.

DISCHARGE

Ms. Smith is discharged from physical therapy after a total of nine physical therapy sessions and attainment of her goals and expectations. These sessions have covered her entire episode of care. She is discharged because she has achieved her goals and expected outcomes.

PSYCHOLOGICAL ASPECTS

It is important to note that the majority of patients who experience acute low back pain recover spontaneously while a small minority of patients go on to become chronic back pain sufferers.[74] It has been shown that recovery from low back pain depends not only on physical factors, but also on psychological factors.[38] Unemployment and compensation are associated with increased psychological factors that

Table 6-6	
WADDELL'S NONORGANIC PHYSICAL SIGNS[49]	
Tenderness	Superficial and/or non-anatomical tenderness
Simulation	Axial loading of the skull, produces report of low back pain
	Passive rotation of shoulders and pelvis produces a report of low back pain of the patient
Distraction	Marked improvement of pain on SLR with distraction
Regional disturbance	A partial cogwheeling "give away" and/or nondermatomal sensory disturbance
Overreaction	Demonstration of disproportionate pain behaviors during examination

affect the patient's perception of his or her low back pain.[38] It has been suggested that there are individual differences in response to a painful experience that have their primary manifestation in terms of a spectrum of fear of pain.[74] This spectrum means that there is a range of fear of pain and a range of consequent behaviors. For example, there are patients who experience severe discomfort, but only have a minimal fear of the pain, are able to confront the pain, and are gradually able to become more functional. There are also patients who experience severe discomfort and have a severe fear of pain. These patients would tend to avoid painful activities.[74] This "fear/avoidance" concept could lead patients to reinforce avoidance behavior and other activities and ultimately reinforce a sick role.[74]

This makes it important for the physical therapist to recognize the many factors involved in a patient's experience of low back pain and also to seek ways to evaluate a patient appropriately. Waddell's nonorganic physical signs (Table 6-6) are a simple clinical screen to identify patients who may require more detailed assessment of psychological factors.[38]

Case Study #2: Spinal Stenosis

Mr. John Zacarro is a 76-year-old male with increasing complaints of difficulty standing up straight and walking for long periods of time.

PHYSICAL THERAPIST EXAMINATION

HISTORY

♦ General demographics: Mr. Zacarro is a 76-year-old white male whose primary language is English. He is right-hand dominant.
♦ Social history: Mr. Zacarro is married and has two children, a daughter age 45 and a son age 42.
♦ Employment/work: He is presently retired. He worked

for many years as a salesman.
♦ Living environment: He lives with his wife in a retirement community in the suburbs.
♦ General health status
  ● General health perception: He reports that his function had been deteriorating of late. He is feeling significant improvement following a series of epidural injections.[75]
  ● Physical function: He reports that he functions relatively well for his age.
  ● Psychological function: Normal.
  ● Role function: Husband, father.
  ● Social function: He enjoys playing golf and cards and reading.
♦ Social/health habits: He reports that he is a non-smoker and enjoys social drinking on weekends.
♦ Family history: His mother is deceased and had a history of OA and cardiac disease. His father is deceased and had a history of hypercholesterolemia and HTN.
♦ Medical/surgical history: He has HTN, hypercholesterolemia, and OA. He received a series of three epidural cortisone injections. The last injection was given 1 month ago.
♦ Prior hospitalizations: He was hospitalized for a hernia repair at age 65.
♦ Preexisting medical and other health-related conditions: He has a history of OA and intermittent chronic back pain.
♦ Current condition(s)/chief complaint(s): Mr. Zacarro is complaining of increasingly poor posture. He is concerned that he has been stooping forward of late and that his walking and standing tolerance have decreased.
♦ Functional status and activity level: He is totally independent in all ADL and IADL. He reports that he likes to walk, especially on the golf course. He has been following a gentle self-designed exercise program for many years.
♦ Medications: He is presently taking Lipitor to regulate his cholesterol level, atenolol to regulate his HTN, and Naprosyn as needed to modulate the pain from his OA.

♦ Other clinical tests: Radiographs revealed mild narrowing of the disc spaces and moderate osteophytes throughout the cervical and lumbar spine. MRI revealed moderate narrowing of the central spinal canal from L4-S1.

SYSTEMS REVIEW

♦ Cardiovascular/pulmonary
  • BP: 140/85 mmHg
  • Edema: None
  • HR: 80 bpm
  • RR: 15 bpm
♦ Integumentary
  • Presence of scar formation: None
  • Skin color: WNL
  • Skin integrity: WNL
♦ Musculoskeletal
  • Gross range of motion: Moderately restricted in flexion, bilateral sidebending and rotation, and severely restricted in extension in the lumbar spine as ascertained from the lower quarter examination. Moderately restricted in flexion, extension, sidebending and rotation bilaterally in the cervical and thoracic spine as ascertained from the upper quarter examination
  • Gross strength: Decreased in abdominals and lumbar extensors
  • Gross symmetry
    ▪ Moderate forward head
    ▪ Mild thoracic kyphosis
    ▪ Reversal of lumbar lordosis
  • Height: 5'10" (1.524 m)
  • Weight: 200 lbs (74.68 kg)
♦ Neuromuscular
  • Standing balance was WFL
  • Ambulating independently
  • Using a straight cane outdoors for safety
  • Independent with transfers and stairs
♦ Communication, affect, cognition, language, and learning style
  • Communication, affect, and cognition: Alert and able to communicate needs
  • Affect: Is visually upset when discussing deteriorating function
  • Learning preferences: Visual leaner

TESTS AND MEASURES

♦ Aerobic capacity/endurance
  • 6-Minute Walk test: He tolerated 4 minutes and completed almost four laps of 40 meters each[76]
♦ Anthropometric characteristics

  • BMI=705 x (body weight [in pounds] divided by height^2 [in inches])
  • Mr. Zacarro's BMI=28.77
  • BMI values between 25 and 30 are considered to be overweight[32]
♦ Assistive and adaptive devices
  • Mr. Zacarro is using a straight cane for ambulation outdoors
♦ Cranial and peripheral nerve integrity
  • Sensation intact to light touch in both LEs
  • SLR test negative but limited length secondary to tight hamstrings bilaterally
♦ Environmental, home, and work barriers
  • Mr. Zacarro is retired so there are no limitations at work
  • His home environment is barrier free
♦ Ergonomics and body mechanics
  • Analysis of body mechanics during self-care, home management, work, community, and leisure actions, tasks, and activities revealed altered posture during all activities
    ▪ Mr. Zacarro leans forward for prolonged periods of time while playing cards in the club house
    ▪ He tends to lean forward while he is walking for pleasure or when on the golf course
    ▪ He tends to slouch when reading novels in his favorite recliner
♦ Gait, locomotion, and balance
  • Gait and locomotion
    ▪ Ambulates independently on level surfaces and stairs in the house
    ▪ Gait pattern becomes increasingly flexed and antalgic secondary to pain after walking for a short period of time
    ▪ He utilizes a straight cane for safety and to maintain balance outdoors
    ▪ His walking speed is decreased
    ▪ He was unable to perform the 6-Minute Walk test, he walked 140 meters in 4 minutes
  • Balance
    ▪ Bilateral static standing balance was WFL with eyes open
    ▪ Bilateral dynamic standing balance required stand-by supervision to contact guarding with eyes closed
    ▪ Unilateral standing balance on a stable surface was limited to 5 seconds for each leg with eyes open
    ▪ Unilateral standing balance was limited to 5 seconds bilaterally with eyes closed requiring contact guarding

♦ Joint integrity and mobility
  ● Joint integrity and mobility assessment entails not only the osteokinematic and arthrokinematic analysis but also the structural integrity of the joint
  ● This includes special tests designed to assess ligamentous stability, compression, distraction tests, impingement tests, and joint play[34]
  ● Cervical spine
    ■ PPIVM testing was moderately restricted, end feel firm and ligamentous in flexion, extension, sidebending and rotation
    ■ PAIVM testing
      ‣ Extension: P/A glide on SPs was moderately restricted with hard end feel
      ‣ Sidebending: Side glide intervertebral mobility was moderately restricted bilaterally with hard end feel
      ‣ Rotation: On articular pillar was moderately restricted bilaterally with firm end feel
      ‣ Distraction of cervical spine was mildly restricted
  ● Thoracic spine
    ■ PPIVM testing was moderately restricted with end feel firm and ligamentous in flexion, extension, sidebending and rotation
    ■ PAIVM testing
      ‣ Extension: P/A glide on SPs was moderately restricted throughout with firm end feel
      ‣ Rotation: Lateral glide on SPs was mildly restricted with firm end feel
  ● Lumbar spine
    ■ PPIVM testing was severely restricted with end feel firm and ligamentous in extension, sidebending, and rotation and mildly restricted in flexion
    ■ PAIVM testing
      ‣ Extension: P/A glide on SPs was severely restricted with hard end feel
      ‣ Rotation: On transverse processes was moderately restricted bilaterally with firm end feel
♦ Motor function
  ● Observation of dexterity, coordination, and agility revealed activities: WNL
♦ Muscle performance
  ● Dynamometry revealed a right grip strength of 65 lbs (normal mean for patient's age is 65.7 lbs), left grip strength 57 lbs (normal mean 55.0)[77]
  ● MMT revealed the following deviations from normal:
    ■ Cervical spine extension=3/5
    ■ Cervical spine flexion=4/5
    ■ Thoracic spine extension=3/5

■ Abdominal=3/5
■ LE=WFL
  ● Muscle tension (palpation)
    ■ Spasm
      ‣ Upper trapezius bilaterally
      ‣ Thoracic and lumbar paraspinals bilaterally
      ‣ Bilateral gluteus medius
♦ Orthotic, protective, and supportive devices
  ● None used
♦ Pain
  ● NPS
    ■ Pain of 8/10 on the NPS (0=no pain and 10=worst possible pain) located in the lumbar spine after walking for 5 minutes, 4/10 across the thoracic and cervical spines
    ■ The patient reports 0/10 at rest in the cervical, thoracic, and lumbar spines
    ■ Downie and associates[35] described a high degree of agreement between the VAS, NPS, and the SDS although they reported that the NPS performed better
    ■ Jensen found the NPS to be the most practical tool[78]
  ● ODQ score was a total of 30/50 for the 10 items included[33]
♦ Posture
  ● Observational assessment done from all perspectives, and grid photographs and plumb line were used
    ■ Lateral view: Mild FHP and mild thoracic kyphosis
    ■ Posterior view: Reversal of lumbar lordosis
    ■ Anterior view: Mild FHP from anterior view
♦ Range of motion
  ● Functional range of motion
    ■ Decreased ability to look up to the ceiling
    ■ Decreased ability to look over either shoulder
    ■ Decreased ability to stand up straight
  ● Joint active and passive movement
    ■ Cervical spine ROM was measured using the CROM instrument
      ‣ Intratester reliability was found to be high (ICC=0.93), and intertester reliability was found to be moderate (ICCs=0.83, 0.775) for CROM measurements[79]
      ‣ Hickey found moderate intertester reliability for both the CROM and the plumb line technique[80]
      ‣ The validity of the CROM measurement was compared to a radiographic measurement, and the Pearson's r correlation was very high between the two methods (flexion r=0.97,

P<0.001, extension r=0.98, P<0.001)[81]
  ▸ Flexion=70 degrees
  ▸ Extension=45 degrees
  ▸ Lateral flexion=20 degrees bilaterally
  ▸ Rotation R=45 degrees and L=45 degrees
  ■ Thoracic spine (inclinometry)
    ▸ Flexion=60 degrees
    ▸ Extension=0 degrees
    ▸ Lateral flexion=15 degrees bilaterally
    ▸ Rotation=30 degrees bilaterally
  ■ Lumbar (inclinometry)
    ▸ Flexion=50 degrees
    ▸ Extension=10 degrees
    ▸ Sidebending=15 degrees bilaterally
    ▸ Rotation=10 degrees bilaterally
  ● Muscle length
    ■ Hamstring tightness bilaterally
    ■ Rectus femoris tightness bilaterally
    ■ Iliopsoas tightness bilaterally
◆ Reflex integrity
  ● DTRs or myotatic reflexes: Right Achilles reflex=1+
  ● All other reflexes WNL
◆ Self-care and home management
  ● Interview concerning ability to safely perform self-care and home management actions, tasks, and activities found they could be done WNL despite mild discomfort
◆ Work, community, and leisure integration or reintegration
  ● Interview concerning ability to safely manage community and leisure actions, tasks, and activities revealed that they could be done, but pain was experienced when standing up straight, walking for prolonged periods of time, and lifting or carrying heavy objects

EVALUATION

Mr. Zacarro's history and risk factors previously outlined indicated that he is a 76-year-old male, non-smoker, overweight, non-vigorous exerciser, with HTN, hypercholesterolemia, OA, intermittent chronic low back pain, and a family history of OA and cardiac disease. He has pain when walking; decreased strength in his cervical, thoracic, and lumbar spines; and decreased ROM throughout his spine. He has difficulty with standing up straight, transferring from sit to stand, and lifting and carrying tasks during his ADL and IADL.

DIAGNOSIS

Mr. Zacarro is a patient with spinal stenosis and pain in the lumbar spine and LEs after walking for 5 minutes and pain across the thoracic and cervical spines. He has impaired: aerobic capacity/endurance; ergonomics and body mechanics; gait, locomotion, and balance; joint integrity and mobility; muscle performance; posture; and range of motion. He is functionally limited in work, community, and leisure actions, tasks, and activities. These findings are consistent with placement in Pattern F: Impaired Joint Mobility, Motor Function, Muscle Performance, Range of Motion, and Reflex Integrity Associated With Spinal Disorders. The identified impairments and functional limitations will be addressed in determining the prognosis and the plan of care.

PROGNOSIS AND PLAN OF CARE

Over the course of the visits, the following mutually established outcomes have been determined:
◆ Ability to perform physical actions, tasks, and activities related to self-care, home management, work, community, and leisure is improved
◆ Fitness is improved
◆ Knowledge of behaviors that foster healthy habits, wellness, and prevention is improved
◆ Muscle length is increased in the hamstring, iliopsoas, and rectus femoris muscles
◆ Muscle performance is increased
◆ Muscle spasm in the upper trapezeii and thoracic and lumbar paraspinals is reduced
◆ Physical capacity is improved
◆ Physical function of the cervical, thoracic, and lumbar spines is improved
◆ Postural control is improved
◆ Risk factors are reduced
◆ Risk of secondary impairment is reduced
◆ ROM is increased in the cervical, thoracic, and lumbar spine
◆ Stress is decreased

To achieve these outcomes, the appropriate interventions for this patient are determined. These will include: coordination, communication, and documentation; patient/client-related instruction; therapeutic exercise; functional training in self-care and home management; functional training in work, community, and leisure integration or reintegration; manual therapy techniques; prescription, application, and, as appropriate, fabrication of devices and equipment; electrotherapeutic modalities; and physical agents and mechanical modalities.

Based on the diagnosis and the prognosis, Mr. Zacarro is expected to require 12 to 14 visits over 12 to 14 weeks. Mr. Zacarro has good social support, is motivated, and follows through with his home exercise program. He is not severely impaired and is healthy.

INTERVENTIONS

RATIONALE FOR SELECTED INTERVENTIONS

Spinal stenosis is a frequently encountered condition, particularly in the elderly, that may lead to significant pain and functional limitations. To understand the rationale for interventions for the patient with spinal stenosis, it is important to understand the pathophysiology of spinal stenosis and the biomechanics of the spine during everyday activities. Spinal stenosis involves the narrowing of one or more of three areas of the spine: the vertebral canal through which the spinal cord and nerve roots run, the area of the intervertebral canal called the lateral recess where the nerve roots branch out from the spinal cord, or the intervertebral foramina through which the spinal nerves exit. Walking is an everyday activity that causes the vertebrae of the lumbar spine to rotate and extend.[82] The overall effect of lumbar extension is a decrease in the cross-sectional area of the vertebral canal.[83] Therefore, extension of the lumbar spine, as occurs with walking and standing, narrows even further an already narrowed vertebral canal, lateral recesses, and/or intervertebral foramina. This causes more pressure or tension on the spinal cord, nerve roots, and/or spinal nerves and leads to increased pain and LE symptoms.[83]

By contrast, the cross-sectional area of the vertebral canal increases in flexion of the lumbar spine[83] thereby increasing the available space for the spinal cord, nerve roots, and spinal nerves and reducing the pressure or tension on these potential pain generating structures. It should also be noted that it is not only increased pressure that may elicit pain from these structures, but also neuroischemia or inflammatory exudate that may cause pain.[2]

The interventions described are an attempt to improve the primary problems caused by spinal stenosis, such as pain and loss of ROM, in addition to the secondary sequelae of spinal stenosis, such as decreased aerobic capacity and endurance and muscle strength. Since the position of flexion of the lumbar spine is usually a position of pain relief, it may be incorporated into all aspects of the patient's program.

Therapeutic Exercise

Aerobic exercise is beneficial in the treatment of patients with spinal stenosis as a method to improve cardiovascular fitness. The patient's fitness level deteriorates as his ability to walk distances decreases due to either pain and/or weakness in the LEs. Pain is worsened during walking due to increased pressure on the spinal cord, nerve roots, or spinal nerves.

Extension of the lumbar spine may also cause pain due to the effects of degenerative changes in the lumbar spine. Pain may be generated by increased load on degenerative zygapophyseal joints. It has also been estimated that patho-logical disc space narrowing may result in some 70% of the axial load being borne by the inferior articular processes and the laminae.[2]

Aerobic exercise in the treatment of patients with spinal stenosis may be used to improve muscular endurance, neuromotor control, and mechanical efficiency. It provides the additional benefits of weight loss and the favorable psychological effects with decreased anxiety and depression.[84] People who are not aerobically fit tend to fatigue rapidly in performing repetitive tasks and therefore are more susceptible to back injury.[84] The most widely cited evidence for the benefits of aerobic exercise is a study of firefighters among whom higher levels of physical fitness predicted a lower risk of subsequent back problems.[35] In this study, fitness was characterized by a combination of data from bicycle ergonometry, muscle strength testing, and spine flexibility. Thus, the particular role of aerobic exercise in the prevention of back injury could not be isolated. By instructing the patient with spinal stenosis to exercise aerobically while keeping the lumbar spine in a more flexed position (eg, using a stationary or recumbent bike), the patient may achieve the benefits of aerobic exercise while minimizing the biomechanical factors that may cause pain.

Flexibility and stretching exercises are designed to improve the extensibility of muscle and other soft tissues to establish normal ROM in the lumbar spine. Of particular importance in the patient with spinal stenosis is the biomechanical dysfunction of the psoas major muscle. This muscle often appears to be shortened and weak due to chronic contraction, and this, in conjunction with abdominal and gluteal weakness, can cause an increase in lumbar lordosis.[10] In the patient with spinal stenosis this can lead to an increase in the pressure on the pain generating structures of the spinal canal and intervertebral foraminae, in addition to those in the posterior part of the vertebra, that is, the posterior disc and zygapophyseal joints.

The lumbopelvic complex has been described as one of the best examples of the intricacies of neuromuscular regulation mechanisms that requires an integration of the lumbar spine, abdomen, and hips.[56] With the spinal musculature removed, the lumbar spine is highly unstable at very low applied loads, which indicates the importance of muscle activity for spinal stability.[85] The different muscle groups of the trunk require different methods for strengthening and improving endurance. For example, the unisegmental muscles of the lumbar spine, such as the intertransversarii and interspinalis, are proposed to function primarily as force transducers, providing feedback on spinal position and movement.[85] In contrast, the abdominal muscles play an important role in generating extensor force during lifting tasks either by increasing intra-abdominal pressure or by creating tension in the thoracolumbar fascia.[2] Many studies have shown that the use of specific exercise interventions results in significant reduction of pain intensity.[86,87]

Manual Therapy Techniques

Bang and Deyle[88] and others[34,60] have demonstrated improvements in ROM, pain, and function associated with manual physical therapy interventions used in the management of patient populations with painful stiff spines and extremity joints.[16,34] Manual therapy techniques include the use of skilled hands to enhance tissue extensibility, joint mobility, modulate pain, decrease spasm, and reduce soft tissue swelling. The reader is referred to Case Study #1 for additional information on rationale on manual therapy.

Electrotherapeutic Modalities

Electrotherapeutic modalities have been documented to decrease pain, muscle spasm, and relax the soft tissue structures. The reader is referred to the rationale for these modalities in Case Study #1 for additional information on rationale for electrotherapeutic modalities.

Physical Agents and Mechanical Modalities

Thermotherapy includes the use of moist heat to enhance tissue perfusion and oxygenation.[65] The reader is referred to the rationale for these modalities in Case Study #1 for additional information on rationale for physical agents and mechanical modalities.

Intermittent mechanical traction may benefit this patient by maximizing the opening between the lumbar vertebrae. Colachis and Strohm[89] found that for maximal posterior separation, the patient should be placed in supine with the knees flexed to 70 degrees and the traction pulling at an 18-degree angle. The authors found the largest degree of posterior separation took place at the L4-5 interspace with the use of 100 lbs of force. Krause and associates,[90] in a review of a number of studies describing the efficacy of traction, outlined the following reasons for the application of traction: normalization of neurological deficit and relief of radicular pain, intervertebral separation, silencing of ectopic impulse generators, reduction of intervertebral disc herniation, altered interdiscal pressure, normalization of conduction, improvement of straight leg raising test, pain relief, and increased joint mobility. They concluded that only separation of the intervertebral space could be established. Van der Heijden and associates,[91] in an analysis of the literature regarding efficacy of traction, concluded that although there is no strong evidence supporting the use of traction, there is also a lack of evidence that determines that it is an ineffective modality. Intermittent pelvic traction has been advocated as a temporary relief in patients with spinal stenosis.[92,93]

COORDINATION, COMMUNICATION, AND DOCUMENTATION

Communication will occur with Mr. Zacarro and his family members to engender support for his exercise program. All elements of the patient's management will be documented. A referral to a nutritionist/dietitian for weight control guidelines will be made to ensure an appropriate diet and weight loss. A plan of care will be developed and discussed with the patient.

PATIENT/CLIENT-RELATED INSTRUCTION

Education regarding his current condition, impairments, and functional limitations will be discussed. The patient will be instructed in appropriate body mechanics, proper posture, and core stabilization. Risk factors will be discussed including a discussion concerning weight management and the influence that poor posture may have on aerobic capacity and functional activities. A nutritional referral will be made. Ergonomic instruction and body mechanics for leisure activities will be addressed.

THERAPEUTIC EXERCISE

- ◆ Aerobic capacity/endurance conditioning
  - Progression for these exercises is time based
  - For example, if the patient tolerates 10 minutes on the stationary bicycle well, he will be started at 8 minutes and then he will increase the time daily by 5% to 10% from this baseline
  - Mode
    - Bicycle[63]
  - Aquatic program
    - Hydrotherapy starting in a warm pool at chest level with a pool-walking program
    - Exercise is progressed by time as described above
- ◆ Balance, coordination, and agility training
  - Sitting on exercise ball in front of a mirror
  - Bouncing on exercise ball
  - Progress to arm raises/leg raises while sitting on the ball
  - Progress from sitting to standing balance
  - Stand on one leg with eyes closed on level ground for proprioceptive retraining
  - Progress to unstable surfaces, such as a balance pad (eg, Airex) or a balance board
  - Unilateral stance on stable surface with perturbations
  - Bilateral standing on an unstable surface (eg, foam rubber cushion)
  - Side gliding
  - Braiding
  - Standing on foam roller
  - Balance beam
  - Obstacle course
- ◆ Body mechanics and postural stabilization
  - Body mechanics training
    - Appropriate sitting posture for leisure activities

- Appropriate lifting and carrying instructions
- Appropriate bending instructions
- Appropriate use of body mechanics while swinging a golf club
- Posture awareness training
  - Verbal cueing and use of a mirror to correct spinal postural impairments
  - Proper alignment of head and cervical, thoracic, and lumbar spines
  - Axial extension to achieve position of no more than 2 inches from the deepest portion of the cervical lordosis to the apex of the thoracic kyphosis[72]
  - Use of mirror for visual input of appropriate alignment
  - Sitting on exercise ball in front of a mirror
  - Standing on foam roller
  - Bilateral standing on foam rubber cushion (eg, Airex)
  - Side gliding
  - Braiding
  - Balance beam
  - Obstacle course
  - Notes all around home and car
- Postural control training
  - Proper alignment of head and cervical, thoracic, and lumbar spines
  - Scapula retraction and depression
  - Transition of position from supine to sitting, standing, and walking
  - Proper postural position during transition:
    - From supine to sitting, standing, and walking
    - From sit to kneel
    - From 1/2 kneel to stand
    - To functional activities at work
  - Transition of position to functional activities at leisure including driving the car and playing golf
- Postural stabilization activities[94]
  - Axial extension starting in supine and progressing to sitting and upright
  - Maintenance of axial extension position with bilateral arm raises
  - Maintenance of pelvic neutral position
  - Maintenance of pelvic neutral position with isolated UE and LE movements starting, for example, with five reps and increasing to three sets of 10 reps
  - Add weights, starting, for example, with a low weight for 8 to 12 reps and increasing accordingly
  - Utilize ball for sitting exercises while learning to control pelvis position

- Control pelvis on ball and isolate extremity movements
- Add reps and weights as described above
- Incorporate the use of the foam roller and unstable surfaces like wobble board or foam rubber cushion in sitting and standing with bilateral and unilateral stance
- Utilize balance beam
- Utilize obstacle course
- Challenge patient out of center of gravity/base of support
- Practice lifting and carrying objects of varying sizes and weights, starting with small, light objects, while maintaining a neutral lumbar spine
- Quadruped, kneeling, sitting, and standing exercises that incorporate postural stabilization with extremity movements

- Flexibility exercises
  - ROM
    - Cervical ROM in all directions
    - Thoracic extension
    - Cat and camel allowing lumbar and thoracic spine to extend to neutral as tolerated
    - Quadruped flexion and extension exercise holding flexion for 5 to 10 seconds, gently moving towards neutral extension if tolerated and holding for 5 to 10 seconds and then repeating the entire sequence three to five times
    - Lumbar AROM in all directions, limiting extension to neutral
    - Hip AROM for extension
  - Stretching
    - Stretching exercises should be done after warming up, using a slow and steady stretch accompanied by deep breathing, and building hold up to 30 to 60 seconds
    - Done two to three times a day, at least two to three repetitions
    - Hamstring stretch
      - Patient is supine with right hip flexed to 90 degrees and hands supporting right posterior thigh
      - Patient extends right knee to tolerance
    - Quadriceps stretching
    - Hip flexor stretching in the Thomas test position
    - Anterior chest wall and shoulder stretching
    - Corner stretch
    - Lumbar flexion with single knee and double knees to chest
- Gait and locomotion training
  - Pool walking initiated for early weightbearing in a warm environment

- Weightbearing progressed by moving to more shallow water depths
- Treadmill walking progressing from supported to unsupported

♦ Relaxation
- Aquatic relaxation techniques
  - Taught in a heated pool to induce muscle relaxation for overworked muscles
- Jacobson relaxation techniques with emphasis on breathing
- Visualization and imagery to induce total relaxation

♦ Strength, power, and endurance training
- Cervical isometric exercises in all directions using a ball between his head and the wall[95]
- Seated push-ups
- Wall push-ups
- Plyometrics with unweighted and weighted ball
- Abdominal strengthening with knees flexed starting with short lever arm and progressing as tolerated
- LE weight training for hip flexion and extension and knee flexion and extension starting, for example, with a low weight for 8 to 12 reps and progressing according to patient's tolerance
- Stool rolling forward and backward

Maintenance of a regular exercise program must be instilled in this patient. To do this there are several key factors that may be helpful in achieving an exercise program that the patient will do on a life-long basis. These tips may be included in part of the patient-related instruction and may include any or all of the following:

♦ Establish a variety of enjoyable activities and alternating activities when possible
♦ Establish a realistic time frame for exercise
♦ Make exercise a family experience when possible
♦ Add exercise to one's weekly schedule (walk whenever feasible, climb up and down several flights of stairs instead of taking the elevator)
♦ Find activities that may be done during the course of the day
♦ Find fun alternative activities for weekends
♦ Allow flexibility
♦ If a scheduled exercise time is missed, work into schedule at another time during the day or week
♦ Use entertainment whenever possible
- Play music when performing weight exercises or while walking outside
- Watch TV while on the treadmill
- Use books on tape at anytime

FUNCTIONAL TRAINING IN SELF-CARE AND HOME MANAGEMENT

♦ ADL training
- Postures and body mechanics instruction for grooming and toileting

♦ Devices and equipment use and training
- Make patient aware of adaptive devices for toileting and grooming and provide information regarding availability if required

♦ Functional training programs
- Make patient aware of back schools that are available in his area and provide referrals as appropriate

♦ Simulated environment
- Review actions, tasks, and activities related to bathing, bed mobility, transfers, and dressing

♦ IADL training
- Review principles of body mechanics as they apply to household chores, shopping, and yard work so that Mr. Zacarro may participate in these activities with his wife

♦ Injury prevention or reduction
- Review proper body mechanics and posture for self care and home management in order to prevent further injury

FUNCTIONAL TRAINING IN WORK, COMMUNITY, AND LEISURE INTEGRATION OR REINTEGRATION

♦ Devices and equipment use and training
- Review proper use of cane on level surfaces, stairs, and curbs

♦ Functional training programs
- Make patient aware of back schools that are available in his area and provide referrals as appropriate
- When patient is ready, simulate golf swings and provide appropriate feedback to modify swing and ball retrieval

♦ Injury prevention or reduction
- Review proper body mechanics and posture for community and leisure actions, tasks, and activities in order to prevent further injury

♦ Leisure and play activities and training
- Instruction and simulation of appropriate positions for reading, watching television, and playing golf emphasizing correct spinal posture

MANUAL THERAPY TECHNIQUES

♦ Massage
- Connective tissue massage/myofascial release[60]

- To upper trapezeii and thoracic and lumbar paraspinals
- ◆ Mobilization/manipulation
  - Soft tissue
    - Anterior chest wall
    - Cervical, thoracic, and lumbar paraspinal muscles
    - Suboccipital muscles
    - Upper trapezius, scaleni, SCM
    - Rhomboids and middle trapezius
    - Hip flexors
    - Hamstrings
  - Spinal joints[16,34]
    - Manual distraction to lumbar spine to increase intervertebral space and improve intervertebral mobility
    - Grades III and IV mobilizations
      - ▸ P/A glide on SPs or articular pillars to increase axial extension of the cervical spine
      - ▸ PAIVM to increase thoracic and lumbar extension
      - ▸ P/A glide of SPs/bilateral transverse processes of thoracic spine to decrease kyphosis and increase mobility
      - ▸ P/A glide of SPs/bilateral transverse processes of lumbar spine to regain lordosis and increase mobility

PRESCRIPTION, APPLICATION, AND, AS APPROPRIATE, FABRICATION OF DEVICES AND EQUIPMENT

- ◆ Straight cane
  - The patient will be provided with and instructed in the use of a straight cane on all surfaces

ELECTROTHERAPEUTIC MODALITIES

- ◆ EMS and TENS to decrease pain and spasm

PHYSICAL AGENTS AND MECHANICAL MODALITIES

- ◆ Sound agents
  - Ultrasound to increase tissue perfusion, oxygenation, and nutrient delivery to the tissues
- ◆ Thermotherapy
  - Hot packs to increase muscle extensibility and decrease spasm in cervical, thoracic, and lumbar spine muscles
- ◆ Traction device
  - Intermittent/static, as indicated, lumbar traction to

increase intervertebral joint space and open nerve root foramen

ANTICIPATED GOALS AND EXPECTED OUTCOMES

- ◆ Impact on pathology/pathophysiology
  - Joint swelling, inflammation, or restriction is reduced by 12% to 15%.
  - Muscle spasm is decreased from moderate to minimal.
  - Neural compression is decreased.
  - Nutrient delivery to tissue is increased.
  - Pain is decreased on the NPS from 8/10 to 5/10 in the lumbar spine and from 4/10 to 1-2/10 in the cervical and thoracic spines while ambulating in the initial stages of treatment. Pain is decreased from 30/50 to 20/50 on the ODQ.
  - Soft tissue inflammation, edema, and restriction are reduced.
  - Tissue perfusion and oxygenation are increased.
- ◆ Impact on impairments
  - Aerobic capacity/endurance is increased from 4 to 5 minutes on the 6-Minute Walk test.
  - Balance is improved. Unilateral standing balance is improved from 5 to 10 seconds with eyes open and bilateral dynamic standing balance with eyes closed requires occasional contact guarding.
  - Energy expenditure per unit of work is decreased.
  - Gait is improved so that gait pattern is normal.
  - Joint integrity and mobility are improved by 10% to 15% in the cervical, thoracic, and lumbar spines.
  - Muscle length is improved by 10% in the hamstrings, iliopsoas, and rectus femoris.
  - Muscle performance (strength, power, and endurance) is increased in the abdominals, in thoracic spine extension, and in cervical spine extension to 4/5.
  - Optimal joint alignment is achieved.
  - Optimal loading on a body part is achieved.
  - Postural control is improved. FHP is reduced. Minimal lumbar lordosis is achieved.
  - Quality of movement between and across body segments is improved.
  - Relaxation is increased.
  - ROM of the cervical, thoracic, and lumbar spines is improved to WFL.
- ◆ Impact on functional limitations
  - Ability to assume or resume required self-care, home management, work, community, and leisure roles is improved.
  - Ability to independently perform physical actions,

tasks, and activities related to ADL/IADL in self-care, home management, work, community, and leisure with or without assistive devices and equipment is increased.

- Level of supervision required for task performance is decreased.
- Tolerance of positions and actions, tasks, and activities is increased—tolerance for sitting in proper posture is increased, tolerance for playing golf is increased, tolerance for walking is increased.

♦ Risk reduction/prevention
- Awareness of precautions and correct resting positions is achieved.
- Pressure on body tissue is reduced.
- Protection of body parts is increased.
- Risk factors are reduced.
- Risk of recurrence of condition is reduced.
- Risk of secondary impairments is reduced.
- Safety is improved.
- Self-management of symptoms is improved.

♦ Impact on health, wellness, and fitness
- Behaviors that foster healthy habits, nutrition, physical activity, wellness, and prevention are acquired. BMI now 28.0.
- Decision making is enhanced regarding health, wellness, and fitness needs.
- Fitness, health status, physical capacity, and physical function are improved.

♦ Impact on societal resources
- Available resources are maximally utilized.
- Documentation occurs throughout patient management and across all settings and follows APTA's *Guidelines for Physical Therapy Documentation.*[58]

♦ Patient/client satisfaction
- Access, availability, and services provided are acceptable to patient/client.
- Case is managed throughout the episode of care.
- Clinical proficiency and interpersonal skills of the physical therapist are acceptable to patient/client.
- Coordination of care is acceptable to patient/client.
- Interdisciplinary collaboration occurs through case conferences.
- Patient's knowledge and awareness of the diagnosis, prognosis, interventions, and understanding of anticipated goals and expected outcomes are increased.
- Sense of well-being is improved.
- Stressors are decreased.

REEXAMINATION

Reexamination is performed throughout the episode of care.

DISCHARGE

Mr. Zacarro is discharged from physical therapy after a total of 14 physical therapy sessions and attainment of his goals and expectations. These sessions have covered his entire episode of service. He is discharged because he has achieved his goals and expected outcomes.

Case Study #3: Anterolisthesis

Ms. Rachel Merlo is a 17-year-old female with an anterolisthesis who has been complaining of left-sided low back pain for 3 weeks.

PHYSICAL THERAPIST EXAMINATION

HISTORY

♦ General demographics: Rachel is a 17-year-old white female whose primary language is English. She is left-hand dominant.

♦ Social history: Rachel lives with her mother and father. She has two siblings, a sister, age 15, and a brother, age 11.

♦ Employment/work: She is presently a junior in high school. She is a member of a gymnastic team. She is required to practice 22 hours per week.

♦ Living environment: She lives with her family in a house in the suburbs.

♦ General health status
- General health perception: She reports to be in good health.
- Physical function: WNL.
- Psychological function: Normal.
- Role function: Daughter, student, gymnast.
- Social function: She enjoys reading and most sports activities.

♦ Social/health habits: She reports that she is a non-smoker and a non-drinker.

♦ Family history: Her mother has low back problems, and her father has gouty arthritis and borderline HTN.

♦ Medical/surgical history: She has a history of chondromalacia and exercise-induced asthma.

♦ Prior hospitalizations: None.

♦ Preexisting medical and other health-related conditions: Rachel has had occasional low back pain after working out at the gym. She reports that she had a similar problem last year but it resolved after resting for 1 week.

- ◆ Current condition(s)/chief complaint(s): She has been complaining of left sided low back pain for the past 3 weeks. She reports that the pain began after learning a new gymnastic skill, a full and one-half on the floor.
- ◆ Functional status and activity level: She is totally independent in all ADL and IADL. However, she experiences pain with any activity that requires twisting and extension. She reports that she practices gymnastics 22 hours a week and is also on the track team.
- ◆ Medications: Advil, arnica, ventalin.
- ◆ Other clinical tests: Radiographs which show a Grade I anterolisthesis of L4 on L5.

SYSTEMS REVIEW

- ◆ Cardiovascular/pulmonary
  - BP: 110/70 mmHg
  - Edema: None
  - HR: 65 bpm
  - RR: 11 bpm
- ◆ Integumentary
  - Presence of scar formation: None
  - Skin color: WNL
  - Skin integrity: WNL
- ◆ Musculoskeletal
  - Gross range of motion
    - ROM in the lumbar spine demonstrates hypermobility secondary to gymnastics as ascertained from the lower quarter examination
  - Gross strength: Decreased in abdominals and lumbar extensors
  - Gross symmetry
    - Mild right thoracic, left lumbar scoliosis
    - Increased lumbar lordosis
    - Genu recurvatum bilaterally
    - Pes planus bilaterally
  - Height: 5'6" (1.67 m)
  - Weight: 115 lbs (52.16 kg)
- ◆ Neuromuscular
  - Bilateral static and dynamic standing balance: WNL
  - Locomotion, transfers, and transitions: WNL
- ◆ Communication, affect, cognition, language, and learning style
  - Communication, affect, and cognition: Alert and able to communicate needs
  - Affect: Normal
  - Learning preferences: Auditory learner

TESTS AND MEASURES

- ◆ Aerobic capacity/endurance
  - She is able to walk/jog 5.5 miles in just under 60 minutes

- ◆ Anthropometric characteristics
  - BMI=705 x (body weight [in pounds] divided by height^2 [in inches])
  - Rachel's BMI=18.61, which is considered to be normal[32]
- ◆ Assistive and adaptive devices
  - Rachel is using an elastic back support during floor exercise at the gym
- ◆ Cranial and peripheral nerve integrity
  - Sensation intact in both LEs
- ◆ Ergonomics and body mechanics
  - Analysis of body mechanics during self-care, home management, work, community, and leisure actions, tasks, and activities revealed poor posture during all activities while sitting on a chair or couch
    - She tends to slouch when reading, doing homework, watching television, and using the computer
- ◆ Gait, locomotion, and balance: WNL
- ◆ Joint integrity and mobility
  - Joint integrity and mobility assessment entails not only the osteokinematic and arthrokinematic analysis but also the structural integrity of the joint. This includes special tests designed to assess ligamentous stability, compression, distraction tests, impingement tests, and joint play[34]
  - Lumbar spine
    - PPIVM testing
      - ▸ Hypermobile, end feel muscular in extension and rotation indicating muscle spasm
      - ▸ All other movements were WNL
    - PAIVM testing
      - ▸ Extension: P/A glide was moderately hypermobile at L4-5, L5-S1 with empty end feel, L1-4 were mildly hypermobile
      - ▸ Rotation: On transverse process was moderately hypermobile bilaterally, L>R, with empty end feel
- ◆ Motor function
  - Observation of dexterity, coordination and agility revealed activities: WNL
- ◆ Muscle performance
  - Dynamometry revealed a right grip strength of 80 lbs and a left grip strength 90 lbs (normal mean for patient's age is not published, the normal mean data for patients ages 20 to 24 are right 70.4 lbs and left 61.0 lbs)[77]
  - MMT revealed the following deviations from normal
    - Thoracic spine extension=4/5
    - Abdominal=4/5
  - Muscle tension (palpation)

- Spasm
  - ▸ Thoracic and lumbar paraspinals bilaterally, L>R
  - ▸ Upper trapezius bilaterally, L>R
  - ▸ Rhomboid and middle trapezius bilaterally, L>R
  - Bony palpation
    - ▸ Step off deformity present at L4-5
- ◆ Orthotic, protective, and supportive devices
  - Elastic lumbar support for use at gym
- ◆ Pain
  - NPS
    - Pain of 6/10 on the NPS (0=no pain and 10=worst possible pain) in the lumbar spine after gymnastic practice
    - The patient reports her pain to be 3/10 in the lumber spine at rest
    - Pain reported at end range extension and left rotation
    - Downie and associates described a high degree of agreement between the VAS, NPS, and the SDS although they reported that the NPS performed better[35]
    - Jensen[78] found the NPS to be the most practical tool
- ◆ Posture
  - Observational assessment done from all perspectives, and grid photographs and plumb line were used (Figure 6-6)
    - Lateral view: Lumbar hyperlordosis, genu recurvatum
    - Posterior view: Mild right thoracic left lumbar scoliosis, lumbar hyperlordosis, pes planus bilaterally
    - Anterior view: Pes planus bilaterally
- ◆ Range of motion
  - Functional range of motion: Increased extensibility in all ranges
  - Joint active and passive movement
    - Lumbar (inclinometry)
      - ▸ Flexion=80 degrees
      - ▸ Extension=70 degrees
      - ▸ Sidebending=45 degrees bilaterally
      - ▸ Rotation=50 degrees bilaterally
  - Muscle length
    - Lower lumbar extensors tight
    - All other muscles demonstrate increased muscle length
- ◆ Reflex integrity
  - DTRs or myotatic reflexes: WNL
- ◆ Self-care and home management
  - She has modified her home activities to eliminate

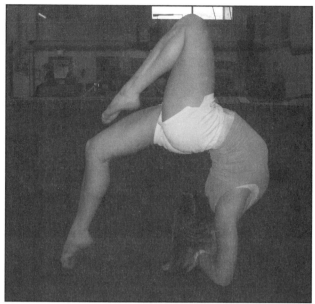

Figure 6-6. Typical gymnastic posture.

rotation and extension
- Interview concerning ability to safely perform self-care and home management actions, tasks, and activities found they could be done, however, all tasks that required excessive extension or rotation were painful
- ◆ Work, community, and leisure integration or reintegration
  - Rachel is excused from gym classes until receiving medical clearance
  - She has modified her gym workout to eliminate activities that require excessive rotation and extension and forceful landings
  - Interview concerning ability to safely manage community and leisure actions, tasks, and activities revealed that they could be done, however, all tasks that required excessive extension or rotation were painful

EVALUATION

Rachel's history and risk factors previously outlined indicated that she is a 17-year-old female, non-smoker, non-drinker, vigorous exerciser, with a 3-week history of left-sided low back pain. She has pain, faulty posture, hypermobility, muscle weakness, muscle spasm, and impaired motor performance in her lumbar spine.

DIAGNOSIS

Rachel is a patient with a diagnosis of anterolisthesis and with left-sided pain in her lumbar spine. She has impaired: ergonomics and body mechanics; joint integrity and mobility; muscle performance; posture; and range of motion. She is functionally limited in self-care, home management, school, community, and leisure actions, tasks, and activities. These findings are consistent with placement in Pattern F: Impaired Joint Mobility, Motor Function, Muscle Performance, Range of Motion, and Reflex Integrity Associated With Spinal Disorders. The identified impairments will be addressed in determining the prognosis and the plan of care.

PROGNOSIS AND PLAN OF CARE

Over the course of the visits, the following mutually established outcomes have been determined:

♦ Fitness is improved
♦ Knowledge of behaviors that foster healthy habits, wellness, and prevention is improved
♦ Muscle length is improved
♦ Muscle performance is increased
♦ Muscle spasm is decreased
♦ Physical capacity is improved
♦ Physical function of the lumbar spine is improved
♦ Postural control is improved
♦ Risk factors are reduced
♦ Risk of secondary impairment is reduced
♦ ROM is improved
♦ Stress is decreased

To achieve these outcomes, the appropriate interventions for the patient are determined. These will include: coordination, communication, and documentation; patient/client-related instruction; therapeutic exercise; functional training in self-care and home management; functional training in work, community, and leisure integration or reintegration; manual therapy techniques; prescription, application, and, as appropriate, fabrication of devices and equipment; electrotherapeutic modalities; and physical agents and mechanical modalities.

Based on the diagnosis and the prognosis, Rachel is expected to require 8 to 12 visits over 6 to 8 weeks. She has good social support and is extremely motivated.

INTERVENTIONS

RATIONALE FOR SELECTED INTERVENTIONS

Therapeutic Exercise

Aerobic exercise is beneficial in the treatment of patients with spondylolisthesis and low back pain to help improve cardiovascular fitness. This may have decreased as the patient has limited her activities due to pain. Aerobic exercise in the treatment of patients with low back pain may improve

muscular endurance, neuromotor control, and mechanical efficiency and provide the additional benefits of weight loss and the favorable psychological effects associated with decreased anxiety and depression.[84] The reader is referred to Case Study #1 for additional information regarding aerobic exercise.

Flexibility and stretching exercises improve the extensibility of muscle and other soft tissues in order to establish normal ROM in the lumbar spine. There is evidence that retraining the deep muscles of the trunk can positively influence the recovery of the muscle in acute low back pain.[9] The reader is referred back to the rationale in Case Study #2 for further clarification.

Lumbar stabilization is designed to help regain control of the muscles needed to protect and support the low back and pelvic region. It relies on the principles of motor learning in order to retrain and facilitate the appropriate muscles required to stabilize the lumbopelvic region. Stabilization exercises incorporate feedback techniques to foster kinesthetic awareness and position sense.[56]

Lumbar stabilization programs begin by having the patient relearn segmental control of the deep trunk musculature (transversus abdominis, multifidus, pelvic floor, and diaphragm). The program is then progressed to include maintaining segmental control while adding closed chain activities and then increasing the gravitational load to open chain functional activities.[56]

Manual Therapy Techniques

Bang and Deyle[88] and others[34,60] have demonstrated improvements in ROM, pain, and function associated with manual physical therapy interventions used in the management of patient populations with painful stiff spines and extremity joints.[16,34] Manual therapy techniques include the use of skilled hands to enhance tissue extensibility, joint mobility, modulate pain, decrease spasm, and reduce soft tissue swelling.[58] The reader is referred to Case Study #1 for additional information on rationale on manual therapy.

Electrotherapeutic Modalities

Electrotherapeutic modalities have been documented to decrease pain, muscle spasm, and relax the soft tissue structures. The reader is referred to the rationale for these modalities in Case Study #1 for additional information on rationale for electrotherapeutic modalities.

Physical Agents and Mechanical Modalities

Thermotherapy includes the use of moist heat to enhance tissue perfusion and oxygenation.[65] The reader is referred to the rationale for these modalities in Case Study #1 for additional information on rationale for physical agents and mechanical modalities.

COORDINATION, COMMUNICATION, AND DOCUMENTATION

Communication will occur with Rachel and her family members to engender support for her exercise program. All elements of the patient's management will be documented. A plan of care will be developed and discussed with the patient.

PATIENT/CLIENT-RELATED INSTRUCTION

Education regarding her current condition, impairments, and functional limitations will be discussed. The patient will be instructed in appropriate body mechanics, proper posture, and core stabilization. Risk factors will be discussed including a discussion concerning the influence that poor posture may have on aerobic capacity and functional activities. Ergonomic instruction and body mechanics for leisure activities will be addressed.

THERAPEUTIC EXERCISE

- ◆ Aerobic capacity/endurance conditioning
  - She will continue with her aerobic workout for the gymnastics and track team
- ◆ Balance, coordination, and agility training
  - Since her balance, coordination and agility abilities were above average because of her gymnastics training, she will continue to work out with the team
- ◆ Body mechanics and postural stabilization
  - Body mechanics training
    - Appropriate sitting posture for school and leisure activities
    - Appropriate use of body mechanics while performing gymnastic maneuvers and while running track
    - Appropriate lifting and carrying instructions
    - Appropriate bending instructions
  - Posture awareness training
    - Verbal cueing and use of a mirror to correct spinal postural impairments
    - Proper alignment of thoracic and lumbar spine
    - Use of mirror for visual input of appropriate alignment
    - Sitting on exercise ball in front of a mirror
    - Standing on foam roller
    - Bilateral standing on foam rubber cushion (eg, Airex)
    - Side gliding
    - Braiding
    - Balance beam
    - Obstacle course
    - Notes all around home and car

- Postural control training
  - Proper alignment of thoracic and lumbar spines
  - Proper postural position with pelvic stabilization during transition:
    - ▸ From supine to sitting, standing, and walking
    - ▸ From sit to kneel
    - ▸ From 1/2 kneel to stand
    - ▸ To functional activities at school and home
  - Transition of position to functional activities at leisure including driving the car, running, and performing gymnastic activities
- Postural stabilization activities[94]
  - Maintenance of pelvic neutral position
  - Maintenance of pelvic neutral position with isolated UE and LE movements starting, for example, with five reps and increasing to three sets of 10 reps
  - Add weights, starting, for example, with a low weight for 8 to 12 reps and increasing accordingly
  - Utilize an exercise ball for sitting exercises while learning to control pelvis position
  - Control pelvis on an exercise ball and isolate extremity movements
  - Add reps and weights as described above
  - Incorporate the use of the foam roller and unstable surfaces like wobble board or foam rubber cushion in sitting and standing with bilateral and unilateral stance
  - Utilize balance beam
  - Utilize obstacle course
  - Challenge patient out of center of gravity/base of support
  - Practice lifting and carrying objects of varying sizes and weights, starting with small, light objects, while maintaining a neutral lumbar spine
  - Quadruped, kneeling, sitting, and standing exercises that incorporate postural stabilization during extremity movements
- ◆ Flexibility exercises
  - Muscle lengthening
    - Cat and camel allowing lumbar and thoracic spine to extend to neutral as tolerated
  - ROM
    - Maintain lumbar ROM since she is already hypermobile
  - Stretching
    - Stretching exercises should be done after warming up, using a slow and steady stretch accompanied by deep breathing, and building hold up to 30 to 60 seconds

- Done two to three times a day, at least two to three repetitions
  - Prayer stretch for lower lumbar extensors
- Relaxation
  - Jacobson relaxation techniques with emphasis on breathing
  - Visualization and imagery to induce total relaxation
- Strength, power, and endurance training
  - Wall push-ups
  - Abdominal strengthening with knees flexed starting with short lever arm and progressing as tolerated
  - Tighten abdominal muscles so spine is in neutral alignment and perform unilateral UE flexion
  - Progress to BUE flexion
  - Progress to unilateral knee to chest
  - Progress to simultaneously flexing one UE and ipsilateral hip and knee to chest
  - Progress to simultaneously flexing one UE and the contralateral hip and knee to chest
  - Use weights or elastic bands to increase resistance

Maintenance of a regular exercise program must be instilled in the patient. To do this there are several keys that may be helpful in achieving an exercise program that the patient will do on a life-long basis. These tips may be included in part of the patient-related instruction and may include any or all of the following:

- Establish a variety of enjoyable activities and alternating activities when possible
- Establish a realistic time frame for exercise
- Make exercise a family experience when possible
- Add exercise to one's weekly schedule (walk to school if possible)
- Find activities that may be done during the course of the day
- Find fun alternative activities for weekends
- Allow flexibility
- If a scheduled exercise time is missed, work into schedule at another time during the day or week
- Use entertainment whenever possible
  - Play music when performing weight exercises or while walking outside
  - Watch TV while on the treadmill
  - Use books on tape at anytime

FUNCTIONAL TRAINING IN SELF-CARE AND HOME MANAGEMENT

- ADL training
  - Make patient aware of maintaining neutral spine with all ADL activities
- Devices and equipment use and training

- Make patient aware of indications for use of elastic back support
- Functional training programs
  - When patient is ready, simulate twisting and extension maneuvers and provide appropriate feedback
- IADL training
  - Review principles of body mechanics as they apply to performing activities including working at the computer, reading, and doing homework
- Injury prevention or reduction
  - Review proper body mechanics and posture for self-care and home management in order to prevent further injury

FUNCTIONAL TRAINING IN WORK, COMMUNITY, AND LEISURE INTEGRATION OR REINTEGRATION

- Devices and equipment use and training
  - Review proper use of elastic lumbar support with gymnastic activities
  - Functional training programs
  - When patient is ready, simulate twisting and extension maneuvers and provide appropriate feedback
  - Injury prevention or reduction
  - Review proper body mechanics and posture for community and leisure actions, tasks, and activities in order to prevent further injury
- Leisure and play activities and training
  - Instruction and simulation of appropriate positions for reading, watching television, and using the computer emphasizing correct spinal posture

MANUAL THERAPY TECHNIQUES

- Massage
  - Connective tissue massage/myofascial release[60]
    - To upper and middle trapezeii, rhomboids, and thoracic and lumbar paraspinals
- Mobilization/manipulation
  - Soft tissue
    - Thoracic and lumbar paraspinal muscles
    - Upper and middle trapezius
    - Rhomboids

PRESCRIPTION, APPLICATION, AND, AS APPROPRIATE, FABRICATION OF DEVICES AND EQUIPMENT

- Elastic lumbar support
  - The patient will be provided with and instructed in the use of an elastic lumbar support while practicing her gymnastic skills

ELECTROTHERAPEUTIC MODALITIES

♦ EMS and TENS to decrease pain and spasm

PHYSICAL AGENTS AND MECHANICAL MODALITIES

♦ Sound agent
  • Ultrasound to increase tissue perfusion, oxygenation, and nutrient delivery to the tissues
♦ Thermotherapy
  • Hot packs to increase muscle extensibility and decrease spasm in cervical, thoracic, and lumbar spine muscles

ANTICIPATED GOALS AND EXPECTED OUTCOMES

♦ Impact on pathology/pathophysiology
  • Muscle spasm is alleviated.
  • Nutrient delivery to tissue is increased.
  • Pain is decreased from a 6/10 to a 3/10 in the lumbar spine after activity from 3/10 to 0/10 at rest.
  • Soft tissue inflammation, edema, and restriction are reduced.
  • Tissue perfusion and oxygenation are increased.
♦ Impact on impairments
  • Energy expenditure per unit of work is decreased.
  • Muscle length of the lumbar extensors is elongated to WNL.
  • Muscle stength is increased to 5/5 in abdominals and thoracic spine extensors.
  • Optimal joint alignment is achieved.
  • Optimal loading on a body part is achieved.
  • Postural control, alignment, and awareness are improved, and she is able to maintain appropriate posture during functional activities.
  • Quality of movement between and across body segments is improved.
  • Relaxation is increased.
  • ROM is maintained.
♦ Impact on functional limitations
  • Ability to assume or resume required self-care, home management, school, community, and leisure roles is improved.
  • Ability to independently perform physical actions, tasks, and activities related to ADL/IADL in self-care, home management, school, community, and leisure with or without assistive devices and equipment is increased.
  • Level of supervision required for task performance is decreased.
  • Patient has resumed gym class at school.

  • Tolerance of positions and actions, tasks, and activities is increased.
♦ Risk reduction/prevention
  • Awareness of precautions and correct resting positions is achieved.
  • Pressure on body tissue is reduced.
  • Protection of body parts is increased.
  • Risk factors are reduced.
  • Risk of recurrence of condition is reduced.
  • Risk of secondary impairments is reduced.
  • Safety is improved.
  • Self-management of symptoms is improved.
♦ Impact on health, wellness, and fitness
  • Behaviors that foster healthy habits, wellness, and prevention are acquired.
  • Decision making is enhanced regarding health, wellness, and fitness needs.
  • Fitness, health status, physical capacity, and physical function are improved.
♦ Impact on societal resources
  • Available resources are maximally utilized.
  • Documentation occurs throughout patient management and across all settings and follows APTA's *Guidelines for Physical Therapy Documentation.*[58]
♦ Patient/client satisfaction
  • Access, availability, and services provided are acceptable to patient/client.
  • Case is managed throughout the episode of care.
  • Clinical proficiency and interpersonal skills of the physical therapist are acceptable to patient/client.
  • Coordination of care is acceptable to patient/client.
  • Patient and family knowledge and awareness of the diagnosis, prognosis, interventions, and understanding of anticipated goals and expected outcomes are increased.
  • Sense of well-being is improved.
  • Stressors are decreased.

REEXAMINATION

Reexamination is performed throughout the episode of care.

DISCHARGE

Rachel is discharged from physical therapy after a total of 10 physical therapy sessions and attainment of her goals and expectations. These sessions have covered her entire episode of service. She is discharged because she has achieved her goals and expected outcomes.

References

1. Williams PL, ed. *Gray's Anatomy*. 38th ed. New York, NY: Churchill Livingstone; 1995.

2. Bogduk N, Twomey LT. *Clinical Anatomy of the Lumbar Spine*. 2nd ed. Melbourne, Australia: Churchill Livingstone; 1991.

3. Grieve GP. *Common Vertebral Joint Problems*. 2nd ed. Edinburgh, England: Churchill Livingstone; 1988.

4. Nachemson A, Morris JM. In vivo measurement of intradiscal pressure. *J Bone Joint Surg*. 1964;46A:1077-1092.

5. Simons DG, Travell JG, Simons LS. *Myofascial Pain and Dysfunction*. 2nd ed. Philadelphia, Pa: Lippincott Williams & Wilkins; 1999.

6. Bogduk N. A reappraisal of the anatomy of the human erector spinae. *J Anatomy*. 1983;131:525-540.

7. Dory MA. Arthrography of the lumbar facet joints. *Radiology*. 1981;140:23-27.

8. Hides JA, Stokes MJ, Saide M, Jull GA, Cooper DH. Evidence of lumbar multifidus wasting ipsilateral to symptoms in patients with acute/subacute low back pain. *Spine*. 1994;19:165-172.

9. Vleeming A, Mooney V, Dorman T, Snijders C, Stoeckart R, eds. *Movement, Stability and Low Back Pain: The Essential Role of the Pelvis*. 1st ed. New York, NY: Churchill Livingstone; 1997.

10. Porterfield C, DeRosa JA. The spine. In: Malone TR, McPoil T, Nitz AJ, eds. *Orthopedic and Sports Physical Therapy*. 3rd ed. St. Louis, Mo: Mosby; 1997.

11. White AA, Panjabi MA. *Clinical Biomechanics of the Spine*. 2nd ed. Philadelphia, Pa: Lippincott; 1990.

12. McKenzie R, May S. *The Lumbar Spine: Mechanical Diagnosis and Therapy*. 2nd ed. Waikanae, New Zealand: New Zealand Publications Inc; 2003.

13. Kapandji IA. *The Physiology of the Joints, Vol 3, The Trunk and the Vertebral Column*. Edinburgh, Scotland: Churchill Livingstone; 1974.

14. Greenman P. *Principles of Manual Medicine*. 2nd ed. Baltimore, Md: Williams & Wilkins; 1996.

15. Lee D. *The Thorax: An Integrated Approach*. 2nd ed. British Columbia, Canada: Churchill Livingstone; 2003.

16. Kaltenborn F, Evjenth O, Laltenborn T, Vollowitz EL. *The Spine Basic Evaluation and Mobilization Techniques*. Minneapolis, Minn: OPTP; 1993.

17. Boisonnault WG. *Examination in Physical Therapy Practice Screening for Medical Disease*. 2nd ed. New York, NY: Churchill Livingstone; 1995.

18. Garrett WE, Nikolauo PK, Ribbeck BM, Glisson RR, Seaber AV. The effect of muscle architecture on the biomechanical failure properties of skeletal muscle under passive extension. *Am J Sports Med*. 1988;16:7-12.

19. Simons DG. Myofascial pain syndromes: where are we? Where are we going? *Arch Phys Med Rehabil*. 1988;69:207-212.

20. Mixter WG, Barr NJS. Rupture of intervertebral disc with involvement of the spinal cord. *N Engl J Med*. 1934;211:210-215.

21. Macnab I. *Backache*. 2nd ed. Baltimore, Md: Williams & Wilkins; 1977.

22. Irani Z, Patel JJ Spondylolisthesis (updated May 3, 2004) http://www.emedicine.com/radio/topic651.htm. Accessed April 30, 2005.

23. Wiltse LL, Newman Ph, Macnab I. Classification of spondylolysis and spondylolisthesis. *Clin Orthop*. 1976;117(June):23-29.

24. Wright IP. Who was Meyerding? *Spine*. 2003;28(7):733-735.

25. Corrigan B, Maitland GD. *Practical Orthopedic Medicine*. 1st ed. London, England: Butterworth and Co; 1983.

26. Scoliosis Research Society Web Site. Available at http//www.srs.org. Accessed June 2003.

27. Agency for Health Care Policy and Research. Acute low back pain. US Department of Health and Human Services. 1994;14:68.

28. Agency for Health Care Policy and Research. Acute low back pain. US Department of Health and Human Services. 1994;14:73.

29. Beattie PF, Meyers SP. MRI in low back pain: general principles and clinical issues. *Phys Ther*. 1998;7:56-71.

30. Boden SD. Abnormal magnetic resonance scans of the lumbar spine in asymptomatic subjects: a prospective investigation. *J Bone Joint Surg*. 1990;72:403-408.

31. Jarvik JG. Rapid MRI vs radiographs for patients with low back pain. *JAMA*. 2003;289(21):2810-2818.

32. USDA Center for Nutrition Policy and Promotion. Body mass index and health. *Nutrition Insight*. 2000;March.

33. Fairbanks JT, Couper J, Davies JB, O'Brien JP. Oswestry Disability Questionnaire. *Physiotherapy*. 1980;66:112-115.

34. Maitland GD, Hengeveld E, Banke K, English K. *Maitland's Vertebral Manipulation*. 6th ed. Oxford, England: Butterworth-Heinemann; 2001.

35. Downie W, Leatham PA, Rhind VM, et al. Studies with pain rating scales. *Ann Rheum Dis*. 1978;37:378-38.

36. Mayer TG, Gatchel RJ. *Functional Restoration for Spinal Disorders: A Sports Medicine Approach*. 1st ed. Philadelphia, Pa: Lea and Febiger; 1988.

37. Sackett DL, Rosenberg WC, Gray MJA, Haynes RB, Richardson WS. Evidence based medicine: what it is and what it isn't. *BMJ*. 1996;312:71-72.

38. Dworkin RH, Handlin DS, Richlin DM, Brand L, Vanusci C. Unravelling the effects of compensation, litigation and employment on treatment response to chronic pain. *Pain*. 1985;23:49-59.

39. Alston W, Carlson KE, Feldman DJ. A quantitative study of muscle factors in the chronic low back pain syndrome. *J Am Geriatr Soc*. 1966;14:1041-1047.

40. Berkson M, Schultz A, Nachemson A. Voluntary strength of male adults with acute low back pain syndrome. *Clin Orthop*. 1977;129:84-87.

41. Cady MD, Bischoff DP, O'Connel ER. Strength fitness and subsequent injuries in firefighters. *Journal of Occupational Medicine*. 1979;21:269-273.

42. Mellin G. Correlations of spinal mobility with the degree of chronic low back pain after correction for age and anthropometric factors. *Spine*. 1987;12:464-468.

43. Boden SD, Davis DO, Dina TS. Abnormal magnetic resonance scans of the lumbar spine in asymptomatic subjects. *J Bone Joint Surg*. 1990;72A:403-408.

44. Delitto A, Erhard RA, Bowling RW. A treatment based classification approach to low back pain syndrome; identifying and staging patients for conservative treatment. *Phys Ther*. 1995;75:470-489.

45. Videman T, Battie MC. Current research of spinal disorders. In: Mayer TG, Gatchel RJ, eds. *Functional Restoration for Spinal Disorders: A Sports Medicine Approach.* 1st ed. Philadelphia, Pa: Lea and Febiger; 1988.

46. Fritz JM, George S. The use of a classification approach to identify subgroups of patients with acute low back pain. *Spine.* 2000;25:106-114.

47. Ito T, Takano Y, Yuasa N. Types of herniated discs. *Spine.* 2001;26(6):648-651.

48. Fritz, JM, Delitto A, Erhard RE. Comparison of classification-based physical therapy with therapy based on clinical practice guidelines for patients with acute low back pain. *Spine.* 2003;28(13):1363-1372.

49. Waddell G, Somerville D, Henderson I, Newton M. Objective clinical evaluation of physical impairment in chronic low back pain. *Spine.* 1992;17:617-628.

50. Mayer TG. Rationale for modern spine care. In: Mayer TG, Mooney V, Gatchel RJ, eds. *Contemporary Conservative Care for Painful Spinal Disorders.* 1st ed. Philadelphia, Pa: Lea and Febiger; 1991.

51. Hazard RG. Functional restoration of the patient with chronic back pain. In: Frymoyer JW, ed. *The Adult Spine: Principles and Practice.* 2nd ed. New York, NY: Raven Press Ltd; 1991.

52. Williams PC. Lumbar spine: reduced lumbosacral joint space; its relation to sciatic nerve root irritation. *JAMA.* 1932;99:1677-1682.

53. Cyriax J. *Textbook of Orthopaedic Medicine, Vol 1: Diagnosis of Soft Tissue Lesions.* 7th ed. London, England: Balliere Tindall; 1978.

54. Sahrmann S. Course notes, muscle imbalances, 1993.

55. Robison R. The new back school prescription: stabilization training part 1. In: White LA, ed. *Back School. Spine State of the Art Review.* Philadelphia, Pa: Hanley & Belfus; 1991.

56. Richardson C, Hodges P, Hides J. *Therapeutic Exercise for Lumbopelvic Stabilization.* 2nd ed. Edinburgh, Scotland: Churchill Livingstone; 2004.

57. Richardson CA, Jull GA. Muscle control-pain control. What exercises would you prescribe? *Man Ther.* 1995;1:2-10.

58. American Physical Therapy Association. Guide to physical therapist practice. 2nd ed. *Phys Ther.* 2001;81:9-744.

59. Evans R, Bronfort G, Nelson B, Goldsmith C. Two-year follow-up of a randomized clinical trial of spinal manipulation, two types of exercise for patients with chronic neck pain. *Spine.* 2002;27(21):2383-2389.

60. Cantu RI, Grodin AJ. *Myofascial Manipulation, Theory and Clinical Application.* 2nd ed. Gaithersburg, Md: Aspen Publishers; 2001.

61. Wyke B. Articular neurology: a review. *Physiotherapy.* 1972;58:94-99.

62. Andersson GB, Lucente T, Davis AM, et al. A comparison of osteopathic spinal manipulation with standard care for patients with low back pain. *N Engl J Med.* 1999;341(19):1426-1431.

63. Koes BW, Bouter LM, van Mameren H, et al. Randomised clinical trial of manipulative therapy and physiotherapy for persistent back and neck complaints: results of a one year follow up. *BMJ.* 1992;304(6827):601-605.

64. Koes BW, Assendelft WJJ, van der Heijden GJMG, Bouter LM. Spinal manipulation for low back pain: an undated systematic review of randomized clinical trials. *Spine.*

1996;21(24):2860-2873.

65. Belánger AY. *Evidence-Based Guide to Therapeutic Physical Agents.* Philadelphia, Pa: Lippincott Williams & Wilkins; 2002.

66. Waddell G. A new clinical model for the treatment of low back pain. *Spine.* 1987;12:632-644.

67. Jones SL, Jones PK, Katz J. Compliance for low back pain patients in the emergency department: a randomized trial. *Spine.* 1988;13(5):553-556.

68. Little P, Roberts L, Blowers H, et al. Should we give detailed advice and information booklets to patients with back pain? A randomized controlled factorial trial of a self management booklet and doctor advice to take exercise for back pain. *Spine.* 2001;26:2065-2072.

69. Indahl A, Velund L, Reikeraas O, Ursin H. Five year follow-up of a controlled clinical trial using light mobilisation and an informative approach to low back pain. *Spine.* 1998;23:2625-2630.

70. Nachemson A, Morris JM. In vivo measurement of intradiscal pressure. *J Bone Joint Surg.* 1964;71(46A):1077-1092.

71. Sato K, Sinichi K, Yonezaha T. In vivo tradiscal pressure measurements in healthy individuals and in patients with ongoing low back problems. *Spine.* 1999;24:2468-2474.

72. Rocabado M. Course notes, temporomandibular joint assessment and treatment, 1982.

73. Morgan D. Concepts in functional training and postural stabilization for the low-back injured. *Topics Acute Care Trauma Rehab.* 1988;April:8-17.

74. Klenerman L, Slade PD, Stanley M, et al. The prediction of chronoicity in patients with an acute attack of low back pain in a general practice setting. *Spine.* 1995;20:478-484.

75. Brotzman SB, Wilk KE *Clinical Orthopaedic Rehabilitation.* 2nd ed. Philadelphia, Pa: Mosby; 2003.

76. American Thoracic Society. ATS statement: guidelines for the Six-Minute Walk test. *Am J Respir Crit Care Med.* 2002;166:111-117.

77. Mathiowetz B, Kashman N, Volland G, et al. Grip and pinch strength, normative data for adults. *Arch Phys Med Rehabil.* 1995;66:71-72.

78. Jensen MP, Karoly P, Braver S. The measurement of clinical pain intensity: a comparison of six methods. *Pain.* 1986;27(1):117-126.

79. Garrett TR, Youdas JW, Madson TJ. Reliability of measuring forward head posture in a clinical setting. *J Orthop Sports Phys Ther.* 1993;17(3):155-160.

80. Hickey ER, Rondeau MJ, Corrente JR, Abysalh J, Seymour CJ. Reliability of the cervical range of motion (CROM) device and plumb-line techniques in measuring resting head posture (RHP). *Journal of Manual and Manipulative Therapy.* 2000;8(1):10-17.

81. Tousignant M, de Bellefeuille L, O'Donoughue S, Grahovac S. Criterion validity of the cervical range of motion (CROM) goniometer for cervical flexion and extension. *Spine.* 2000;25(3):324-330.

82. Lee D. *The Pelvic Girdle.* 2nd ed. Edinburgh, Scotland: Churchill Livingstone; 1998.

83. Butler DS. *Mobilization of the Nervous System.* 1st ed. Melbourne, Australia: Churchill Livingstone; 1991.

84. Deyo RA, Tsui-Wu Y. Descriptive epidemiology of low back pain and its related medical care in the United States. *Spine.*

1987;12:264-268.

85. Fritz JM, Erhard RE, Hagen BF. Segmental instability of the lumbar spine. *Phys Ther.* 1998;78:889-896.

86. Stankovic R, Johnell O. Conservative treatment of acute low back pain: a five year follow-up study of two methods of treatment. *Spine.* 1995;20:469-472.

87. Manniche C, Helsoloe G, Bentzen K, Christensen I, Lunberg E. Clinical trial of intensive muscle training for chronic low back pain. *Lancet.* 1988;2:1473-1476.

88. Bang MD, Deyle GD. Comparison of supervised exercise with and without manual physical therapy for patients with shoulder impingement. *J Orthop Sports Phys Ther.* 2000;30:126-137.

89. Colachis SC, Strohm BR Effects of intermittent traction on separation of lumbar vertebra. *Arch Phys Med Rehabil.* 1969;May:251-258.

90. Krause M, Refshauge KM, Dessen, M, Boland R. Lumbar spine traction evaluation of effects and recommended application for treatment. *Man Ther.* 2000;5(2):72-81.

91. Van der Heijden G, Beurskens A, Koes BW Assendelft W, de Vet H, Bouter LM. The efficacy of traction for back and neck pain: a systematic, blinded review of randomized clinical trial methods. *Phys Ther.* 1995;75:93-104.

92. Cailliet R. *Low Back Pain Syndrome.* 5th ed. Philadelphia, Pa: FA Davis Co; 1995.

93. Fritz, JM, Delitto A, Welch WC, Erhard RE. Lumbar spinal stenosis: a review of current concepts in evaluation, management, and outcome measurements. *Arch Phys Med Rehabil.* 1998;79(June):700-708.

94. Morgan D. Concepts in functional training and postural stabilization for the low back injured. *Topics Acute Care Trauma Rehab.* 1988;April:8-17.

95. Axen K, Haas F, Schicchi J, Merrick J. Progressive resistance neck exercises using a compressible ball coupled with an air pressure gauge. *J Orthop Sports Phys Ther.* 1992;16(6):275-279.

Impaired Joint Mobility, Muscle Performance, and Range of Motion Associated With Fracture (Pattern G)

Joshua A. Cleland, PT, DPT, PhD, OCS

Matthew B. Garber, PT, DSc, OCS, FAAOMPT

ANATOMY

The skeletal system is a multifaceted organ that is comprised of 206 interconnected bones of varying sizes and shapes that serve as the structure that determines the physical attributes of the body. The complexity of the skeletal system is exemplified by its ability to perform several functions essential to the production of movement and the maintenance of homeostasis.

The skeletal system as a whole provides protection for many of the body's vital organs including the spinal cord, brain, heart, and reproductive systems. Individual bones serve as attachment sites for muscles, ligaments, tendons, and a variety of other connective tissues and act as lever systems that assist with providing joint stability and facilitating movement. The skeletal system also serves as a reservoir for critical ions (calcium, phosphorus, sodium, potassium, zinc, magnesium) that can be distributed throughout the body as necessary.[1] The yellow marrow of bone provides a storage site for lipids, an important source of chemical energy. The red marrow carries out the function of hematopoiesis, the production of red blood cells.[2] The anatomy and physiology of bone are also detailed in Pattern A: Primary Prevention/Risk Reduction for Skeletal Demineralization.

BIOCHEMICAL COMPOSITION

Similar to other connective tissues, bone consists of an extracellular matrix (30% to 35%), inorganic components (65%), and water (found within the ground substance and surrounding the collagen fibers). The distinguishing feature between bone (osseous tissue) and other connective tissues is the ground substance, which is mineralized in bone. In other connective tissues, the ground substance is composed of a higher percentage of water and glycoaminoglycans. The tough organic components of osseous tissue, specifically the collagen fibers, provide strength in tension, whereas the calcified inorganic matrix provides strength in compression.[3]

The extracellular organic matrix of bone consists of 90% to 95% collagen fibers with the remaining percent composed of ground substance. Type I collagen predominates and provides a great deal of multidirectional strength.[4] The ground substance surrounding the collagen fibers consists primarily of extracellular fluid and PGs, including chondroitin sulfate and hyaluronic acid.

The inorganic components deposited in bone primarily consist of calcium and phosphorous. The major crystalline salt being hydroxyapatite $[CA_{10}(PO_4)_6(OH)_2]$. Hydroxyapatite is the mineral that provides strength and hardness. It provides the storage for 99% of the body's calcium, 80% of the body's phosphorus, and 65% of the body's sodium and magnesium.[5] The hydroxyapatite is intermingled within the Type I collagen and the ground substance of the extracellular matrix. The extracellular matrix combined with the inorganic salts becomes mineralized giving bone significant rigidity and strength.

MICROSCOPIC STRUCTURE

A variety of bone forming and bone resorption cells located within osseous tissue contribute to the functional unit. The bone forming cells located in cavities within the matrix known as lacunae include osteoprogenitors, osteoblasts, and osteocytes. These each have a distinct role in the formation and synthesis of the organic matrix components, as well as bone maintenance. Also located in the lacunae are osteoclasts that are primarily responsible for bone resorption and the remodeling of osseous tissue.

The bone forming cells each have separate and distinct functions. Osteoprogenitor cells are located near the bones' surface and have the ability to produce osteoblasts. They are essential to the growth and repair of bone. Osteoblasts are responsible for the synthesis, transport, and arrangement of the organic matrix. The osteoblasts also initiate the mineralization process. Depending on the osteoblasts production of collagen and PGs, bone can be classified as either immature (woven) if deposited in random weave fashion or mature (lamellar) if deposited in a layered fashion.[5]

As osteoblasts become surrounded by newly formed matrix and encased in bone, they are known as osteocytes. The primary responsibility of the osteocytes, although not as metabolically active as the osteoblasts, is maintenance of the bony matrix. The osteocytes communicate with other cells though an intricate network of tiny tunnels known as canaliculi. The canaliculi allow for the transportation of nutrients to the osteoclasts from regional blood supply. Arteries enter the bones through the periosteum and travel obliquely through Volkmann's canals (perforating canals) to reach the Haversian canal (the central canal that runs longitudinally through bone).

The primary function of the osteoclast that is located on the bony surface is bone resorption. Osteoclasts release a multitude of enzymes that not only facilitate the disassembly of matrix proteins but also activate growth factors. Thereby they assist with the break down of bone into its elemental units while releasing substances that facilitate its renewal.[5]

MACROSCOPIC STRUCTURE

Bone, a specialized type of connective tissue, is frequently thought of as a single unit, or collectively (skeleton) as a metabolically active physiological organ.[3] Bone is not completely solid. Between the calcified matrices exist channels that allow for the passage of blood vessels and nerves, lacunae that house osteocytes, and air space. Depending upon its extent and distribution, bone tissue is structurally defined as being either compact or cancellous. It has been determined that compact bone is only 5% to 30% nonmineralized or porous, whereas cancellous bone is 30% to 90% porous.[6] All bones will have a component of both cancellous and compact tissue. The ratio of these will vary depending on the shape and type of bone.

In cancellous bone, patterns of irregular latticework of thin plates called trabeculae are recognized. The spaces between the trabeculae are filled with blood vessels, nerve fibers, adipose tissue, and hemopoietic tissue (red marrow that is responsible for producing red blood cells).[3] This classification of osseous tissue primarily exists in short flat irregular shaped bones and in the epiphysis of long bones. A layer of compact (cortical) bone with a concentric lamella structure and a greater percentage of mineralized tissue typically surrounds cancellous bone. The concentric lamella structure surrounds the Haversian canals that pass longitudinally through the bone and allow for the passage of nerves and lymph/blood vessels. Each central canal, along with its associated concentric lamella, lacunae, osteocytes, and caniculi, is referred to as an osteon.[2] The osteon, considered to be the structural unit of bone, is only found within matured compact bone.

A dense, white, tough fibrous membrane with two layers called the periosteum covers the cortical bone. The outer fibrous layer consists of connective tissue that contains blood vessels, lymphatic vessels, and nerves that supply the respective bone. The inner osteogenic layer contains elastic fibers and osteoprogenitor cells.[2] The periosteum is bound to the bone by periosteal collagen called Sharpey's fibers.[7] Deep to the periosteum is a layer of connective tissue and osteoprogenitor cells called the endosteum. Both the periosteum and endosteum function to provide nutrients to osseous tissue and provide a constant supply of osteoblasts for repair and growth.

PHYSIOLOGY

BONE MAINTENANCE AND REMODELING

Although bone growth is completed when skeletal maturity is reached, remodeling of bone continues throughout life. Skeletal maintenance is achieved by simultaneous breakdown and renewal of new bone during the remodeling process. Osteoclasts remove bone while osteoblasts produce new bone. During early adulthood, the rates of bone resorption and bone formation are in equilibrium. The normal remodeling process is dependent upon a number of factors including quantities of calcium and phosphorus, sufficient amounts of vitamins (A, B_{12}, C, and D) and the proper amount of growth hormones.[2] However, after the third decade of life, the amount of bone resorbed begins to exceed the amount of bone being formed. This results in a steady decrement of skeletal mass.[5]

Bone remodeling also occurs as a result of physical

demands. Bone is deposited along lines of stress and resorbed where there is little or no stress.[3] This principle, known as Wolff's law, refers to the ability of osseous tissues to adapt to the mechanical demands placed upon it. This is exemplified by cortical thickenings on the concave side of a curved bone as well as the alignment of the trabeculae system within the neck of the femur.[3]

PATHOPHYSIOLOGY

The fact that osseous tissue has the capability to respond to the stresses applied upon it (Wolff's law) was discussed above. However, if the mechanical forces (shear, bending, torsion, compression) applied to bone exceed the bone's ability to contain the force, a fracture will result. Fracture is defined as "a break in the surface of the bone, either across its cortex or through its articular surface."[8] It has been documented that the yearly incidence of fractures in the United States exceeds 6.2 million.[9] Given these statistics it is expected that physical therapists will frequently encounter patients either after bone healing has occurred or prior to diagnosis of a fracture when the patient enters the health care system through the physical therapist.

The magnitude and type of fracture is widely dependant on the extent of the force applied to the tissue and the direction in which the force was applied. However, there are predictable patterns in which fractures occur.[10] Numerous classifications of fractures have been defined in Table 7-1.[2,3,10]

The degree of mineralization of bone can significantly influence the type of fracture that occurs with trauma. For example, in the adult population, a bone that is subjected to excessive bending forces may fracture completely. Yet in a child, the forming bone, that at the time is still a large percent cartilage, may simply bend without fracturing. This phenomenon is known as plastic deformation of bone.[3]

Children are also susceptible to fractures of the cartilaginous epiphyseal plate. These injuries present unique complications and may cause disturbance of bone growth, possibly resulting in bony deformity. Fortunately however, 85% of epiphyseal fractures do not result in bony deformity.[11] The Salter-Harris classification is used to describe epiphyseal plate fractures. This schema classifies the fractures according to their relationship to the epiphyseal plate.[11]

FRACTURE MANAGEMENT

According to Salter,[3] the four basic goals of fracture management are to: 1) relieve pain; 2) obtain and maintain satisfactory fracture position; 3) allow and encourage bony union; and 4) restore optimum function. Other factors, such as the patient's age, the nature of the fracture (intra- vs extra-articular), the displacement and stability of the fracture, the degree of comminution, and the extent of soft-tissue injury, may significantly influence management strategies.[12] A number of conservative treatment techniques, such as protection, immobilization, and closed reduction, can be successfully utilized with uncomplicated fractures.

If the fracture site is stable, it is possible that protection alone will be an adequate management strategy. This may take the form of non-weightbearing in the LE or sling support in the UE. If the fracture is not aligned, it may be managed with closed reduction. Closed reduction refers to manipulation of the fracture site in an attempt to achieve reduction. Once reduction is achieved, the site is frequently immobilized through the application of a cast, splint, or brace. Traction may occasionally be utilized for the purpose of maintaining fracture continuity.

REPAIR AND HEALING RESPONSE

Unlike other soft tissues that heal by poorly organized scar tissue, bone is regenerated rather than repaired, and the properties of the preexisting bone are largely restored.[6,13] Fracture healing is a complicated cascade of events that

Table 7-1	
CLASSIFICATION OF FRACTURES[2,3,10]	
Type of Fracture	*Definition*
Avulsion	A fracture in which fragments of bone are pulled away by force exerted through a tendon or ligament
Closed	A fracture in which the bone does not penetrate the skin
Comminuted	A fracture consisting of multiple fragments
Compression	A fracture in which one fracture surface is impacted into the opposing fracture surface
Greenstick	A partial fracture in which one side of the bone breaks while the other bends
Oblique	A fracture that extends across the bone at an oblique angle
Open	A fracture in which the fractured end of the bone protrudes through the skin
Spiral	A fracture that usually results from twisting of the bone
Stress	A fatigue fracture as a result of repetitive stresses applied to a bone
Transverse	A fracture line that extends in the transverse plane, perpendicular to the long axis of the bone

involves two different stages: primary and secondary healing. Primary healing occurs when the fracture segments are intimately related and involves an attempt from osteoblasts to bridge the fracture gap. This form of healing requires complete and rigid immobilization that is most often only accomplished by surgical fixation and will be further detailed in Pattern I: Impaired Joint Mobility, Motor Function, Muscle Performance, and Range of Motion Associated With Bony or Soft Tissue Surgery.

Secondary healing is more common and involves both intramembranous and endochondral ossification. Five distinct phases are involved in the healing of osseous tissues: 1) the initial stage in which a hematoma is formed, 2) a subsequent stage in which angiogenesis develops and cartilage begins to form, 3) cartilage calcification, 4) cartilage removal and bone formation, and 5) bone remodeling.[13]

At the time of the initial injury, periosteal and medullary blood vessels are ruptured producing a localized hemorrhage within 6 to 8 hours after the injury. This hematoma forms a fibrin mesh that assists with sealing off the fracture site and is a precursor to the influx of inflammatory cells and ingrowth of fibroblasts and capillary buds. Soon macrophages, phagocytes, and osteoclasts invade the area and begin clearing out the cellular debris. As necrotic tissue is removed from the fracture site, radiographically the fracture line becomes more visible.[12]

Intramembranous ossification begins to occur within 7 days and osteoblasts located adjacent to the fracture site begin synthesizing new bony matrix. Within 7 to 10 days, along with the ingrowth of blood vessels, the fracture site is invaded by chondroblasts that begin to form a soft callus. The soft tissue callus provides continuity between the two ends of the fracture but offers no structural stability.[5] The periosteum and endosteum around the fracture site begin to produce large amounts of osteoprogenitor cells that in turn begin rapidly producing osteoblasts. The osteoblasts begin synthesizing trabeculae of woven (immature) bone that approach the fracture site. The cartilage that occupied the fracture site begins to undergo endochondral ossification forming a hard callus. As the hard callus mineralizes, the strength of the bone increases to the point where controlled weightbearing can be tolerated.[5] Complete mineralization of the callus can take up to 4 to 16 weeks depending on the type of bone (long, short, trabecular, etc), type of fracture, and location of the fracture.[14]

The remodeling phase that begins about 6 weeks after the inciting event may take years to complete.[8] This process involves simultaneous removal and replacement of bone. It is the function of the osteoclasts to break down the immature bone while osteoblasts lay down lamellar bone forming a new osteon.[15] The soft callus that had previously occupied the marrow cavity is removed.[14] Radiographically, a fracture is considered healed when there is progressive callus formation and the fracture line is no longer visible.[12]

The time of union, the point at which the structural repair of the fractured bone has regenerated enough strength and stiffness to function without external support, will vary depending on the bone involved.[16] Table 7-2 shows the fracture healing time for respective bones as adapted from Compere and associates.[17] If bony union does not occur within the expected time frame, it will be considered "delayed union." Delayed union may be attributed to a number of factors including the nature of injury, post-injury tissue response, the pre-injury limb status, and the overall systemic status of the patient.[18] In these circumstances evidence suggests that low-intensity pulsed ultrasound is beneficial in enhancing fracture healing.[19] In the case where bone osteogenesis is outweighed by bone resorption, the fracture is classified as nonunion.[16] Nonunion fractures will require bony fixation and this is discussed in Pattern I: Impaired Joint Mobility, Motor Function, Muscle Performance, and Range of Motion Associated With Bony or Soft Tissue Surgery.

IMAGING

All of the methods used to determine the presence of a fracture and to assess the continuity of bone or stage of osseous healing include:

- Radiographs, which are the most common method and first attempt to assess disorders of the skeletal system. The radiograph should include the entire length of the bone and at least two projections, taken at right angles to each other, to diagnose a fracture.[3,10]
- CT, which may be beneficial in detecting subtle fractures or to assist with detecting metabolic bone disorders, assessing BMD, and detecting fractures that may be difficult to visualize with radiographs, such as those involving the spine and pelvis.[3]
- A radionucleide bone scan, which may be of use in recognizing disorders that cannot be captured through the use of conventional radiographs. These images appear to be most beneficial in recognizing stress fractures.[10]

PHARMACOLOGY

The following pharmacological agents may be utilized in the management of patients who have sustained a fracture. Depending on the severity of the fracture, patients may be placed on medications to control pain. These can range from NSAIDs, in mild cases, to opioid analgesics in the case of severe pain. If the fracture is compound or is at risk for infection, the patient may be given pharmacological agents, such as antibiotics, to combat or prevent infection.

If delayed or nonunion of the fracture occurs, other pharmacological agents may be prescribed and will be described in detail in Pattern I: Impaired Joint Mobility, Motor Function, Muscle Performance, and Range of Motion

	Table 7-2	
HEALING TIMES FOR COMMON SPINE AND EXTREMITY FRACTURE SITES[17]		
Fracture Site	*Adult Healing Times (in weeks)*	*Children's Healing Times (in weeks)*
Femur		
Intracapsular	24	16
Intertrochanteric	10 to 12	6
Shaft	18	8 to 10
Supracondylar	12 to 15	6 to 8
Tibia		
Proximal	8 to 10	6
Shaft	14 to 20	8 to 10
Malleolus	6	6
Calcaneus	12 to 16	10
Metatarsal	6	6
Phalanx	3 to 5	3
Humerus		
Supracondylar	8	6
Midshaft	8 to 12	6
Proximal (impacted)	3 (early motion)	3
Proximal (displaced)	6 to 8	6
Radius and Ulna	10 to 12	6 to 8
Scaphoid	10 or more until x-ray reveals union	Rare
Carpal	6	Rare
Metacarpal	6	6
Clavicle	6 to 10	4
Pelvis	6	4
Vertebra	16	16

Associated With Bony or Soft Tissue Surgery. If the fracture was a result of insufficient bone strength, the patient may be placed on a variety of other medications in an attempt to maximize bone density and strength. For a detailed description of these, the reader is referred to Pattern A: Primary Prevention/Risk Reduction for Skeletal Demineralization. In addition, the reader is referred to *Pharmacology in Rehabilitation*[20] for further information regarding the use of pharmacological management of this patient population.

Case Study #1: Humeral Head Fracture

Mr. John Skelly is a 48-year-old male who fell off a ladder 12 weeks ago landing on his right elbow, resulting in an impacted humeral head fracture (Figure 7-1).

PHYSICAL THERAPIST EXAMINATION

HISTORY

♦ General demographics: Mr. Skelly is a 48-year-old white male. He did not complete high school but received his General Education Diploma in 1982.

♦ Social history: Mr. Skelly is married with two children, a 12-year-old boy and a 15-year-old girl. He is the sole income provider for the family and needs to return to work at full capacity.

♦ Employment/work: He has been employed as a house painter for 30 years.

♦ General health status
   • General health perception: Mr. Skelly's perception is that his general health is fair for his age.
   • Physical function: He reports that he stopped exercising regularly when his second child was born.
   • Psychological function: Normal.
   • Role function: House painter, husband, father.

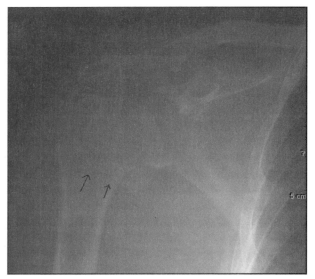

Figure 7-1. Radiograph of Mr. Skelly's right impacted humeral head fracture immediately following the injury.

- Social function: He enjoys canoeing with his children and playing an occasional game of basketball with his friends.
- Social/health habits: Mr. Skelly is a non-smoker and social drinker.
- Family history: His father died of lung cancer at 58.
- Medical/surgical history: He denies any episodes requiring hospitalization or surgery.
- Current condition(s)/chief complaint(s): Following the humeral head fracture, Mr. Skelly's physician elected to immobilize the fracture site with the use of a sling. Mr. Skelly remained in the sling and out of work for 8 weeks to allow the fracture site to heal. He was instructed to begin weaning out of the sling after 3 weeks but was to refrain from shoulder abduction and elevation, as this could result in angular deformity of the humerus.[21] The patient was instructed to attend physical therapy by his primary care physician. However, the patient neglected the doctor's orders and simply returned to work. After attempting to work for 3 weeks and being unable to perform all work-related activities secondary to pain and restricted motion, he scheduled a physical therapy visit.
- Functional status and activity level: He was unable to perform his job duties secondary to an increase in symptoms when lifting his arm above shoulder level. He reported no deficits with ADL or performing tasks around the house.
- Medications: At the time of the evaluation he was not taking any medications.
- Imaging/diagnostic tests: Radiographs taken at 8 weeks post-injury revealed that the fracture was well healed (Figure 7-2).

SYSTEMS REVIEW

- Cardiovascular/pulmonary
  - BP: 128/87 mmHg
  - Edema: None noted
  - HR: 76 bpm
  - RR: 18 bpm
- Integumentary
  - Presence of scar formation: None
  - Skin color: WNL
  - Skin integrity: WNL
- Musculoskeletal
  - Gross range of motion: Limitations right shoulder
  - Gross strength: WNL except for the right upper quadrant
  - Gross symmetry: Visible atrophy right deltoids
  - Height: 6'2" (1.88 m)
  - Weight: 190 lbs (86.18 kg)
- Neuromuscular
  - Gross coordinated movements (balance, locomotion, transfers, and transitions): WNL
- Communication, affect, cognition, language, and learning style
  - Communication, affect, cognition: WNL
  - Learning preferences: Demonstration and practice

TESTS AND MEASURES

- Aerobic capacity/endurance: WNL
- Anthropometric characteristics
  - BMI=24.3, which is normal (weight [in kg] divided by height^2 [in meters])
  - No visible edema noted
- Assistive and adaptive devices: None
- Cranial and peripheral nerve integrity
  - Although the patient did not complain of any neurological symptoms, it is reported that fractures of the diaphysis of the humerus may also be associated with radial nerve lesions,[12] therefore reflex and sensory integrity and upper limb neural provocation were tested and all found to be WNL
- Ergonomics and body mechanics
  - Demonstrates abnormal right SH rhythm (scapula elevation and decreased upward rotation of the glenoid fossa) when simulating an overhead painting task
- Gait, locomotion, and balance
  - The patient exhibited decreased arm swing on the right during gait
- Joint integrity and mobility
  - Joint integrity and mobility assessment entails not only the osteokinematic and arthrokinematic analy-

sis, but also assessing the structural integrity of the joint. This includes performing special tests, such as compression, distraction tests, impingement tests, joint play, and assessing ligament integrity

- Passive joint mobility
  - Demonstrated moderately hypomobile inferior and posterior gliding of the right GH joint
  - Revealed decreased glide of distal clavicle at the right AC joint
- PPIVM and PAIVM of the cervical and thoracic spine revealed:
  - Moderate hypomobility of C5, C7, and T1-T3[22]
- The stage of fracture healing will dictate which special tests are utilized. The patient demonstrated a positive Hawkins and Kennedy test.[23] The sensitivity and specificity of detecting shoulder impingement utilizing the Hawkins and Kennedy test have been well documented in the literature (sensitivity 0.62 to 0.92 and specificity 0.25 to 0.76)[24-26]

♦ Motor function
- Dexterity, coordination, and agility: Altered SH rhythm noted with active GH abduction and flexion above 60 degrees on the right

♦ Muscle performance
- The intrarater reliability of muscle testing has been shown to be between moderate and good for measurements obtained with MMT (ICC=0.63 to 0.98)[27]
- MMT revealed the following strength deficits on the right:
  - Deltoids=4/5
  - Supraspinatus=4-/5
  - Infraspinatus and teres minor=4-/5
  - Subscapularis=4/5
  - Bicep brachii=4+/5
  - Triceps=4/5
  - Serratus anterior=4-/5
  - Middle and lower trapezius=4-/5
  - Rhomboids=4/5

♦ Pain
- 1-2/10 on the NPS at rest, escalating to a 5/10 with overhead work. A strong correlation exists between the VAS and NPS[28]
- His major complaint was lifting his right arm over his head secondary to restricted motion and pain

♦ Posture
- Static postural observation using a plumb line revealed:
  - Forward head
  - Forward right shoulder
  - Right elevated shoulder
  - Mild increased upper to mid-thoracic spine

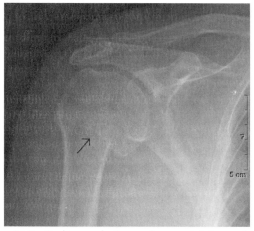

Figure 7-2. Radiograph 8 weeks post-injury showing healing through surgical neck of the humerus.

kyphosis
- Visual observation also revealed considerable atrophy of the deltoids and rotator cuff musculature on right

♦ Range of motion
- Visual estimation of AROM
  - Cervical spine revealed a 25% decrease in cervical sidebending left and cervical rotation right
- Joint AROM of the right GH joint
  - Goniometric measurements have demonstrated poor to good intratester (ICC=0.74 to 0.99) and intertester reliability (ICC=0.32 to 0.97) depending on the joints measured[29]
    - Flexion=0 to 120 degrees
    - Abduction=0 to 98 degrees
    - ER=0 to 47 degrees
    - IR=0 to 57 degrees
- PROM
  - The intrarater agreement of end feel testing of the elbow is between 75% and 80%[30]
  - Motion restriction with capsular end feels in all planes
  - Decreased flexibility of right pectoralis major

♦ Self-care and home management
- Patient reports the ability to safely perform all self-care and home management actions, tasks, and activities, despite mild discomfort with any activities requiring lifting (lifting trash bag out of the trash can)

♦ Work, community, and leisure integration or reintegration
- Interview concerning the ability to safely manage work actions, tasks, and activities revealed limitations that included the inability to paint at shoulder

level or higher without a significant increase in his symptoms

- Patient reports the ability to perform all leisure activities despite mild discomfort with any activities requiring lifting

EVALUATION

Mr. Skelly's history previously outlined indicated that he is a 48-year-old male non-smoker who was injured during a fall at work. The fall resulted in an impacted right humeral head fracture requiring immobilization in a sling for 8 weeks. As a result of the immobilization he has developed decreased joint mobility, muscle performance, and ROM associated with fracture. In addition, his posture is altered, and he is unable to perform his job duties. He also has difficulty performing any task requiring lifting or shoulder movements greater than 90 degrees of flexion or abduction.

DIAGNOSIS

Mr. Skelly is a patient who sustained an impacted fracture of the right humeral head. He has impaired: ergonomics and body mechanics; gait, locomotion, and balance; joint integrity and mobility; motor function; muscle performance; posture; and range of motion. He is functionally limited in self-care and home management and in work, community, and leisure actions, tasks, and activities. These findings are consistent with placement in Pattern G: Impaired Joint Mobility, Muscle Performance, and Range of Motion Associated With Fracture. The identified impairments and functional limitations will be addressed in determining the prognosis and the plan of care.

PROGNOSIS AND PLAN OF CARE

Over the course of the visits, the following mutually established outcomes have been determined:

- Ability to perform home management and work actions, tasks, and activities is improved
- Ability to perform physical actions, tasks, and activities is improved
- Gait is improved
- Joint integrity and mobility are improved
- Motor function and muscle performance are improved
- Pain is decreased
- Physical function is improved
- Postural control is improved
- ROM is improved
- Self-management of symptoms is improved

To achieve these outcomes, the appropriate interventions for this patient are determined. These will include: coordi-nation, communication, and documentation; patient/client-related instruction; therapeutic exercise; functional training in self-care and home management; functional training in work, community, and leisure integration or reintegration; and manual therapy techniques.

Based on the diagnosis and prognosis, Mr. Skelly is expected to require between 10 to 12 visits over an 8-week period of time. Mr. Skelly has good social support, is moti-vated, and follows through with his home exercise program. He is not severely impaired and is generally healthy.

INTERVENTIONS

RATIONALE FOR SELECTED INTERVENTIONS

Therapeutic Exercise

Patients with a fracture may exhibit impairments as a primary result of the fracture or as a secondary result of soft tissue injury that may have occurred at the time of the event. It is also likely that these patients will have impairments that result directly from the immobilization period necessary to assure optimal fracture healing. The effects of immobiliza-tion on connective tissue, bone, muscle, and nervous tissue have been well documented.[6,31-34] Immobilization of bone may cause changes in the rate of bone turnover and result in the initiation of osteoporosis.[6,33] Marchetti and associates[32] have demonstrated that significant BMD decreases occur in the humeral head and neck (between 6% to 14%) fol-lowing 6 weeks of immobilization (as a result of soft tissue surgery). Frequently, in combination with immobilization following a fracture of the LE, a decrease in weightbearing is also required during the initial stages of bone healing. The absence of weightbearing will reduce the remodeling of bone associated with Wolff's law. Therapeutic exercise has been demonstrated to assist with bone remodeling and articular cartilage repair following remobilization and return to weightbearing status.[35-37]

The effects of immobilization on muscle tissues depend on a number of factors, including the position of immobi-lization and the length of time in the immobilized position. Immobilization, regardless of the position, results in muscle atrophy. However, it is purported that immobilization in the shortened position is the most detrimental.[33] This not only results in a reduction in the number of sarcomeres, but also starts a cascade of events that leads to a change in muscle fibers of SO to FG muscle fiber properties. It has been demonstrated in the human model that muscle fiber size decreases up to 17% during the first 72 hours of immobilization.[6,38] Studies[31,34] have demonstrated that 4 to 6 weeks of LE immobilization results in significant reduc-tions in quadriceps cross-sectional area (14% to 21%) with a concomitant decrease in force production (25% to 53%) in healthy subjects.[31,34]

Shaffer and associates[39] investigated the effects of 8 weeks of immobilization in 10 patients following an ankle fracture. Immediately following immobilization, the group exhibited a significant reduction in peak plantarflexor torque as compared to a group of age- and sex-matched controls. This also correlated with functional impairments as recorded by timed walks of 20, 50, and 100 feet. However, after following a physical therapy program three times per week for 10 weeks including moist heat, posterior talar mobilizations, passive gastrocnemius and soleus stretching, resistance training, and ambulation training, postoperative peak torque and functional performance returned to control levels.[39]

Manual Therapy Techniques

Bang and Deyle[40] and others[41,42] have demonstrated improvements in ROM, pain, and function associated with incorporation of manual physical therapy interventions into the management of patient populations with painful, stiff shoulders. Manual techniques include the use of skilled hands to enhance tissue extensibility, joint mobility, modulate pain, decrease spasm, and reduce soft tissue swelling.

Maitland[43] reported that fracture of the proximal humerus may damage the GH ligaments and capsule and progressively lead to a stiff joint. In addition, during periods of immobilization, the normal weave pattern of collagen becomes disorganized.[33] Connective tissue, similar to bone, will respond to the mechanical forces placed upon it. Therefore, it is essential to stress connective tissue structures (capsule, ligaments) through controlled movement following remobilization. PROM techniques, joint mobilization, or STM techniques may be beneficial in these circumstances.[44]

In addition, immobilization of a joint renders it susceptible to biomechanical changes within the synovium and articular cartilage. Studies in the animal model have shown that during immobilization, portions of the articular cartilage are replaced with fibrocartilage that significantly hinders motion of the joint.[45] Immobilization also adversely affects periarticular structures and synovial joints.[35,36,46] PROM and joint mobilization may be beneficial in maximizing the supply of nutrients to the synovial fluid and enhancing joint mobility.

It has also been postulated that joint mobilization might be an effective method to facilitate and enhance bone healing at a fracture site.[43] Two types of motion may occur at a fracture site: elastic and plastic. Elastic motion is minute displacement of the fracture site that reverses after the load is removed. This type of motion may facilitate healing. Plastic motion occurs when the fracture fragment is displaced and does not return once the load is removed. This type of motion is obviously detrimental to the fracture healing process.[21]

COORDINATION, COMMUNICATION, AND DOCUMENTATION

Communication will occur with Mr. Skelly and his wife regarding all components of his care and to engender support for his program. This will begin in the hospital and continue at home through his return to work and leisure activities. All elements of the patient's management will be documented.

PATIENT/CLIENT-RELATED INSTRUCTION

The patient will be instructed in appropriate activity modification to avoid placing stress on soft tissue structures that are currently impaired. Mr. Skelly will be instructed in proper postural habits and body mechanics during self-care, home management, work, community, and leisure actions, tasks, and activities. Mr. Skelly will be educated about impairments identified during the examination, plan of care, and prognosis. He will be educated on the stages of tissue healing that will include advice about avoiding any painful activities.

THERAPEUTIC EXERCISE

- ◆ Body mechanics and postural stabilization
  - Postural awareness in front of mirror for visual feedback
  - Scapula depression and adduction seated and during all exercise activities
  - Supine with patient retracting chin
  - Sitting with back against wall and performing chin retraction activities
  - Neuromuscular reeducation of the middle and lower trapezius muscles prone
  - Seated scapular retraction with elastic band resistance and proper chin and cervical spine positioning
- ◆ Flexibility exercises
  - Stretching exercises should be done after warming up, using a slow and steady stretch accompanied by deep breathing, and building hold up to 30 to 60 seconds
  - Cervical muscle stretching seated starting with active cervical sidebending progressing to assistance from the UEs
  - Stretching into right cervical rotation progressing to assistance from the UEs
  - Right GH PROM and AROM starting supine and progressing to standing, ensuring that patient demonstrates proper SH rhythm
  - Stretching into GH abduction by having patient walk fingers up the wall or using cane/pulley for assistance
  - Stretching into GH flexion by having patient walk

fingers up the wall or using cane/pulley for assistance
- Stretching into horizontal adduction
- Stretching into ER and IR of the GH joint, supine, using cane for assistance
- Right scapular PROM and AROM into retraction and depression starting in the seated position and progressing to prone
- Pectoralis stretch in doorway or corner

♦ Gait and locomotion training
- Reciprocal arm swing with gait in front of mirror
- Marching in place using verbal cues for proper arm swing

♦ Strength, power, and endurance training
- Supine deep neck flexor exercises with chin retraction
- Chair push-ups
- Seated scapula retraction with elastic band resistance
- Elastic band resistance during shoulder flexion, abduction, extension, and adduction activities
- Push-ups on static surface progressing to dynamic surfaces (trampoline, Physioball)
- PNF techniques to BUE starting supine and progressing to standing, with resistance starting with a low weight
- Neuromuscular reeducation of serratus anterior muscle leaning against wall
- Rhythmic stabilization activities to RUE and scapula in open-kinetic-chain (OKC) position
- Rhythmic stabilization activities in CKC position with patients hand against the wall
- Rhythmic stabilization activities in quadruped position
- Quadruped exercises with weight shifts
- Upper body ergometer starting with short duration (2 minutes) and increasing according to patient's subjective reports, RR, and pulse
- Rotator cuff strengthening with elastic resistance in the sitting and standing positions
- Progress to increased shoulder abduction with rotator cuff strengthening
- Hold shoulder abduction position for increasing periods of time
- Serratus push-ups standing with patient's arms on wall progressing to an incline and eventually to the horizontal position
- Medicine ball toss against trampoline
- Overhead ball toss against trampoline

FUNCTIONAL TRAINING IN SELF-CARE AND HOME MANAGEMENT

♦ Self-care and home management
- Review all actions, tasks, and activities and postural alignment for self-care and home management

FUNCTIONAL TRAINING IN WORK, COMMUNITY, AND LEISURE INTEGRATION OR REINTEGRATION

♦ Work
- Review all actions, tasks, and activities and postural alignment for work

MANUAL THERAPY TECHNIQUES

♦ Soft tissue mobilization addressing tight right pectoralis major
♦ Peripheral and spinal mobilization/manipulation
- Joint mobilization to the right GH joint in an inferior and posterior direction starting with Grades I and II and progressing to III and IV
- Joint mobilizations to the right distal clavicle in an inferior direction starting with Grades III and IV
- Joint mobilization/manipulation of restricted cervical and thoracic segments in a P/A direction starting with Grade III and progressing to Grades IV and V as appropriate
♦ Passive range of motion
- PROM to right shoulder in flexion, extension, abduction, and IR/ER providing a low load prolonged stretch at the end range of all planes
- PROM to right scapula in the inferior and medial (vertebral) directions

ANTICIPATED GOALS AND EXPECTED OUTCOMES

♦ Impact on pathology/pathophysiology
- Pain is decreased from a 1-2/10 at rest to 0/10 at rest in 3 to 4 weeks. Pain is decreased from a 5/10 during work activities to a 1/10 in 3 to 4 weeks.
♦ Impact on impairments
- AROM is improved to the following: Shoulder flexion 160 degrees, shoulder abduction 150 degrees, ER 70 degrees, and IR 75 degrees in 4 weeks.
- Patient will demonstrate proper SH rhythm during work-related activities including tasks over shoulder height in 3 to 4 weeks.
- Patient will exhibit improved coordination of RUE during activities over shoulder height in 3 to 4 weeks.

- Strength of the right upper quarter musculature will improve to the following: Deltoids 5/5, supraspinatus 4+/5, infraspinatus and teres minor 4+/5, subscapularis 5/5, bicep brachii 5/5, triceps 5/5, serratus anterior 4+/5, middle and lower trapezius 4+/5, and rhomboids 5/5 in 4 to 6 weeks.
- The patient will exhibit improvements in arthrokinematic motion of the shoulder in the direction of a posterior and inferior glide. Patient will also achieve improved mobility of the C-T spine in 3 to 4 weeks.

◆ Impact on functional limitations
  - Patient will be able to perform all job duties required of a house painter, including activities requiring shoulder flexion greater than 90 degrees, for 6 to 8 hours per day, in 4 to 6 weeks.

◆ Risk reduction/prevention
  - Patient achieved an understanding and demonstrates behavioral changes regarding proper postures that will alleviate excessive stress on soft tissue structures in 2 weeks.
  - Patient will achieve an understanding of risk factors associated with improper SH mechanics and activities above shoulder height. Risk factors are reduced in 2 weeks.

◆ Impact on health, wellness, and fitness
  - Mr. Skelly will understand the importance of exercise and will develop a plan to return to his exercise program that was ceased at the time his second child was born.
  - Physical function is improved, including the ability to maintain shoulder in a position of over 90 degrees of flexion while performing work-related activities.

◆ Impact on societal resources
  - Resources available to Mr. Skelly are maximally utilized.
  - Documentation occurs throughout the patient management and across settings and follows APTA's *Guidelines for Physical Therapy Documentation*.[47]

◆ Patient/client satisfaction
  - Patient and family become knowledgeable and aware of the diagnosis, prognosis, interventions, and understanding of anticipated goals and expected outcomes.

REEXAMINATION

Reexamination is performed throughout the episode of care.

DISCHARGE

Mr. Skelly is discharged from physical therapy after a total of 12 physical therapy sessions and attainment of his goals and expectations. These sessions have covered his entire episode of care. He is discharged because he has achieved his goals and expected outcomes.

Case Study #2: Radius and Ulnar Styloid Process Fracture

Mrs. Schult is a 68-year-old female who sustained a fracture to her left distal radius and ulnar styloid process (Figure 7-3) and had her left wrist and forearm immobilized in a cast for 10 weeks.

PHYSICAL THERAPIST EXAMINATION

HISTORY

◆ General demographics: Mrs. Schult is a 68-year-old white female whose primary language is English. She is right-side dominant. She graduated from high school.

◆ Social history: Mrs. Schult is a widow with two married children and three grandchildren (3 months and 2- and 4-years-old). Her husband passed away 5 years ago as a result of a cardiac event.

◆ Employment/work: She is a retired secretary.

◆ Living environment: Mrs. Schult lives independently in a two-story condominium in close proximity to her daughter's house (3 miles).

◆ General health status
  - General health perception: Mrs. Schult reports that she is in good health.
  - Physical function: Her reported physical function has been normal for her age prior to the event.
  - Psychological function: Normal.
  - Role function: Mother, grandmother.
  - Social function: Mrs. Schult enjoys playing cards and cribbage with her friends two nights per week.

◆ Social/health habits: She is a non-smoker and does not drink alcohol.

◆ Family history: Both parents and her two siblings are still living and are in good health. She reports that her mother also has osteoporosis.

◆ Medical/surgical history: Mrs. Schult reports a history of mild osteoporosis.

◆ Prior hospitalizations: She was hospitalized twice for the

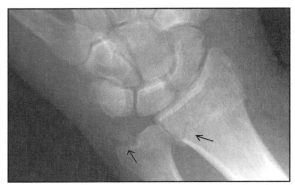

Figure 7-3. Radiograph of Mrs. Schult's left distal radial and ulnar styloid fracture immediately following the injury.

births of her two children.

♦ Preexisting medical and other health-related conditions: Other than the previously indicated osteoporosis, she has no other preexisting conditions.

♦ Current condition(s)/chief complaint(s): Mrs. Schult reports the injury occurred when she tripped over one of her grandson's toys and fell, landing on her left wrist in an extended position. Immediately after the fall she began to complain of pain and swelling in her wrist and forearm. She was taken by her daughter to the emergency room and evaluated by the physician on duty. Radiographs revealed a fracture of the left distal radius and ulnar styloid process. The fracture was reduced by closed manipulation and the forearm was immobilized with a fiberglass cast with the wrist in slight extension and neutral forearm position. She was immobilized in the cast for 10 weeks. Her current complaints are of mild discomfort (2-3/10 on the 0-10 NPS, with 0 indicating no pain and 10 indicating the worst pain imaginable) when attempting to use the arm for light functional activities (washing her hair), but her main complaint is stiffness and inability to move her wrist or forearm. She continues to live at home independently, but "has been using her right hand" for all functional activities.

♦ Functional status and activity level: Mrs. Schult is independent with all ADL and IADL for self-care and home management. She exercises regularly and walks 3 miles, 5 days per week. She reports that she has been walking ever since being diagnosed with osteoporosis 4 years ago.

♦ Medications: She is currently taking bisphosphanates and calcium and vitamin D supplements.

♦ Imaging/diagnostic tests: Adequate healing was confirmed via radiographs prior to removal of the cast (Figure 7-4).

SYSTEMS REVIEW

♦ Cardiovascular/pulmonary
  ● BP: 138/86 mmHg
  ● Edema: Moderate edema noted left hand and dorsal/volar forearm
  ● HR: 77 bpm
  ● RR: 15 bpm
♦ Integumentary
  ● Presence of scar formation: No visible scarring noted
  ● Skin color: Mild bluish discoloration of left hand and fingers
  ● Skin integrity: WNL
♦ Musculoskeletal
  ● Gross range of motion: WNL except for LUE distal to the elbow
  ● Gross strength: WNL except for the LUE with which she demonstrated reduced strength of the wrist flexors and extensors, as well as decreased grip and pinch strength
  ● Gross symmetry: Moderate atrophy of the dorsal and volar forearm musculature and hypotrophy of the thenar and hypothenar muscles
  ● Height: 5'0" (1.52 m)
  ● Weight: 128 lbs (58 kg)
♦ Neuromuscular
  ● Gross coordinated movements (balance, locomotion, transfers, and transitions): WNL
♦ Communication, affect, cognition, language, and learning style
  ● Communication, affect, cognition, and language: WNL
  ● Learning preferences: Visual learner

TESTS AND MEASURES

♦ Aerobic capacity/endurance
  ● 6-Minute Walk test graded as WNL
♦ Anthropometric characteristics
  ● BMI=25,[1] which is overweight (weight [in kg] divided by height[2] [in meters])
  ● Visual inspection revealed swelling of digits 2 to 5
  ● Volumetric measurements confirmed swelling (left 279 mL and right 244 mL); the accuracy of a standard commercial volumeter has been shown to have a SD of 4.26 mL for edematous hands[48]
  ● Moderate atrophy of the dorsal and volar forearm musculature
  ● Hypotrophy of the thenar and hypothenar muscles
♦ Assistive and adaptive devices: None used
♦ Cranial and peripheral nerve integrity

- Although none of the subjective complaints indicated neurological involvement, given the frequent complication of carpal tunnel syndrome in this population,[10,12] peripheral nerve testing was performed and was found to be negative throughout
♦ Ergonomics and body mechanics
  - Demonstrated poor postural habits during the history gathering, including a forward head and bilateral abducted scapula
♦ Gait, locomotion, and balance: WNL
♦ Joint integrity and mobility
  - Joint mobility assessment revealed moderate hypomobility of volar and dorsal glide at the left radiocarpal and midcarpal joints
  - Proximal and distal radioulnar joints also exhibited moderate hypomobility in both posterior and anterior directions
♦ Motor function
  - Dexterity, coordination, and agility
    - Coordination was assessed with the use of the Purdue Pegboard (test-retest reliability ranging from 0.37 to 0.70)[49] and she scored a 16 with the right hand and an 8 with the left hand
    - Analysis of the LUE during leisure activities (playing cribbage and shuffling cards) revealed considerable coordination and dexterity deficits of the left wrist, hand, and fingers
♦ Muscle performance
  - Muscle performance assessment utilizing MMT revealed strength deficits on the left within the available ROM to be the following:
    - Extensor carpi radialis longus=4-/5
    - Extensor carpi radialis brevus=4/5
    - Flexor carpi ulnaris=4/5
    - Flexor pollicis longus=4/5
    - Extensor pollicis longus=4-/5
    - Extensor digitorum=4/5
    - Flexor digitorum superficialis and profundus=4-/5
    - Supination and pronation of the forearm=4/5
    - Biceps and triceps=4/5 and 4+/5, respectively
  - Grip strength, assessed with a dynamometer, revealed the following:
    - 11 lbs on the left and 29 lbs on the right
    - The intrarater reliability has been shown to be between moderate and good for measurements obtained with both MMT (ICC=0.63 to 0.98) and hand-held dynamometry (ICC=0.69 to 0.90)[27]
    - Grip strength has been demonstrated to be superior to functional questionnaires[50] in detecting change in a patient population with distal radial

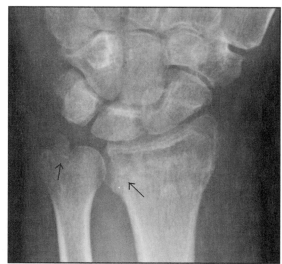

Figure 7-4. Radiograph 6 weeks post-injury showing healed distal radial and ulnar styloid fracture.

fractures treated with closed manipulation
  - Pinch strength was also assessed with a dynamometer and revealed the following deficits:
    - Key pinch (2 lbs left vs 6 lbs right)
    - Jaw pinch (3 vs 7 lbs)
    - Tip pinch (3 vs 9 lbs)
♦ Pain
  - 3/10 on the NPS when attempting to use her left hand to lift anything heavier than 1 lb
♦ Posture
  - Static postural observation using a plumb line revealed:
    - Forward head
    - Increased thoracic kyphosis
    - Decreased lumbar lordosis
    - Cervical spine slightly sidebends left
    - Right elevated clavicle and scapula
♦ Range of motion
  - Active goniometric measurements of the left wrist were limited in the following pattern:
    - Extension=0 to 38 degrees
    - Flexion=0 to 29 degrees
    - Radial deviation=0 to 7 degrees
    - Ulnar deviation=0 to 12 degrees
    - According to Cyriax,[51] this pattern of limitation at the wrist is suggestive of a capsular pattern. However, the reliability and validity of Cyriax's capsular classifications has recently been challenged for other joints[52]
    - Finger flexion was also limited in digits 2 through 5 at the proximal interphalangeal (PIP) joints and

DIP joint ranging between 0 to 50 degrees and 60 degrees for all
- Supination was limited=0 to 43 degrees
- Pronation was limited=0 to 47 degrees
- PROM measurements were consistent with the active limitations and were recorded as followed
  - Wrist extension=0 to 42 degrees
  - Flexion=0 to 34 degrees
  - Radial deviation=0 to 10 degrees
  - Ulnar deviation=0 to 14 degrees
  - Passive supination of the forearm=0 to 50 degrees
  - Passive pronation of the forearm=0 to 56 degrees
  - End feels were determined to be tissue stretch in all directions
- Self-care and home management
  - Interview with Mrs. Schult concerning ability to safely perform self-care and home management actions, tasks, and activities revealed that they could be performed
  - She had difficulty performing grooming, hygiene, and dressing as a result of decreased ROM and strength
- Work, community, and leisure integration or reintegration
  - The patient scored a 60% on the Disability of the Arm, Shoulder, and Hand questionnaire (DASH), which has been demonstrated to be more responsive in detecting change in this patient population than non-specific functional questionnaires, such as the SF-36[50]

EVALUATION

Mrs. Schult's history and risk factors previously outlined indicated that she is a retired white female status post left distal radius and ulnar styloid fracture with a history of mild osteoporosis. She has a number of impairments associated with the fracture and the immobilization period that followed. She demonstrated decreased ROM of the forearm, wrist, and fingers as well as strength deficits of the RUE, including grip and pinch. These impairments contributed to her functional limitations.

DIAGNOSIS

Mrs Schult is a patient who sustained a fracture of her left distal radius and ulnar styloid and had her wrist and forearm immobilized in a cast for 6 weeks. She has pain in her left wrist and has impaired: anthropometric characteristics, ergonomics and body mechanics, joint integrity and mobility, motor function, muscle performance, posture, and range of motion.

She is functionally limited in self-care and home management and in work, community, and leisure actions, tasks, and activities. These findings are consistent with placement in Pattern G: Impaired Joint Mobility, Muscle Performance, and Range of Motion Associated With Fracture. These impairments and functional limitations will be addressed in determining the prognosis and the plan of care.

PROGNOSIS AND PLAN OF CARE

Over the course of the visits, the following mutually established outcomes have been determined:
- Ability to perform physical actions, tasks, and activities related to self-care and home management are increased
- Joint integrity and mobility are improved
- Motor function is improved
- Muscle performance is improved
- Pain is decreased
- Performance of and independence in ADL and IADL are improved
- Postural control is improved
- ROM is improved
- Soft tissue swelling is reduced

To achieve these outcomes, the appropriate interventions for this patient are determined. These will include: coordination, communication, and documentation; patient/client-related instruction; therapeutic exercise; functional training in self-care and home management; functional training in work, community, and leisure integration or reintegration; and manual therapy techniques.

Based on the diagnosis and prognosis, Mrs. Schult is expected to require between 12 to 14 visits over a 12-week period. Mrs. Schult has good social support, is motivated, and follows through with her home exercise program. She is not severely impaired and is generally healthy.

INTERVENTIONS

RATIONALE FOR SELECTED INTERVENTIONS

Therapeutic Exercise

The importance of physical therapy in this patient population should not be underestimated. Byl and associates[53] demonstrated that following closed reduction and cast immobilization, patients with distal radial fractures exhibited significant impairments in ROM, mid-forearm girth, and grip strength. The results of a recent randomized controlled trial demonstrated that a group of patients, all of whom had sustained a Colles' fracture, who received physical therapy (exercises, patient education, and joint mobilization) for an average of five visits over a 6-week time period, achieved a significantly greater increase in active wrist extension and grip strength as compared to a control group (home exercise sheet).[54]

Manual Therapy Techniques

These techniques should only be used once radiographic evidence has demonstrated that the fracture is well healed. Immobilization results in biological changes within capsular and ligamentous tissues since the newly synthesized matrix is haphazardly organized.[55] Immobilization has a dramatic effect on muscle tissue and results in a reduction of muscle strength, endurance, cross-sectional area, and muscle fiber diameter.[34] In addition, it has been demonstrated that immobilization of muscle results in an increase in connective tissue in shortened muscle (the wrist extensors with this patient).[56] Applying controlled forces to these structures with manual therapy (stretching and mobilization) can assist with facilitating proper organization of the collagen links and restoring interstitial fluid content to within normal levels.[44] Perhaps providing greater support for the use of manual therapy in this population are the results of a randomized controlled trial that compared the effects of conventional physical therapy (heat, TENS, and exercise) to conventional physical therapy techniques with manual therapy directed at the joint and soft tissues.[57] Results revealed that although both groups demonstrated a statistically significant reduction in pain and increase in ROM, the group receiving the manual therapy exhibited a statistically significant increase in ROM and did so more efficiently in fewer visits.[57]

COORDINATION, COMMUNICATION, AND DOCUMENTATION

Communication will occur with Mrs. Schult and her family regarding all components of her care and to engender support for her program. This will begin in the outpatient setting and continue at home through her return to leisure activities. All elements of the patient's management will be documented.

PATIENT/CLIENT-RELATED INSTRUCTION

The patient will be provided with information about her current condition, including impairments and functional limitations. She will also be instructed in proper postural techniques that would assist with the prevention of further musculoskeletal impairments. Mrs. Schult will also be educated about risk factors associated with osteoporosis and possible means by which she can make lifestyle changes to assist with slowing the rate of progression of osteoporosis.

THERAPEUTIC EXERCISE

♦ Balance, coordination, and agility training

- Purdue Pegboard activities including placing pegs in holes and placing washers on pegs
- Timed Purdue Pegboard activities assessing the number of pegs and washers that are completed in 60 seconds
- Finger dexterity exercises including rapid alternate finger to finger movements and snapping of fingers
- Playing jacks
- Shuffling a deck of cards
- "O" pinching activities with clothes pin for resistance, eventually progressing to increasing the resistance with an elastic band around the clothespin

♦ Body mechanics and postural stabilization
- Postural central training and postural stabilization activities
- Postural activities in front of mirror for visual feedback
- Postural activities seated against wall with emphasis on chin and scapula retraction

♦ Flexibility exercises
- Stretching exercises should be done after warming up, using a slow and steady stretch accompanied by deep breathing, and building hold up to 30 to 60 seconds
- Stretching of supinator and pronator muscles with patient seated and elbow supported on plinth
- Stretching wrist flexor and extensor muscles with patient seated and elbow in a flexed and extended position
- Stretching of finger flexor and extensor muscles both with wrist flexed and extended
- AROM of all involved joints with prolonged hold at end range
- PROM of all involved joints with prolonged low load hold at end range
- Quadruped weightbearing activities first, with proximal phalanges with a closed fist and then progressing to a position of wrist and finger extension
- Tendon glides with the patient seated and elbow supported on the table
  - The patient will stabilize four of her fingers in extension with the contralateral hand and then move the digit that is not stabilized in extension repeatedly

♦ Strength, power, and endurance training
- Strengthening activities began as non-resisted straight plane motions and then progressed to resistive exercises
- Putty exercises having the patient use an "O"
- Concentric and eccentric wrist exercises with resistance (elastic band or weights)
- Squeeze a tennis ball

- Supination and pronation with weights, extending the lever arm and as patient can tolerate, increased resistance
- Wring out a wet towel
- Pull putty apart
- Quadruped weightbearing activities
- Lift a crate with light weights initially, progressing within patient tolerance
- Lift weighted crate to different heights (waist, shoulder, overhead)

FUNCTIONAL TRAINING IN SELF-CARE AND HOME MANAGEMENT

- ◆ Self-care and home management
  - Review all actions, tasks, and activities for self-care and home management
  - Use left hand increasingly for or to assist as many self-care (eg, washing hair) and home management activities as possible

FUNCTIONAL TRAINING IN WORK, COMMUNITY, AND LEISURE INTEGRATION OR REINTEGRATION

- ◆ Leisure
  - Review all leisure actions, tasks, and activities (spending time with grandchildren and playing cards and cribbage)
  - Stress use of left hand increasingly for as many of these activities as practical

MANUAL THERAPY TECHNIQUES

- ◆ Massage
  - Retrograde massage for edema control
- ◆ Mobilization/manipulation
  - Joint mobilization directed at hypomobile intercarpal joints in both a dorsal and volar direction, beginning with Grades I and II and progressing to Grades III and IV
  - Joint mobilization directed at hypomobile radiocarpal joint in both an anterior and posterior direction, beginning with Grades I and II and progressing to Grades III and IV
  - Joint mobilization directed at hypomobile proximal and distal radioulnar joints in both an anterior and posterior direction, beginning with Grades I and II and progressing to Grades III and IV
- ◆ Passive range of motion
  - PROM into wrist flexion, extension, and radial and ulnar deviation with low load prolonged hold at end ranges of motion

- PROM into supination and pronation with low load prolonged hold at end ranges

ANTICIPATED GOALS AND EXPECTED OUTCOMES

- ◆ Impact on pathology/pathophysiology
  - Edema in the left hand and dorsal/volar forearm is reduced in 2 weeks.
  - Pain is decreased from a 2-3/10 to 0/10 in 4 weeks.
- ◆ Impact on impairments
  - AROM of the LUE is improved to the following: wrist extension 55 degrees, wrist flexion 60 degrees, radial deviation 15 degrees, ulnar deviation 15 degrees, forearm supination 70 degrees, and forearm pronation 70 degrees in 4 to 6 weeks.
  - Coordination will improve, and Mrs. Schult will be able to score at least a 15 on the Purdue Pegboard test, with the left hand in 4 to 6 weeks.
  - Grip strength on the left will improve to 20 lbs in 6 weeks.
  - Patient will achieve improved mobility of volar and dorsal glides at the radiocarpal joint. Patient will also achieve improved mobility at the proximal and distal radioulnar joints in 3 to 4 weeks.
  - Patient will achieve the same ability as RUE to shuffle a deck of cards in 6 weeks.
  - Pinch strength on the left will improve to the following: key pinch 4 lbs, jaw pinch 5 lbs, and tip pinch 7 lbs in 6 weeks.
  - Strength of the LUE will improve as follows: extensor carpi radialis longus 4+/5, extensor carpi radialis brevus 5/5, flexor carpi ulnaris 5/5, flexor pollicis longus 5/5, extensor pollicis longus 4+/5, extensor digitorum 5/5, flexor digitorum superficialis and profundus 4+/5, supination and pronation of the forearm 5/5, biceps and triceps 5/5 in 6 weeks.
- ◆ Impact on functional limitations
  - Patient will achieve the ability to use her left hand for grooming, hygiene, and dressing in 4 weeks.
  - Patient will achieve the ability to play cards with her LUE in 6 weeks.
- ◆ Impact on disabilities
  - Mrs. Schult will achieve the ability to return to her social and recreational activities including playing cribbage with her friends in 6 weeks.
- ◆ Risk reduction/prevention
  - Mrs. Schult will achieve an understanding of the risk factors of osteoporosis and make behavioral changes to reduce these in 3 to 4 weeks.
- ◆ Impact on health, wellness, and fitness
  - Mrs. Schult increases her exercise regimen to foster

healthy habits and slow the progression of osteoporosis.

♦ Impact on societal resources
  • Resources available to Mrs. Schult are maximally utilized.
  • Documentation occurs throughout patient management and across all settings and follows APTA's *Guidelines for Physical Therapy Documentation.*[47]
  • Utilization of physical therapy services is optimized.

♦ Patient/client satisfaction
  • Patient and family are knowledgeable and aware of the diagnosis, prognosis, interventions, and understanding of anticipated goals and expected outcomes.

REEXAMINATION

Reexamination is performed throughout the episode of care.

DISCHARGE

Mrs. Schult is discharged from physical therapy after a total of 14 physical therapy sessions and attainment of her goals and expectations. These sessions have covered her entire episode of care. She is discharged because she has achieved her goals and expected outcomes.

Case Study #3: Jones' Fracture

Mr. Bryan is a 28-year-old male who tripped while descending stairs and sustained a minimally displaced transverse fracture at the junction of the diaphysis and metaphysis of his right proximal fifth metatarsal (Jones' fracture).

PHYSICAL THERAPIST EXAMINATION

HISTORY

♦ General demographics: Mr. Bryan is a 28-year-old white male whose primary language is English. He is right-leg dominant.

♦ Social history: Mr. Bryan is married with an 18-month-old toddler and a 175-pound Great Dane.

♦ Employment/work: Mr. Bryan is a physician's assistant who works at a local teaching hospital. He works full-time and is on-call once per week and every other weekend.

♦ Living environment: He lives in a two-story house with all bedrooms upstairs and a railing on the right side of the stairs. There are two steps to the front entry of the house and one step at all other entries. There is a tub and shower combination in all bathrooms.

♦ General health status
  • General health perception: Mr. Bryan reports being in excellent health.
  • Physical function: His reported function is normal for his age.
  • Psychological function: Normal.
  • Role function: Health care provider, father, husband.
  • Social function: He is an avid triathlete who also enjoys camping, hiking, and hunting.

♦ Social/health habits: Mr. Bryan is a non-smoker and moderate, but regular drinker (seven to 10 drinks per week).

♦ Family history: Mr. Bryan's parents and four grandparents are alive and healthy and live in various regions of the country.

♦ Medical/surgical history: He reports that his medical history is nonsignificant except for mitral valve prolapse. Surgical history includes a left inguinal hernia repair 3 years ago and a right knee arthroscopy and debridement 1 year ago.

♦ Prior hospitalizations: Day surgery for each of the above surgeries, otherwise no prior hospitalizations.

♦ Preexisting medical and other health-related conditions: Mitral valve prolapse.

♦ Current condition(s)/chief complaint(s): Mr. Bryan sustained a Jones' fracture of his right proximal fifth MT when he tripped over his dog while descending stairs causing him to misstep and land on the lateral border of his right foot. He was treated for 8 weeks in a non-weightbearing short leg cast, with x-rays taken at 4 and 8 weeks. The follow-up x-rays at 8 weeks revealed minimal fracture healing, but clinically he had no pain at the fracture site. He was subsequently allowed weightbearing as tolerated in a fracture brace and referred to physical therapy.

♦ Functional status and activity level: Mr. Bryan is totally independent in all ADL and IADL. Immediately following the injury he took 1 week off from work and then returned to work on a full-time basis. Initially he had been using crutches, but he now ambulates without an assistive device.

♦ Medications: None.

♦ Imaging/diagnostic tests: No other imaging has been performed other than the initial and follow-up x-rays.

SYSTEMS REVIEW

♦ Cardiovascular/pulmonary

- BP: 120/78 mmHg
- Edema: Mild edema noted right ankle and foot
- HR: 64 bpm
- RR: 10 bpm
- ◆ Integumentary
  - Presence of scar formation: None
  - Skin color: WNL
  - Skin integrity: Dry, scaly skin on RLE, over area previously covered by short leg cast
- ◆ Musculoskeletal
  - Gross range of motion: WNL except for right ankle that visually demonstrates limitations in plantarflexion, dorsiflexion, inversion, and everison
  - Gross strength: WNL except for right ankle, as patient has difficulty standing on toes and heel
  - Gross symmetry: Mild atrophy noted of the right anterior tibialis and gastrocnemius/soleus
  - Height: 5'10" (1.78 m)
  - Weight: 155 lbs (70.3 kg)
- ◆ Neuromuscular
  - Balance: Unable to balance on RLE more than 5 seconds prior to using hands to grasp chair
  - Balance, locomotion, transfers, and transitions: Ambulates weightbearing as tolerated without assistive device in fracture brace, without antalgia
- ◆ Communication, affect, cognition, language, and learning style
  - Communication, affect, cognition, and language: WNL
  - Learning preferences: Visual learner

TESTS AND MEASURES

- ◆ Aerobic capacity/endurance:
  - Mild deficits as determined by the 6-Minute Walk test
- ◆ Anthropometric characteristics
  - BMI=22.17, which is normal (weight [in kg] divided by height^2 [in meters])
  - Mild pitting edema noted in right foot
  - Significant atrophy noted in right calf with girth measurements demonstrating a 2-cm difference at the mid calf level and mild atrophy noted in right thigh
- ◆ Assistive and adaptive devices
  - Fracture brace used for RLE that fits well without evidence of skin breakdown
- ◆ Environmental, home, and work barriers
  - Potential barriers include steps at all entrances to his home and stairs leading to bedrooms on second floor of home
- ◆ Gait, locomotion, and balance

- Exhibits decreased toe push-off on the RLE
- Slight favoring of RLE with ambulation and stair climbing
- ◆ Integumentary integrity
  - Skin intact
  - Dry, scaly skin noted on right foot and lower leg
- ◆ Joint integrity and mobility
  - Joints not involving the fifth MT bone were assessed. The fifth MTP and TMT joints would only be assessed after the fracture site was well healed.
  - Joint mobility assessment revealed:
    - Decreased mobility of the talocrural joint in dorsiflexion
    - Marked hypomobility of subtalar inversion and eversion, intermetatarsal (I-IV) anterior to posterior glides, and intertarsal joint anterior to posterior glides on the right
    - Mild restriction noted with anterior to posterior and posterior to anterior glides of the talocrural and subtalar joints on the right
- ◆ Motor function
  - Agility testing: Difficulty performing carioca and tandem walking
  - Dexterity of UEs and LLE: WNL
  - Lack of coordination during proprioceptive and kinesthetic assessment
    - RLE was tested with the One-Legged Stance test
    - He was able to stand on his left leg for 20 seconds with eyes open and closed for each of the five trials, but only 5 seconds with eyes open on the right and 3 seconds with eyes closed on the right, for each of the five trials
- ◆ Muscle performance
  - MMT revealed the following right leg deviations from normal:
    - Hip abduction=4+/5
    - Hip extension=4+/5
    - Knee flexion=4+/5
    - Extension=4+/5
    - Ankle dorsiflexion=4-/5
    - Ankle plantarflexion=4-/5
    - Ankle inversion=4-/5
    - Ankle eversion=4-/5
- ◆ Pain
  - Pain in the right ankle during full weight shift to the RLE, when ascending and descending stairs, was rated at 0-1/10 on the NPS
  - Pain with palpation over the proximal fifth MT was rated as a 2/10 on the NPS
- ◆ Posture
  - Right iliac crest was slightly elevated in standing secondary to fracture brace

- Forward head
♦ Range of motion
  - Active limitations of the right ankle included the following:
    - Plantarflexion=0 to 25 degrees
    - Dorsiflexion=0 to 5 degrees
    - Inversion=0 to 5 degrees
    - Eversion=0 to 10 degrees
  - Passive limitations of the right ankle ROM were as follows:
    - Plantarflexion=0 to 30 degrees
    - Dorsiflexion=0 degrees
    - Inversion=0 to 10 degrees
    - Eversion=0 to 10 degrees
  - Goniometric measurements of ankle ROM for plantarflexion and dorsiflexion have demonstrated good (ICC=0.86 to 0.09) intratester reliability, yet the intratester reliability for inversion and eversion measurements is poor (ICC=0.22 to 0.30)[58]
  - Passive muscle flexibility testing revealed decreased extensibility of the right hamstrings, ankle plantarflexors, and toe extensors
♦ Self-care and home management
  - Interview concerning ability to safely perform self-care and home management actions, tasks, and activities reveals that he is independent with all basic ADL
♦ Sensory integrity: WNL
♦ Work, community, and leisure integration or reintegration
  - Interview concerning ability to safely perform work, community, and leisure actions, tasks, and activities reveals that he has continued to work full-time except for the first week after his injury
  - Leisure activities not yet possible

EVALUATION

Mr. Bryan's history previously outlined indicated that he is a young white male who sustained a fracture of his right proximal fifth MT when he misstepped and landed on the lateral aspect of his right foot. He was subsequently placed in a non-weightbearing cast for 8 weeks. He lives with his wife, toddler, and large dog in a two-story home. Mr. Bryan is independent in his normal daily activities and has continued to work full-time. He has altered posture and decreased motor and muscle performance, ROM, and balance of his RLE. He is currently ambulating without an assistive device. His physician has approved gait progression as tolerated to include progression of agility and endurance exercises.

DIAGNOSIS

Mr. Bryan is a patient who has sustained a Jones' fracture of his right fifth MT and has some pain over the fifth MT. He has impaired: anthropometric characteristics; gait, locomotion, and balance; integumentary integrity; joint integrity and mobility; motor function; muscle performance; posture; and range of motion. He is functionally limited in leisure actions, tasks, and activities. These findings are consistent with placement in Pattern G: Impaired Joint Mobility, Muscle Performance, and Range of Motion Associated With Fracture. The identified impairments and functional limitations will be addressed in determining the prognosis and the plan of care.

PROGNOSIS AND PLAN OF CARE

Over the course of the visits, the following mutually established outcomes have been determined:
♦ Aerobic capacity and endurance are increased
♦ Balance is improved
♦ Joint mobility is improved
♦ Motor function is improved
♦ Muscle performance is increased
♦ Pain is decreased
♦ Passive muscle flexibility is improved
♦ Physical function is improved
♦ Postural control is improved
♦ ROM is improved
♦ Self-management of symptoms is improved

To achieve these outcomes, the appropriate interventions for this patient are determined. These will include: coordination, communication, and documentation; patient/client-related instruction; therapeutic exercise; functional training in work, community, and leisure integration or reintegration; and manual therapy techniques.

Based on the diagnosis and prognosis, Mr. Bryan is expected to require between six and eight visits within a 6-month time frame. Mr. Bryan has good social support, is motivated, and follows through with his home exercise program. He is not severely impaired and is generally healthy.

INTERVENTIONS

RATIONALE FOR SELECTED INTERVENTIONS

Therapeutic Exercise

The effects of immobilization on strength and torque of the triceps surae muscle group, ROM, and function have been well documented in the literature.[39,59-62] For specific details regarding the effects of ankle immobilization and evidence for the therapeutic benefits of exercise the readers are referred to Pattern I: Impaired Joint Mobility, Motor Function, Muscle Performance, and Range of Motion Associated With Bony or Soft Tissue Surgery.

Manual Therapy Techniques

As previously discussed, patients who underwent a rehabilitation program consisting of ambulation, strengthening, proprioceptive retraining, and joint mobilization made significant improvements in functional performance and returned to control levels.[39] A pilot study by Wilson demonstrated exercise plus manual therapy (joint mobilization and traction to hypomobile joints) was superior to exercise therapy alone in increasing ROM and function in a group of patients who had been immobilized for 6 weeks following an ankle fracture.[63] For further evidence regarding the use of manual therapy following ankle immobilization, the reader is referred to Pattern I: Impaired Joint Mobility, Motor Function, Muscle Performance, and Range of Motion Associated With Bony or Soft Tissue Surgery.

COORDINATION, COMMUNICATION, AND DOCUMENTATION

Communication will occur with Mr. Bryan and his wife regarding all components of his care and to engender support for his program. This began in the hospital and continued at home through his return to work and leisure actions, tasks, and activities. All elements of the patient's management will be documented.

PATIENT/CLIENT-RELATED INSTRUCTION

The patient will be provided with information about his current condition including impairments and functional limitations. He will be instructed in ways of enhancing his performance, health, wellness, and fitness. He will also be informed of the plan of care.

THERAPEUTIC EXERCISE

- ◆ Aerobic capacity/endurance conditioning
  - Parameters for aerobic capacity/endurance conditioning
    - Begin, for example, at 10 minutes and increase within patient tolerance to 30 minutes
    - Intensity will be 60% to 80% of THR and Borg scale will be used to determine perceived exertion (see Pattern A: Primary Prevention/Risk Reduction for Skeletal Demineralization)
    - Frequency will be three to four times per week
  - Mode
    - Start with stationary bicycle and progress to elliptical trainer or stair stepper then walking and running as tolerated

- Progression of exercises is determined by Mr. Bryan's response to these activities
- Once he is able to tolerate weightbearing activity on the elliptical trainer or stair stepper without increased pain or swelling in his foot or ankle he can progress both the time and intensity of his exercise
- Any increase in pain or swelling should result in a modification of the exercise program until he can progress without these clinical signs
- Likewise, depending on his response to the exercise progression, it may be necessary to communicate with Mr. Bryan's physician for additional radiographs or other imaging, if pain and/or swelling persist
  - Pool exercises to include deep water running
- ◆ Balance, coordination, and agility training
  - Gait progression forward and backward, eyes open and closed
  - Single leg balance activities, first on static surface, progressing to dynamic surface
  - Single leg stance with external perturbations, first on static surface, then progressing to mini trampoline
  - Progress to agility drills such as carioca, lateral shuffles, figure-eights
  - Hopping and jumping on trampoline with eyes open then progressing to eyes closed
  - Similar to the aerobic conditioning exercises, progression is based on the patient's response to the activity
- ◆ Body mechanics and postural stabilization
  - Body mechanics training
    - Lifting techniques with verbal cues for proper form
  - Postural control training and postural stabilization exercises
    - Proper sitting techniques with chin retraction
    - Chin retraction with all exercises
- ◆ Flexibility exercises
  - Stretching exercises should be done after warming up, using a slow and steady stretch accompanied by deep breathing, and building hold up to 30 to 60 seconds
  - Gastrocnemius and soleus stretching in long sitting, with assistance from strap or towel wrapped around foot with 30-second holds
  - Gastrocnemius and soleus stretching leaning against a wall, in tandem stance with 30-second holds
  - Gastrocnemius and soleus stretching on slant board with 30-second holds
  - Manual stretching of the toe extensors with 30-second holds

- Hamstring stretching may be included to address general LE flexibility; supine, with the hip flexed 90 degrees and knee extended with 30-second holds
- Seated and doorway stretch for hamstring muscle on the right with 30-second hold

- ◆ Gait and locomotion training
  - Gait in front of mirror for visual cues
  - Forward and backward walking with eyes open and closed
  - Gait on treadmill
  - Gait on uneven terrain
  - Progress to light jogging activities as appropriate
  - Gait around obstacles
  - Gait up and down stairs
- ◆ Strength, power, and endurance training
  - Ankle AROM, all planes, with elastic band resistance
  - Toe raises with UE support, progressing from bilateral to unilateral
  - Heel raises with UE support, progressing from bilateral to unilateral
  - Bridging on static surface
  - Bridging on therapeutic ball
  - Mini squats
  - Lunges
  - Step-ups; starting with 2-inch height, progressing to the height of a normal stair (approximately 8 inches)
  - One leg squats progressing to an uneven surface (foam pad)
  - Hamstring curls
  - Ankle inversion and eversion with elastic band for resistance

FUNCTIONAL TRAINING IN WORK, COMMUNITY, AND LEISURE INTEGRATION OR REINTEGRATION

- ◆ Work
  - Review all actions, tasks, and activities and postural alignment for work
- ◆ Leisure
  - Training for return to sport activities when appropriate (eg, triathalons, camping, hiking, and hunting)

MANUAL THERAPY TECHNIQUES

As indicated in the joint integrity tests and measures, the fifth MTP and TMT joints would only be treated with manual therapy after the fracture site was well healed.

- ◆ Mobilization/manipulation
  - Joint mobilization Grades IV to IV+, anterior to

posterior and posterior to anterior, for talocrural and subtalar joints
  - Joint mobilization/manipulation of right intertarsal joints using Grades IV to IV+ for anterior to posterior accessory glides
  - A distraction manipulation targeted at the subtalar and talocrural joints may also be considered if graded mobilizations do not produce the desired outcome
- ◆ Passive range of motion
  - PROM of right foot into ankle plantarflexion, dorsiflexion, inversion, and eversion
  - Passive MTP flexion and extension of digit 5
  - SLR to stretch right hamstrings
  - Hip flexed to 90 degrees, while performing passive knee extension, to stretch right hamstrings

ANTICIPATED GOALS AND EXPECTED OUTCOMES

- ◆ Impact on pathology/pathophysiology
  - Pain is eliminated with ambulation and palpation of fifth MT in 1 to 2 weeks.
  - Patient will be educated on healing times for his particular fracture.
- ◆ Impact on impairments
  - Balance is improved to single leg stance of 60 seconds in 2 to 3 weeks.
  - Full AROM and PROM equal to the left side in 4 to 6 weeks.
  - Gait is normal, including toe push off, in 2 to 3 weeks.
  - Normal strength, via MMT, for the RLE in 6 weeks.
- ◆ Impact on functional limitations
  - Ability to participate in recreational activities including hiking and running up to 3 miles, without pain, in 8 to 12 weeks.
  - Return to triathalon competition in 6 to 9 months.
- ◆ Impact on disabilities
  - None identified during examination, no goals indicated.
- ◆ Impact on health, wellness, and fitness
  - Fitness, health status, and physical capacity are returned to same level as prior to injury.
  - Physical function is improved, including the ability to participate in triathalons.
- ◆ Patient/client satisfaction
  - Coordination of care is acceptable to patient/client.
  - Patient and family knowledge and awareness of the diagnosis, prognosis, interventions, and understanding of anticipated goals and expected outcomes are increased.

REEXAMINATION

Reexamination is performed throughout the episode of care.

DISCHARGE

Mr. Bryan is discharged from physical therapy after a total of seven physical therapy sessions and attainment of his goals and expectations. These sessions have covered his entire episode of care. He is discharged because he has achieved his goals and expected outcomes.

ACKNOWLEDGMENTS

The authors would like to graciously thank a number of individuals for assisting with the preparation of this chapter. We would first like to extend our gratitude to Jessica Palmer, SPT, for her assistance and diligence with the formatting and referencing of the chapter. We are also greatly indebted to Mary Ley, Jill Wixom, Beth Pollock, and Andrea Torrisi from the Franklin Pierce College Library, Rindge, New Hampshire, for their efforts and countless hours spent searching for and acquiring references through interlibrary loan. In addition, acquisition of the figures for this chapter would not have been possible without the assistance of the Physical Therapy Staff at Brooke Army Medical Center, Ft. Sam Houston, Texas, and Dr. Liem Mansfield, Department of Radiology, Brooke Army Medical Center, Ft. Sam Houston, Texas.

REFERENCES

1. Enoka RM. Single-joint system components. In: Enoka RM, ed. *Neuromechanics of Human Movement.* 3rd ed. Champaign, Ill: Human Kinetics; 2002:211-239.
2. Tortora GL, Anagnostakos NP. Skeletal tissue. In: Tortora GL, Anagnostakos NP, eds. *Principles of Anatomy and Physiology.* 6th ed. New York, NY: Harper and Row; 1990:141-158.
3. Salter RB. Normal structure and function of musculoskeletal tissues. In: Salter RB, ed. *Textbook of Disorders and Injuries of the Musculoskeletal System.* Baltimore, Md: Lippincott Williams & Wilkins; 1999:7-33.
4. Culav EM, Clark CH, Merrilees MJ. Connective tissues: matrix composition and its relevance to physical therapy. *Phys Ther.* 1999;79:308-319.
5. Rosenberg AE. Skeletal system and soft tissue tumors. In: Cotran RS, Kumar V, Robbins SL, eds. *Robbins Pathologic Basis of Disease.* 5th ed. Philadelphia, Pa: WB Saunders Co; 1994:1213-1229.
6. Engles M. Tissue response. In: Donatelli RA, Wooden MJ, ed. *Orthopaedic Physical Therapy.* 3rd ed. New York, NY: Churchill Livingstone; 2001:1-24.
7. Junqueira LC, Carneiro J, Kelley RO. Bone. In: Junqueira LC, Carneiro J, Kelley RO, eds. *Basic Histology.* 9th ed. Stamford, Conn: Appleton and Lange; 1998:134-151.
8. Heckman JD, Dingle RV, eds. *The Netter Collection of Medical Illustrations, Vol 8, The Musculoskeletal System.* Summit, NJ: Novartis Pharmaceuticals Corp; 1997.
9. Praemer A, Furner S, Price OP. *Musculoskeletal Conditions in the United States.* Rosemont, Ill: American Academy of Orthopaedic Surgeons; 1992:85-91.
10. McKinnis LN. *Fundamentals of Orthopaedic Radiology.* Philadelphia, Pa: FA Davis Co; 1997.
11. Salter RB. Specific fractures and joint injuries in children. In: Salter RB, ed. *Textbook of Disorders and Injuries of the Musculoskeletal System.* Baltimore, Md: Lippincott Williams & Wilkins; 1999:499-560.
12. Hoppenfeld S, Murthy VL. *Treatment and Rehabilitation of Fractures.* Philadelphia, Pa: Lipincott Williams & Wilkins; 2000.
13. Einhorn TA. The cell and molecular biology of fracture healing. *Clin Orthop.* 1998;355S:S7-S21.
14. Nitz AJ, Kitzman PH. Bone injury and repair. In: Placzek JD, Boyce DA, eds. *Orthopaedic Physical Therapy Secrets.* Philadelphia, Pa: Hanley and Belfus; 2001:22-27.
15. Perry CR, Elstrom JA. *Handbook of Fractures.* 2nd ed. New York, NY: McGraw-Hill, Inc; 2000.
16. Marsh DR, Gang Li. The biology of fracture healing: optimizing outcome. *Br Med Bull.* 1999;55:856-869.
17. Compere EL, Banks SW, Compere CL. *Pictorial Handbook of Fracture Treatment.* 5th ed. Chicago, Ill: Yearbook Medical Publishers, Inc; 1963:72.
18. Hayda RA, Brighton CT, Esterhai JL. Pathophysiology of delayed healing. *Clinical Orthop.* 1998;355S:S31-S40.
19. Busse JW, Bhandari M, Kulkarni AV, Tunks E. The effect of low-intensity pulsed ultrasound therapy on time to fracture healing: a meta-analysis. *CMAJ.* 2002;166:437-441.
20. Ciccone CD. *Pharmacology in Rehabilitation.* 2nd ed. Philadelphia, Pa: FA Davis Co; 1996.
21. Sarmiento A, Waddell J, Latta LL. Diaphyseal humeral fractures: treatment options. *J Bone Joint Surg (Am).* 2001;83A:1566-1579.
22. Maitland G, Hengeveld E, Banks K, English K. *Maitland's Vertebral Manipulation.* 6th ed. Oxford, England: Butterworth-Heinemann; 2001.
23. Magee DJ. *Orthopaedic Physical Assessment.* 3rd ed. Philadelphia, Pa: WB Saunders Co; 1997.
24. Bak K, Faunl P. Clinical findings in competitive swimmers with shoulder pain. *Am J Sports Med.* 1997;25:254-260.
25. Calis M, Akgun K, Birtane M, Karacan F, Calis H, Tuzun F. Diagnostic values of clinical diagnostic tests in subacromial impingement syndrome. *Ann Rheum Dis.* 2000;59:44-47.
26. Rupp S, Berininger K, Hopf T. Shoulder problems in high level swimmers-impingement, anterior instability, muscular imbalance? *Int J Sports Med.* 1995;16:557-562.
27. Wadsworth CT, Krishnan R, Sear M, Harrold J, Nielsen DH. Intrarater reliability of manual muscle testing and hand-held dynametric muscle testing. *Phys Ther.* 1987;67:1342-1347.
28. Paice JA, Cohen FL. Validity of a verbally administered numeric rating scale to measure cancer pain intensity. *Cancer Nurs.* 1997;20:88-93.
29. Rothstein JM, Miller PJ, Roettger RF. Goniometric reliability in a clinical setting. Elbow and knee measurements. *Phys Ther.* 1983;63:1611-1615.

30. Patla CE, Paris SV. Reliability of interpretation of the Paris classification of normal end feel for elbow flexion and extension. *Journal of Manual and Manipulative Therapy.* 1993;1:60-66.

31. Berg HE, Larsson L, Tesch PA. Lower limb skeletal muscle function after 6 wk of bed rest. *Applied Physiology.* 1997;81(1):182-188.

32. Marchetti ME, Houde JP, Steinberg GG, Crane GK, Goss TP, Baran DT. Humeral bone density losses after shoulder surgery and immobilization. *J Shoulder Elbow Surg.* 1996;5:471-476.

33. Olson VL. *Connective Tissue Response to Injury, Immobilization, and Mobilization.* La Crosse, Wisc: Orthopaedic Section, American Physical Therapy Association; 2001.

34. Veldehuizen JW, Verstappen FTJ, Vromen JPAM, Kuipers H, Greep JM. Functional and morphological adaptations following four weeks of knee immobilization. *Int J Sports Med.* 1993;14:283-287.

35. Haapala J, Arkoski JPA, Hyttinen MM, et al. Remobilization does not fully restore immobilization induced articular cartilage atrophy. *Clin Orthop.* 1999;362:218-229.

36. Kaneps AJ, Stover SM, Lane E. Changes in canine and cortical and cancellous bone mechanical properties following immobilization and remobilization with exercise. *Bone.* 1997;21:419-423.

37. Vandenborne K, Elliott MA, Walter GA, et al. Longitudinal study of skeletal muscle adaptations during immobilization and rehabilitation. *Muscle Nerve.* 1998;21:1006-1012.

38. Lindboe CF, Platou CS. Effect of immobilization of short duration on the muscle fibre size. *Clinical Physiology.* 1984;4:183-188.

39. Shaffer MA, Okereke E, Esterhai J, et al. Effects of immobilization on plantar-flexion torque, fatigue, resistance, and functional ability following an ankle fracture. *Phys Ther.* 2000;80:769-780.

40. Bang MD, Deyle GD. Comparison of supervised exercise with and without manual physical therapy for patients with shoulder impingement. *J Orthop Sports Phys Ther.* 2000;30:126-137.

41. Nicholson GG. The effects of passive joint mobilization on pain and hypomobility associated with adhesive capsulitis. *J Orthop Sports Phys Ther.* 1985;6:238-246.

42. Schneider G. Restricted shoulder movement: capsular contracture or cervical referral—a clinical study. *Aust J Physiother.* 1989;35:97-100.

43. Maitland GD. *Peripheral Manipulation.* 3rd ed. London, England: Butterworth-Heinemann; 1991.

44. Threlkeld JA. The effects of manual therapy on connective tissue. *Phys Ther.* 1992;72:893-902.

45. Finsterbush A, Freidman B. Reversibility of joint changes produced by immobilization in rabbits. *Clin Orthop.* 1975;111:290-298.

46. Jortikka MO, Inkinen RI, Tammi MI, et al. Immobilisation causes long lasting matrix changes both in the immobilized and contralateral joint cartilage. *Ann Rheum Dis.* 1997;56:255-261.

47. American Physical Therapy Association. Guide to physical therapist practice. 2nd ed. *Phys Ther.* 2001;81:9-744.

48. Waylett-Rendall J, Seibly DS. A study of the accuracy of a commercially available volumeter. *J Hand Ther.* 1991;January-March:10-13.

49. Buddenberg LA, Davis C. Test-retest reliability of the Purdue pegboard test. *Am J Occup Ther.* 2000;54:555-558.

50. MacDermaid JC, Richards RS, Donner A, Bellamy N, Roth JH. Responsiveness of the short form-36. Disability of the arm, shoulder, and hand questionnaire, patient-rated wrist evaluation, and physical impairment measurements in evaluating recovery after a distal radius fracture. *J Hand Surg (Am).* 2000;25A:330-340.

51. Cyriax JH. *Textbook of Orthopaedic Medicine.* 8th ed. London, England: Baillere Tindall; 1998.

52. Klassbo M, Ringdahl-Harms K, Larsson G. Examination of passive ROM capsular patterns in the hip. *Physiother Res Int.* 2003;8:1-12.

53. Byl NN, Kohlhase W, Engel G. Functional limitation immediately after cast immobilization and closed reduction of distal radius fractures. *J Hand Ther.* 1999;12:201-211.

54. Watts CF, Taylor NF, Baskus K. Do Colles' fracture patients benefit from routine referral to physiotherapy following cast removal? *Arch Orthop Trauma Surgery.* 2000;120(7-8):413-415.

55. Buckwalter JA, Grodzinsky AJ. Loading and healing of bone, fibrous tissue, and muscles: implications for orthopaedic practice. *J Am Acad Orthop Surg.* 1999;7:291-299.

56. Williams PE, Catanese T, Lucey EG, Goldspink G. The importance of stretch and contractile activity in the prevention of connective tissue accumulation in muscle. *Anatomy.* 1998;158:109-114.

57. Can F, Erden Z, Yuceturk A. The effect of manual therapy in the rehabilitation of distal radius fractures [Turkish]. *Fizyoterapi Rehabilitasyon.* 2001;12(3):99-104.

58. Eleveru RA, Rothstein JM, Lamb RL. Goniometric reliability in a clinical setting: subtalar and ankle joint measurements. *Phys Ther.* 1988;68:672-677.

59. Dogra AS, Rangan A. Early mobilsation versus immobilization of surgically treated ankle fracture. Prospective randomized control trial. *Injury.* 1999;30:417-419.

60. Duchateau J. Bed rest induces neural and contractile adaptations in triceps surae. *Med Sci Sports Exerc.* 1995;27:1581-1589.

61. Geboers JFM, van Tuijl, Seelen HAM, Drost MR. Effect of immobilization on ankle dorsiflexion strength. *Scand J Rehab Med.* 2000;32:66-71.

62. Tropp H, Norlin R. Ankle performance after ankle fracture: a randomized study of early mobilization. *Foot Ankle Int.* 1995;16:7-83.

63. Wilson FM. Manual therapy versus traditional exercise in mobilizations of the ankle post-ankle fracture: a pilot study. *New Zealand Journal of Physiotherapy.* 1991;Dec:11-16.

Impaired Joint Mobility, Motor Function, Muscle Performance, and Range of Motion Associated With Joint Arthroplasty (Pattern H)

Karen A. Fritzsche, PT
Susan Collura Schiliro, PT, DPT, CHT

ANATOMY

HIP

The hip joint is a multiaxial ball and socket type of synovial joint. It is formed by the head of the femur and the acetabulum of the pelvis. The head of the femur is covered with hyaline cartilage. The joint allows for flexion/extension in the sagittal plane, abduction/adduction in the frontal plane, and IR/ER in the transverse plane.[1] Stability in the hip comes from the muscles, the capsule, and the strong intrinsic ligaments. Knowledge of the muscle groups is important in considering the surgical procedure and resulting impairments. A summary of the muscles and their motions are found in Table 8-1.[2]

The acetabulum is deepened by the fibrocartilaginous acetabular labrum. The ligaments of the hip joint are the transverse, articular capsular, iliofemoral, ligamentum teres, ischiofemoral, and the pubofemoral. The transverse acetabular ligament completes the rim of the acetabulum. The articular capsule encompasses the hip joint and most of the neck of the femur and functions to hold the head of the femur in the acetabulum. The iliofemoral ligament is an accessory band of fibers that connects with the articular capsule and covers the anterior aspect of the hip joint. It

helps to strengthen the capsular ligament and functions to prevent hyperextension during standing, abduction, and ER. The ligamentous teres femoris (ligament of the head of the femur) is a triangular band from the head of the femur blending into the transverse acetabular ligament. It is a weak ligament and functions as a guide for the artery to the head of the femur. The ischiofemoral ligament blends with the capsule and acts as a check to IR. Finally, the pubofemoral ligament joins the iliofemoral ligament and functions to check abduction.[1,2]

It is important to note that the articular capsule is either excised or saved for later repair during a posterolateral total hip arthroplasty (THA). This approach provides good visualization without disturbing the abductor mechanism.[3]

KNEE

The knee complex consists of both the tibiofemoral and patellofemoral joints. These joints are contained within one joint capsule. The distal femoral condyles and the proximal tibial condyles make up the tibiofemoral articulation. The knee joint anatomy allows for flexion and extension with slight medial and lateral rotation when the knee is in flexion. The patellofemoral joint is the articulation between the patella and the femur, and it allows for sliding of the patella on the femur.

Table 8-1
HIP MUSCLES AND THEIR ACTIONS[2]

Flexion	Extension	Abduction	Adduction	Internal Rotation	External Rotation
Iliopsoas	Gluteus maximus	Gluteus medius	Adductor magnus	Gluteus medius	Piriformis
Sartorius	Semitendinosus	Gluteus minimus	Adductor longus	Gluteus minimus	Obturator internus
Pectineus	Semimembranosus	Tensor fascia latae	Adductor brevis	Tensor fascia latae	Gemilli
Rectus femoris	Biceps femoris	Piriformis	Gracilis	Adductor magnus	Obturator externus
Adductor longus	Adductor magnus (posterior portion)	Sartorius	Pectineus		Quadratus femoris
Adductor brevis			Obturator externus		Gluteus maximus
Adductor magnus (anterior portion)			Quadratus femoris		Adductors (all)
Tensor fascia latae					

The knee joint is surrounded by a fibrous capsule that is strengthened by the surrounding ligaments. The capsule helps to maintain joint integrity and is lined with synovium. The ligaments prevent or control excessive movement. The function of the ligaments is as follows: the patellar ligament provides anterior reinforcement to the joint capsule; the fibular or lateral collateral ligament resists varus stresses across the knee joint; the tibial or medial collateral ligament resists valgus stresses across the knee joint and checks ER of the tibia; the posterior oblique ligament (POL) resists ER; and the arcuate popliteal ligament (APL) complex, or posterolateral corner, reinforces the lateral side of the knee and is a secondary restraint to posterior tibial translation. Both the POL and APL reinforce the capsule posteriorly. The cruciate ligaments are located within the articular capsule but outside the synovial cavity. The posterior cruciate prevents anterior displacement of the femur on the tibia and checks IR of the tibia on the femur. The anterior cruciate prevents anterior movement of the tibia on the femur and hyperextension and IR of the tibia on the femur.[1,2]

The menisci are fibrocartilagenous and are located on the tibial condyles. They function to distribute weightbearing forces, deepen the articular surfaces, and increase joint congruency of the tibia. The internal edges of the menisci are poorly vascularized and therefore do not heal well.[4]

The muscle that provides the most stability to the knee joint is the quadriceps femoris. A list of the muscles surrounding the knee joint and their motions are found on Table 8-2.[1]

SHOULDER

The shoulder joint is a ball and socket synovial joint in which the head of the humerus articulates with the glenoid. The glenoid fossa is a shallow cavity that covers approximately one-third of the humeral head. The cavity is deepened by the glenoid labrum. The humeral head is covered with hyaline cartilage that is thickest centrally and thinnest peripherally. Conversely, the glenoid fossa is lined by hyaline cartilage that is thickest peripherally and thinnest centrally.

The anatomy of the GH joint allows for the largest amount of range of any joint in the body, including flexion/extension, abduction/adduction, and IR/ER. With this increased ROM comes decreased stability.[1]

Stability of the joint is provided by the static and dynamic stabilizers. The static stabilizers consist of the capsule, the labrum, and the ligaments. The dynamic stabilizers are the four rotator cuff muscles (supraspinatus, infraspinatus, teres minor, and subscapularis [SITS muscles]).[1]

The joint is surrounded by a thin, fibrous capsule that arises from the glenoid cavity and attaches to the anatomical neck of the humerus. The capsule is taut in abduction and relaxed in adduction. The inferior portion is the weakest. Superiorly it encloses the long head of the biceps.[1,2]

There are multiple ligaments that help to provide stability to the shoulder joint. The GH ligaments are thickenings of the anterior portion of the capsule that help to stabilize the anterior and inferior portions of the capsule. The transverse humeral ligament passes from the lesser to the greater tuberosity and helps hold the tendon of the long head of the biceps as it emerges from the capsule. The coracohumeral ligament arises from the coracoid process and blends into the supraspinatus. It provides stability by strengthening the superior portion of the capsule. There is a protective arch, known as the coracoacromial arch (made up of the coracoid process, coracoacromial ligament, and the acromion) that prevents displacement of the humeral head superiorly from the glenoid cavity.[1,2]

The rotator cuff muscles help to center and hold the head of the humerus in the glenoid cavity and provide the most stability to the shoulder in abduction. The supraspinatus and the coracoacromial arch provide stability superiorly; the infraspinatus and teres minor provide stability posteriorly;

and the subscapularis provides stability anteriorly. The least stability is provided inferiorly and thus is the direction in which the shoulder is most likely to dislocate.[1] Table 8-3 describes the muscles of the shoulder and their motions.[2] It is important to note that although the deltoid is a strong abductor of the shoulder, it cannot initiate the movement. The supraspinatus is critical in the early phases of shoulder abduction.

METACARPOPHALANGEAL JOINT

The MCP joint is a condyloid synovial joint. It is formed by the distal end of the head of the metacarpal (MC) bone and the proximal end of the adjoining base of the proximal phalanx. A fibrous capsule that has a synovial membrane lining encapsulates this joint.[5] The collateral ligaments originate from both sides of the MC head and travel in a volar and oblique direction distally to both sides of the respective proximal phalanx base. These ligaments fuse together on the anterior (palmar) side of the MCP joint and form a thick fibrocartilaginous structure called the palmar or volar plate. The collateral ligaments serve to strengthen and stabilize the lateral sides of the MCP joint when positioned in flexion.[6]

The extensor digitorum communis muscle originates from the lateral epicondyle of the humerus within the fourth extensor compartment.[5] This compartment accommodates the four tendon slips of the extensor digitorum communis

and the more deeply situated and functionally independent extensor indicis proprius muscle. The four tendons of the extensor digitorum communis flatten as they pass deep to the extensor retinaculum at the wrist, enter the dorsal surface of the hand and continue distally over each of the four finger MCs. On the dorsal surface of the hand, the extensor digitorum communis tendons are interconnected by tendinous communications that preclude its independent action on a single finger.[6] Each extensor tendon flattens again at the level of the MCP joint and forms the extensor expansion which is a triangular tendinous aponeurosis that wraps around the sides of each MC and the proximal portion of the proximal phalanx. This is anchored by the palmar ligament. The extensor expansion is responsible for maintaining the extensor digitorum tendon in a central position on the top of the MC head. The extensor tendon continues distally over the proximal phalanx and inserts dorsally at the central slip at the base of the middle phalanx. This insertion is called the central slip. The extensor digitorum communis tendon is a prime mover for extension of both the MCP joint and PIP joint.[6]

TRAPEZIOMETACARPAL JOINT

This region is referred to as the basal joint complex. It is comprised of the four articulations of the trapezium bone—the thumb MC, the scaphoid and trapezoid, and the

Table 8-2
KNEE MUSCLES AND THEIR ACTIONS[1]

Flexion	Extension	Internal Rotation	External Rotation
Semimembranosus	Quadriceps femoris	Popliteus	Biceps femoris
Semitendinosus	Tensor fascia latae	Semimembranosus	
Biceps femoris		Semitendinosus	
Sartorius		Sartorius	
Gracilis		Gracilis	
Popliteus			
Gastrocnemius			
Plantaris			

Table 8-3
SHOULDER MUSCLES AND THEIR ACTIONS[2]

Flexion	Extension	Abduction	Adduction	Internal Rotation	External Rotation
Pectoralis major	Latissimus dorsi	Deltoid	Pectoralis major	Pectoralis major	Infraspinatus
Deltoid	Teres major	Supraspinatus	Latissimus dorsi	Latissimus dorsi	Teres minor
Coracobrachialis	Deltoid		Teres major	Teres major	Deltoid
Biceps	Triceps		Subscapularis	Deltoid	
			Triceps		

Table 8-4

INTRINSIC MUSCLES OF THE THUMB AND THEIR ACTIONS[5]

Muscle	Action
Abductor pollicis brevis	Abduction of thumb
Flexor pollicis brevis	Flexion and rotation of thumb
Opponens pollicis	Rotation of first metacarpal toward palm

radial facet of the index MC.[7] The actual anatomical trapeziometacarpal (TM) joint is composed of two reciprocally opposed, tightly fitting, saddle-shaped articulations and is commonly referred to as the basal joint or CMC joint.[8] This anatomical arrangement affords the thumb a great amount of mobility and versatility, allowing for a wide arc of motion. However, the basal joint has very little intrinsic stability and is therefore dependent upon extrinsic soft tissue restraints for stability. The five major ligaments that provide stability to this joint are the ACL, also referred to as the beak ligament because of its attachment to the beak of the thumb MC; the intermetacarpal ligament; the ulnar collateral ligament; the POL; and the dorsal radial ligament.[9] Thumb mobility is necessary for hand dexterity. Conversely, thumb stability is necessary for a pain-free, powerful, pinch.[10]

The muscles of the thumb and their actions are outlined in Table 8-4.[5]

KINESIOLOGY

HIP

The hip joint is a very large and stable joint. The intrinsic stability is aided by strong surrounding musculature and the articular capsule. Arthrokinematically, the convex femoral head glides within the concave acetabulum allowing for the femoral head to glide in the opposite direction of the distal end of the femur. Both spin and glide occur in the hip.[11]

Hip motion occurs in three planes: sagittal, frontal, and transverse. Normal hip ROM is as follows: 10 to 30 degrees of extension, 120 to 135 degrees of flexion (with the knee bent), 30 to 50 degrees of abduction, 10 to 30 degrees adduction, 30 to 45 degrees of IR, and 45 to 60 degrees of ER.[11]

Normal gait requires 30 to 40 degrees of hip flexion, 10 degrees of extension, 5 degrees of abduction and adduction, and 5 degrees of IR and ER.[5] During gait the greatest degree of hip flexion is achieved during late swing, as the LE moves forward for heel strike. The greatest degree of hip extension occurs at toe off. There is minimal abduction during late swing, and adduction occurs at heel strike into late stance. ER occurs throughout the swing phase, and IR occurs just before heel strike.

A study by Bergmann examined the body weight forces present during a variety of activities (Table 8-5). Bergmann referenced earlier studies by Pauwels, Blount, and Denham that described the use of a cane on the contralateral side as reducing force on the femoral head.[12]

Johnston studied the ROM requirements at the hip for various ADL and functional activities. The results can be found in Table 8-6.[13]

KNEE

The knee joint is an important part of the kinematic chain providing mobility and also support for the body weight statically and dynamically. The knee joint sustains high forces. Although the primary motions at the knee joint are flexion and extension, motions also occur in the frontal and transverse planes. Normal ROM is 5 to 10 degrees of hyperextension to 130 to 140 degrees of flexion. Approximately 60 degrees of knee flexion and 0 degrees of knee extension are required during the gait cycle. The position of the hip can influence knee ROM because of the presence of many two-joint muscles.[11] Kettelkamp described the degree of ROM of knee flexion required to perform various functional activities (Table 8-7).[14]

There is an asymmetry in the size of the medial and lateral condyles causing incongruence at these joints. In the closed chain position, terminal medial rotation of the femur occurs in the final degrees of extension placing the knee joint in the close-packed position. This is known as the screw home mechanism. The femur must laterally rotate before the knee unlocks and flexion can resume. In an open chain position, the tibia laterally rotates on the fixed femur to lock the knee and medially rotates the tibia on the femur to unlock the knee.[11]

Table 8-5

BODY WEIGHT FORCES ON HIP JOINT DURING ACTIVITY[12]

Activity	Body Weight Forces
Single leg stance	2x BW
SLR	1.5 to 1.8x BW
Stair climbing	2 to 3.5x BW
Jogging	5x BW
Level walking	2.7x BW
Cycling	Very little, 2.7x BW quick acceleration
Carrying load ipsilateral side	Reduced the force transmitted

Table 8-6

HIP RANGE OF MOTION REQUIREMENTS DURING ACTIVITIES[13]

Activity	Hip ROM Requirements
Tying shoes	120 degrees flexion
Sitting/average seat	112 degrees flexion
Stooping	125 degrees flexion
Squatting	115 degrees flexion
	20 degrees abduction
	20 degrees IR
Ascending stairs	67 degrees flexion
Descending stairs	36 degrees flexion
Putting foot on	120 degrees flexion
opposite thigh	20 degrees abduction
	20 degrees ER
Putting on pants	90 degrees flexion

SHOULDER

The shoulder joint is made up of multiple articulations that allow for the arm to be positioned in space and perform many functional activities. The shoulder is in the close-packed position when it is abducted and externally rotated. The GH joint has three degrees of freedom: flexion/extension, abduction/adduction, and IR/ER. To obtain full abduction the humerus must be externally rotated so the greater tubercle can pass under or behind the acromion. There is less restriction of movement because the capsule is less taut when the humerus moves in the plane of the scapula. In this position, ER of the humerus is not needed to help the greater tubercle clear the acromion. The arthrokinematics allow for rolling and gliding of the humeral head on the glenoid fossa in a direction opposite to movement of the shaft of the humerus. The muscles of the GH joint help to move the humerus, provide gliding, and maintain apposition of the joint surfaces.[11] The shoulder allows for 180 degrees of forward flexion, 60 degrees of extension, 180 degrees of abduction, and 90 degrees of IR/ER.

METACARPOPHALANGEAL JOINT

The MCP joints of the index, middle, ring, and small fingers are classified as condyloid. The convex surface of the MC head articulating with the concave surface of the base of the respective proximal phalanx allows for movement in two planes: flexion/extension in the sagittal plane and abduction/adduction in the frontal plane.[15] The close-packed position of the MCP joint is full flexion (90 degrees). The lateral motions of abduction and adduction cannot occur while the joint is in the close-packed position because of the tightness of the collateral ligaments. The collateral ligaments are redundant when

the joint is in full extension, which allows abduction to be relatively free. Passive accessory motions of distraction, rotation, dorsal, volar, medial, and lateral glides have the greatest motion in this position. This allows the fingers to span apart as in the grasp of a large cylindrical object.

TRAPEZIOMETACARPAL JOINT

The CMC joint is considered the weightbearing joint of the UE. The first CMC joint of the thumb is the articulation between the first MC and the trapezium bone. It is unique in that it is a saddle joint with two degrees of freedom: flexion/extension and abduction/adduction. It also allows for a combination of motions, which are referred to as axial rotation.

The axes of motion are oblique due to the natural configuration of the carpal bone arch.[15] Flexion and extension occur around an oblique coronal axis allowing them to be almost completely parallel to the palm (frontal plane) and abduction and adduction nearly perpendicular to the palm (sagittal plane). This is directly opposite to the rest of the finger motions.

Kinesiologically and functionally, the most important motion of the thumb is opposition.[16] Opposition is a combination of thumb abduction, coupled with rotation at the CMC joint that allows the thumb to move towards the tip of the little finger. Flexion of the thumb MP and IP joints helps to bring the thumb tip closer to the fingertips.[16] Abduction and adduction may be performed during any position of opposition, which creates versatility in the function of the thumb. The uniqueness of this joint and its ability to perform multiple motions at the same time is due to its saddle-type joint configuration. The analogy of this can be made to a rider on a horse shifting from side to side in the saddle in various positions of forward and backward tipping. The muscles activated for abduction/adduction will vary based upon the exact degree of opposition.[17]

The compressive forces exerted at the CMC joint and on its stabilizing structures during lateral pinch (thumb pulp to side/tip of index finger) are magnified 10 to 15 times.[18] Picking up a full glass of water would require approximately

Table 8-7

KNEE RANGE OF MOTION REQUIREMENTS DURING ACTIVITIES[14]

Activity	Knee ROM Requirements
Tying shoes	0 to 106 degrees flexion
Sitting down	0 to 93 degrees flexion
Ascending stairs	0 to 83 degrees flexion
Descending stairs	0 to 90 degrees flexion
Swing phase of gait	0 to 67 degrees flexion

2 lbs of pinch strength, while the forces exerted on the CMC joint during this motion is 20 to 30 lbs.

PATHOPHYSIOLOGY

Arthritis is a leading cause of disability in the United States with OA being the most common form.[19,20] Primary OA is a progressive degenerative disease of the joints of unknown etiology. Weightbearing joints such as the hip, knee, and lumbar spine are most commonly affected. Characteristics of primary OA are the destruction of articular cartilage and osteophyte formation resulting in impaired function.

Secondary OA more commonly affects only one joint and is the result of incongruity between the joint surfaces (eg, OA that occurs as a result of developmental dysplasia of the hip or trauma to a joint).[3]

Early stages of OA are often treated conservatively through nonpharmacologic and pharmacologic interventions.[20] Nonpharmacologic treatment interventions include patient education, weight loss (that is often hindered by the inability to walk distances secondary to pain), activity restriction, support groups, aquatic exercise programs, and physical and occupational therapy. Physical therapy includes education of the patient; strengthening of the muscles around the joint and throughout the extremity; providing appropriate assistive, adapted, supportive, and protective devices; and instruction in joint protection.

HIP

Hip OA has been cited to occur in 0.5/1000 people per year.[19] Characteristics of hip OA include groin pain, anterior or lateral thigh pain, stiffness in the morning, leg length discrepancy, and limitations and/or pain with motion at the hip.[20] The pain is often chronic, persistent, and progressive. Pain at night may interfere with sleep and is often present with motion and weightbearing. Ambulation quality and distance decrease as pain increases.

Leg length discrepancy may be seen if the femoral head or acetabulum is worn or deformed. The affected extremity is usually slightly shortened, flexed, externally rotated, and adducted. Resulting muscle shortening or contractures of the hip flexors and adductors may also be found. Other joint abnormalities, such as contractures of the knee and scoliosis of the spine, must also be analyzed in order to determine the source of the possible leg length discrepancy.

The American College of Rheumatology uses the following classification criteria for diagnosis of hip OA: the presence of hip pain in addition to two out of the following three items: 1) erythrocyte sedimentation rate (ESR) <20 mm/hour, 2) evidence of radiographic femoral or acetabular osteophytes, and 3) evidence of radiographic joint space narrowing.[21]

KNEE

OA is the most common form of arthritis of the knee.[2] Symptoms of knee OA include pain, stiffness, and swelling. Pain is worse in the morning and with activities such as walking, kneeling, and stairs. Common deformities include genu varum and valgum and knee flexion contractures. Genu valgum is associated with arthritis of the lateral compartment and genu varum with the medial compartment. Post-traumatic arthritis is also a common diagnosis successfully treated by total knee arthroplasty (TKA).

SHOULDER

OA of the shoulder is characterized by pain, stiffness, loss of motion, and grinding or grating within the joint. The head of the humerus flattens and becomes enlarged. There is also wear of the glenoid posteriorly as the head of humerus displaces posteriorly. As a whole, the capsule becomes contracted but more so in the anterior portion, resulting in IR contractures. The rotator cuff may be contracted from chronic restriction of motion, but is not usually torn. Upon physical examination, tenderness can be elicited along the posterior line, and there is a flattening of the anterior shoulder and fullness posteriorly. Forward flexion, ER, and IR may be painful, and ROM becomes restricted as pain increases. Early in the arthritic process pain is worse in the morning, worsens with activity, and lessens with rest. As the disease progresses, pain becomes constant. Strength of the external rotators is not often affected because the rotator cuff is usually intact. As in the hip and knee, osteophyte formations may occur.[22-24]

OA is the most common cause for total shoulder arthroplasty (TSA). Other diseases associated with TSA may include RA, post-traumatic arthritis, osteonecrosis, and septic arthritis.[23]

METACARPOPHALANGEAL JOINT

The extensor digitorum communis tendons, the collateral ligaments, the accessory collateral ligaments, and the volar plate help to stabilize and prevent volar subluxation or dislocation of the MCP joint during active motion.[25] The progressive rheumatoid process damages these stabilizing structures and the articular surface of the affected joint. The destructive process of the articular surface of the MCP joint occurs in the space between the MC head and the origin of the collateral ligament. This destructive process begins as proliferative synovitis that stretches the joint capsule and its stabilizing ligamentous structures.[26] This process may also result in fraying of the collateral ligaments.

The normal MCP joint is most stable in full flexion and allows for little lateral motion in this position. However, in the rheumatoid hand, the flexed MCP joint may often be laterally deviated as much as 45 degrees. Flatt[27] believed that the laxity of the collateral ligaments at the MCP joint in the rheumatoid hand significantly reduced its inherent stability. This is one of the early factors that leads to the progressive ulnar drift deformity commonly seen in the rheumatoid hand. Proliferative synovitis is also responsible for damage of the stabilizing structures of the dorsal extensor expansion. This disruption allows the extensor digitorum tendon to sublux in an ulnar direction off of the MC head and is another contributing factor to the ulnar drift pattern of the fingers (Figure 8-1).

TRAPEZIOMETACARPAL JOINT

OA of the basal joint is commonly found in the aging population, affecting 25% of women and 8% of men between the ages of 50 and 70 years. Post-menopausal women are afflicted 10 to 20 times more commonly than their male counterparts.[7] The shallow concavity of the basal joint, coupled with its ligamentous laxity, and the relative thinness of its cartilage in women predisposes it to high shear stresses and subsequent degeneration. The primary stabilizer of the joint is the anterior oblique ligament (beak ligament).[28] If this ligament becomes attenuated by trauma or by internal factors, it may fray or subsequently detach initiating the degeneration process of the basal joint.[28]

Progressive basal joint arthritis leads to imbalance with predictable deformation of the entire thumb ray (MC and respective phalanges). Dorsal radial subluxation of the CMC joint results in a characteristic and disabling adduction posture of the first MC that is clinically seen as a diminished thumb-index web angle. This imbalance produces a compensatory hyperextension posture at the thumb MP joint and flexion at the IP joint (zigzag deformity).[28]

The prominence or shoulder sign[29] is another common deformity in progressive basal joint arthritis and is seen at

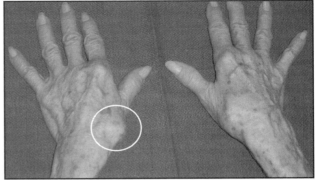

Figure 8-2. Left hand presents with shoulder sign. Right hand is postoperative.

the level of the base of the first MC. This deformity is caused by dorsal subluxation of the thumb MC over the trapezium bone (Figure 8-2).

The grind test is a specific evaluative test that helps make a clinical diagnosis of CMC OA by identifying isolated cartilage damage.[30] It is performed by palpation of the patient's CMC joint with the examiner's thumb while compressing and circumducting the first MC on the trapezium bone.[30] A positive grind test would produce pain at the CMC joint level directly under the examiner's thumb.

ARTHROPLASTY AS TREATMENT FOR OSTEOARTHRITIS

Failure of conservative therapies for OA, pain, and loss of function may lead to the need for surgical intervention. Total joint arthroplasty (TJA) is a highly successful procedure for replacing arthritic, painful, and deteriorated joints. OA is the leading cause of hip, knee, and shoulder joint arthroplasties.

The goals of TJA are to relieve pain and increase mobility while maintaining stability and improving function.

HIP

Impairments that may be found with OA of the hip are loss of functional ROM, decreased ability to perform ADL/IADL, decreased strength, and the inability to work. Loss of ROM in the hip may lead to the inability to tie shoelaces, put socks on independently, and cut toenails.

THA is an operative procedure where the diseased hip joint is resected and replaced with an artificial acetabulum, femoral component, and polyethylene liner. The components are fixated by bone cement (polymethylmethacrylate) or bone ingrowth. According to the most recent statistics available from the American Academy of Orthopaedic Surgeons, there were an estimated 75,000 THA surgeries performed in 1982, 134,000 in 1995, and 217,000 in 2003.[31]

Other disorders that may successfully be treated with THA include avascular necrosis, certain types of hip frac-

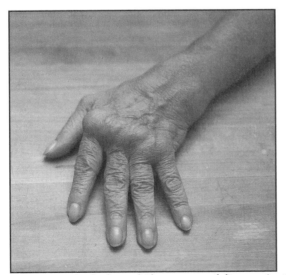

Figure 8-1. Typical ulnar drift pattern of fingers in the rheumatoid hand.

tures, bone tumors, other forms of arthritis (eg, RA, juvenile RA), Paget's disease, and ankylosing spondylitis.

The age range of patients appropriate for THA has expanded over the past two decades. Traditionally the best candidates were considered to be patients between 60 and 75 years of age who were less active and therefore would put less mechanical stress on the implants. Outcomes of alternative procedures performed on younger populations have not proven to be more effective than THA. In the elderly population, it appears that poor outcomes are related to factors such as multiple co-morbidities, not age.[32]

Contraindications to performing a THA include local or systemic infection, medical instability, a neuropathic or Charcot joint, rapidly progressive neurologic diseases, and absent or insufficient musculature in the abductors and quadriceps. Despite concerns about mechanical failure in the obese population, the long-term outcome of reduced pain and disability are similar to the general population.[32]

Dislocation is a serious complication following THA. The overall incidence has been reported to be 2% to 3%, of which 75% to 81% was reported to occur within the first 3 months after surgery when the soft tissues are their weakest.[33,34] There is no consensus as to how long precautions should be maintained. Total hip precautions following a posterolateral approach are no hip flexion past 90 degrees, no IR beyond neutral, and no adduction past midline. Late dislocation is generally related to intrinsic instability of the prosthetic joint.

Early dislocation factors may be categorized into three areas: 1) patient-related, including patient compliance, revision hip arthroplasty, and patients with neurological deficits; 2) surgeon-related, including the type of approach, the experience of the surgeon, and orientation of the acetabular component (cup malposition); and 3) miscellaneous, including infection, trauma, and profound weight loss with resulting loss of muscle mass. Factors not found to be significant include age, height, weight, obesity, and preoperative diagnosis.[33,34]

Other complications following THA include DVT, pulmonary embolism, HO, periprosthetic fracture, nerve injury, leg length discrepancy, infection, and loosening.[33]

KNEE

TKA is an operative procedure where the diseased knee joint is resected and replaced with an artificial tibial and femoral component and a polyethylene liner. The patella may or may not be replaced or lined with polyethylene. The components are fixated by bone cement (polymethylmethacrylate) or bone ingrowth. The most recent statistics available from the American Academy of Orthopaedic Surgeons, estimate 160,000 TKA surgeries were performed in 1991, 216,000 in 1995, and 402,000 in 2003.[31]

Statistics from the American Academy of Orthopaedic

Surgeons indicate the average age of patients in 1999 was 67 years. Sixty-eight percent of all TKA surgeries performed were on people over 65 years of age.[31] TKA surgical candidates followed a trend similar to that of the THA population. The age range of patients having TKA over the past 20 years continues to expand. Physicians are weighing the possibility of revision surgery in the future against physical disability that can occur while waiting 5 to 10 years for a TKA. Patients in the fourth and fifth decade, who fail conservative treatment, are now considered possible candidates for TKA. TKA is also performed on patients well into their 80s who do not have contraindications and where functional mobility and quality of life may be improved. Careful patient selection is necessary for any successful outcome following surgery. Contraindications to TKA include local or systemic infection, medical instability, neuropathic or Charcot joint, rapidly progressive neurologic diseases, and absent or insufficient musculature in the quadriceps.

Complications following TKA include DVT, pulmonary embolism, periprosthetic fracture, nerve injury, loosening, infection, and joint stiffness.

Many patients affected with OA and RA experience bilateral joint disease. This requires a decision regarding whether to perform simultaneous bilateral TKA or a staged procedure, either within one or two hospitalizations. Simultaneous bilateral TKA is associated with a higher number of complications including hypoxia, DVT, arrhythmia, congestive heart failure, confusion, ileus, and increased blood loss requiring a greater number of blood transfusions. Reported benefits of simultaneous bilateral TKA include greater patient satisfaction, lower overall recovery time, similar functional improvement, decreased time until relief of pain is gained, and decreased costs for both the patient and facility.[35,36] Ultimately, this is a decision that requires clearance by the medical and surgical team and a desire by the patient to have only one surgical episode.

SHOULDER

TSA includes the resection of the humeral head and replacement with a humeral head, glenoid component, and a polyethylene liner. Components can be cemented or uncemented and constrained, semi-constrained, or unconstrained.

Indications include pain that no longer responds to conservative treatment and loss of function. Stiffness alone is not considered to be an indication for TSA.[23] Contraindications include an active or recent infection, a neuropathic joint, a noncompliant patient, and a combination of loss or paralysis of the rotator cuff and deltoid muscles. Loss of either muscle alone may be managed during surgery with soft tissue procedures and/or muscle transfers.[23]

The most common complication following TSA is postoperative instability that occurs most often with unconstrained TSAs. Instability that is demonstrated by sub-luxation or dislocation of the humeral head may occur anteriorly, posteriorly, superiorly, or inferiorly. Posterior instability is most common because of the asymmetric wear of the glenoid. There is the potential for the glenoid component to be placed in too much retroversion, allowing the humeral component to slide down the face of the glenoid. Anterior instability usually occurs secondary to a rupture of the repaired subscapularis and capsule. Superior instability is associated with rotator cuff pathology and inferior instability is associated with muscle atrophy or incorrect humeral length.[22,23,37]

The second most common complication is postoperative rotator cuff tears.[38] Small tears result in minimal symptoms that may often be corrected with physical therapy. Larger rotator cuff tears are associated with poor outcomes.[22]

Component loosening is more common on the glenoid side. Postoperative x-rays must be taken periodically to evaluate for loosening. Radiolucent lines around the glenoid are common, but actual clinical worsening is infrequent. Mechanical failure is more common with constrained designs.[22,23]

Other complications include tubercle nonunion or malunion (for arthroplasties related to proximal humeral fractures), periprosthetic fracture, infection, nerve injury, deltoid rupture, humeral loosening, impingement, and heterotopic bone formation.[22]

Soft tissue balancing during surgery has an important affect on the degree of shoulder stiffness following TSA. If the subscapularis is shortened or overtightened the joint may be stiff. It is important to release all adhesions intraoperatively, surgically address capsular tightness, and lengthen the subscapularis. If an acceptable ROM is achieved intraoperatively, then subsequent stiffness is probably related to inadequate rehabilitation.[23] A joint that is overstuffed with components that are too large may result in difficulty achieving ROM, especially ER.[22]

METACARPOPHALANGEAL JOINT

MCP joint replacement typically is reserved for the patient with severe RA and specifically for those who demonstrate joint space narrowing, ulnar drift, volar subluxation, and/or intrinsic tightness. In 1953, Brannon and Klein[39] introduced the first titanium intramedullary stemmed flexible hinged prosthesis. Since that time, many different types of MCP joint implants have been introduced, however, all may be classified into three categories of prostheses that include: the hinged prosthesis, the flexible prosthesis, and the surface prosthesis. In 1961, Flatt[27] developed a newer metal-hinged implant improving on the original hinged design. However, inherent in this design was a high fracture rate. A solution to this problem led to the development of the flexible hinged prosthesis. In 1966, Swanson introduced

the first silastic flexible hinged prosthesis to be used in MCP joint implant arthroplasty.[40] In 1986, Swanson improved upon the molecular structure of the silastic to reduce the high fracture rate.

As revolutionary as the introduction of silastic was to the surgical repertoire of implant arthroplasty, complications, such as transplant fracture, dislocation, loosening, and recurrent ulnar deviation, continued to occur. Swanson and his associates[41] attempted to address these problems with the use of a titanium grommet as a bone liner to protect the actual implant. In 1987, the Sutter prosthesis was introduced. This prosthesis incorporated collars with the intent of stopping bony outgrowths.[42] Since that time, an extensive variety of designs have been developed and used surgically. Many have challenged the Swanson silastic hinge implant design, but today this design is still the most commonly used prosthesis for finger joint and wrist arthroplasty.

In implant arthroplasty, the flexible hinge implant acts as a dynamic spacer[26] within the joint. The implant becomes encapsulated by a newly forming fibrous pseudocapsule that maintains the implant in place. The formation of the new capsule is referred to as the encapsulation process.[43]

The encapsulation process of the implant begins 3 to 5 days following surgery. The tensile strength of the collagen increases during the next 6 to 8 weeks, however, is not considered to be fully mature until 1 year following surgery.[43] During the first 3 to 4 postoperative weeks, it is imperative that all finger motion is controlled to protect the newly forming joint capsule. The newly formed collagen fibers orient toward the desired longitudinal direction when influenced by controlled stress.[26] The sole purpose of the prolonged, continued use of a dorsal outrigger splint is to direct and control collagen fiber orientation. When motion is delayed or is not controlled by splinting, the collagen fibers tend to form in a disorganized pattern, which impedes proper joint stabilization and results in limited ROM of the newly forming joint[26] (Figure 8-3).

TRAPEZIOMETACARPAL JOINT

Silicone implant arthroplasty was popularized by Swanson[44] and Niebauer[45] in the 1960s. The silicone polymers that have the silicone properties of rubber are referred to as elastomers.[44] The original silastic prostheses of Swanson,[44] Niebauer,[45] and others experienced problems of fragmentation, collapse, and loosening.[46] Subsequently, a high-molecular-weight polymer called silastic high performance was introduced to resolve these problems.[9] The silastic high performance implant generated a fibrous response, resulting in capsular formation ("encapsulation process").[43] The same biological process of encapsulation described for the MCP joint develops and encapsulates the CMC joint following arthroplasty surgery.

Basal joint implant arthroplasty experienced multiple

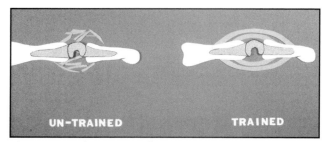

Figure 8-3. The encapsulation process.

problems, including the development of bone cysts, as a direct result of a destructive synovial response caused by "silicone synovitis."[47] The cyclic and shear forces generated at the basal joint resulted in microparticulate debris from shedding from the implant. This debris resulted in an intense inflammatory response that led to progressive destructive bony changes and the formation of bone cysts.[48] Increased recognition of the severity and frequency of complications associated with the use of silicone implants resulted in the steady decline of their use.[28] However, the dissatisfaction with the silicone implant renewed the enthusiasm for the traditional surgical techniques for CMC arthritis (ie, trapezium excision), with or without soft tissue augmentation. This surgical technique was initially reported in 1949 by Gervis[49] and again in 1973.[50] Although elimination of disabling pain was achieved with the original surgical procedure, joint instability with resultant loss of pinch strength proved to be a frequent disadvantage of the "simple" excision (trapeziectomy).[51] Froimson,[52] Carroll,[53] and others[54,55] modified this procedure by interposing rolled autogenous tendon or fascia at the site of the excision to enhance thumb stability. In 1985, Eaton[56] and in 1986, Burton[57] emphasized the efficacy of ligament reconstruction to provide greater stability of the thumb with either a partial or total trapezial excision. Outcomes have shown the direct correlation between increased thumb stability and increased pinch power resulting in improvement in the functional use of the thumb.[7]

Depending on the surgical technique performed, either half or the entire trapezium is excised, and also the flexor carpi radialis tendon or the superficial portion of the abductor pollicis longus tendon is used for ligament stabilization. If the flexor carpi radialis tendon is used, one half of its width from the forearm to the second MC is harvested and used as a "pseudo" ligament for stability. The remaining flexor carpi radialis tendon is rolled in an anchovy fashion and inserted in place of the excised trapezium bone to allow for spacing and cushioning. Elimination of the surrounding arthritic surfaces are routinely performed, and the joint capsule is then closed.[57]

Although there is a continued controversy concerning which surgical technique is most favorable, it is clearly accepted that ligament reconstruction tendon interposition (LRTI) arthroplasty is the treatment of choice for patients who demonstrate Stage III or IV osteoarthritic changes at the basal joint.[7]

Melone,[28] in one of the largest basal joint arthroplasty studies to date, routinely excised the entire trapezium and used a slip of the superficial portion of the abductor pollicis longus tendon instead of the flexor carpi radialis for soft tissue stabilization and ligament reconstruction. Melone and others[58-61] favor using the abductor pollicis longus tendon because of its consistent availability as a substantive source of tissue, the strategic location of its attachment at the CMC joint, and the ease of access requiring a relatively limited dissection. An additional benefit is that procurement of the abductor pollicis longus tendon necessitates division of the first dorsal extensor tendon compartment. Since de Quervain's stenosing tenosynovitis is frequently seen as a concurrent problem in patients with basal joint arthritis, it can be surgically addressed simultaneously using this technique.[28,29,62-64] Melone also felt that sacrificing the flexor carpi radialis tendon (a major wrist flexor) creates weakness of the wrist and therefore may impede postoperative recovery.

In the event that hyperextension laxity of the thumb MP joint is greater than 30 degrees, the joint should be surgically stabilized by arthrodesis. Lesser degrees (<30) of hyperextension at the thumb MP joint may be managed by temporary pinning of the MP joint in 30 degrees of flexion for 4 weeks. Limiting the propensity for hyperextension at the MP joint and effectively unloading the CMC joint protects the arthroplasty and ligament reconstruction against recurrent collapse deformity of the entire thumb.[28] LRTI arthroplasty is now the surgical treatment of choice for basal joint arthritis in Stages III and IV (Table 8-8).[65]

IMAGING

HIP

Roentgenograms are used to confirm the diagnosis of OA and joint destruction. Roentgenograms of the hips, spine, and knees are most common. The individual surgeon will decide which sets of films are needed. Roentgenograms may include A/P and lateral views of the hip and femoral shaft, true or frog lateral, and A/P of the lumbar spine. Some patients may have standing A/P roentgenograms of the hip, knee, and ankle to determine weightbearing alignment and any varus or valgus deformity that may need correction.[3]

Preoperative x-rays are used for diagnosing and templating. Templating aids in selection of the type and size of the implant to insure best fit and neck length.[3]

Postoperative x-rays are used to confirm prosthetic position and are taken in the recovery room and at various inter-

	Table 8-8		
EATON AND GLICKEL RADIOGRAPHIC STAGE TREATMENT OPTIONS[65]			
Stage	*Description*	*Treatment*	*Surgery*
I	Increased TM joint space, subluxation, synovitis, looks relatively normal	Rest, splinting, NSAIDs thenar strengthening	Ligament reconstruction
II	Narrowed TM joint space, osteophyte <2 mm, sclerosis	Rest, splinting, NSAIDs, thenar strengthening	Ligament reconstruction
III	Narrowed or absent TM joint, osteophyte >2 mm, sclerosis, normal ST joint	Rest, splinting, NSAIDs	LRTI arthroplasty, hemi or complete trapeziectomy
IV	Absent or narrowed TM joint, ST joint space changes, pan trapezial arthrosis	Rest, splinting, NSAIDs	LRTI, complete trapeziectomy

TM=trapeziometacarpal joint, ST=scaphoid trapezial joint

vals thereafter. For example, x-rays are commonly taken at the 6-week postoperative follow-up appointment and yearly thereafter. Repeated x-rays are used to identify signs of aseptic loosening and osteolysis (bone resorption).

KNEE

Roentgenograms may include a standing A/P view, a lateral view, and Merchant views. Long leg standing A/P views may also be helpful. The medial and lateral compartments are examined for narrowing. Films are also examined for varus/valgus deformity, osteophyte formation, patella position, and subchondral surface condition. Templating is performed with the use of preoperative roentgenograms.

Postoperative x-rays are used to confirm prosthetic position and are taken in the recovery room and at various intervals thereafter. Repeated x-rays are used to identify signs of aseptic loosening and osteolysis (bone resorption) over time.

SHOULDER

Common views taken during the diagnostic process and prior to surgery include an A/P view of the GH joint, axillary lateral, and scapular lateral or "Y" views. The AC joint should also be examined radiographically.[22]

In an osteoarthritic joint the A/P view shows GH joint narrowing, humeral head elevation, tubercle position, GH wear, subluxation, and osteophyte formation. The axillary view confirms joint space narrowing and the condition of the glenoid. The "Y" view shows the position of the humeral head in the glenoid and the direction of humeral head dislocation.[23,24,33]

CT scans are used to show detailed bony images. Although not done routinely, a CT scan may be used to clarify the position of the tuberosities or look in greater detail at the wear of the glenoid. MRI is used for soft tissue images and may be used to check the status of the rotator cuff. Rotator cuff tears are not common in the patient with

OA of the shoulder.[23]

Postoperatively x-rays are used to determine prosthetic position and signs of loosening or osteolysis.

METACARPOPHALANGEAL JOINT

Both an A/P and a lateral view of the MCP joint are typically taken during the diagnostic process and prior to surgical intervention of the rheumatoid hand. The degree of ulnar deviation is measured on the A/P view. The degree of volar subluxation is assessed using the lateral view. Clinical deformities are usually consistent with the degree of radiographic change.[66] CT and MRI are not routinely performed, unless soft tissue assessment is warranted.

Alter and associates[66] developed a classification system using reference radiographs for various anatomical areas. The patient's radiographs are compared to the standard set of these films. This classification system uses the following grading system:

♦ Grade 0 is a normal joint
♦ Grade I indicates slight joint changes, such as soft tissue swelling, osteoporosis, and mild joint space narrowing
♦ Grade II indicates definite early changes, such as joint space narrowing
♦ Grade III indicates medium destructive changes, such as joint space narrowing and erosion in all joints
♦ Grade IV indicates severe destructive changes, such as loss of joint spaces and bony deformity

TRAPEZIOMETACARPAL JOINT

Three radiographic views of the thumb are routinely performed to determine the degree of OA at the basal joint. They are the A/P, lateral, and oblique views. Eaton and Glickel[65] developed a classification system using a lateral view that is based on the extent of radiographic involvement of the TM joint (see Table 8-8). The lateral view, with the thumb positioned in abduction, gives the clearest picture of the CMC joint. This grading system is useful in determining if conservative management and/or which surgical options would be appropriate for intervention. Stage I radiographs may reveal increased joint space that is indicative of active synovitis, but the films have a relatively normal appearance. Stage II demonstrates classic radiographic signs of osteoarthritic joint "overload" with joint space narrowing and the presence of osteophytes that are less than 2 mm in diameter. Stage III disease reveals more advanced TM involvement with joint narrowing, severe sclerosis, and osteophytes greater than 2 mm in diameter, but without radiographic evidence of scaphoid trapezial disease. Stage IV includes all the properties found in Stage III with the addition of radiographic evidence of scaphoid trapezial involvement.[65]

Diagnostic tools such as MRI, CT, and ultrasound are not routinely used unless other soft tissue problems are suspected.

PHARMACOLOGY

PREOPERATIVE

Pharmacologic intervention is utilized for the relief of pain but cannot reverse any structural or biochemical changes associated with OA.[20] Drug therapies include: non-opioid analgesics such as acetaminophen, NSAIDs such as ibuprofen, opioid analgesics such as codeine, and COX-2 inhibitors such as celecoxib.

NSAIDs are an alternative class of compounds for pain management. These drugs act by reducing prostaglandin synthesis by inhibiting one or both of the COX isoenzymes. They have analgesic activity both locally and centrally and are synergistic with opioids. A serious disadvantage to using NSAIDs is the risk of toxicity and upper gastrointestinal complications. NSAID-related complications are responsible for the hospitalization of more than 100,000 patients and the death of 16,500 patients annually in the United States.[67]

The term opioids refers to synthetic narcotics resembling opiates, but is often used to describe both opiates and synthetic narcotics. Opioids, including morphine, codeine, hydrocodone, and oxycodone, are used as analgesics. These drugs dull the senses, relieve pain, and induce sleep. They are used for exacerbations but are not recommended for long-term use as they are habit forming. Side effects include constipation, dry mouth, nausea, vomiting, dizziness, sweating, and itching.[67]

COX-2 inhibitors (eg, celecoxib) have been found to have an analgesic efficacy similar to NSAIDs. The COX-2 inhibitors have been believed to offer better gastric protection and therefore reduced incidence of gastrointestinal events including perforation, obstruction, symptomatic ulcers, and upper gastrointestinal bleeding.[67] In addition, with their lack of antiplatelet activity at therapeutic dosages, they were

purported to allow patients to continue taking the COX-2 inhibitors throughout the perioperative period. These helped decrease inflammation and pain, prevented exacerbation of arthritic pain in other joints, and allowed greater participation in postoperative rehabilitation.[67]

POSTOPERATIVE

Postoperative pharmacology is focused on pain management as well as managing any preoperative medications. The most common forms of pain management are patient-controlled analgesia (PCA) via epidural or intravenous initially, progressing to oral medication within 1 to 2 days. Medications commonly found alone or in combination in epidural PCAs are opioids (eg, Dilaudid and fentanyl) and local anesthetics (eg, bupivicaine). Opioids are used for intravenous PCAs. Oral medications include opioids and COX-2 inhibitors. COX-2 inhibitors have been found to reduce opioid use while not reducing platelet aggregation.[68] Anti-inflammatory medications are avoided secondary to their blood-thinning properties.

Case Study #1: Total Hip Arthroplasty

Mr. John Williams is a 68-year-old male who has undergone a left hybrid total hip arthroplasty. The case will begin in the acute phase and continue through discharge to home, home care, and outpatient services.

PHYSICAL THERAPIST EXAMINATION

HISTORY

♦ General demographics: Mr. John Williams is a 68-year-old white male whose primary language is English. He is right-hand dominant. He is a college graduate with an MBA.

♦ Social history: Mr. Williams is married and has three children who range in age from 32 to 40 years. He is also the grandfather of five grandchildren.

♦ Employment/work: Mr. Williams works approximately 50 hours per week as a business executive.

♦ Living environment: He lives in a single-family home with stairs leading into the house. His bedroom is on the second floor as is a bathroom with a walk-in shower stall. There is also a bathroom downstairs, but there is no shower/tub available. All stairs in and outside the home have at least one rail.

♦ General health status
  • General health perception: Mr. Williams reports

being in good health.

- Physical function: Mr. Williams reported a limitation in his ability to walk long distances prior to surgery.
- Psychological function: Normal.
- Role function: Business executive, husband, father, grandfather.
- Social function: He is involved in a mentoring program for high school students twice a month.

♦ Social/health habits: Mr. Williams is a non-smoker who drinks socially, approximately two to three drinks per week.

♦ Family history: His father had arthritic knees that were never treated. His father died at 75 of a stroke. His mother is alive and relatively healthy at 91.

♦ Medical/surgical history: Mr. Williams is in generally good health but his past medical history is significant for HTN and high cholesterol. His past surgical history is significant for left THA status post 1 day, right knee arthroscopy/medial menisectomy status post 8 years.

♦ Prior hospitalizations: His only hospital experience prior to the current hospitalization was for ambulatory right knee surgery 8 years ago. A partial menisectomy was performed for a medial meniscal tear.

♦ Preexisting medical and other health-related conditions: His OA affects primarily his left hip. He has early arthritic changes in his right knee, but they are not consistently symptomatic.

♦ Current condition(s)/chief complaint(s): Preoperatively Mr. Williams was able to ambulate approximately 10 city blocks (1/2 mile) without a device, but with pain. He negotiated stairs nonreciprocally. He has had pain for the last 3 years with a significant increase in pain over the last 3 months. He had pain at night and with ambulation. The pain was primarily located in his groin and radiated to his knee. He participated in physical therapy approximately 2 months ago for 3 to 4 weeks, twice a week, with no relief of pain.

♦ Functional status and activity level: Preoperatively he was independent in ADL except for the inability to easily don his socks or tie his shoes on his LLE. He was independent in all IADL. Mr. Williams enjoyed recreational doubles tennis and golf and exercised at the gym two to three times per week. He was no longer able to walk the golf course during a round of golf. He stopped skiing approximately 8 years ago, before his hip became painful.

♦ Medications: Mr. Williams takes Celebrex, Lipitor, atenolol, and a multivitamin every day.

♦ Imaging/diagnostic tests: A preoperative frontal radiograph of the pelvis and frontal and frog lateral views of the left hip were obtained. The radiographs showed moderate narrowing of the superior portion of the left

hip joint space with flattening of the femoral head. Small osteophytes were also present.

SYSTEMS REVIEW

♦ Cardiovascular/pulmonary
- BP
  - Hypotension related to intraoperative blood loss and epidural anesthesia is very common[69]
  - BP at rest 110/75 mmHg, postoperative day 1 (POD #1)
  - BP normalized to Mr. Williams' baseline of 130/85 mmHg by POD #3
- Edema: Swelling noted in left lateral/posterior hip and thigh region
- HR: 76 bpm
- RR: 14 bpm

♦ Integumentary
- Presence of scar formation
  - Staples are intact until POD #10
  - At that time staples are removed and steri-strips applied
  - The wound is healing and scar formation has started
- Skin color
  - Redness and ecchymosis noted around area of incision postoperatively
  - By POD #4 the redness has diminished and the ecchymosis is fading
- Skin integrity
  - A compression dressing and constavac drain are in place immediately postoperatively
  - The drain is removed POD #1, and on POD #2 the compression dressing is removed
  - As of POD #2 the incision is noted to be clean, dry, and intact
  - No evidence of drainage is noted

♦ Musculoskeletal
- Gross range of motion: BUE and RLE ROM is WFL, and impairment is noted in his left hip that will require further testing
- Gross strength: BUE and RLE strength is 5/5, his LLE strength is impaired and will require further testing
- Gross symmetry
  - Preoperatively, the LLE externally rotated when compared to the RLE
  - Postoperatively, the LLE remains externally rotated
  - Leg length will be measured for any discrepancy under anthropometric tests and measures
- Height: 5'11" (1.8 m)

- Weight: 189 lbs (85.73 kg)
- ◆ Neuromuscular
  - Balance: Impaired
  - Locomotion, transfers, and transitions: Gross coordinated movements are all impaired
- ◆ Communication, affect, cognition, language, and learning style
  - Mr. Williams is able to make all his needs known
  - Mr. Williams is oriented to person, place, and time
  - His expected emotional/behavioral response is normal
  - No barriers to learning noted
  - Mr. Williams states he learns best by listening and demonstration

TESTS AND MEASURES

- ◆ Aerobic capacity/endurance
  - Measured walkways
    - Phase I: Acute phase, postoperative days 1 to 4
      - HR, BP, and RR are measured pre- and post-ambulation for short measured distances (as tolerated)
    - Phase II: Postoperative weeks 2 to 6, reexamination
      - By postoperative week 4, Mr. Williams completes 1320 feet (0.25 mile) in a 6-Minute Walk test[70]
      - Norms for seniors in a community center setting were as follows[70]:
        - ○ Mean (SD): 1629 ± 313 feet
        - ○ Range: 777 to 2353 feet
- ◆ Anthropometric characteristics
  - BMI=705 x (body weight [in pounds] divided by height^2 [in inches])
    - Mr. Williams' BMI=26.43
    - This is considered to be overweight
  - Tape measure assessment for leg length discrepancy
    - Phase I: Acute phase, postoperative days 1 to 4
      - Per Mr. Williams, he had a minor leg length discrepancy prior to his THA, his left leg being shorter than his right
      - No orthotic device or lift was worn prior to surgery
      - Now that the surgery has been performed he feels the change in leg length is reversed
      - His perception is that his LLE is longer than his RLE
      - Tape measurement reveals there is an apparent leg length discrepancy but no true leg length discrepancy
    - Phase II: Postoperative weeks 2 to 6, reexamination

- Mr. Williams feels less difference between the legs
- There is no change in true leg length but the apparent leg length values have decreased
  - Phase III: Postoperative weeks 6 to 12, reexamination
    - Mr. Williams no longer complains of a difference in leg length
    - Tape measurements show no true or apparent leg length discrepancies
- ◆ Assistive and adaptive devices
  - Observation
    - Phase I: Acute phase, postoperative days 1 to 4
      - Walker for 3 days
      - Straight cane from POD #3 on
    - Phase II: Postoperative weeks 2 to 6 (precautions adherence)
      - Straight cane indoors until 3 weeks postoperatively
      - Straight cane outdoors until 5 to 6 weeks postoperatively
  - Interview
    - Phase I: Acute phase, postoperative days 1 to 4
      - Due to his posterior hip precautions Mr. Williams demonstrates the need for adaptive devices such as a long-handled reacher, long-handled shoe horn, long-handled sponge, sock aid, and elevated toilet seat
      - Mr. Williams did not need a tub chair since he has a stall shower which he can walk into, and his balance was adequate for standing in the shower
    - Phase II: Postoperative weeks 2 to 6, reexamination
      - As above
      - Adaptive devices must be used continuously until precautions are lifted by the surgeon
    - Phase III: Postoperative weeks 6 to 12, reexamination
      - Hip precautions are lifted at 6 weeks, per Mr. Williams' surgeon
      - Mr. Williams is allowed to begin a gradual return to bathing and dressing without the use of adaptive equipment as his available ROM allows
  - Safety during use of devices and equipment
    - Phase I: Acute phase, postoperative days 1 to 4
      - Mr. Williams demonstrates good safety awareness regarding the use of the assistive/adaptive devices prior to discharge from the hospital
    - Phase II: Postoperative weeks 2 to 6, reexamination

- ▸ Mr. Williams continues to demonstrate good safety awareness
  - ■ Phase III: Postoperative weeks 6 to 12, reexamination
    - ▸ Hip precautions are lifted at 6 weeks
    - ▸ Gradual discontinuation of adaptive devices as ROM returns to normal
- ◆ Environmental, home, and work barriers
  - ● Current and potential barriers
    - ■ Phase I: Acute phase, postoperative days 1 to 4
      - ▸ Upon interviewing Mr. Williams, it is found that he has stairs at home leading up to his bedroom
      - ▸ There is a bathroom on the first floor of the house without a tub/shower
    - ■ Phase II: Postoperative weeks 2 to 6, reexamination
      - ▸ Interviewing of Mr. Williams reveals the following findings regarding his office
        - ○ No stairs to be negotiated
        - ○ There is a handicapped bathroom
        - ○ His desk chair can have two pillows added to raise the seat height
- ◆ Ergonomics and body mechanics
  - ● Specific work conditions or activities
    - ■ Phase II: Postoperative weeks 2 to 6, reexamination
      - ▸ Mr. Williams is at risk for postural stress secondary to his altered posture while sitting in a raised chair at his desk
- ◆ Gait, locomotion, and balance
  - ● Observation
    - ■ Phase I: Acute phase, postoperative days 1 to 4 (physician referral for weightbearing as tolerated)
      - ▸ Balance during functional activities with/without devices
      - ▸ Within 4 days the patient is found to have good balance during functional activities such as washing at the sink, brushing his teeth, and shaving using an assistive device (walker then straight cane)
      - ▸ Static and dynamic balance with/without device
        - ○ Within 4 days static and dynamic balance are good with a device (walker then cane, with bilateral stance)
      - ▸ Gait and locomotion during functional activities with/without device
        - ○ Mr. Williams requires the use of a walker for 3 days
        - ○ While standing, the patient is noted to have increased weightbearing in his UEs and his RLE secondary to increased pain in his left hip
        - ○ On POD #3 he progresses to a straight cane
        - ○ By POD #4 he is independent with the cane
      - ▸ Gait and locomotion with/without device
        - ○ Observation will be the test and measure used initially to examine balance, locomotion, and gait
        - ○ Initially balance is altered secondary to pain, weakness, and possible dizziness
        - ○ Gait observation reveals altered step rhythm, decreased step length and stance time on the LLE, and decreased speed
        - ○ Decreased excursion through the available ROM at the hip and knee is also noted
      - ▸ Safety during gait, locomotion, and balance
        - ○ Mr. Williams is able to follow proper sequencing and shows a good awareness of his environment and potential hazards
    - ■ Phase II: Postoperative weeks 2 to 6, reexamination
      - ▸ Balance during functional activities with/without device
        - ○ After week 3, Mr. Williams no longer needs the cane indoors
        - ○ He is able to shower and prepare a simple meal demonstrating good balance
      - ▸ Static and dynamic balance with/without device
        - ○ Mr. William's single support balance continues to improve
      - ▸ Gait and locomotion during functional activities with/without device
        - ○ Mr. Williams requires the use of the cane for approximately 3 weeks postoperatively
        - ○ After 3 weeks he is able to safely ambulate in his home environment without a device
        - ○ It is not until postoperative week 5 to 6 that he is safe to walk outdoors on uneven surfaces without his cane
      - ▸ Safety during gait, locomotion, and balance
        - ○ Mr. Williams continues to demonstrate good safety awareness
  - ● Berg Balance scale (balance static/dynamic)[71]
    - ■ Phase II: Postoperative weeks 2 to 6, reexamination
      - ▸ Mr. Williams scores a 40/56 when tested at home 2 weeks after surgery
        - ○ By 6 weeks Mr. Williams scores 56/56

○ Precautions are maintained throughout testing

▸ General population norms for 247 older community dwellers are 55/56[71]

- Functional reach test (dynamic balance)[72]
  - Phase II: Postoperative weeks 2 to 6, reexamination
    ▸ Mr. Williams is able to reach 8 inches when tested at home 2 weeks after surgery
    ▸ By 6 weeks he is able to reach 12 inches
    ▸ General population norms are as follows[72]:
      ○ 20 to 40 years of age
        Males 16.73 inches ± 1.94
        Females 14.64 inches ± 2.18
      ○ 41 to 69 years of age
        Males 14.98 inches ± 2.21
        Females 13.81 inches ± 2.2
      ○ 70 to 87 years of age
        Males 13.16 inches ± 1.55
        Females 10.47 inches ± 3.5

- Single Leg Stance test (balance static)[73]
  - Phase I: Acute phase, postoperative days 1 to 4
    ▸ Mr. Williams is able to stand unsupported on his operated side with his eyes open for approximately 10 seconds
  - Phase II: Postoperative weeks 2 to 6, reexamination
    ▸ Mr. Williams is able to stand unsupported on his operated side with his eyes open for 1 minute by 4 weeks
    ▸ He is able to stand on his operated side for 30 seconds with his eyes closed by 4 weeks

◆ Integumentary integrity
- Observation of the skin and wound
  - Phase I: Acute phase, postoperative days 1 to 4
    ▸ Redness, warmth, and ecchymosis are noted once the compression bandage was removed POD #1
    ▸ No drainage or bleeding is noted at the time of discharge from the hospital
  - Phase II: Postoperative weeks 2 to 6, reexamination
    ▸ Staples removed at home POD #10
    ▸ Steri-strips are applied to the wound
    ▸ No drainage noted
    ▸ Ecchymosis is faded
    ▸ There is no increase in redness or warmth

◆ Muscle performance
- MMT
  - Phase I: Acute phase, postoperative days 1 to 4
    ▸ Gross testing of BUE is performed supine in bed and found to be WNL
    ▸ Isometric testing of bilateral extensor hallicus longus, gastrocnemius, and anterior tibialis are WNL
    ▸ Right knee extension=5/5
    ▸ Right hip flexion=5/5
    ▸ Right hip abduction at least=2+/5 (Patient cannot lie on affected hip for appropriate test position)
    ▸ Left knee extension=3+/5
    ▸ Left hip abduction=2-/5
    ▸ Left hip flexion, staying below 90 degrees=3-/5
  - Phase II: Postoperative weeks 2 to 6, reexamination
    ▸ Left knee extension=5/5
    ▸ Left hip abduction=4/5
    ▸ Left hip flexion, staying below 90 degrees=4/5

- Functional testing
  - Phase I: Acute phase, postoperative days 1 to 4
    ▸ LLE: Isometrically the patient is able to perform a quadriceps set and a gluteal set
    ▸ Actively the patient is able to perform a heel slide through part of his available motion in supine POD #1
    ▸ He is unable to perform a SLR secondary to decreased strength
    ▸ He is unable to perform active abduction in supine until POD #3, secondary to decreased strength
  - Phase II: Postoperative weeks 2 to 6, reexamination
    ▸ By POD #7 the patient is able to perform five repetitions of a SLR without any pain

◆ Orthotic, protective, and supportive devices
- No orthotic device was needed in this case
- Mr. Williams did not have a true leg length discrepancy, and his perception of a discrepancy resolved

◆ Pain
- The NPS of 0 to 10 (with 0 being no pain and 10 the worst pain ever) was utilized
  - Phase I: Acute phase, postoperative days 1 to 4
    ▸ Pain levels were assessed daily just prior to the initiation of physical therapy, during activity, and after the activity had ended
    ▸ Pain levels varied from 0-5/10
  - Phase II: Postoperative weeks 2 to 6, reexamination
    ▸ Mr. Williams no longer complained of pain (0/10)
    ▸ Chief complaint was stiffness in the morning

♦ Posture
  • Observation of postural alignment and position (static and dynamic) of the shoulders, spine, pelvis (standing and sitting), and LEs revealed:
    ■ Phase I: Acute phase, postoperative days 1 to 4
      ‣ Postural alignment and position
        ○ It is noted that he avoids weight on his left side when he sits and he must be cued to try to evenly distribute weight on both ischial tuberosities
        ○ Pain and apprehension can cause this shift to the right
        ○ The patient is observed to be standing flexed slightly forward and requires cues to stand straight, extend his hips and knees, and not to look at the floor
        ○ He also requires cues to increase weightbearing on his LLE to full weightbearing
        ○ Mr. Williams is noted to rest with his LLE in hip ER, hip abduction, and slight knee flexion while in supine
    ■ Phase II: Postoperative weeks 2 to 6, reexamination
      ‣ Postural alignment and position
        ○ Mr. Williams is able to sit with weight evenly distributed on his ischial tuberosities by the end of 7 to 10 days
        ○ Mr. Williams is able to evenly bear weight on BLE in standing, but tends to bear less weight on his LLE
        ○ He requires cues to evenly distribute his weight
      ‣ Specific body part
        ○ Mr. Williams rests while supine with his LLE in slight ER, similar to that of his RLE
  • Leg length tests: See anthropometric characteristics above
♦ Range of motion
  • ROM testing of the left hip is limited because of adherence to total hip precautions, and these precautions will be maintained per physician's orders for 6 weeks
  • Observation during functional activities
    ■ Phase I: Acute phase, postoperative days 1 to 4
      ‣ Functional ROM: Supine in bed
        ○ Left hip flexion is limited actively in supine secondary to decreased strength and pain
        ○ He is able to perform a heel slide to approximately 45 to 50 degrees of hip flexion in supine

        ○ He is able to achieve active neutral hip rotation while supine
      ‣ Functional ROM: Sitting
        ○ Left hip flexion is limited actively by decreased strength and pain
        ○ Although allowed to flex to 90 degrees, Mr. Williams can only actively flex to approximately 75 degrees by POD #3
        ○ Hip flexion is performed in a raised chair leaning his back against the backrest or sitting on a bed leaning back on his hands
  • Goniometry
    ■ Phase I: Acute phase, postoperative days 1 to 4
      ‣ Goniometry is not performed during the acute phase for Mr. Williams
      ‣ Functional testing is adequate at this time
    ■ Phase II: Postoperative weeks 2 to 6, reexamination
      ‣ Mr. Williams is able to actively achieve 90 degrees of hip flexion, 0 degrees of IR, and 25 degrees of abduction
    ■ Phase III: Postoperative weeks 6 to 12, reexamination
      ‣ Hip flexion is 110 degrees, IR is 15 degrees, and abduction is 30 degrees
  • Muscle length, soft tissue extensibility, and flexibility
    ■ Phase II: Postoperative weeks 2 to 6, reexamination
      ‣ A modified Thomas test (with left hip not flexing past 90 degrees) is negative bilaterally
      ‣ SLR test reveals 70 degrees left and 75 degrees right
♦ Self-care and home management
  • Interview
    ■ Phase I: Acute phase, postoperative days 1 to 4
      ‣ Mr. Williams is interviewed to determine barriers that exist at and in his home
      ‣ Mr. Williams has stairs outside and inside the home, but is independent with ascending/descending stairs by POD #4
  • Observation
    ■ Phase I: Acute phase, postoperative days 1 to 4
      ‣ Ability to perform self-care is observed in the hospital during treatment sessions
      ‣ Mr. Williams is able to stand long enough to shower/sponge bath
      ‣ He is able to manipulate faucets and necessary equipment, but requires assistance for set up
      ‣ He also requires assistance with dressing at this time

➤ He is discharged home with a reacher, sock aid, long-handled sponge, and long-handled shoe horn

■ Phase II: Postoperative weeks 2 to 6, reexamination

➤ Mr. Williams is now independent with showering and dressing and can perform set up independently

➤ He is safe and continues to use appropriate devices to assist with self-care, but no longer needs the assistance of his wife

➤ Items he uses include a reacher, sock aid, long-handled sponge, and long-handled shoe horn

◆ Work, community, and leisure integration or reintegration

● Interview

■ Phase I: Acute phase, postoperative days 1 to 4

➤ Mr. Williams is not returning to work at this time

➤ Mr. Williams is not returning to community and leisure actions, tasks, and activities at this time

■ Phase II: Postoperative weeks 2 to 6, reexamination

➤ Mr. Williams would like to return to work at 4 weeks postoperatively

■ Phase III: Postoperative weeks 6 to 12, reexamination

➤ Mr. Williams would like to resume sports when cleared by the physician

➤ The estimated time of return to golf and doubles tennis per his physician is 12 weeks

● Transportation assessments

■ Phase II: Postoperative weeks 2 to 6, reexamination

➤ Mr. Williams is not cleared by his physician to drive until 6 weeks after surgery

➤ Since he wishes to return to work after 4 weeks he has arranged for his wife to drive him to the office

● Physical capacity tests

■ Phase III: Postoperative weeks 6 to 12, reexamination

➤ Mr. Williams will be assessed during outpatient physical therapy for his ability to return to desired activities, such as golf and doubles tennis

➤ Sport-specific activities will be integrated into treatments during Phase III

EVALUATION

A summary of the examination reveals a 68-year-old male with OA, HTN, and elevated cholesterol. He is married and works full-time. He was active in recreational sports prior to his surgery. Following a left THA, he has been found to have decreases in ROM and strength in his LLE and faulty posture, gait and locomotion, and ADL/IADL.

DIAGNOSIS

Mr. Williams is a patient with OA, HTN, and elevated cholesterol who has undergone a left THA. He has impaired: aerobic capacity/endurance; gait, locomotion, and balance; muscle performance; posture; and range of motion. He is functionally limited in self-care and home management and in work, community, and leisure actions, tasks, and activities. These findings are consistent with placement in Pattern H: Impaired Joint Mobility, Motor Function, Muscle Performance, and Range of Motion Associated With Joint Arthroplasty. The identified impairments and functional limitations will be addressed in determining the prognosis and the plan of care.

PROGNOSIS AND PLAN OF CARE

Over the course of the visits, the following mutually established outcomes have been determined:

◆ Ability to perform physical actions, tasks, and activities related to self-care, home management, work, community, and leisure is improved

◆ Aerobic capacity is improved

◆ Balance is increased

◆ Endurance is increased

◆ Gait, locomotion, and balance are improved

◆ Muscle performance is increased

◆ Physical capacity is improved

◆ Physical function is improved

◆ Postural control is improved

◆ Quality and quantity of movement between and across body segments are improved

◆ Risk factors are reduced

◆ ROM is increased

◆ Weightbearing status is improved

To achieve these outcomes, the appropriate interventions for this patient are determined. These will include: coordination, communication, and documentation; patient/client-related instruction; therapeutic exercise; functional training in self-care and home management; functional training in work, community, and leisure integration or reintegration; prescription, application, and, as appropriate, fabrication of devices and equipment; and physical agents and mechanical modalities.

Based on the diagnosis and prognosis, Mr. Williams is expected to require between 21 and 24 visits. An example of how those visits may be broken down can be seen in Table 8-9. The total duration of physical therapy services is 21 visits, over an 11-week period of time. Outpatient physical therapy was not begun until the posterior hip precautions were lifted, following his first follow-up visit with his orthopedic surgeon, at 6 weeks postoperative.

Mr. Williams has good social support, is motivated, and follows through with his home exercise program. He is not severely impaired and is generally healthy.

INTERVENTIONS

RATIONALE FOR SELECTED INTERVENTIONS

Therapeutic Exercise

Patients with OA are more likely to have lower levels of muscle strength, decreased tolerance to exercise, and reduced aerobic capacity. Mobility decreases as pain increases with the progression of OA.[74] A review of the literature shows that physical therapy is initiated from the day of surgery to POD #2. Protocols including exercises such as quad sets, glut sets, ankle pumps, and active hip flexion are commonly found. Hip abductor strength is also addressed early in the rehabilitation process. There are many protocols and exercise programs, but there are no prospective randomized controlled trials that have determined the most effective exercise program following THA.

Early mobilization has been recognized as a key component in achieving functional mobility after THA.[75] The evidence suggests that early intensive rehabilitation can be tolerated by even the elderly population. This leads to fewer days in the hospital and lower costs. It has also been shown that physical therapy intervention during acute hospitalization results in decreasing the cost of care.[76]

Gilbey and associates looked at exercise and its affect on early functional recovery after THA. This study included an 8-week preoperative exercise program and a postoperative program. The control group received no exercise other than that received from routine in-hospital physical therapy. The results showed that patients receiving the additional therapy had significant improvements in hip strength and ROM prior to surgery. Postoperatively the hip strength data suggested that the exercise program led to a greater rate of improvement and accelerated the rate of rehabilitation. Significantly better physical function scores and better patient satisfaction scores were noted for the group who participated in the exercise program pre-and postoperatively.[74]

An understanding of forces through the hip is necessary as therapists design exercise programs for patients and guide them back to more demanding activities. Body weight forces during different activities are described in the kinesiology section of this chapter.

Common activity ROM requirements are important to consider as interventions are designed. Many common activities require more than 90 degrees of hip flexion. Various degrees of hip flexion ROM were described in the kinesiology section of this chapter.

Adherence to total hip precautions will require that patients use various assistive and adaptive devices and equipment. Orthotic devices might be needed if a true leg length discrepancy exists. It must be noted that pelvic obliquity, muscle imbalance, soft tissue contractures, a tight capsule, and other joint abnormalities may give the appearance of leg length inequity. Shoe lifts are not recommended until 6 months after surgery.[77]

Participation in high impact athletic activity increases the risk for joint-bearing surface wear and loosening of implant fixation and are therefore discouraged. Low contact and low impact activities are recommended after THA. Table 8-10 delineates the peak joint forces that occur at the hip with various activities.[78] Table 8-11 provides the results of a survey of the members of the Hip Society regarding recommendations for return to sports following THA.[79]

COORDINATION, COMMUNICATION, AND DOCUMENTATION

Communication will occur with Mr. Williams and his wife regarding all components of his care and to engender

Table 8-9
PHYSICAL THERAPY VISITS FOR MR. WILLIAMS (THA)

Setting	Frequency	Duration	Number of PT Visits
Acute care hospital	Daily	4 days	4
Home care	3x/week	3 weeks	9
Interlude between home care and beginning of outpatient program		2 weeks	
Outpatient	2x/week	4 weeks	8

Table 8-10
HIP JOINT PEAK FORCES DURING ACTIVITY[78]

Activity	Peak Forces
Walking at 1.5 m/s	2.5x BW
Running at 3.5 m/s	3.5x BW
Skiing (long turns)	4.1x BW
Skiing (short turns)	7.8x BW
Cross country skiing	4.0x BW

BW=body weight

support for his program. This will begin in the hospital and continue at home through his return to work and leisure activities. All elements of the patient's management will be documented.

♦ Coordination with agencies including:
  ● Equipment suppliers
    ■ High chair rental
    ■ Raised toilet seat (one for home, one for the office)
    ■ Straight cane
    ■ Reacher, shoe horn, sock aid, long-handled sponge
    ■ Raised tub chair is not needed as Mr. Williams is safe to stand while showering
  ● Home care agencies
    ■ Home care physical therapy is arranged for Mr. Williams while he is in the hospital

  ■ The initial visit is to be the day after he returns home
♦ Documentation across settings including:
  ● Changes in impairments, functional limitations, and disabilities as Mr. Williams is reexamined
  ● Elements of patient management including examination, evaluation, diagnosis, prognosis, and interventions
  ● Changes in interventions over the entire episode of care
  ● Outcomes of interventions throughout the entire episode of care

PATIENT/CLIENT-RELATED INSTRUCTION

Instruction began for Mr. Williams preoperatively with a THA education class provided by the hospital where his surgery was performed. Preoperative education classes allowed him to learn about the procedure and expectations following surgery. It also allowed his primary caregivers to learn what their role and responsibilities would be and allowed for early discharge planning discussions.

Total hip replacement precautions were explained to Mr. Williams in the physician's office, during the preoperative class, and by the physical therapist during treatment. These precautions are essential for avoiding hip dislocation. Posterior hip precautions and functional adjustments need to be followed by all patients who undergo a THA, with a posterolateral approach. These include:
♦ No hip flexion past 90 degrees
  ● Sit on elevated chairs or a chair with two pillows or 4-inch firm cushion

Table 8-11
RECOMMENDATIONS FOR RETURN TO SPORTS FOLLOWING THA[79]

Allowed	Allowed With Experience	Not Recommended	No Conclusion
Ballroom dancing	Bowling	Baseball	Downhill skiing
Croquet	Canoeing	Basketball	Fencing
Doubles tennis	Cross country skiing	Football	Roller blading
Golf	Hiking	Gymnastics	Rowing
Horseshoes	Horseback riding	Handball	Speed walking
Shooting	Low impact aerobics	High impact aerobics	Stationary skiing
Shuffleboard	Road bicycling	Hockey	Weight lifting
Stationary bicycle		Jogging	Weight machines
Swimming		Lacrosse	
Walking		Racquetball	
		Rock climbing	
		Singles tennis	
		Soccer	
		Squash	
		Volleyball	

- Keep knees lower than hips when sitting
- Use of elevated toilet seat
- Do not bend forward when sitting in a chair
♦ No adduction past the mid-line
  - Avoid crossing legs (even at the ankles) in lying, sitting, and standing
  - Keep a pillow or abduction wedge/pillow between his legs in supine
  - Lie on non-operated side with two full-length pillows or abduction wedge/pillow between his legs
♦ No IR past neutral
  - Keep legs pointing forwards or slightly rotated out
  - No pivoting on operated extremity during ambulation/standing
  - When turning during ambulation, turn away from the side of the operation
  - When turning toward the operated side, lead with the operated leg before turning the rest of the body

The patient and family will be instructed and educated about the risk factors associated with posterior hip precautions. This instruction will include the posterior hip precautions as outlined above and the daily activity modifications necessary to maintain the hip precautions. The length of time that the hip precautions should be followed will be detailed and will be a minimum of 6 weeks, which is the time when Mr. Williams will have his first follow-up appointment with his surgeon.

The patient and family will understand the importance of his home exercise program and the outcomes that can be expected. Mr. Williams will receive ongoing instruction/ modification of his exercise and home exercise program. Mrs. Williams will have an understanding of: the need to be supportive, ways to remind Mr. Williams of his hip precautions and exercises, and ways she can participate in his physical therapy program by walking with him for exercise and reminding him to premedicate himself prior to exercise. Together they will be educated in his individual plan of care, risk factors, and his overall health, wellness, and fitness over his entire episode of care.

Education regarding abnormal wound healing will include knowledge of the signs of:
♦ Infection, including fever, chills, redness, swelling, drainage, and pain
♦ DVT, including Homans' sign, redness, and increased temperature
♦ Neurovascular impairment, including loss of sensation or movement of the affected LE

THERAPEUTIC EXERCISE

♦ Aerobic capacity/endurance conditioning
  - Phase I: Acute phase, postoperative days 1 to 4
    - Walking to tolerance within the acute care hospital setting

- Inpatient goal of 100 feet, three times per day is reached by POD #3
- Phase II: Postoperative weeks 2 to 6
  - Walking program: Indoor/outdoor, even/uneven surfaces, flat surfaces/hills
    ▸ Mr. Williams will begin by ambulating within his home initially upon discharge
    ▸ He progresses to outdoor ambulation using a cane on flat, even surfaces beginning by walking 5 minutes, three times per day, and increasing by 2 to 3 minutes each day as tolerated
    ▸ Mr. Williams begins graded surfaces once he is able to comfortably ambulate 15 to 20 minutes, three times per day
    ▸ With the supervision of the home care therapist, he begins uneven surfaces, including grass and patio stones
  - Aquatic programs (once wound is fully healed, generally within 3 to 4 weeks)
    ▸ Mr. Williams has access to a swimming pool and walks the length of the pool, as allowed by the depth of the water, for 15 minutes per session, two times per week
  - Treadmill
    ▸ Mr. Williams uses the treadmill at home when the weather does not allow him to walk outside
    ▸ He begins with no grade, at 2 miles per hour, increasing the speed as tolerated
    ▸ The grade is increased once he is able to ambulate 15 to 20 minutes
    ▸ Time frames follow that of his outdoor walking program
  - Elliptical trainer
    ▸ Mr. Williams returns to the gym 4 weeks after his THA
    ▸ He replaces one walking session with the elliptical trainer on the days he goes to the gym
    ▸ Mr. Williams uses the elliptical trainer on the lowest ramp setting available with no resistance for 5 minutes increasing the time by 2 to 3 minutes per session
    ▸ The ramp is not increased until his precautions are lifted, and he can tolerate 15 to 20 minutes
    ▸ Resistance is increased as tolerated once he can tolerate 15 to 20 minutes unresisted
- Phase III: Postoperative weeks 6 to 12
  - Walking program, aquatics, treadmill, and elliptical trainer all continue as outlined above
  - Bicycling

▸ Precautions are lifted at 6 weeks, and there are no restrictions

▸ Mr. Williams may resume stationary bicycling at this time if he so chooses to do (Mr. Williams did not bicycle outdoors prior to his surgery)

▸ He begins with 10 minutes with no resistance and increases the time by 2 to 3 minutes each session

▸ Resistance is increased after he tolerates 15 to 20 minutes

♦ Balance, coordination, and agility training
  ● Phase I: Acute phase, postoperative days 1 to 4
    ■ Postural awareness
      ▸ Equal weightbearing on ischial tuberosities in sitting and on both LEs in standing
  ● Phase II: Postoperative weeks 2 to 6
    ■ Single leg stance
      ▸ Eyes open progressed to eyes closed
    ■ Side stepping (maintaining hip precautions)
    ■ Task specific performance
      ▸ Reaching for items from low/high surfaces
      ▸ Transfers in/out of tub/shower
      ▸ Picking up items from the floor (maintaining hip precautions by extending LLE behind him as he reaches down)
  ● Phases II and III: Postoperative weeks 2 to 12
    ■ Standing on the involved LE
      ▸ Single stance hip extension with and without resistance (elastic band)
    ■ Standing on the involved LE
      ▸ Single stance abduction with and without resistance (elastic band)
    ■ Step up (progression 4-6-8 inches)
    ■ Step down (progression 4-6-8 inches)
    ■ Balance board
    ■ KAT 1000

♦ Body mechanics and postural stabilization
  ● Postural alignment awareness during ambulation
    ■ Head up, shoulders gently down, stomach in, and buttocks together
  ● Abdominal strengthening (see strength, power, and endurance training)
  ● Standing "W" position of arms, slide up wall

♦ Flexibility exercises (maintaining posterior hip precautions until lifted by physician)
  ● Stretching exercises should be done after warming up, using a slow and steady stretch accompanied by deep breathing, and building hold up to 30 to 60 seconds
  ● AAROM progressed to AROM

■ IR to neutral
■ Hip flexion to 90 degrees
■ Hip abduction
■ Stationary bicycle after hip precautions are lifted

♦ Gait and locomotion training
  ● Gait training with a device
  ● Gait training without a device

♦ Strength, power, and endurance training
  ● LE exercise training to include AAROM, AROM, resisted range of motion (RROM) (concentric/eccentric, isometric/isotonic/isokinetic, and aquatic programs)
  ● Progression guidelines are based on pain, quality of movement, ability to maintain appropriate postures, and the ability to stand with equal weightbearing for bilateral closed chain activities
  ● Exercises may be progressed or modified based on the patient's status at the time of treatment
  ● Hip flexion less than 90 degrees until 6 weeks when precautions are lifted by the surgeon
    ■ Heel slides
    ■ Sitting hip flexion
      ▸ Patient is seated in an elevated chair or regular chair with two pillows, leaning against the back of the chair to keep the hip at less than 90 degrees
    ■ SLR (if patient is weightbearing as tolerated and SLR produces no groin pain)
    ■ Standing hip flexion with knee bent or knee straight
  ● Hip abduction
    ■ Isometric abduction, hooklying position
    ■ Abduction in supine and standing
    ■ Progress to sidelying as strength allows
      ▸ Progress from knee bent to knee straight
    ■ Hip extension
      ▸ Standing hip extension
      ▸ Prone hip extension when patient is able to safely assume a prone position (with and without assistance)
      ▸ Bridging
  ● Abdominals
    ■ Abdominal sets
    ■ Single knee to chest (less than 90 degrees of hip flexion until hip precautions are lifted) while maintaining abdominal stabilization
  ● Knee extension
    ■ Sitting knee extension
  ● Knee flexion
    ■ Standing knee flexion
    ■ Prone knee flexion when patient is able to safely

assume a prone position (with and without assistance)

- Ankle plantarflexion
  - Heel raises (bilateral to unilateral)
- Multiple muscle groups
  - Wall squats
  - Mini squats without wall
  - Sit to stand from high chair without UE assistance
  - Step up/down (progression from 4-6-8 inch step)
  - Note: The patient must have good control during the bilateral activities listed above before progressing to step up/down and step up is initiated prior to step down
  - Resisted walking with Sportcord
    - Backward/forward
    - Side to side
- Simulated sports activity (postoperative weeks 10 to 12)
  - Tennis
    - Mr. Williams will bring in his tennis racquet and simulate forehand/backhand/serve
    - Mr. Williams will simulate court mobility, forward/back and side/side
  - Golf
    - Mr. Williams will practice his swing

FUNCTIONAL TRAINING IN SELF-CARE AND HOME MANAGEMENT

Adherence to total hip precautions will require that patients use various assistive and adaptive pieces of equipment.

The following interventions related to ADL and IADL for this patient may be included in his overall program.

- ◆ Functional training in self-care and home management
  - Much of Mr. Williams' physical therapy in Phase I will focus on his bed mobility and transfers
  - He will receive bed mobility and transfer training to be independent in these activities before his discharge to home
  - Assistive devices for ambulation will include a walker and cane
  - Dressing will be assisted by the use of reacher, long-handled shoe horn, and sock aid
  - Bathing will be assisted by the use of a long-handled sponge
- ◆ IADL training
  - During Phase I Mr. Williams will be in the hospital and will not be participating in IADL activities
  - During Phases II and III Mr. Williams will slowly

resume household chores that he performed prior to his THA

- Strict adherence to his posterior hip precautions must be maintained for 6 weeks
- Taking the trash out of the house
  - Mr. Williams will be instructed to carry trash on the ipsilateral side, since studies have shown this decreases the stresses applied to the abductors[12]
- Assisting in grocery shopping
  - Mr. Williams will be instructed to carry bags on the ipsilateral side
- Light yard work
  - Mr. Williams no longer mows his own lawn, but he does do some clean up about the yard and gardening
  - Mr. Williams will be instructed in proper techniques for bending and lifting
  - He will also receive instruction for positions for gardening
- ◆ Injury prevention or reduction
  - Mr. Williams will receive education on principles to prevent violation of his posterior hip precautions during self-care and home management and to improve his safety awareness
  - A hip abduction wedge or regular pillow will be used to remind Mr. Williams of his precautions when in bed
    - A regular bed pillow folded over while patient is supine or two full-length pillows while sidelying is acceptable and often more comfortable than off-the-shelf wedges
    - There is no evidence to support the use of an abduction wedge over regular pillows

FUNCTIONAL TRAINING IN WORK, COMMUNITY, AND LEISURE INTEGRATION OR REINTEGRATION

These following interventions will occur during Phases II and III of Mr. Williams' recovery.

- ◆ Device and equipment use and training
  - Mr. Williams uses a straight cane in his home for approximately 3 weeks
  - He receives instruction to continue using his cane in the community for approximately 5 to 6 weeks, when his balance and gait are appropriate for ambulation without a device
- ◆ IADL training
  - See functional training interventions in self-care and home management and IADL training above
- ◆ Injury prevention or reduction

- Instruction given in prevention of postural stresses as Mr. Williams returns to work at week 4
  - Office chair to have two pillows or special cushion on it to maintain hip flexion precautions
  - Computer and keyboard to be raised to accommodate higher seating
  - Chair wheels to be locked to keep from rolling
  - Mrs. Williams will drive him to work until his hip precautions are lifted, and he can safely drive
- Leisure
  - Before returning to sports Mr. Williams must be cleared by his surgeon and demonstrate the following:
    - Adequate ROM in all joints for specific activity
    - 5/5 muscle strength
    - Adequate flexibility in all joints
    - Adequate aerobic capacity
  - Sport-specific activities to prepare Mr. Williams to return to doubles tennis and golf

PRESCRIPTION, APPLICATION, AND, AS APPROPRIATE, FABRICATION OF DEVICES AND EQUIPMENT

- Adaptive devices utilized for 6 weeks until hip precautions are lifted
  - Raised toilet seat
  - High chair or regular chair with two pillows or cushion
  - Pillows or abduction wedge
- Assistive devices utilized as needed until his precautions are lifted
  - Walker used in the hospital for 3 days until Mr. Williams was independent with the straight cane
  - Cane was used for 3 weeks indoors and 5 to 6 weeks in the community
  - Reacher, sponge, sock aid, and shoe horn were used until precautions were lifted after 6 weeks
- In the examination it was found that Mr. Williams' perception of leg length inequity resolved by 6 weeks after surgery. No orthotic intervention was necessary because there was no true leg length discrepancy

PHYSICAL AGENTS AND MECHANICAL MODALITIES

- Cryotherapy (cold packs)
  - Phase I
    - Cold packs 20 minutes every 3 hours
  - Phase II
    - Cold packs are recommended three times per day initially and decreased to application after exercise

ANTICIPATED GOALS AND EXPECTED OUTCOMES

- Impact on pathology/pathophysiology
  - Joint swelling, inflammation, or restriction is reduced, so that joint swelling and inflammation dissipate during Phase II.
  - Pain is decreased, and pain is consistently 0/10 as the patient continues through Phase II.
  - Soft tissue inflammation, edema, and restriction are reduced, and edema continues to dissipate during Phase II with only occasional episodes of swelling in Phase III.
- Impact on impairments
  - Aerobic capacity is increased, and the patient will be able to ambulate for ¼ mile by postoperative week 4 which is in Phase II.
  - Balance is improved, so that during Phase II the patient will be able to reach for items from high/low surfaces without losing his balance. During Phase III the patient will be able to stand on the involved LE while performing exercise on the uninvolved LE and perform exercises on the balance board and KAT 1000.
  - Endurance is improved, and the patient will be able to ambulate for ¼ mile by postoperative week 4 which is in Phase II.
  - Energy expenditure per unit of work is decreased during the end of Phase II and throughout Phase III.
  - Gait and locomotion are improved, so that the patient no longer uses an ambulatory device by the end of Phase II inside the home or outdoors.
  - Integumentary integrity is improved, and complete scar healing occurs during Phase II.
  - Joint integrity and mobility are improved, and there are no episodes of subluxation or dislocation. Hip precautions are maintained for 6 weeks.
  - Motor function is improved, particularly during Phases II and III when the patient gains much of his motor function. Highest level activities (return to sports) does not occur until after Phase III.
  - Muscle performance is increased throughout all three phases of healing. MMT reveals good to normal strength returning by the end of Phase II. The patient is ready to return to sports, such as doubles tennis and golf, after the end of Phase III (12 weeks) when strength now tests as normal throughout his LE.
  - Optimal joint alignment is achieved, and apparent leg length discrepancy resolved during Phase II. There was not a true leg length discrepancy.
  - Optimal loading/weight on a body part is achieved during Phase II.

- Postural control is achieved during Phase II.
- ROM is improved with AROM not exceeding hip precaution limitations during the early weeks of Phase II, and AROM beyond the hip precautions occurs during Phase III.
- Weightbearing status is weightbearing as tolerated in Phase I. Patient is off his cane before the end of Phase II.

♦ Impact on functional limitations
- Ability to independently perform physical actions, tasks, and activities related to ADL/IADL in self-care, home management, work, community, and leisure with or without assistive devices and equipment is increased. Patient is independent in self-care during the early weeks of Phase II (weeks 2 to 3).
- Level of supervision required for task performance is decreased, and the patient is independent in self-care during the early weeks of Phase II (weeks 2 to 3).
- Necessary equipment and home care are in place when patient arrives home from the hospital by the end of Phase I.

♦ Impact on disabilities
- Ability to assume or resume required self-care, home management, work, community, and leisure roles is improved, so that the patient is independent in self-care during the early weeks of Phase II; returns to household chores during the early weeks of Phase III (6 to 8 weeks); returns to work at 4 weeks postoperatively (Phase II), with adaptations made to his seating height for the chair and toilet; begins driving during the early weeks of Phase III (weeks 6 to 7); and returns to doubles tennis and golf approximately 3 months after surgery, which is after Phase III has ended.

♦ Risk reduction/prevention
- Postoperative complications are reduced throughout all three phases of healing.
- Risk factors are reduced, and dislocation precautions are lifted at 6 weeks, at the end of Phase II.
- Risk of recurrence of condition is reduced, and dislocation precautions are lifted at 6 weeks, at the end of Phase II.
- Risk of secondary impairments is reduced throughout all three phases of healing.
- Safety is improved throughout all three phases of healing.
- Self-management of symptoms is improved throughout all three phases of healing.

♦ Impact on health, wellness, and fitness
- Behaviors that foster healthy habits, wellness, and prevention are acquired throughout all three phases of healing.

- Decision making is enhanced regarding health, wellness, and fitness needs throughout all three phases of healing.
- Fitness, health status, physical capacity, and physical function are improved throughout all three phases of healing.

♦ Impact on societal resources
- Available resources are maximally utilized throughout all three phases of healing.
- Documentation occurs throughout patient management, throughout all three phases of healing, and across all settings and follows APTA's *Guidelines for Physical Therapy Documentation*.[80]
- Utilization of physical therapy services is optimized throughout all three phases of healing.
- Utilization of physical therapy services results in efficient use of health care dollars throughout all three phases of healing.

♦ Patient/client satisfaction
- Access, availability, and services provided are acceptable to patient throughout all three phases of healing.
- Case is managed throughout the episode of care throughout all three phases of healing.
- Clinical proficiency and interpersonal skills of the physical therapist are acceptable to patient throughout all three phases of healing.
- Coordination of care is acceptable to patient throughout all three phases of healing.
- Patient and family knowledge and awareness of the diagnosis, prognosis, interventions, and understanding of anticipated goals and expected outcomes are increased throughout all three phases of healing.
- Sense of well-being is improved throughout all three phases of healing.

REEXAMINATION

Reexamination is performed throughout the episode of care, particularly as the setting of care changes and as hip precautions are lifted.

DISCHARGE

Mr. Williams is discharged from physical therapy after a total of 21 physical therapy sessions and attainment of his goals and expectations. These sessions have covered his entire episode of care, beginning in the acute care hospital, to his transfer home with home care, and after 4 weeks of outpatient physical therapy. He is discharged because he has achieved his goals and expected outcomes.

Case Study #2: Total Knee Arthroplasties

Evelyn Johnson is a 72-year-old female who has undergone bilateral total knee arthroplasties. This case begins in the acute phase and continues through inpatient rehabilitation, discharge to home, home care, and outpatient services.

PHYSICAL THERAPIST EXAMINATION

HISTORY

♦ General demographics: Mrs. Evelyn Johnson is a 72-year old black American female whose primary language is English. She is right-hand dominant. She is a high school graduate.

♦ Social history: Mrs. Johnson is a widow with two children who are 46 and 48 years of age. She is the grandmother of four grandchildren.

♦ Employment/work: Mrs. Johnson cares for two of her grandchildren after school for approximately 15 hours per week.

♦ Living environment: Mrs. Johnson lives in an apartment building on the first floor. There are two steps into the building. There are rails on both sides of the stairs. There is one bathroom with a shower in the tub.

♦ General health status
  • General health perception: Mrs. Johnson reported having had "bad knees," HTN, and diabetes.
  • Physical function: Mrs. Johnson was unable to walk more than one block and required a straight cane for outdoor walking prior to surgery. She had difficulty rising from chairs and climbing into the bathtub. She could not climb stairs reciprocally.
  • Psychological function: Normal.
  • Role function: Mother, grandmother, caretaker.
  • Social function: Mrs. Johnson attends church weekly.

♦ Social/health habits: Mrs. Johnson is a non-smoker and does not drink alcohol.

♦ Family history: Her mother died following a cerebrovascular accident (CVA) at 76, and her father died of a heart attack at 50.

♦ Medical/surgical history: Mrs. Johnson has a past medical history significant for HTN and Type 2 DM. Her past surgical history is significant for a left knee arthroscopy, medial meniscectomy (status post 2 years), and cataract surgery. Her past surgical history is also significant for bilateral TKA status post 1 day.

♦ Prior hospitalizations: Mrs. Johnson has been previously hospitalized for HTN and DM management on two separate occasions. She also had two ambulatory surgery admissions for her knee arthroscopy and cataract surgery.

♦ Preexisting medical and other health-related conditions: Mrs. Johnson had OA in both of her knees.

♦ Current condition(s)/chief complaint(s): Preoperatively Mrs. Johnson was able to ambulate only one city block with a straight cane and with significant pain. She negotiated stairs non-reciprocally. She had pain for the last 5 years with a significant increase in pain over the last 6 months. Her pain was worse in the morning and with ambulation. The pain was primarily located in her knees. She received physical therapy after her left knee arthroscopy for approximately 1 month. She had not performed her home exercise program since shortly after her discharge from therapy. Prior to having bilateral TKA her range was as follows:
  • Right knee flexion=95 degrees
  • Left knee flexion=100 degrees
  • Right knee extension=lacking 10 degrees
  • Left knee extension=lacking 12 degrees

♦ Functional status and activity level-preoperatively: She was independent in ADL. Her family had been assisting her with housework for the past 2 years. Mrs. Johnson does not participate in any sports. She was unable to walk to the grocery store, and her family had been doing her grocery shopping.

♦ Medications: Insulin injections, ibuprofen, and atenolol.

♦ Other clinical tests: Preoperative radiographs revealed significant narrowing of the medial compartment in both knees with mild varus. There were small osteophytes present in the left knee. Effusion was also present in the left knee.

SYSTEMS REVIEW

♦ Cardiovascular/pulmonary
  • BP
    ▪ Hypotension related to intraoperative blood loss and epidural anesthesia is very common[69]
    ▪ BP at rest 95/65 mmHg on POD #1
    ▪ BP normalized to Mrs. Johnson's baseline of 135/85 mmHg by POD #3
  • Edema: Swelling noted in both knees
  • HR: 80 bpm
  • RR: 17 bpm
♦ Integumentary
  • Presence of scar formation
    ▪ Staples are intact until POD #14
    ▪ At that time staples are removed and steri-strips applied
    ▪ The wounds are healing and scar formation has started

- Skin color
  - Redness and ecchymosis noted around area of incisions immediately postoperatively
- Skin integrity
  - Compression dressings and constavac drains are in place immediately postoperatively
  - The drains are removed POD #1, and on POD #2 the compression dressings are removed
  - Anterior mid-line knee incisions
  - As of POD #2 the incisions are noted to have pin-point bloody drainage from a few of the staples in each LE
  - No other evidence of drainage is noted
- Musculoskeletal
  - Gross range of motion: BUE ROM is WFL, and impairment is noted in both knees and will require further testing
  - Gross strength
    - BUE strength is 5/5
    - Both LEs have impaired strength and will require further testing
  - Gross symmetry
    - Preoperatively bilateral knee flexion contractures and bilateral varus deformities
    - Postoperatively bilateral knee flexion contractures
  - Height: 5'2" (1.57 m)
  - Weight: 170 lbs (77.11 kg)
- Neuromuscular
  - Gross coordinated movements (balance, locomotion, transfers, and transitions) are all impaired
  - No impairment in motor function is noted
- Communication, affect, cognition, language, and learning style
  - Mrs. Johnson is able to make all her needs known
  - Mrs. Johnson is oriented to person, place, and time
  - Her expected emotional/behavioral response is normal
  - No barriers to learning are noted
  - Educational needs include safety, use of devices/equipment, ADL, and exercise program
  - Mrs. Johnson states she learns best by demonstration

TESTS AND MEASURES

- Aerobic capacity/endurance
  - Measured walkways
    - Phase I: Acute phase, postoperative days 1 to 4
      - HR, BP, and RR are measured pre- and post-ambulation for short measured distances (as tolerated)

- Phase II: Postoperative weeks 2 to 6, reexamination
  - Mrs. Johnson completes 1056 feet (0.2 mile) in a 6-Minute Walk test[70]
  - Norms for seniors in a community center setting were as follows[70]:
    - Mean (SD): 1629 (313) feet
    - Range: 777 to 2353 feet
- Anthropometric characteristics
  - BMI=705 x (body weight [in pounds] divided by height^2 [in inches])
    - Her BMI is 31.18
    - Patient is considered to be obese
  - Tape measure assessment for edema
    - Phase I: Acute phase, postoperative days 1 to 4
      - Edema is noted surrounding both knees and distally
      - Measurements are taken 1 inch cephalad to the superior aspect of the patella
      - Right=17.5 inches
      - Left=17.75 inches
    - Phase II: Postoperative weeks 2 to 6, reexamination
      - Edema is present, but steadily decreasing
      - Right=17.25 inches
      - Left=17.5 inches
- Assistive and adaptive devices
  - Observation
    - Phase I: Acute phase, postoperative days 1 to 4
      - Walker for ambulation weightbearing as tolerated
    - Phase II: Postoperative weeks 2 to 6, reexamination
      - Progression from walker to Lofstrand crutches week 2
      - Progression to two straight canes week 3
      - Progression to one straight cane week 4
  - ADL/IADL scales
    - Phase I: Acute phase, postoperative days 1 to 4
      - Mrs. Johnson demonstrates the need for adaptive devices, such as a long-handled reacher, long-handled shoe horn, long-handled sponge, sock aid, and elevated toilet seat
      - A tub chair will also be needed for the home
    - Phase II: Postoperative weeks 2 to 6, reexamination
      - As above until Mrs. Johnson will begin gradual discontinuation of equipment as her ROM improves
  - Safety during use of equipment/device

- Phase I: Acute phase, postoperative days 1 to 4
  - Mrs. Johnson requires assistance in the use of the assistive/adaptive devices prior to discharge from the hospital
- Phase II: Postoperative weeks 2 to 6, reexamination
  - Mrs. Johnson demonstrates good safety awareness regarding the use of the assistive/adaptive devices prior to discharge from inpatient rehabilitation
  - Gradual discontinuation of adaptive devices as ROM, strength, and balance improve

- Environmental, home, and work barriers
  - Current and potential barriers
    - Phase I: Acute phase, postoperative days 1 to 4
      - Mrs. Johnson is being discharged from the acute care hospital to an inpatient rehabilitation center
    - Phase II: Postoperative weeks 2 to 6, reexamination
      - Upon interviewing Mrs. Johnson it is found that she has stairs at home leading into the apartment building
      - There is a tub with a shower in Mrs. Johnson's bathroom

- Gait, locomotion, and balance
  - Observation will be used initially to examine gait, locomotion, and balance
    - Phase I: Acute phase, postoperative days 1 to 4 (physician referral for weightbearing as tolerated)
      - Balance during functional activities with/without devices
        - Mrs. Johnson requires assistance and guarding secondary to decreased balance during functional activities, such as bathing at the sink and brushing her teeth
      - Static and dynamic balance with/without device
        - Mrs. Johnson requires guarding for static balance and assistance for dynamic balance with a walker
      - Gait and locomotion during functional activities with/without device
        - Mrs. Johnson will leave the acute care hospital ambulating with a walker and assistance
        - Mrs. Johnson is found to ambulate with significantly reduced knee flexion excursion bilaterally
        - She also does not achieve full extension secondary to knee flexion contractures
        - She demonstrates decreased step length and speed

- Her balance is altered secondary to pain, weakness, and possible dizziness
  - Safety during gait, locomotion, and balance
    - Mrs. Johnson is able to follow proper sequencing and shows good awareness of her environment and potential hazards
- Phase II: Postoperative weeks 2 to 6, reexamination
  - Balance during functional activities with/without device continues to improve
  - After 2 weeks she is able to perform functional activities with the walker without assistance
  - Static and dynamic balance with/without device
    - Mrs. Johnson can stand statically on both feet without the use of an assistive device by the end of 2 weeks
    - She still requires the use of a device for dynamic balance
  - Gait and locomotion during functional activities with/without device
    - Mrs. Johnson requires the use of the walker for approximately 2 weeks postoperatively
    - After 2 weeks in the acute rehabilitation center, she is able to safely ambulate in her home environment with a walker and crutches
    - It is not until postoperative week 3 that she is safe to walk with two canes and then one cane at week 4
    - Outdoor ambulation on uneven surfaces with her canes is begun week 3
    - Mrs. Johnson continues to use one cane indoors until 8 weeks postoperatively. She uses the cane outdoors for her entire episode of care
  - Safety during gait, locomotion, and balance
    - Mrs. Johnson continues to demonstrate good safety awareness
- Berg Balance scale (static/dynamic balance)
  - Phase II: Postoperative weeks 2 to 6, reexamination
    - At 7 days postoperatively Mrs. Johnson is given the Berg Balance scale
    - She scores 26/56, which places her at a high risk for falls
    - At 2 weeks postoperatively she scores 38/56
  - Phase III: Postoperative weeks 6 to 12, reexamination
    - At 6 weeks postoperatively she scores 56/56
    - Population norms based on 247 older community dwellers in an inner city[71] are 53/56
- Functional reach test (dynamic balance)[72]

- Phase II: Postoperative weeks 2 to 6, reexamination
  - At 2 weeks postoperatively she is able to reach 5 inches
- Phase III: Postoperative weeks 6 to 12, reexamination
  - At 6 weeks postoperatively she is able to reach 10 inches
  - General population norms are as follows[72]:
    - ○ 20 to 40 years of age
      Males 16.73 inches ± 1.94
      Females 14.64 inches ± 2.18
    - ○ 41 to 69 years of age
      Males 14.98 inches ± 2.21
      Females 13.81 inches ± 2.2
    - ○ 70 to 87 years of age
      Males 13.16 inches ± 1.55
      Females 10.47 inches ± 3.5
- Single Leg Stance (static balance)[73]
  - Phase II: Postoperative weeks 2 to 6, reexamination
    - At 2 weeks postoperatively she is able to stand on one leg 30 seconds with her eyes open with UE support
  - Phase III: Postoperative weeks 6 to 12, reexamination
    - At 6 weeks postoperatively she is able to stand on one leg 30 seconds with her eyes closed and 60 seconds with her eyes open without UE support

- ◆ Integumentary integrity
  - Observation of the skin and wound
    - Phase I: Acute phase, postoperative days 1 to 4
      - Redness, warmth, and ecchymosis are noted once the compression bandages were removed POD #2
      - Pinpoint bloody drainage is noted along both incisions that increases with knee flexion
    - Phase II: Postoperative weeks 2 to 6, reexamination
      - Staples removed at the inpatient rehabilitation center on POD #14
      - Steri-strips are applied to the wounds
      - No drainage or bleeding is noted
      - Ecchymosis is faded bilaterally
      - There is no increase in redness or warmth
      - The wounds are healing uniformly
- ◆ Muscle performance
  - MMT
    - Phase I: Acute phase, postoperative days 1 to 4
      - Gross testing of BUE is performed supine in

bed and found to be WNL
- Isometric testing of bilateral extensor hallicus longus, gastrocnemius, and anterior tibialis are WNL
- Left hip flexion=3/5, limited by pain
- Right hip flexion=3-/5, limited by pain and weakness
- Left hip abduction=3-/5
- Right hip abduction=2/5
- Knee flexion and extension are not tested at this time
- Phase II: Postoperative weeks 2 to 6, reexamination
  - Left hip flexion=4/5
  - Right hip flexion=3+/5
  - Left hip abduction=4/5
  - Right hip abduction=3+/5
  - Bilateral knee extension=3+/5
  - Left knee flexion=3/5
  - Right knee flexion=3-/5
  - Bilateral plantarflexion=4/5
- Phase III: Postoperative weeks 6 to 12, reexamination
  - Bilateral hip flexion=5/5
  - Left hip abduction=5/5
  - Right hip abduction=4/5
  - Bilateral knee extension=4/5
  - Left knee flexion=4/5
  - Right knee flexion=3+/5
  - Bilateral plantarflexion=5/5
- Functional testing
  - Phase I: Acute phase, postoperative days 1 to 4
    - BLE: The patient is able to perform isometric quadriceps and gluteal muscle contractions
    - Actively the patient is unable to initially perform a heel slide
    - By POD #3 the patient is able to perform heel slides through part of her available range
    - She is unable to perform a SLR on either leg secondary to decreased strength and pain
    - She is able to perform mid range AROM in sitting with her foot supported on the floor starting POD #1. She can perform the activity with her foot dangling unsupported by POD #4, with the other leg supported during the activity
  - Phase II: Postoperative weeks 2 to 6, reexamination
    - By POD #7 she is able to comfortably tolerate sitting with both legs unsupported and perform AROM, knee flexion/extension, through

her available range

- ▸ By POD #10 the patient is able to perform five repetitions of a SLR with minimal pain

♦ Pain

- A NPS of 0 to 10, with 0 being no pain and 10 the worst pain ever, was utilized
  - ■ Phase I: Acute phase, postoperative days 1 to 4
    - ▸ Pain levels were assessed daily just prior to the initiation of physical therapy, during activity, and after the activity had ended
      - ○ Pain levels at rest ranged from 2-4/10
      - ○ Pain levels during activity ranged from 5-8/10
  - ■ Phase II: Postoperative weeks 2 to 6, reexamination
    - ▸ Mrs. Johnson reports pain of 3/10 primarily with activity (ie, ROM and sit to stand)
    - ▸ Mrs. Johnson reports increased stiffness in the morning

♦ Posture

- Observation
  - ■ Phase I: Acute phase, postoperative days 1 to 4
    - ▸ Postural alignment and position
      - ○ In standing, the patient is noted to have increased weightbearing on her UEs related to increased pain and decreased strength in her LEs
      - ○ The patient is observed to be standing flexed slightly forward and requires cues to stand straight, extend her hips and knees, and not to look at the floor
      - ○ She also requires cues to increase weightbearing on her LEs as her pain decreases and strength increases
  - ■ Phase II: Postoperative weeks 2 to 6, reexamination
    - ▸ Postural alignment and position
      - ○ Mrs. Johnson continues to stand and ambulate with knee flexion, related to her lack of full extension
      - ○ As she tires, she tends to flex more at the hips and knees

♦ Range of motion

- Observation during functional activities
  - ■ Phase I: Acute phase, postoperative days 1 to 4
    - ▸ Her knee flexion is severely limited secondary to pain, swelling, and muscle guarding
    - ▸ She is unable to sit with her feet under her knees
    - ▸ Knee extension is also limited
    - ▸ She walks with knees slightly bent

- ▸ When supine her knees remain slightly flexed

- Goniometry
  - ■ Phase I: Acute phase, postoperative days 1 to 4
    - ▸ Goniometric measurements are taken in sitting for flexion and supine for extension
    - ▸ Initial ROM on POD #1
      - ○ Left knee flexion=60 degrees
      - ○ Right knee flexion=55 degrees
      - ○ Left knee extension=-15 degrees from full extension
      - ○ Right knee extension=-10 degrees from full extension
  - ■ Phase II: Postoperative weeks 2 to 6, reexamination
    - ▸ Goniometry reveals that Mrs. Johnson is able to consistently achieve 90 degrees of knee flexion by POD #7 on her left leg and by POD #10 on her right
    - ▸ Extension by POD #10 is 10 degrees from full extension on her left and 5 degrees on her right
  - ■ Phase III: Postoperative weeks 6 to 12, reexamination
    - ▸ By the end of week 12, Mrs. Johnson has 105 degrees of left knee flexion, 100 degrees of right knee flexion, and lacks 5 degrees from full extension bilaterally

- Muscle length, soft tissue extensibility and flexibility
  - ■ Phase II: Postoperative weeks 2 to 6, reexamination
    - ▸ Thomas test is positive bilaterally (hip flexor length)
    - ▸ Ely test cannot be properly performed secondary to pain, muscle guarding and lack of ROM (rectus femoris length)
    - ▸ Straight leg raising test (hamstring length)
      - ○ Left=60 degrees
      - ○ Right=65 degrees
    - ▸ Dorsiflexion
      - ○ Knee extended
        Left=5 degrees
        Right=5 degrees
      - ○ Knee flexed
        Left=15 degrees
        Right=20 degrees
    - ▸ Tensor fascia latae
      - ○ Ober test is negative bilaterally
    - ▸ Patellar glide test
      - ○ Negative bilaterally

♦ Self-care and home management

- Interview
  - Phases I and II
    - Mrs. Johnson is interviewed to determine barriers that exist at and in her home
    - Mrs. Johnson has stairs outside the home
    - She will be discharged from the acute care hospital to an inpatient rehabilitation center
    - She will be able to negotiate stairs before discharge from the inpatient rehabilitation center
- Observation
  - Phase I: Acute phase, postoperative days 1 to 4
    - Ability to perform self-care is observed in the hospital during treatment sessions
    - Mrs. Johnson requires assistance with LE bathing and dressing
  - Phase II: Postoperative weeks 2 to 6, reexamination
    - Mrs. Johnson receives therapy for 2 weeks while in the inpatient rehabilitation center
    - She is able to shower sitting on a tub seat and dress independently at the time of discharge
    - She uses ADL devices, such as a long-handled sponge, long-handled shoe horn, reacher, and sock aid
    - She requires assistance with activities, such as laundry, grocery shopping, and house cleaning
    - Home care services including physical therapy and a home health aide will be arranged upon her discharge to home
    - Her family will also assist with grocery shopping and house cleaning
- ◆ Work, community, and leisure integration or reintegration
  - Interviews
    - Phase II: Postoperative weeks 2 to 6, reexamination
      - Mrs. Johnson will not be caring for her two grandchildren until she feels safe and comfortable
      - Mrs. Johnson resumes independent outdoor walking approximately at week 5
    - Phase III: Postoperative weeks 6 to 12, reexamination
      - Mrs. Johnson resumes after school care of her grandchildren 8 weeks after her bilateral knee replacement
  - Transportation assessments
    - Phases II and III: Postoperative weeks 2 to 12, reexamination
      - Mrs. Johnson does not drive

- She takes buses or is driven by family members to most activities
- She is unable to negotiate a bus step until week 8 secondary to decreased strength and ROM
- She is able to transfer in and out of a car by the time she is discharged from the inpatient rehabilitation center

EVALUATION

A summary of the examination reveals a 72-year-old female with OA, HTN, and DM. She is a widow and cares for two of her grandchildren after school. She was not active in recreational sports prior to her surgery. Following bilateral TKA she has been found to have decreased ROM and strength and faulty posture, gait, balance, and locomotion. She is limited in her ADL/IADL.

DIAGNOSIS

Mrs. Johnson is a patient with OA, HTN, and DM who has undergone bilateral TKA with pain in both knees. She has impaired: aerobic capacity/endurance; anthropometric characterstics; gait, locomotion, and balance; integumentary integrity; muscle performance; posture; and range of motion. She is functionally limited in self-care and home management and in work, community, and leisure actions, tasks, and activities. These findings are consistent with placement in Pattern H: Impaired Joint Mobility, Motor Function, Muscle Performance, and Range of Motion Associated With Joint Arthroplasty. The identified impairments and functional limitations will be addressed in determining the prognosis and the plan of care.

PROGNOSIS AND PLAN OF CARE

Over the course of the visits, the following mutually established outcomes have been determined:
- ◆ Ability to perform physical actions, tasks, and activities related to self-care, home management, work, community, and leisure is improved
- ◆ Aerobic capacity is improved
- ◆ Balance is increased
- ◆ Endurance is increased
- ◆ Gait, locomotion, and balance are improved
- ◆ Muscle performance is increased
- ◆ Physical capacity is improved
- ◆ Physical function is improved
- ◆ Postural control is improved
- ◆ Quality and quantity of movement between and across body segments are improved
- ◆ Risk factors are reduced

♦ ROM is increased

♦ Weightbearing status is improved

To achieve these outcomes, the appropriate interventions for this patient are determined. These will include: coordination, communication, and documentation; patient/client-related instruction; therapeutic exercise; functional training in self-care and home management; functional training in work, community, and leisure integration or reintegration; manual therapy techniques; prescription, application, and, as appropriate, fabrication of devices and equipment; electrotherapeutic modalities; and physical agents and mechanical modalities. Since there are no ROM restrictions after an uncomplicated primary TKA, the common activity ROM requirements (see Table 8-7) are important to consider as you design your goals and interventions.

Based on the diagnosis and prognosis, Mrs. Johnson is expected to require between 45 and 48 visits. An example of how those visits may be broken down can be seen in Table 8-12. The total duration of physical therapy services will be over a 10-week period of time. Mrs. Johnson has DM, but her wounds healed well, and there were no complications. Mrs. Johnson had good family support upon her return home.

INTERVENTIONS

RATIONALE FOR SELECTED INTERVENTIONS

Therapeutic Exercise

ROM exercises are incorporated immediately following TKA. Ninety degrees is considered the minimum amount of functional knee flexion necessary following a TKA. However, a range of 0 to 105 degrees is more functional because ADL, such as tying shoes, requires approximately 106 degrees of flexion. This is especially important if both knees are involved. Factors affecting postoperative ROM include preoperative ROM, postoperative pain, arthrofibrosis, and technical errors during surgery. The ROM of the knee required for various activities are seen in Table 8-7.[14]

All postoperative rehabilitation exercise programs are designed to increase mobility, strength, ROM, flexibility, and ultimately functional independence. Exercise programs should address the quadriceps, hamstrings, hip, and ankle weakness, as well as flexibility of the lateral retinaculum, ITB, hamstrings, and gastrocnemius. There are no universally accepted exercise protocols following TKA.

As with the THA population, persistent strength deficits exist following a TKA. Berman and associates performed isokinetic testing on 68 patients who had undergone a TKA. Hamstring peak torque values matched the non-operated knee by 7 to 10 months postoperatively. However, the quadriceps continued to show a deficit at the 2-year follow-up testing.[21] Lorentzen studied 30 patients who underwent isokinetic and isometric testing 1 week prior to surgery and then 3 and 6 months after surgery. Isokinetic testing showed significant and increasing strength in the flexor muscle group at 30 degrees per second and 120 degrees per second. Limited gains in extensor strength were also noted. Isometric flexion peak torque, at 75 degrees of knee flexion, initially showed a decrease at 3 months postoperatively. By 6 months postoperatively patients were at preoperative levels of flexor strength.[81]

Quadriceps weakness may persist following a TKA. Stevens and associates assessed quadriceps strength and voluntary activation before and after TKA in a prospective study with 28 subjects who underwent TKA for primary OA. Quadriceps strength and voluntary activation was completed on an average of 10 days prior to surgery and 26 days after surgery. A supramaximal electric stimulus was applied on a maximum voluntary contraction. Results showed that the quadriceps muscle on the involved side was significantly weaker than that on the uninvolved side both prior to and after surgery. Normalized quadriceps strength was decreased by an average of 60% on the involved leg. Voluntary muscle activation was significantly reduced on the involved side after surgery, but not before surgery. They concluded that a major cause of quadriceps muscle weakness after TKA was the inability to fully activate the quadriceps muscle.[82]

Weightbearing recommendations must be adhered to for each individual patient. Unlike the hip, the majority of TKA are cemented and can be weightbearing as tolerated from the onset.

As discussed in the hip case, participation in high impact athletic activity increases the risk for joint-bearing surface wear and loosening of implant fixation. Therefore low contact and low impact activities are recommended following

Table 8-12			
PHYSICAL THERAPY VISITS FOR MRS. JOHNSON (TKA)			
Setting	Frequency	Duration	Number of PT Visits
Acute care hospital	Daily	4 days	4
Inpatient rehabilitation	5x/week, BID	2 weeks	20
Home care	3x/week	3 weeks	9
Outpatient	3x/week	4 weeks	12

Table 8-13			
RECOMMENDATIONS FOR RETURN TO SPORTS FOLLOWING TKA[79]			
Allowed	*Allowed With Experience*	*Not Recommended*	*No Conclusion*
Bowling	Bowling	Basketball	Downhill skiing
Croquet	Canoeing	Football	Fencing
Dancing	Cross country skiing	Gymnastics	Roller blading
Golf	Doubles tennis	Handball	Weight lifting
Horseback riding	Hiking	Hockey	
Low impact aerobics	Ice skating	Jogging	
Shuffleboard	Road bicycling	Lacrosse	
Stationary bicycle	Rowing	Racquetball	
Swimming	Speed walking	Rock climbing	
Walking	Stationary skiing	Singles tennis	
	Weightbearing	Soccer	
		Squash	
		Volleyball	

TJA.[79] Table 8-13 provides the results of a survey of the members of the Knee Society regarding recommendations for return to sports following TKA.[79]

Electrotherapeutic Modalities

Electrical stimulation may be utilized to help increase strength and function of the quadriceps muscle. Avramidis and associates showed a statistically significant increase in walking speed following TKA in groups treated with EMS of the vastus medialis. EMS was utilized for 2 hours, twice a day, beginning on POD #2 and continued for 6 weeks. At 6 and 12 weeks postoperatively, walking speed was greater than that of the group that received the same physical therapy protocol, but without the EMS. Hospital for Special Surgery Knee Scores and Physiological Cost Index showed no difference between the groups.[83]

Gotlin and associates performed a study on patients who had a TKA utilizing EMS with continuous passive motion (CPM) for 1 hour twice a day and measuring its effect on extensor lag and length of stay. Extensor lag was measured preoperatively and prior to hospital discharge. The difference between the two groups, in postoperative lag scores, was significant at the 0.01 confidence level. The experimental group reached hospital discharge criteria at a faster rate than the control group with differences that were significant at $p<0.05$.[84]

Physical Agents and Mechanical Modalities

Controversy exists regarding the use of CPM following TKA. Reported benefits include early increased knee flexion, decreased pain, and decreased need for manipulation. Reported disadvantages include increased wound complications, bleeding, and pain. Long-term ROM does not appear to be affected by use of the CPM.[19] Although use of the CPM remains controversial, it is accepted as a cost-effective

intervention that has been found to help facilitate early knee flexion. The most appropriate length and duration of use has not been determined.

Kumar used the "drop and dangle" method versus the CPM in a prospective study of 37 patients. This method consisted of the patient putting his foot on the floor and moving his body forward until 90 degrees of knee flexion is achieved. Both groups also received 2 hours of physical therapy per day. Patients in the drop and dangle group were discharged 1 day earlier, had significantly better extension range at 6 months, and had significantly less wound drainage. The drop and dangle method was not found to significantly increase flexion by 6 months postoperatively. Kumar also reported that postoperative ROM was directly related to preoperative ROM.[85] Worland compared home physical therapy versus CPM after discharge from the acute care hospital, in 103 patients who underwent TKAs. The CPM was used 3 hours per day for 10 days. The home physical therapy group received physical therapy for 1 hour, three times per week, for 2 weeks. At 2 weeks knee flexion scores were similar, and at 6 months there was no statistical significance between the two groups.[86]

Chen and associates performed a prospective study on the use of CPM in the inpatient rehabilitation setting. Fifty-one patients at an inpatient rehabilitation center were assigned to two groups. Group 1 received CPM plus physical therapy, and group 2 received only physical therapy. They concluded there was no statistical or clinical significance between the two groups relating to passive knee flexion.[87]

COORDINATION, COMMUNICATION, AND DOCUMENTATION

Communication will occur with Mrs. Johnson regarding all components of her care and to engender support for her program that will begin in the hospital and continue at home through her return to caring for her grandchildren. All elements of the patient's management will be documented.

- ◆ Coordination with agencies including:
  - Equipment suppliers
    - Raised toilet seat
    - Walker, crutches, and two straight canes
    - Reacher, long-handled shoe horn, sock aid, long-handled sponge
    - Raised tub chair
  - Home care agencies
    - Home care physical therapy is arranged for Mrs. Johnson while she is in the inpatient rehabilitation center
    - The initial visit is to be the day after she returns home
- ◆ Referral will be made to a nutritionist
- ◆ Documentation across settings including:
  - Changes in impairments, functional limitations, and disabilities as Mrs. Johnson is reexamined
  - Elements of the patient management including examination, evaluation, diagnosis, prognosis, interventions
  - Changes in interventions over the entire episode of care
  - Outcomes of interventions throughout the entire episode of care

PATIENT/CLIENT-RELATED INSTRUCTION

Instruction for Mrs. Johnson begins preoperatively. Many hospitals now hold preoperative education classes or give out instructional material prior to surgery, although there are no data to support the benefit of these types of programs with this specific population.[19] Mrs. Johnson attended a TKA preoperative education class 1 week prior to her surgery.

The long-term impact of activity and exercise must also be discussed with the patient. Proper exercise, general fitness principles, and the effects on implant longevity must also be conveyed to the patient. Appropriate activities will be discussed under functional training in leisure activities.

The patient/family will understand the importance of her home exercise program and the outcomes that can be expected. Mrs. Johnson will receive ongoing instruction/modification of her exercise program.

Mrs. Johnson's family will have an understanding of:
- ◆ The need to be supportive
- ◆ Ways to remind the patient of the importance of her exercise program
- ◆ Ways to participate in her physical therapy program by walking with her for exercise and reminding her to premedicate herself prior to exercise
- ◆ Together they will be educated in her individual plan of

care, risk factors, and her overall health, wellness, and fitness over her entire episode of care

Education will be provided on appropriate nutrition. Education regarding abnormal wound healing will include knowledge of the signs of:
- ◆ Infection: Fever, chills, redness, swelling, drainage, pain
- ◆ DVT: Homans' sign, redness, increased temperature
- ◆ Neurovascular impairment: Loss of sensation or movement in the affected LE

THERAPEUTIC EXERCISE

- ◆ Aerobic capacity/endurance conditioning
  - Phase I: Acute phase, postoperative days 1 to 4
    - Walking to tolerance with a walker within the acute care hospital setting
    - Inpatient goal of 50 feet, two times per day is reached by POD #4
  - Phase II: Postoperative weeks 2 to 6, reexamination
    - Walking program: Indoor/outdoor, even/uneven surfaces, flat surfaces/hills
      - ▸ Mrs. Johnson is ambulating 300 feet with a walker by her discharge from the acute rehabilitation center
      - ▸ She has also been progressed to Loftstrand crutches on level surfaces by the end of week 2 and can ambulate 150 feet
      - ▸ By week 3 she progressed to two canes, and by week 4 she is using only one cane on level surfaces
      - ▸ She progresses to outdoor ambulation on flat, even surfaces, at 3 weeks postoperatively beginning with 5 minutes, three times per day and increasing by 2 to 3 minutes each day, as tolerated, using two canes
      - ▸ Mrs. Johnson begins graded surfaces once she is able to comfortably ambulate 15 to 20 minutes, three times per day
      - ▸ With the supervision of the home care therapist, she begins uneven surfaces, including grass and patio stones, at the third postoperative week
    - Stationary bicycling (short crank initially while at the acute rehabilitation center)
      - ▸ She begins with 5 minutes with no resistance and increases the time by 2 to 3 minutes each session
  - Phase III: Postoperative weeks 6 to 12, reexamination
    - Treadmill
      - ▸ Mrs. Johnson has access to a treadmill in the acute rehabilitation center and her outpatient physical therapy center

- ▸ She begins with no grade, at 2 miles per hour
- ▸ Speed is increased as tolerated
- ▸ Grade is increased once she is able to ambulate 15 to 20 minutes
- ▸ Increases in time frames follow that of her outdoor walking program
  - ■ Aquatic programs (once her wounds are fully healed, generally 3 to 4 weeks postoperatively)
    - ▸ Since she has access to a swimming pool in her outpatient physical therapy center, she walks two times per week in the water
    - ▸ She walks the length of the pool, as allowed by the depth of the water, walking 15 minutes per session
  - ■ Stationary bicycling
    - ▸ Once Mrs. Johnson has adequate ROM she switches from the short crank bicycle to the regular stationary bicycle
    - ▸ She begins with no resistance for 10 minutes and increases by 2 to 3 minutes until she can tolerate 15 to 20 minutes
    - ▸ Resistance can then be added as tolerated
- ◆ Balance, coordination, and agility training
  - ● Phase II: Postoperative weeks 2 to 6, reexamination
    - ■ Postural awareness
      - ▸ Equal weightbearing on BLE with UEs used for support and progressing to no UE support
    - ■ Single leg stance
      - ▸ Progressing from eyes open to eyes closed
    - ■ Side stepping
    - ■ Stepping over objects (eg, book)
    - ■ Task specific performance
      - ▸ Reaching for items from low/high surfaces
      - ▸ Transfers in/out of tub/shower
      - ▸ Picking up items from the floor
  - ● Phases II and III: Postoperative weeks 2 to 12, reexamination
    - ■ Standing on BLE, single terminal knee extension against resistance (elastic band)
    - ■ Standing on each LE, abduction with and without resistance (elastic band)
    - ■ Step ups (progression from 2-4-6-8 inches)
    - ■ Step downs (progression from 2-4-6-8 inches)
    - ■ Balance board
    - ■ KAT 1000
    - ■ BAPS board
- ◆ Body mechanics and postural stabilization
  - ● Postural alignment awareness during ambulation
    - ■ Head up, shoulders gently down, stomach in, and buttocks together

- ● Standing "W" position of arms, slide arms up wall
- ● Use of a mirror for feedback during exercise
- ◆ Flexibility exercises (Phases I, II, and III)
  - ● Stretching exercises should be done after warming up, using a slow and steady stretch accompanied by deep breathing, and building hold up to 30 to 60 seconds
  - ● Muscle lengthening
    - ■ Hamstring stretch (supine, seated, standing)
    - ■ Calf stretch (standing)
    - ■ Hip flexor stretch (supine, standing)
  - ● ROM
    - ■ Heel slides in supine
    - ■ Sitting knee flexion/extension
    - ■ Standing knee flexion
    - ■ Prone knee flexion
    - ■ Stationary bicycle (short crank initially)
  - ● Stretching
    - ■ Stair stretch for knee flexion
      - ▸ Holding on to the handrails, step up one step with one extremity and while keeping the other extremity on the ground with the knee straight, lean forward until a stretch is felt in the up knee
    - ■ Prone towel stretch for knee flexion
      - ▸ Lie prone on the table and use a sheet or towel around the ankle to assist with knee flexion
    - ■ Towel under heel/ankle in long sitting or supine, for knee extension
      - ▸ Lie supine and place a small pillow or towel roll under the ankle/heel
      - ▸ This position can be used for a prolonged stretch
    - ■ Prone hangs over end of bed/plinth for knee extension
      - ▸ Lie prone on a plinth with the lower legs off the end of the plinth
      - ▸ A light weight may be placed at the ankles
      - ▸ Gravity will assist in achieving extension
- ◆ Gait and locomotion
  - ● Gait training with a device
    - ■ Phase I: Acute phase, postoperative days 1 to 4
      - ▸ Walker
    - ■ Phase II: Postoperative weeks 2 to 6, reexamination
      - ▸ Progression form walker to Lofstrand crutches (2 weeks)
      - ▸ Progression from Lofstrand crutches to two canes (3 weeks)
      - ▸ Progression from two canes to one cane (4 weeks)

- Gait training without a device
  - Phase III: Postoperative weeks 6 to 12, reexamination
    - Progression from 1 cane to no device, indoors only (8 weeks)
- Treadmill walking as above
- Retrograde walking on treadmill to promote extension
- Muscle performance
  - LE exercise training to include AAROM, AROM, RROM (concentric/eccentric, isometric/isotonic, and aquatic programs)
  - Exercises are added, eliminated, and modified according to the progress of each LE individually
    - Hip flexion
      - Heel slides
      - Sitting hip flexion
      - SLR
      - Standing hip flexion with knee bent or knee straight
    - Hip abduction
      - Isometric abduction
      - Abduction in supine and standing, progressed to sidelying
    - Hip extensors
      - Standing hip extension
      - Prone hip extension
      - Bridging
    - Knee extensors
      - Sitting knee extension
      - Standing end range extension with elastic band resistance
    - Knee flexors
      - Sitting knee flexion
      - Standing knee flexion
      - Prone knee flexion
    - Ankle plantarflexion
      - Heel raises (bilateral to unilateral)
    - Multiple muscle groups (gluts, quads)
      - Wall squats
      - Mini squats without wall
      - Sit to stand, without UE assistance, progressing from higher seat levels to lower seat levels
      - Step ups (progression from 4-6-8 inch step)
      - Step downs (progression from 4-6-8 inch step)
      - Leg press
      - Total gym
      - Retrograde treadmill

FUNCTIONAL TRAINING IN SELF-CARE AND HOME MANAGEMENT

- ADL training and devices
  - Dressing will be assisted by the use of a reacher, long-handled shoe horn, and sock aid
  - Bathing will be assisted by the use of a long-handled sponge and tub chair
- IADL training
  - Phase I: Acute phase, postoperative days 1 to 4
    - Mrs. Johnson will be in the hospital and will not be participating in IADL activities
  - Phase II: Postoperative weeks 2 to 6, reexamination
    - Mrs. Johnson will begin to participate in IADL activities
    - She will have assistance of a home health aide and her family upon discharge home
  - Phase III: Postoperative weeks 6 to 12, reexamination
    - Mrs. Johnson will slowly resume household chores she performed prior to her bilateral TKA, including:
      - Taking the trash down the hall
      - Grocery shopping
      - House cleaning
        - Mrs. Johnson will be instructed in proper techniques for bending and lifting
        - She will also receive instruction for positions for cleaning low places such as the floors and tub
- Injury prevention or reduction
  - Mrs. Johnson will receive education on principles to prevent injury during self-care and home management and to improve her safety awareness

FUNCTIONAL TRAINING IN WORK, COMMUNITY, AND LEISURE INTEGRATION OR REINTEGRATION

- Phases II and III: Postoperative weeks 2 to 12
  - Device and equipment use and training
    - Mrs. Johnson begins using two straight canes outdoors at 3 weeks
    - At 4 weeks she uses one cane
    - She continues to use one cane outdoors in the community throughout her entire episode of care
    - Although she does not use the cane indoors, Mrs. Johnson likes the sense of security it provides for her in the community
  - IADL training
    - See functional training interventions in self-

care and home management and IADL training above

- Injury prevention or reduction
  - Instruction given for proper techniques for bending and lifting when caring for her grandchildren
  - Ensuring she has adequate ROM for bending
  - Ensuring she has adequate strength for bending and lifting

MANUAL THERAPY TECHNIQUES

- Phase II: Postoperative weeks 2 to 6, reexamination
  - Scar tissue massage once wound is fully healed
  - Patella mobilizations medially/laterally and superiorly/inferiorly performed with knee extended
  - Soft tissue mobilization of the quadriceps, hamstrings, gastrocnemius, and retinaculum

PRESCRIPTION, APPLICATION, AND, AS APPROPRIATE, FABRICATION OF DEVICES AND EQUIPMENT

- Adaptive devices utilized for 6 to 8 weeks
  - Raised toilet seat
  - Tub chair
- Assistive devices
  - Walker used in the hospital for 1 to 2 weeks
  - Lofstrand crutches weeks 2 to 3
  - Two canes weeks 3 to 4
  - One cane indoors weeks 4 to 8
  - Reacher, sponge, sock aid, and shoe horn were used as needed for 6 to 8 weeks

ELECTROTHERAPEUTIC MODALITIES

- EMS
  - Phase I: Acute phase, postoperative days 1 to 4
    - EMS with CPM
      - 4 to 6 hours per day with CPM, in 2-hour intervals
      - Ramp time 3 seconds
      - Pulse width of 300 microseconds
      - Frequency of 40 Hz
      - Hold for 15 seconds and rest for 10 seconds
      - Electrode placement over the distal vastus medialis and the lateral side of the thigh
  - Phase II: Postoperative weeks 2 to 6, reexamination
    - EMS continued without CPM
      - Used two times daily in inpatient rehabilitation center
      - Used three times per week as an outpatient
      - Discontinued by 6 weeks

PHYSICAL AGENTS AND MECHANICAL MODALITIES

- CPM
  - Phase I: Acute phase, postoperative days 1 to 4
    - 4 to 6 hours per day in 2-hour intervals
    - 0 to 60 degrees as tolerated, applied in the recovery room 1 to 2 hours after surgery
    - ROM progressed as tolerated daily during acute hospitalization
    - CPM discontinued following acute hospitalization
- Cryotherapy (cold packs)
  - Phase I: Acute phase, postoperative days 1 to 4
    - Cold packs 20 minutes every 3 hours
  - Phase II: Postoperative weeks 2 to 6, reexamination
    - Cold packs are recommended three times per day initially and decreased to application after exercise

ANTICIPATED GOALS AND EXPECTED OUTCOMES

- Impact on pathology/pathophysiology
  - Joint swelling, inflammation, or restriction dissipates during Phases II and III.
  - Pain is decreased, and as Phase II progresses, the patient is comfortable at rest and has minimal pain with activity.
  - Soft tissue inflammation, edema, and restriction are reduced, and edema continues to dissipate during Phases II and III with only occasional episodes of swelling after Phase III.
- Impact on impairments
  - Aerobic capacity is increased, and during Phase III the patient will achieve a walking distance during a 6-Minute Walk test equal to age-related norms.
  - Balance is improved, and the patient ambulates independently with a variety of devices during Phase II. She achieves her preoperative functional state during this phase. She achieves age-related norm values for the Berg Balance and Functional Reach tests during Phase III.
  - Endurance is improved during Phase III.
  - Energy expenditure per unit of work is decreased during Phase III.
  - Gait and locomotion are improved, and the patient ambulates independently with a variety of devices during Phase II. She achieves her preoperative functional state during this phase.
  - Integumentary integrity is improved, and complete scar healing occurs during Phase II.

- Joint integrity and mobility are improved, and there are no episodes of subluxation or dislocation.
- Muscle performance is increased throughout all three phases of healing. During Phase III she achieves good to normal values in most of her MMT scores.
- Optimal joint alignment is achieved, and there are no issues with leg length during Phase II.
- Postural control is achieved during Phase II.
- ROM improvement occurs during all three phases of healing. It takes until Phase III to achieve knee flexion greater than 100 degrees.
- Weightbearing status is improved during Phase II where the patient moves off the walker, progresses to crutches, two canes, and finally one cane.

♦ Impact on functional limitations
- Ability to assume or resume required self-care, home management, work, community, and leisure roles occurs during Phases II and III.
- Ability to independently perform physical actions, tasks, and activities related to ADL/IADL in self-care, home management, work, community, and leisure with or without assistive devices and equipment is increased and required self-care and home management roles are resumed during Phases II and III.
- Level of supervision required for task performance is decreased during Phase II.
- Necessary equipment and home care are in place when patient arrives home from the inpatient rehabilitation center early in Phase II.

♦ Risk reduction/prevention
- Postoperative complications are reduced during all three phases of healing.
- Risk factors are reduced during all three phases of healing.
- Risk of secondary impairments is reduced during all three phases of healing.
- Safety is improved during all three phases of healing.
- Self-management of symptoms is improved during all three phases of healing.

♦ Impact on health, wellness, and fitness
- Behaviors that foster healthy habits, wellness, and prevention are acquired during all three phases of healing.
- Decision making is enhanced regarding health, wellness, and fitness needs during all three phases of healing.
- Fitness, health status, physical capacity, and physical function are improved during all three phases of healing.

♦ Impact on societal resources
- Available resources are maximally utilized during all

three phases of healing.
- Documentation occurs throughout patient management and across all settings and follows APTA's *Guidelines for Physical Therapy Documentation*.[80]
- Utilization of physical therapy services is optimized during all three phases of healing.
- Utilization of physical therapy services results in efficient use of health care dollars during all three phases of healing.

♦ Patient/client satisfaction
- Access, availability, and services provided are acceptable to patient/client during all three phases of healing.
- Case is managed throughout the episode of care during all three phases of healing.
- Clinical proficiency and interpersonal skills of the physical therapist are acceptable to patient during all three phases of healing.
- Coordination of care is acceptable to patient during all three phases of healing.
- Patient and family knowledge and awareness of the diagnosis, prognosis, interventions, and understanding of anticipated goals and expected outcomes are increased during all three phases of healing.
- Sense of well-being is improved during all three phases of healing.
- Smooth transition from the inpatient rehabilitation center to home to full independence is achieved during Phase III.

REEXAMINATION

Reexamination is performed throughout the episode of care, particularly as the setting of care changes.

DISCHARGE

Mrs. Johnson is discharged from physical therapy after a total of 45 physical therapy sessions and attainment of her goals and expectations. These sessions have covered her entire episode of care, beginning with 4 days in the acute care hospital, 2 weeks in the acute rehabilitation center, 3 weeks of home care physical therapy, and 4 weeks of outpatient physical therapy. She is discharged because she has achieved her goals and expected outcomes.

Case Study #3: Total Shoulder Arthroplasty

Joseph Smith is a 70-year-old male who has undergone a left total shoulder arthroplasty. This case study will begin in the acute phase and continue through discharge to home and outpatient services.

PHYSICAL THERAPIST EXAMINATION

HISTORY

♦ General demographics: Mr. Joseph Smith is a 70-year-old white male whose primary language is English. He is left-hand dominant.

♦ Social history: Mr. Smith is married and has two children, ages 35 and 37. He is also the grandfather of two young grandchildren.

♦ Employment/work: Mr. Smith was a plumber by trade and retired 3 years ago.

♦ Living environment: He lives in a condominium with stairs leading into the house. His bedroom is on the second floor. There are bathrooms on the main and bedroom levels. The bathroom on the bedroom level has a tub/shower set up. There is no shower in the downstairs bathroom. There are rails on the left side of the stairs going up.

♦ General health status
  ● General health perception: Mr. Smith reports being in good health.
  ● Physical function: Mr. Smith reported a limitation in his ability to use his left arm for overhead activities and had pain with basic ADL and while sleeping.
  ● Psychological function: Normal.
  ● Role function: Husband, father, grandfather.
  ● Social function: Mr. Smith plays bridge and bowls.

♦ Social/health habits: Mr. Smith is a non-smoker who drinks socially, approximately one to two drinks per week.

♦ Family history: His father died of a heart attack at the age of 58. His mother died of natural causes at the age of 88.

♦ Medical/surgical history: Mr. Smith is in generally good health but his past medical history is significant for HTN, high cholesterol, and past episodes of gout. His past surgical history is significant for an inguinal hernia repair and a right Achilles tendon repair. His past surgical history is also significant for left TSA status post 1 day

♦ Prior hospitalizations: Inguinal hernia repair and Achilles tendon repair, both over 30 years ago.

♦ Preexisting medical and other health-related conditions: His OA primarily affected his left shoulder.

♦ Current condition(s)/chief complaint(s)
  ● Preoperatively Mr. Smith had constant pain. He had grinding with shoulder flexion and abduction. His ROM was limited as follows:
    ▪ Shoulder flexion=85 degrees
    ▪ Shoulder abduction=80 degrees
    ▪ Shoulder ER=20 degrees
    ▪ Shoulder IR=To the gluteal cleft

♦ Functional status and activity level: Preoperatively he was independent in ADL/IADL. Mr. Smith enjoys bridge and bowling.

♦ Medications: Mr. Smith takes Aleve, Lipitor, and atenolol every day. He also takes a daily multivitamin.

♦ Other clinical tests: Preoperative radiographs: A/P, "Y," and axillary lateral views were obtained and showed flattening of the humeral head, moderate osteophyte formation, subchondral sclerosis, and pseudocyst formation.

SYSTEMS REVIEW

♦ Cardiovascular/pulmonary
  ● BP
    ▪ Hypotension related to intraoperative blood loss and epidural anesthesia is very common[69]
    ▪ BP at rest 100/70 mmHg, POD #1
    ▪ BP normalized to Mr. Smiths' baseline of 140/85 mmHg by postoperative day POD #2
  ● Edema: Minimal swelling noted in shoulder region and in the hand
  ● HR: 76 bpm
  ● RR: 14 bpm

♦ Integumentary
  ● Presence of scar formation
    ▪ Staples are intact until POD #10
    ▪ At that time staples are removed and steri-strips applied
    ▪ The wound is healing and scar formation has started
  ● Skin color
    ▪ Redness and ecchymosis noted around area of incision postoperatively
  ● Skin integrity
    ▪ A bulky dressing is applied in the operating room and is reduced to a smaller dressing on POD #1
    ▪ As of POD #2, the incision is noted to be clean, dry, and intact
    ▪ No evidence of drainage is noted

♦ Musculoskeletal
  ● Gross range of motion: BLE and RUE ROM is

WFL, and impairment is noted in his LUE and will require further testing

- Gross strength: BLE and RUE strength is 5/5, and his LUE strength is impaired and will require further testing
- Gross symmetry
    - Preoperatively, a decrease in muscle mass is noted in his left shoulder region
    - Postoperatively, in addition to the decrease in muscle mass of the left shoulder region, Mr. Smith demonstrates left shoulder hiking
- Height: 5'9" (1.80 m)
- Weight: 195 lbs (88.45 kg)
- Neuromuscular
    - Gross coordinated movements (balance, locomotion, transfers, and transitions) are all impaired
- Communication, affect, cognition, language, and learning style
    - Mr. Smith is able to make all his needs known
    - Mr. Smith is oriented to person, place, and time
    - His expected emotional/behavioral response is normal
    - No barriers to learning noted
    - Educational needs include safety, use of devices/equipment, ADL, and exercise program
    - Mr. Smith states he learns best by listening and demonstration

TESTS AND MEASURES

- Anthropometric characteristics
    - BMI=705 x (body weight [in pounds] divided by height^2 [in inches])
        - BMI=28.87
        - Patient is considered to be overweight
    - Palpation for pitting edema
        - Phase I: Acute phase, postoperative days 1 to 2
            - 1+ (barely detectable)
        - Phase II: Postoperative weeks 1 to 6, reexamination
            - None noted
        - Phase III: Postoperative weeks 6 to 12, reexamination
            - None noted
- Assistive and adaptive devices
    - Observation
        - Phase I: Acute phase, postoperative days 1 to 2
            - Cane for 1 week to improve balance
    - ADL/IADL scales
        - Phase I: Acute phase, postoperative days 1 to 2
            - Due to restrictions of his LUE, Mr. Smith demonstrates the need for assistance in don-

ning/doffing his sling and for dressing.
- Phase II: Postoperative weeks 1 to 6, reexamination
    - Mr. Smith is now able to don and doff his sling independently
    - He can also dress and perform ADL independently
- Safety during use of equipment/device
    - Phase I: Acute phase, postoperative days 1 to 2
        - Mr. Smith demonstrates good safety awareness regarding the use of the assistive/adaptive devices and his sling prior to discharge from the hospital
    - Phase II: Postoperative weeks 1 to 6, reexamination
        - Mr. Smith continues to demonstrate good safety awareness
- Environmental, home, and work barriers
    - Current and potential barriers
        - Phase I: Acute phase, postoperative days 1 to 2
            - Upon interviewing Mr. Smith, it is found that he has stairs at home leading up to his bedroom
            - There is a bathroom on the first floor of the house, without a tub/shower
            - Mr. Smith is retired so there are no work barriers
- Gait, locomotion, and balance
    - Observation
        - Phase I: Acute phase, postoperative days 1 to 2
            - Balance during functional activities with/without devices
                - Within 2 days the patient is found to have good balance during functional activities, such as bathing at the sink, brushing his teeth, and shaving using the counter for balance as needed
            - Static and dynamic balance with/without device
                - Initially balance is altered secondary to pain, weakness, and possible dizziness
                - Within 2 days static and dynamic balance are good with a cane
            - Gait and locomotion during functional activities with/without device
                - Mr. Smith required the use of a cane for approximately 1 week in his home environment
                - He continued to use the cane in the community for 2 more weeks
            - Gait and locomotion with/without device

○ Gait observation reveals altered step rhythm, decreased step length, and decreased speed
  ▸ Safety during gait, locomotion, and balance
    ○ Mr. Smith is able to follow proper sequencing and shows a good awareness of his environment and potential hazards
- Phase II: Postoperative weeks 1 to 6, reexamination
  ▸ Balance during functional activities with/without a device
    ○ After 1 week, Mr. Smith no longer needs the cane indoors
    ○ He is able to shower and prepare a simple meal demonstrating good balance
  ▸ Static and dynamic balance with/without a device
    ○ By the end of 1 week, static and dynamic balance are good without a device
  ▸ Gait and locomotion during functional activities with/without a device
    ○ Mr. Smith requires the use of the cane outdoors for approximately 2 weeks postoperatively
    ○ After 2 weeks he is able to safely ambulate in his home environment and in the community without a device
  ▸ Safety during gait, locomotion, and balance
    ○ Mr. Smith continues to demonstrate good safety awareness

♦ Integumentary integrity
  • Observation of the skin and wound
    - Phase I: Acute phase, postoperative days 1 to 2
      ▸ Redness, warmth, and ecchymosis are noted once the bulky bandage was removed POD #1
      ▸ No drainage or bleeding is noted at the time of discharge from the hospital
    - Phase II: Postoperative weeks 1 to 6, reexamination
      ▸ Staples are removed at the doctor's office POD #10
      ▸ Steri-strips are applied to the wound
      ▸ No drainage noted
      ▸ Ecchymosis is fading
      ▸ No increase in redness or warmth

♦ Muscle performance
  • MMT
    - Phase I: Acute phase, postoperative days 1 to 2
      ▸ Gross testing of BLE is performed supine in bed and found to be WNL
      ▸ Gross testing of his RUE is WNL

▸ Isometric testing of left elbow flexion and extension is performed and is slightly limited secondary to pain
▸ Left wrist strength for flexion and extension is 5/5 and grip strength is good
▸ Left shoulder strength is not tested
▸ Scapula retraction=3/5
▸ Scapula elevation=3/5
- Phase II: Postoperative weeks 1 to 6, reexamination at the end of week 6
  ▸ Left shoulder flexion=3-/5
  ▸ Left shoulder extension=4-/5
  ▸ Left shoulder abduction=3-/5
  ▸ Left shoulder ER=3+/5 (with limit to 20 degrees)
  ▸ IR not tested: No active IR allowed until week 6
  ▸ Scapula retraction=4/5
  ▸ Scapula protraction=4/5
  ▸ Scapula elevation=4/5
  ▸ Elbow flexion=4/5
  ▸ Elbow extension=4-/5
- Phase III: Postoperative weeks 6 to 12, reexamination at the end of week 12
  ▸ Left shoulder flexion=4/5
  ▸ Left shoulder extension=5/5
  ▸ Left shoulder abduction=4/5
  ▸ Left shoulder ER=4/5
  ▸ Left shoulder IR=4/5
  ▸ Scapula retraction=5/5
  ▸ Scapula protraction=5/5
  ▸ Scapula elevation=5/5
  ▸ Elbow flexion=5/5
  ▸ Elbow extension=5/5

♦ Orthotic, protective, and supportive devices
  • A sling is used postoperatively for 6 weeks
  • Initially it is on at all times except for periods of exercise and ADL
  • Use of the sling is continued during sleep and is used to avoid overuse of the LUE and when the patient is out in the community
  • The sling may be removed for periods of time during the day
  • The involved LUE may not be used for heavy activity

♦ Pain
  • The NPS of 0 to 10, with 0 being no pain and 10 the worst pain ever, was utilized
    - Phase I: Acute phase, postoperative days 1 to 2
      ▸ Pain levels were assessed daily just prior to the initiation of physical therapy, during activity,

and after the activity had ended
- ▸ Pain levels varied from 3-6/10
  - ■ Phase II: Postoperative weeks 1 to 6, reexamination
    - ▸ Mr. Smith reported pain levels between 2-4/10
    - ▸ Chief complaint was stiffness in the morning and pain with ROM activities
  - ■ Phase III: Postoperative weeks 6 to 12, reexamination at the end of week 12
    - ▸ Mr. Smith reports discomfort only during stretching/exercise

♦ Posture
- ● Observation
  - ■ Phase I: Acute phase, postoperative days 1 to 2
    - ▸ Postural alignment and position
      - ○ Initially Mr. Smith was noted to sit and stand with his left shoulder elevated
      - ○ Pain and apprehension can lead to increased muscle tension and posturing
      - ○ With cues Mr. Smith is able to reduce this posturing
    - ▸ Specific body part
      - ○ The sling is set so that the elbow is at approximately 90 to 100 degrees of flexion
      - ○ The shoulder is in IR and slight flexion
      - ○ Mr. Smith is educated to adjust the sling multiple times per day, as needed
  - ■ Phase II: Postoperative weeks 1 to 6, reexamination
    - ▸ Postural alignment and position
      - ○ By the end of 7 to 10 days Mr. Smith no longer needs verbal cues to relax his left shoulder region
      - ○ His shoulders are of equal height in sitting and standing
      - ○ Mr. Smith continues to require cues to avoid shoulder hiking during exercise
      - ○ Mr. Smith now has a good understanding of proper elbow and sling positioning

♦ Range of motion
- ● Initially ROM testing is limited by pain in the left shoulder
- ● External ROM is limited by the surgeon because of the subscapularis lengthening that was performed to address preoperative contractures
- ● IR is not measured for 6 weeks to allow for subscapularis healing
- ● There was no additional rotator cuff or biceps involvement during the surgery
- ● Observation during functional activities

- ■ Phase I: Acute phase, postoperative days 1 to 2
  - ▸ ROM not measured since Mr. Smith is in a sling
  - ▸ In the sling the LUE is positioned in elbow flexion, shoulder IR, slight scapula protraction, and elevation
- ■ Phase II: Postoperative weeks 1 to 6, reexamination
  - ▸ Functional ROM of the LUE is tested actively
    - ○ Mr. Smith is able to use his LUE at 4 weeks for activities such as feeding, dressing, self-care, and stabilizing objects
    - ○ These activities allow for elbow flexion/extension, scapula protraction/retraction, and ER (not going beyond his 20-degree limitation)
    - ○ Mr. Smith remains in the sling
- ■ Phase III: Postoperative weeks 6 to 12, reexamination
  - ▸ Mr. Smith is now able to use his LUE fully for ADL and is no longer wearing the sling
  - ▸ He is able to perform activities, such as combing his hair, reaching into his back pocket for his wallet, and putting his belt through the back loops of his pants
  - ▸ Mr. Smith performs IR sliding his hand up his back toward the end of Phase III

- ● Goniometry
  - ■ ROM is measured supine, without a pillow under the head, with the UE in 35 to 45 degrees of abduction and a towel roll under the humerus
  - ■ IR is initially measured in the same position
  - ■ Performed while stabilizing the scapula to obtain GH motion only
  - ■ Phase I: Acute phase, postoperative days 1 to 2
    - ▸ Goniometry is utilized to obtain baseline ROM data
      - ○ Shoulder flexion=75 degrees
      - ○ Shoulder ER=20 degrees (limited to 20 degrees by physician)
      - ○ Shoulder abduction=60 degrees
      - ○ Shoulder IR=35 degrees
  - ■ Phase II: Postoperative weeks 1 to 6, reexamination at the end of 6 weeks
    - ▸ As the patient progresses through the phases of healing, goniometry reveals the following ranges of motion:
      - ○ Shoulder flexion=110 degrees
      - ○ Shoulder ER=20 degrees (limited to 20 degrees by physician)
      - ○ Shoulder abduction=90 degrees

○ Shoulder IR=40 degrees
- Phase III: Postoperative weeks 6 to 12, reexamination at the end of 12 weeks
  - In Phase III IR will be measured functionally by having the patient slide his hand up the posterior aspect of the spine, and measurements are recorded at the vertebral level at which the tip of the thumb rests
    ○ Shoulder flexion=160 degrees
    ○ Shoulder ER=40 degrees
    ○ Shoulder abduction=140 degrees
    ○ Shoulder IR=To the T8 level
- Palpation
  - Phase I: Acute phase, postoperative days 1 to 2
    - The scapula is palpated during retraction to assess mobility and is found to have minimal limitations in mobility
  - Phase II: Postoperative weeks 1 to 6, reexamination
    - The scapula is palpated during scapula AROM/PROM to assess mobility
    - Mobility improves throughout the 6 weeks
    - The scapula is palpated during AROM abduction to assess scapulothoracic motion
    - ST motion is found to be present and improving throughout the 6 weeks
    - While sitting and having the patient shrug his shoulders, the SC joint is palpated bilaterally to compare height and location, and no differences are noted
    - While seated and extending the shoulder, the AC joint is palpated, and no tenderness is noted
- ◆ Self-care and home management
  - Interview
    - Phase I: Acute phase, postoperative days 1 to 2
      - Mr. Smith is interviewed to determine barriers that exist at and in his home
      - Mr. Smith has stairs outside and inside the home
      - He is independent with ascending/descending stairs with the assistance of a cane by POD #2
  - Observation
    - Phase I: Acute phase, postoperative days 1 to 2
      - Ability to perform self-care is observed in the hospital during treatment sessions
      - Mr. Smith is able to stand long enough to shower/sponge bath
      - He is able to manipulate faucets and necessary equipment using his RUE

- He requires assistance with dressing at this time
- He is discharged home with a reacher and long-handled shoe horn
- Phase II: Postoperative weeks 1 to 6, reexamination
  - Mr. Smith is now independent with showering
  - He is safe and continues to use appropriate devices to assist with self-care and no longer requires the assistance of his wife
◆ Work, community, and leisure integration or reintegration
- Interviews
  - Phase I: Acute phase, postoperative days 1 to 2
    - Mr. Smith is retired and will not be returning to work
    - Mr. Smith is not returning to leisure actions, tasks, and activities at this time
  - Phase II: Postoperative weeks 1 to 6, reexamination
    - Mr. Smith is able to return to playing bridge
  - Phase III: Postoperative weeks 6 to 12, reexamination
    - Mr. Smith would like to resume bowling when cleared by the surgeon
    - The estimated time of return to bowling, per his surgeon, is 12 to 16 weeks
- Transportation assessments
  - Phase II: Postoperative weeks 1 to 6, reexamination
    - Mr. Smith is not cleared by his physician to drive until 6 weeks after surgery
    - At that point he will no longer be taking pain medication that may interfere with his ability to drive, and the sling is discontinued at 6 weeks
    - Mr. Smith drives an automatic transmission car
- Physical capacity tests
  - Phase III: Postoperative weeks 6 to 12, reexamination
    - Mr. Smith will be assessed during outpatient physical therapy for his ability to return to desired activities, such as yard work and bowling
    - Sport-specific activities will be integrated into therapeutic exercise during Phase III

EVALUATION

A summary of the examination reveals a 70-year-old male with a history of OA of his left shoulder, HTN, high cholesterol, and gout. He is married and is a retired plumber. He was active in bridge, bowling, and yard work prior to his surgery. Following a left TSA he has been found to have decreased ROM and strength and faulty posture, gait, balance, and locomotion. He has difficulty with ADL/IADL.

DIAGNOSIS

Mr. Smith is a patient who has undergone a left TSA with pain in that shoulder. He has impaired: gait, locomotion, and balance; muscle performance; posture; and range of motion. He is functionally limited in self-care and home management and in work, community, and leisure actions, tasks, and activities. These findings are consistent with placement in Pattern H: Impaired Joint Mobility, Motor Function, Muscle Performance, and Range of Motion Associated With Joint Arthroplasty. The identified impairments and functional limitations will be addressed in determining the prognosis and the plan of care.

PROGNOSIS AND PLAN OF CARE

Over the course of the visits, the following mutually established outcomes have been determined:
♦ Ability to perform physical actions, tasks, and activities related to self-care, home management, community, and leisure is improved
♦ Gait, locomotion, and balance are improved
♦ Muscle performance is increased
♦ Physical function is improved
♦ Postural control is improved
♦ Quality and quantity of movement between and across body segments are improved
♦ Risk factors are reduced
♦ ROM is increased

To achieve these outcomes, the appropriate interventions for this patient are determined. These will include: coordination, communication, and documentation; patient/client-related instruction; therapeutic exercise; functional training in self-care and home management; functional training in work, community, and leisure integration or reintegration; manual therapy techniques; prescription, application, and, as appropriate, fabrication of devices and equipment; and physical agents and mechanical modalities.

Based on the diagnosis and prognosis, Mr. Smith is expected to require between 32 and 35 visits. An example of how those visits may be broken down can be seen in Table 8-14. The total duration of physical therapy services is 32 visits, over a 14- to 15-week period of time. Mr. Smith has good family support and motivation, and there were no postoperative complications.

INTERVENTIONS

RATIONALE FOR SELECTED INTERVENTIONS

Therapeutic Exercise

In contrast to THA and TKA, little evidence exists regarding rehabilitation following TSA. Rehabilitation programs are based on the surgical procedure that was performed, soft tissue quality, bone quality, and the time needed for adequate healing of repaired structures. During the surgical procedure the anterior structures of the shoulder (anterior capsule and subscapularis) are divided and then surgically repaired. Presurgical contractures of the anterior capsule are common and may result in the need for capsule or subscapularis lengthening. IR strengthening is restricted for approximately 6 weeks while the subscapularis heals. Limits on ER ROM may also be restricted during this time.[37] It is also important for the physical therapist to know if a rotator cuff repair was performed and if there were any resulting restrictions for ER strengthening.[23] In this case presentation the rotator cuff was intact, but the subscapularis and anterior capsule were lengthened.

A review of the literature shows a progression from passive/active and assisted exercise to active exercise. Finally, aggressive stretching and strengthening are allowed. Early mobilization within the constraints of healing is essential. Prolonged immobilization and inadequate rehabilitation

Table 8-14			
PHYSICAL THERAPY VISITS FOR MR. SMITH (TSA)			
Setting	Frequency	Duration	Number of PT Visits
Acute care hospital	Daily	2 days	2
Outpatient	3x/week	6 weeks	18
Outpatient	2x/week	4 weeks	8
Outpatient	1x/week	4 weeks	4

Table 8-15			
RECOMMENDATIONS FOR RETURN TO SPORTS FOLLOWING TSA[79]			
Allowed	*Allowed With Experience*	*Not Recommended*	*No Conclusion*
Bowling	Downhill skiing	Football	Baseball/softball
Canoeing	Golf	Gymnastics	Fencing
Croquet	Ice skating	Hockey	Handball
Cross country skiing	Shooting	Rock climbing	High impact aerobics
Dancing			Horseback riding
Doubles tennis			Lacrosse
Horseshoes			Racquetball, squash
Low impact aerobics			Roller or inline skating
Road and stationary			Rowing
bicycling			Singles tennis
Shuffleboard			Soccer
Speed walking/jogging			Weight training
Stationary skiing (Nordic track)			
Swimming			

may result in shoulder stiffness and decreased ROM, while being too aggressive may compromise the healing of the subscapularis.[77,88,89]

It is also important to remember that the shoulder complex is made up of multiple joints. In addition to the GH joint, the ST, AC, and SC joints must all be considered. It is essential to work in the plane of the scapula in order to minimize capsular stresses, optimize the length tension relationship, center the humeral head in the glenoid, and maximize elevation.[22,88,89] It is also important to assess the scapula because ST motion is necessary for abduction of the shoulder. Normalizing the ST and SH rhythm is imperative.

The rotator cuff, deltoids, trapezius, rhomboids, serratus anterior, levator scapulae, latissimus dorsi, and pectoralis major and minor should be assessed by the physical therapist for strength and muscle length when rehabilitating patients following a TSA.

Isokinetic equipment may be utilized on the passive setting for PROM, similar to a CPM, in the outpatient setting. This modality can be used in the clinic to assist with ROM.

It is important to consider proprioception in addition to ROM and strength. Proprioception may be worked on either on land or in the water. Neuromuscular control can be achieved with rhythmic stabilization and PNF exercises.

Hydrotherapy may be used to assist with support of the UE for ROM, provide proprioception, and increase strength. The buoyancy of the water may help to assist the UE for ROM. The slower the movement is through the water the less resistance there will be. Warm water may help increase muscle relaxation allowing for greater ROM. Increasing the velocity of the movement may provide resistance for muscle strengthening.[90]

Healy performed a literature review regarding safe and appropriate activities following TJA, including TSA. As with THA and TKA, high-impact loading sports should be avoided. In the case of the total shoulder replacement, the loading of the GH joint needs to be considered. It is also important to think about whether it is the dominant or the non-dominant arm when considering return to sports. Table 8-15 provides the results of a survey of the members of The American Shoulder and Elbow Surgeons Society regarding recommendations for return to sports following TSA.[79]

Functional Training in Self-Care and Home Management

Loss of ROM prior to and immediately after TSA may result in difficulty with self-care. Loss of IR may cause difficulty with toileting, putting on a belt, and tucking a shirt into pants. Loss of ER makes reaching for items, dressing, and hair combing difficult.[21] The use of the sling following surgery increases the difficulty with self-care.

Physical Agents and Mechanical Modalities

Cryotherapy may be used to control pain and swelling. Although deep tissues may not adequately be cooled with ice, gel packs, or Cryo Cuff devices, relief of pain may be felt secondary to cooling of the cutaneous and subcutaneous tissue.[91]

The use of CPM has not been well documented for TSA. Craig reported results on two groups, one receiving CPM following a variety of shoulder surgeries and the other group not receiving CPM. The CPM group achieved the same ROM as the control group at an earlier rate. He also reported less postoperative pain in the CPM group. He concluded there was no adverse effect of using the CPM following shoulder surgery.[92]

COORDINATION, COMMUNICATION, AND DOCUMENTATION

Communication will occur with Mr. Smith and his wife regarding all components of his care and to engender support for his program. This will begin in the hospital and continue through his outpatient rehabilitation and return to community and leisure activities. A referral will be made to a nutritionist. All elements of the patient's management will be documented.

- Coordination with agencies, including:
  - Equipment suppliers
    - Straight cane
    - Reacher and shoe horn
    - Pulleys
- Documentation across settings, including:
  - Changes in impairments, functional limitations, and disabilities as Mr. Smith is reexamined
  - Changes in interventions over the entire episode of care
  - Outcomes of interventions throughout the entire episode of care

PATIENT/CLIENT-RELATED INSTRUCTION

Instruction begins preoperatively. Mr. Smith was given reading material related to TSA by his physician prior to surgery. Mr. Smith also participated in 1 month of physical therapy prior to deciding to have the surgery. He was instructed in ROM and strengthening exercises while participating in outpatient physical therapy. Preoperative physical therapy provides the opportunity to demonstrate the postoperative program, educate the patient, and begin the process of setting goals and expectations.

Proper exercise and general fitness principles and compliance with the home exercise program must be discussed. The effects of activity on implant longevity must also be conveyed to the patient. Appropriate activities will be discussed under functional training in leisure activities.

The inability to sleep comfortably is a common complaint before and after surgery. Instruction in alternative sleep positions to decrease discomfort will be offered to Mr. Smith.

The patient and family will understand the importance of Mr. Smith's home exercise program and the outcomes that can be expected. They will be educated in his individual plan of care, risk factors, and his overall health, wellness, and fitness over his entire episode of care. Mr. Smith will receive ongoing instruction/modification of his exercise program. Mr. Smith's wife will have an understanding of:

- The need to be supportive
- Ways to remind the patient of the importance of his exercise program

Education regarding abnormal wound healing will include knowledge of the signs of:

- Infection, including fever, chills, redness, swelling, drainage, and pain
- Neurovascular impairment, including loss of sensation or movement of the affected UE

Education regarding alternative sleep positions immediately following surgery will include:

- Sleeping in a partially reclined position instead of supine
- Support under the humerus with a towel roll or pillow

Education regarding the use of the sling, proper application, and positioning will be provided. The patient will also receive education regarding proper diet.

THERAPEUTIC EXERCISE

In this case there are ER ROM limitations immediately postoperatively. The physician referral outlines the following postoperative considerations: ER is limited to 20 degrees for 6 weeks and no active IR for 6 weeks. The sling is required for 6 weeks.

Although there are phases of healing that may help guide the physical therapist through a proper progression of exercise and ROM, it is always necessary to progress patients based on reexamination and the meeting of previous goals.

- Aerobic capacity/endurance conditioning
  - Phases II and III: Postoperative weeks 1 to 12, reexamination
    - Walking program to maintain or increase aerobic capacity
      - Increasing ambulation as tolerated by distance or time
    - Stationary bicycle to maintain or increase aerobic capacity
      - Increasing as tolerated by distance or time
- Body mechanics and postural stabilization
  - Phase II: Postoperative weeks 1 to 6, reexamination
  - Postural alignment awareness
    - Relaxation to avoid left shoulder hiking
    - Mirror during exercise for proper shoulder position (ie, avoiding shoulder hiking)
  - Scapula mobility
    - Scapula protraction/retraction, elevation/depression
    - Progress from active assisted to active to resisted
- Flexibility exercises
  - Stretching exercises should be done after warming up, using a slow and steady stretch accompanied by deep breathing, and building hold up as tolerated, ideally 30 seconds
  - Phase I: Acute hospitalization, postoperative days 1 to 2

- AROM elbow, forearm, wrist, and hand
- Codman's (pendulum) exercises: Keeping the UE relaxed to allow for momentum to move the arm through the motions initiated by the trunk
  - ▸ Starting position: Standing, bend forward at the hips and move the body in order to allow for forward/backward, side to side, circles clockwise, and circles counterclockwise of the involved UE
- PROM/AAROM forward flexion in the plane of the scapula
  - ▸ Starting position: Supine, maintaining the plane of the scapula, with a towel roll under humerus to keep it from dropping into extension
  - ▸ The motion of forward flexion will be assisted by the therapist, a family member, or with the patient's hands clasped or holding a cane
- PROM ER limited to 20 degrees in the plane of the scapula
  - ▸ Starting position: Supine, maintaining the plane of the scapula, with a towel roll under humerus to keep it from dropping into extension
  - ▸ ER will be assisted by the therapist, family member, cane, or contralateral UE
- PROM abduction
  - ▸ Starting position: Supine, with a towel roll under humerus to keep it from dropping into extension
  - ▸ Abduction is assisted by the therapist, family member, or a cane
- AROM scapula retraction
  - ▸ Starting position: Sitting in a chair, wearing the sling
  - ▸ Pull the scapula together into retraction
- Phase II: Postoperative weeks 1 to 6, reexamination
  - Continue distal AROM
  - Continue Codman's (pendulum) exercises
  - Continue PROM in forward flexion, ER, and abduction
    - ▸ Observe for scapula motion with abduction
  - Scapula AROM
    - ▸ Scapula protraction/retraction and elevation/depression
    - ▸ Sidelying
      - ○ Progressing from active-assisted to active
      - ○ Assessment of scapula mobility
  - Pulleys
    - ▸ Facing the pulleys with emphasis on no shoulder hiking, trunk sidebending, or arching of the back and maintaining the plane of the scapula

- Late Phase II: Postoperative weeks 4 to 6
  - Hydrotherapy
    - ▸ ROM exercises may be performed in a pool with water covering the shoulders
    - ▸ Incision must be fully healed
  - Airdyne bicycle for warm-up
    - ▸ No resistance
    - ▸ Begin 2 to 3 minutes, increasing to 10 minutes as tolerated
  - Upper body ergometer for warm-up
    - ▸ No resistance
    - ▸ Begin 2 to 3 minutes, increasing to 10 minutes as tolerated
- Phase III: Postoperative weeks 6 to 12, reexamination
  - ER ROM restrictions are lifted at 6 weeks
    - ▸ May begin gentle stretching past 20 degrees and progress as tolerated
  - Begin IR PROM and AROM
    - ▸ Begin in supine with the extremity in abduction as tolerated
    - ▸ Progress to standing functional stretch up the back
  - End range stretching as motions improve and are tolerated
  - Posterior capsule stretching
    - ▸ Sitting or standing, pulling arm across the chest (horizontal adduction)
    - ▸ 30-second hold
- ◆ Gait and locomotion training
  - Phase I: Acute hospitalization, postoperative days 1 to 2
    - Gait training with a straight cane
  - Phase II: Postoperative weeks 1 to 6, reexamination
    - Gait training without a device
- ◆ Muscle performance
  - Phase I: Acute hospitalization, postoperative days 1 to 2
    - No strengthening at this time
  - Phase II: Postoperative weeks 1 to 6, reexamination
    - Initiate submaximal isometrics
      - ▸ Standing, push against wall, elbow flexed to 90 degrees (forward flexion, extension, abduction, and ER)
    - Scapula ROM progressing to manual resistance
      - ▸ Scapula protraction, retraction, elevation, and depression
      - ▸ Sidelying
        - ○ Assisted by therapist initially
        - ○ Actively performed by patient
        - ○ Resistance applied by therapist during treatment sessions

- Late Phase II: Postoperative weeks 4 to 6
  - Elastic band exercises
    - Shoulder flexion, extension, abduction, and ER
    - Scapula retraction
  - Isotonic exercise with light weights
    - Shoulder shrugs bilaterally
    - Elbow flexion
    - Elbow extension
    - Wrist flexion and extension
    - Forearm pronation and supination
  - Scapula stabilization
    - Begin on stable surface (plinth) progressing to unstable surface (exercise ball), weightbearing through BUE
    - Begin with minimal forward flexion and progress to positions of increased forward flexion
- Phase III: Postoperative weeks 6 to 12, reexamination
  - Allowed to begin active IR
  - Progress to IR strengthening
    - Begin with isometrics (submaximal)
    - Progress to elastic band
    - Weights
  - PRE
    - Forward flexion
    - ER
    - IR
    - Chest press
    - Row
    - Cable column
    - Latissimus dorsi pull down
  - Continue to progress scapula stabilization exercises as tolerated
  - PNF patterns provide motion at the scapula, shoulder, elbow, forearm, wrist, and fingers
    - Motion begins distally and moves proximally, begin supine progressing to sitting or standing or in the water
    - PNF patterns are begun without resistance, progressing to resistance
    - D1 flexion
      - Motions at the shoulder: Flexion, adduction, ER
      - Motions at the scapula: Elevation, abduction, upward rotation
    - D1 extension
      - Motions at the shoulder: Extension, abduction, IR
      - Motions at the scapula: Depression, adduction, downward rotation
    - D2 flexion
      - Motions at the shoulder: Flexion, abduction, ER
      - Motions at the scapula: Elevation, adduction, upward rotation
    - D2 extension
      - Motions at the shoulder: Extension, adduction, IR
      - Motions at the scapula: Depression, abduction, downward rotation
    - Rhythmic stabilization
      - Patient must have adequate ROM prior to beginning these exercises
      - Work at various degrees of range, starting close to the body and then moving it away from the body into flexion and abduction
      - Force is applied by the therapist and a counter force by the patient
      - Progression is from supine to sitting to standing
  - Push-ups
    - Begin against wall, progress to plinth
    - Mr. Smith does not progress to push-ups on the floor
  - Sport-specific training
    - Simulation of bowling using a medicine ball
    - Throwing and catching using a medicine ball utilizing various degrees of ROM

FUNCTIONAL TRAINING IN SELF-CARE AND HOME MANAGEMENT

- ◆ Self-care and home management
  - Dressing will be assisted by the use of a reacher and long-handled shoe horn
  - Mr. Smith will be instructed in donning/doffing the sling for ADL
  - Mr. Smith will use a cane for ambulation in the house for approximately 1 week
  - He will sponge bathe until his staples are removed 10 days postoperatively
  - After that he will stand and shower, tub seat and long-handled sponge are no longer necessary
- ◆ IADL training
  - During Phase I Mr. Smith will be in the hospital and will not be participating in IADL activities
  - During Phase II Mr. Smith will begin to participate in IADL activities
  - During Phase III Mr. Smith will slowly resume household chores he performed prior to his TSA that include:
    - Taking the trash out

- Watering the outdoor plants
♦ Injury prevention or reduction
  - Mr. Smith will receive education on principles to prevent injury during self-care and home management and to improve his safety awareness

FUNCTIONAL TRAINING IN WORK, COMMUNITY, AND LEISURE INTEGRATION OR REINTEGRATION

These following interventions will occur during Phases II and III of Mr. Smith's recovery.
♦ Device and equipment use and training
  - Mr. Smith uses a cane when out in the community for a total of 3 weeks
♦ IADL training
  - See functional training interventions in self-care and home management and IADL training above
♦ Leisure activities and training
  - Before returning to sports or leisure activities Mr. Smith must be cleared by his surgeon and demonstrate the following:
    - Adequate ROM in all joints for specific activity
    - 5/5 muscle strength
    - Adequate flexibility in all joints
  - Sport-specific activities to prepare Mr. Smith to return to bowling and gardening (see sport-specific therapeutic exercise interventions)

MANUAL THERAPY TECHNIQUES

♦ Phases II and III: Postoperative weeks 1 to 12, reexamination
  - Soft tissue mobilization of the pectoralis major, deltoid, trapezius, and latissimus dorsi muscles

PRESCRIPTION, APPLICATION, AND, AS APPROPRIATE, FABRICATION OF DEVICES AND EQUIPMENT

♦ Sling
  - Phase I: Acute hospitalization, postoperative days 1 to 2
    - Sling is applied immediately following surgery
    - Removed only for exercise and bathing
    - Mr. Smith and his wife are educated regarding the use of the sling and proper application and positioning
  - Phase II: Postoperative weeks 1 to 6, reexamination
    - The sling is used for 6 weeks postoperatively
    - Removed for exercise and ADL

PHYSICAL AGENTS AND MECHANICAL MODALITIES

♦ Cryotherapy
  - Phase I: Acute hospitalization, postoperative days 1 to 2
    - Cryotherapy 20 minutes every 3 hours
  - Phase II: Postoperative weeks 1 to 6, reexamination
    - Cryotherapy is recommended three times per day initially and decreased to application after exercise
♦ CPM
  - Phase I: Acute hospitalization, postoperative days 1 to 2
    - Settings according to physician limits
    - 4 to 6 hours per day
  - Phase II: Postoperative weeks 1 to 6, reexamination
    - Increase settings as tolerated within physician limits
    - Home CPM is discontinued after 1 week
♦ Isokinetic PROM
  - Phase II: Postoperative weeks 1 to 6, reexamination
    - Increase settings as tolerated within physician limits
    - Discontinued as the patient's ROM improves

ANTICIPATED GOALS AND EXPECTED OUTCOMES

♦ Impact on pathology/pathophysiology
  - Edema, lymphedema, or effusion is reduced during Phase II.
  - Joint swelling, inflammation, or restriction is reduced during Phase II.
  - Pain is decreased during the second half of Phase II at which time the patient reports early morning stiffness with minimal pain.
  - Soft tissue inflammation, edema, and restriction are reduced during Phase II.
♦ Impact on impairments
  - Aerobic capacity is increased during Phase II.
  - Balance is improved, and the patient no longer uses a cane during early Phase II.
  - Endurance is improved during Phase II.
  - Gait and locomotion are improved, and a cane is used for 1 to 2 weeks and then discontinued.
  - Integumentary integrity is improved, and the incision is fully healed during Phase II.
  - Joint integrity and mobility are improved during all three phases of healing.
  - Joint stability is improved, and there are no episodes of subluxation or dislocation.

- Muscle performance is increased, so that good to normal strength is achieved during Phase III.
- Optimal joint alignment is maintained for 6 weeks with a sling.
- Optimal loading on a body part is achieved in late Phase II and Phase III.
- Postural control is improved during Phase II.
- ROM is improved during all three phases of healing.

♦ Impact on functional limitations
  - Ability to independently perform physical actions, tasks, and activities related to ADL/IADL in self-care, home management, work, community, and leisure with or without assistive devices and equipment is increased during Phases II and III.
  - Level of supervision required for task performance is decreased during Phases II and III.
  - Necessary equipment and outpatient services are in place when patient arrives home during Phase I.
  - Ability to assume or resume required self-care, home management, work, community, and leisure roles is improved during Phases II and III.

♦ Risk reduction/prevention
  - Postoperative complications are reduced during all three phases of healing.
  - Protection of body parts is increased during all three phases of healing.
  - Risk factors are reduced during all three phases of healing.
  - Risk of recurrence of condition is reduced during all three phases of healing.
  - Risk of secondary impairments is reduced during all three phases of healing.
  - Safety is improved during all three phases of healing.
  - Self-management of symptoms is improved during all three phases of healing.

♦ Impact on health, wellness, and fitness
  - Behaviors that foster healthy habits, wellness, and prevention are acquired during all three phases of healing.
  - Decision making is enhanced regarding health, wellness, and fitness needs during all three phases of healing.
  - Fitness, health status, physical capacity, and physical function are improved during all three phases of healing.

♦ Impact on societal resources
  - Available resources are maximally utilized during all three phases of healing.
  - Documentation occurs throughout patient management and across all settings and follows APTA's *Guidelines for Physical Therapy Documentation.*[80]
  - Utilization of physical therapy services is optimized during all three phases of healing.
  - Utilization of physical therapy services results in efficient use of health care dollars during all three phases of healing.

♦ Patient/client satisfaction
  - Access, availability, and services provided are acceptable to patient/client during all three phases of healing.
  - Case is managed throughout the episode of care during all three phases of healing.
  - Clinical proficiency and interpersonal skills of the physical therapist are acceptable to patient/client during all three phases of healing.
  - Coordination of care is acceptable to patient/client during all three phases of healing.
  - Patient and family knowledge and awareness of the diagnosis, prognosis, interventions, and understanding of anticipated goals and expected outcomes are increased during all three phases of healing.
  - Sense of well-being is improved during all three phases of healing.
  - Smooth transition from the hospital to home to full independence is achieved during all three phases of healing.
  - Stressors are decreased during all three phases of healing.

REEXAMINATION

Reexamination is performed throughout the episode of care, particularly as the setting of care changes and as ROM restrictions are lifted.

DISCHARGE

Mr. Smith is discharged from physical therapy after a total of 32 physical therapy sessions and attainment of his goals and expectations. These sessions have covered his entire episode of care, beginning in the acute care hospital to his transfer home and after outpatient physical therapy. He is discharged because he has achieved his goals and expected outcomes.

Case Study #4: Metacarpophalangeal Joint Implant Arthroplasty

Ruth Solomon is a 56-year-old, right-hand dominant female who has rheumatoid arthritis and has undergone right metacarpophalangeal joint (II-V) implant arthroplasties and arthrodesis of the right proximal interphalangeal joints of all fingers.

PHYSICAL THERAPIST EXAMINATION

HISTORY

♦ General demographics: Ruth Solomon is a 56-year-old, right-hand dominant white Jewish female. She is a college graduate and her primary language is English.

♦ Social history: She is married and has two daughters, ages 25 and 27, and has two grandchildren. Both daughters and their families live within a 10-mile radius of their parents.

♦ Employment/work: Mrs. Solomon is a retired fifth grade teacher. She is an active board member in a Jewish community group. Her interests include traveling with her husband, spending time with her daughters and her grandchildren, and playing a weekly bridge game.

♦ Living environment: She lives with her husband in a one-family, ranch-style home in Bayside, New York. There is a handrail on the left side while ascending the basement stairs.

♦ General health status
  • General health perception: Mrs. Solomon reports being in good health. She was diagnosed with RA at the age of 46. But other than taking prednisone (10 mg) daily for the past 10 years, she does not report any interference with her lifestyle until 6 months ago.
  • Physical function: Mrs. Solomon reports that she was totally independent in all ADL until 6 months ago. She has become increasingly more dependent and now requires assistance with tasks that necessitate bilateral fine motor skills, such as with buttons, snaps, and ties. She is experiencing increased foot pain, making it difficult to walk and negotiate stairs.
  • Psychological function: Normal.
  • Role function: Wife, mother, grandmother, community board member.
  • Social function: She enjoys and takes pride in her leadership role in the community. She enjoys traveling with her husband.

♦ Social/health habits: She reports being a non-smoker and non-drinker.

♦ Family history: Both parents are deceased secondary to cardiac-related problems. Her mother was an insulin dependent diabetic for 14 years. She reports no known history of other family members with RA.

♦ Medical/surgical history: She has had RA for 10 years.

♦ Prior hospitalizations: She reports that she was hospitalized for the birth of her two daughters, and both were caesarean deliveries.

♦ Preexisting medical and other health-related conditions: Concurrent with increased bilateral hand pain, edema, and deformity, Mrs. Solomon states that she is experiencing pain, edema, and deformity in both of her feet.

♦ Current condition(s)/chief complaint(s): Within the past 6 months she has experienced increased pain, edema, and deformity of both her hands, specifically localized to the MCP joints and wrists, right greater than left. Within the past 2 months, she has noticed that her fingers have shifted towards the fifth finger (ulnarly). She has found it increasingly more difficult to perform fine motor tasks, especially while grooming. Pain and deformity are the primary reasons for seeking the help of a hand surgeon. She has undergone right MCP joint (II-V) implant arthroplasties and arthrodesis of the right PIP joints of all fingers.

♦ Functional status and activity level: Preoperatively, she required moderate assistance in ADL that necessitated bilateral fine motor skills. She is unable to ambulate more than one city block because of bilateral foot pain.

♦ Medications: She has been taking daily prednisone (10 mg) for the past 10 years.

♦ Other clinical tests: Radiographs, frontal, and lateral views, were taken. Lateral views revealed moderate volar MCP joint subluxation, right hand greater than left hand, ring and small fingers greater than index and middle fingers. Frontal view radiographs revealed grade III proliferative synovitis at the MCP joint level of the index, middle, ring, and small fingers.

SYSTEMS REVIEW

♦ Cardiovascular/pulmonary
  • BP: 100/85 mmHg
  • Edema: Moderate dorsal edema of the right hand and fingers
  • HR: 85 bpm
  • RR: 12 bpm
♦ Integumentary
  • Presence of scar formation
    ▪ The incisions transverse the dorsal aspect of the hand at the MC head level of the index, middle, ring, and small fingers (II-V) (Figure 8-4)

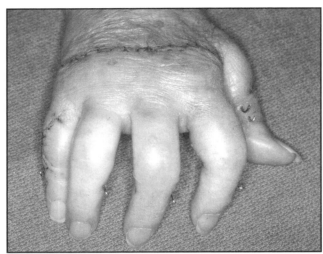

Figure 8-4. Postoperative hand following MCP joint implant arthroplasty and K-wire stabilizations.

- Sutures are in situ and will be removed 10 to 12 days post surgery
- Kirschner (K) wires are subcutaneous across the MP joint of the thumb and PIP joints of the fingers; they are removed between the 4th to 6th postoperative week
- The incisions are clean and dry
- The wounds are in the inflammatory phase of wound healing
  - Skin color: Redness and mild ecchymosis are localized to the surgical sites
  - Skin integrity: Thinness of the skin noted on the dorsum of the hand
- ◆ Musculoskeletal
  - Gross range of motion
    - Restricted cervical spine rotation to the right
    - Bilateral shoulder and elbow AROM is WNL
    - All left wrist motions are WNL
    - Impairment noted in the right wrist and will require further testing
  - Gross strength
    - BLE were WFL
    - Left grip strength weak
    - RUE not tested at this time
  - Gross symmetry: Relatively symmetrical
  - Height: 5'4" (1.62 m)
  - Weight: 170 lbs (63.45 kg)
- ◆ Neuromuscular
  - Gross coordinated movements (balance, locomotion, transfers, and transitions) are all WFL
  - No impairment in motor function is noted

- ◆ Communication, affect, cognition, language, and learning style
  - Mrs. Solomon is oriented to time, place, and person and able to express herself and make her needs known to others
  - Mrs. Solomon states she learns best by visual demonstration
  - No barriers to learning are noted nor expected

TESTS AND MEASURES

- ◆ Aerobic capacity/endurance during functional activities was not tested at this time
- ◆ Anthropometric characteristics
  - BMI=705 x (body weight [in pounds] divided by height^2 [in inches])
  - Mrs. Solomon's BMI=29.26
  - BMI values between 25 and 30 are considered to be overweight[93]
  - Edema
    - Circumferential measurement around the right MCP joint level was 30 cm as compared to the left MCP joint level at 20 cm
    - Edema was boggy to touch
- ◆ Assistive and adaptive devices
  - Preoperatively, Mrs. Solomon was fitted with a custom fabricated, dorsally based, dynamic outrigger splint with both a dorsal bar and radial bar attachments (Figure 8-5)
- ◆ Cranial and peripheral nerve integrity
  - Cranial nerves were intact
  - Peripheral nerve tests included light touch, deep touch, moving touch, and two-point static touch
    - All tests were WNL proximal to the incision on

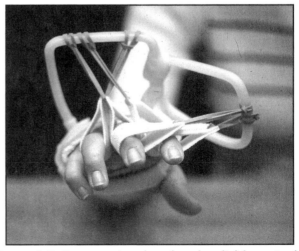

Figure 8-5. Preoperative dorsal and radial bar attachments with slings for outrigger splint.

the right hand, but are diminished distal to the incision
- Sensory testing on the left hand was WNL
♦ Environmental, home, and work barriers
- She has been experiencing increased difficulty negotiating the stairs to her basement where her washer and dryer are located
- There are no work barriers since Mrs. Solomon is retired
♦ Ergonomics and body mechanics
- Dexterity and coordination during leisure activities are restricted at this point in the rehabilitation
♦ Gait, locomotion, and balance
- She has been unable to ambulate more than one city block prior to surgery because of bilateral foot pain
- She does not require the use of an assistive device at this time
♦ Integumentary integrity
- Associated skin
  - Skin characteristics
    - Very sensitive and fragile at the wound margins, temperature is slightly warm to touch
    - Skin is slightly red and ecchymotic
- Wound
  - Signs of infection
    - No signs of acute infection are noted
    - K-wire sites are clean and dry
    - Sutures are in situ, and no drainage noted
- Left hand was WNL
♦ Motor function
- Hand function
  - Not tested at this time, on left
  - The right hand is in the dorsal outrigger splint full-time and cannot be functionally used at this time
♦ Muscle performance
- MMT: Not done at this time
  - Gross grip and pinch strength are not tested on the right hand at this time but will be tested at 6 weeks post surgery
- Left grip strength was tested using a Jamar dynamometer
  - The Jamar dynamometer is the most common instrument used to evaluate grip strength
  - Its reliability is based on the condition that it is calibrated annually[94]
  - Grip and pinch strength were tested according to the recommendations of the American Society of Hand Therapists[95]
    - Testing position
    - Shoulder adducted, next to side of body, elbow

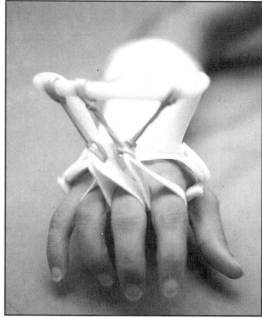

Figure 8-6. Preoperative dorsal bar and sling attachments for outrigger splint.

flexed to 90 degrees, forearm in neutral rotation, wrist between 0 to 30 degrees of extension and in slight ulnar deviation
- The dynamometer is on the "second" handle position
- The test is performed three times with a short rest period allowed between readings so that the results are not affected by fatigue[95]
- Left grip strength averaged 28 lbs over three trials
  - Normal is 47.3 lbs for the non-dominant side of a 56-year-old woman[96]
- Left key pinch strength, was tested using a Jamar pinch gauge and averaged 9 lbs over three trials
  - Normal is 14.7 lbs. for the non-dominant side of a 56-year old woman[96]
♦ Orthotic, protective, and supportive devices
- Preoperatively, Mrs. Solomon was fitted with a custom fabricated, dorsally based, dynamic outrigger splint with dorsal bar and radial bar attachments
  - For adequate support of the two outrigger attachments, the base of the outrigger splint must extend proximally two-thirds the length of the forearm and distally to the level of the MC heads
  - All four fingers are dynamically supported at the level of the proximal phalanx by slings that are attached to the dorsal bar of the outrigger by rubber bands (Figure 8-6)

- These slings position the fingers in the neutral position, which is 0 degrees of flexion and extension at the MCP joint
- Another two slings are attached by rubber bands to the radial bar of the outrigger and are positioned at the level of the middle phalanx of the index and middle fingers and provide lateral (radial) support (see Figure 8-5)
- The force couple, created on the index and middle fingers by the slings from the dorsal bar and the slings from the radial bar, positions the MCP joints of these two fingers in neutral and supination
- Supination is an accessory motion of the MCP joint that allows for pad-to-pad pinch between the index and middle fingers and the thumb
- Placement of both sets of slings requires extreme care and precision for proper formation of this force couple into the newly forming fibrous pseudocapsule
- The base of the outrigger splint is secured to the forearm and hand using three Velcro straps, the most proximal strap wraps circumferentially around the upper forearm securing the proximal part of the outrigger base to the forearm
- Mrs. Solomon's wrist had a tendency toward radial deviation, therefore, the second Velcro strap held the wrist in a neutral position, helping reduce the ulnar forces on the fingers. When a joint is postured in one position, the next most distal joint will be postured in the extreme opposite position: this is commonly referred to as a zigzag deformity[26]
- The base of the second and third MCs are firmly anchored to the carpus forming the CMC joints and have little mobility at this level
- In contrast to this, the fourth and fifth MCs have a great degree of mobility at this level. This mobility is necessary for cupping of the hand and convergence of the ring and small fingers with full flexion, allowing for power grasp and creation of the palmar arch[6]
- The palmar arch of the hand is supported well below the distal palmar crease of the hand with the third Velcro strap. This is padded and helps prevent flattening of the palmar arch
- A flattened arch restricts mobility between the MC heads of the ring and small fingers which interferes, and ultimately limits, active flexion of these fingers while in the outrigger
- On the fourth postoperative day, the surgical compression bandages are replaced with a light gauze dressing

- Compression wraps (coban) are used to control excessive dorsal edema of the hand
- A light dressing and coban wrap remains in place over the surgical site until the sutures are removed, usually between 12 to 14 days postoperatively, or when the incision is completely closed. This prevents the outrigger splint from creating direct pressure on the wound
- Full-time use of the outrigger splint is encouraged until 6 weeks postoperatively
- Patients who are on corticosteroids or immunosuppressant medications have a tendency to have thin, sensitive skin and heal more slowly.[26] Therefore, the application of the custom splint should be delayed 5 to 7 days or until the wound has shown a greater degree of healing

◆ Pain
- Pain at rest was 4/10 on the NPS with 0=no pain and 10=the worst pain possible[97]
- Pain with motion was 6/10 on the NPS at the surgical site

◆ Posture
- Mrs. Solomon has a mild FHP, thoracic kyphosis, bilateral genu valgus, pronated feet, and hallux valgus

◆ Range of motion
- AROM and PROM (goniometry)
- Cervical spine (CROM)
  ‣ Flexion: WFL
  ‣ Extension: WFL
  ‣ Rotation to the right: 45 degrees
  ‣ Rotation to the left: WFL
  ‣ Lateral flexion to right and left: WFL
- AROM of all fingers on the right hand was tested within the confines of the outrigger splint
  ‣ AROM of the right MCP joints: limited in both terminal flexion and extension and will require further testing
  ‣ AROM of the left MCP joints
    ○ Composite flexion of all fingers is WNL
    ○ Terminal extension is limited and will require further testing
  ‣ Active motion of the right PIP joints are unable to be tested due to pinning. The DIP joints: WNL
  ‣ The left middle and ring fingers are beginning to show signs of swan-neck deformities and will require further testing
  ‣ Ulnar drift of the left ring and small finger is noted and will require further testing
    ○ Measurements for ulnar drift are taken on the dorsal aspect of the MCP joint using a standard goniometer

- ► Thumb opposition
  - ○ Incomplete to the tip of the index finger on the right
  - ○ WNL on the left
- ■ Right elbow AROM
  - ► Flexion: WFL
  - ► Extension: WFL
- ■ Right forearm AROM
  - ► Supination: 0 to 70 degrees
  - ► Pronation: 0 to 75 degrees
- ■ Right forearm PROM
  - ► Supination: 0 to 70 degrees
  - ► Pronation: 0 to 75 degrees
- ■ Right wrist AROM
  - ► Extension: 0 to 40 degrees
  - ► Flexion: 0 to 45 degrees
  - ► Ulnar deviation: 0 to 5 degrees
  - ► Radial deviation: 0 to 25 degrees
- ■ Right wrist PROM
  - ► Extension: 0 to 55 degrees
  - ► Flexion: 0 to 50 degrees
  - ► Ulnar deviation: 0 to 25 degrees
  - ► Radial deviation: 0 to 35 degrees
- ■ Right thumb AROM
  - ► MP joint K-wires across joint at 15 degrees, therefore not tested
  - ► IP joint: +15 to 30 degrees
  - ► Opposition: To index finger tip, not tested
- ■ Right thumb PROM
  - ► MP joint K-wires across joint at 15 degrees, therefore not tested
  - ► IP joint: +20 to 40 degrees
  - ► Opposition: To index finger tip, not tested
- ■ Right fingers (tested in outrigger splint) AROM
  - ► MCP joints (II-V): 0 to 30 degrees
  - ► PIP joints (II-V): Pinned
  - ► DIP joints (II-V): 0 to 40 degrees
- ■ Right fingers (tested in outrigger splint) PROM
  - ► MCP joints (II-V): 0 to 60 degrees
  - ► PIP joints (II-V): Pinned
  - ► DIP joints (II-V): 0 to 50 degrees
- ◆ Reflex integrity
  - ● Deep reflexes are WNL
  - ● Superficial reflexes are WNL
- ◆ Self-care and home management
  - ● An interview concerning the ability to safely perform self-care and home management actions, tasks, and activities revealed that bilateral tasks required minimal to moderate assistance
- ◆ Work, community, and leisure integration or reintegration

- ● An interview concerning the ability to safely manage community and leisure actions, tasks, and activities revealed the need for assistance if the task was bilateral

EVALUATION

Mrs. Solomon's history previously outlined indicated that she is a 56-year-old, right-hand dominant female, who is a retired fifth grade teacher. She does not smoke or drink. She was diagnosed with RA 10 years ago, and until 6 months ago, reported to be essentially pain free and fully functional at home, in self-care, and in the community. She is 4 days post right MCP joint implant arthroplasties of the index, middle, ring, and small fingers (II-V) and arthrodesis of the PIP joints of the fingers and the MP joint of the right thumb. K-wires are in situ. AROM and PROM of the small joints of the right hand are limited in terminal flexion and extension. The wrist is limited in all terminal ranges of motion. She reports pain at the surgical sites at rest (4/10) and increased pain with attempted active finger motion (6/10).

DIAGNOSIS

Mrs. Solomon is a patient who is 4 days postoperative right MCP joint (II-V) implant arthroplasties and arthrodesis of the right PIP joints of all fingers and the right MP joint of the thumb, with pain. She has impaired: anthropometric characteristics; cranial and peripheral nerve integrity; gait, locomotion, and balance; integumentary integrity; motor function; muscle performance; posture; and range of motion. She is functionally limited in self-care and home management and in work, community, and leisure actions, tasks, and activities. In addition, she has environment, home, and work barriers. She is using an orthotic device. These impairments, functional limitations, and barriers will be addressed in determining the prognosis and the plan of care.

PROGNOSIS AND PLAN OF CARE

Over the course of the visits, the following mutually established outcomes have been determined:
- ◆ Ability to perform bilateral ADL is increased
- ◆ Ability to perform home management, community, and leisure actions, tasks, and activities independently is increased
- ◆ AROM is improved
- ◆ Coordination is improved
- ◆ Deformity is decreased
- ◆ Endurance during fine motor activities is improved
- ◆ Gross grip strength is improved
- ◆ Key pinch strength is improved
- ◆ Joint edema and inflammation are reduced

♦ Pain is reduced
♦ Patient and family members' knowledge of techniques of joint conservation is increased
♦ PROM is improved

To achieve these outcomes the appropriate interventions for this patient are determined. These will include: coordination, communication, and documentation; patient/client-related instruction; therapeutic exercise; functional training in self-care and home management; functional training in work, community, and leisure integration or reintegration; manual therapy techniques; prescription, application, and, as appropriate, fabrication of devices and equipment; integumentary repair and protection techniques; and physical agents and mechanical modalities.

Based on the diagnosis and prognosis, Mrs. Solomon is expected to require between 32 and 35 visits over a 14- to 15-week period of time. Mrs. Solomon has good family support and motivation, and there were no postoperative complications.

Patients should be reevaluated on their 1-year anniversary of surgery. At this time, a prospective splinting schedule for the next year should be developed. Generalizations cannot be made when patients are discharged from therapy. Their schedule is solely dependent upon their assessment at 1 year. If the patient's fingers have the tendency toward recurrent ulnar drift when held unsupported, continued nighttime splinting in the volar splint would be recommended for at least the next 6 to 9 months. However, if the patient's fingers demonstrate good alignment when held unsupported, nighttime splinting should be discontinued. Post-surgical patients should be encouraged to continue exercising to strengthen the radial intrinsic muscles (radial walk against resistance) to retard recurrent ulnar drift of fingers.

INTERVENTIONS

RATIONALE FOR SELECTED INTERVENTIONS

Therapeutic Exercise

Swanson developed the post operative rehabilitation program for patients who undergo implant arthroplasty concurrently with the development of the actual implant design.[41] Swanson described the concept of silastic implant as "bone resection+implant+encapsulation=functional joint."[43] The postoperative rehabilitation program that Mrs. Solomon followed was based upon the Swanson protocol.[98] The rationale for the specific postoperative exercise program and the rationale for the prolonged use of the dynamic outrigger splint following MCP joint implant arthroplasty has been well documented by Swanson,[98] Madden,[99] and The Hand Rehabilitation Center of Indiana.[100] The specific

exercise program established for patients with this diagnosis is based on the different wound healing stages.[26] These stages include:

♦ Fragile or inflammatory stage (PO 1 to 5 days)
♦ Early fibroplastic or remolding stage (PO 5 to 10 days)
♦ Late fibroplastic stage (PO 10 days to 3 to 4 weeks)
♦ Transitional stage (PO 4 to 6 weeks)
♦ Early scar maturation stage (PO 6 weeks to 6 months)
♦ Late scar maturation stage (PO 6 months to 1 year)

During the inflammatory and early fibroplastic stages (0 to 10 days PO) the focus of the exercise program is to achieve maximum AROM at the MCP joints.[43] Following suture removal and wound closure, a variety of primary modalities may also be used. The radial walk exercise is initiated very early in the postoperative exercise program and is the one exercise that is continued past the 1-year anniversary of surgery. The radial walk exercise is performed by placing the palm and fingers flat on a table. Beginning with the index finger, slide it on the table toward the thumb; then do the same for the middle, ring, and small fingers. This exercise helps to strengthen the radial intrinsic muscles of the hand. These muscles usually require strengthening because of years of being stretched into ulnar deviation. Strong radial intrinsic muscles will reinforce good alignment of the fingers and help prevent recurrent ulnar drift of the fingers. At 6 weeks postoperative, gentle strengthening is initiated.[99] Therapy putty is an excellent medium to use since the resistance may be periodically upgraded to allow for progressive strengthening. It allows the therapist to be creative and develop exercises for strengthening of the extensor muscles, radial intrinsics, and the flexor muscles.

Manual Therapy Techniques

The patient is instructed in massage techniques, including fluid flushing, gentle cross friction, and deep circular massage. These techniques are incorporated into the home program at different stages. The fluid flushing massage is used to reduce the postoperative edema of the fingers, hand, and wrist.[101] The patient is instructed to perform this massage on the first postoperative visit. The second massage technique, cross friction massage, is introduced about 1 week following suture removal, when the wound margins can tolerate the pressure. A deep circular massage is used after the third postoperative week. Cross friction and deep circular massage techniques are used to reduce the propensity of the incision to adhere to the underlying extensor tendons.[101] Adherence of these two tissues will ultimately limit extensor tendon excursion and MCP joint extension.

Prescription, Application, and, as Appropriate, Fabrication of Devices and Equipment

During the fragile or inflammatory stage (PO 1 to 5 days) an outrigger splint is worn full-time except for when the hand is supported on a tabletop during wound care and to allow for performing the radial walk exercise. The newly forming collagen fibers orient towards the desired longitudinal direction when influenced by controlled stress. The sole purpose of the prolonged, continued use of the dorsal outrigger splint is to direct and control collagen fiber orientation. Collagen fibers tend to form in a disorganized fashion when not controlled by splinting. A disorganized collagen capsule will limit ROM of the joint and decrease necessary joint stabilization.[26]

The base of the outrigger splint generally needs to be modified to accommodate for the bulky surgical dressing and to alleviate pressure on the surgical site. The underside of the splint is padded using adhesive-backed foam to prevent shearing forces on the incision. The slings on the dorsal outrigger bar are applied to each proximal phalanx at a 90-degree angle of pull.[98-100] The slings from the radial bar are placed on the index and middle fingers at the middle phalanx level. The force couple created by the dorsal sling and the radial sling positions the index and middle fingers in supination to allow for pad-to-pad pinch with the thumb (Figure 8-7). The tension on the dorsal rubber bands is tight enough to support the MCP joints in zero degrees extension (neutral) but allows for 70 to 75 degrees of active MCP joint flexion.

During the early fibroplastic or remolding stage (PO 5 to 10 days) the outrigger continues to be worn full-time. Radial and dorsal slings are adjusted during each therapy session to maintain the force couple of supination of the index and middle fingers and neutral extension of the MCP joints.[43]

At the end of the late fibroplastic stage (PO 10 days to 3 to 4 weeks) weaning from the splint begins for 15-minute intervals.[98] Use of the hand is restricted to very light ADL, avoiding all pinching activities (turning a key, tying laces, etc). Volar slings that originate from the flexion cuff are applied to the ring and small fingers. The flexion cuff sling is rarely used on the index finger because this finger requires stability in extension over mobility. These slings are worn in 30-minute intervals, followed by active flexion exercises of the MCP joints.

During the transitional stage (PO 4 to 6 weeks) a volar resting splint that is used to position the fingers in neutral alignment replaces the outrigger for nighttime use. The volar resting splint is only worn during the day with severe joint instability.[98] The outrigger is used periodically during the day for rest and exercise.

During the early scar maturation stage (PO 6 weeks to 6 months) most patients will be out of the outrigger splint all day, and the volar resting splint is worn at night.[98]

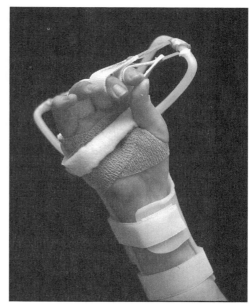

Figure 8-7. Supination of index and middle fingers in outrigger splint.

During the late scar maturation stage (PO 6 months to 1 year) nighttime splinting is continued.

At the time of the 1-year postoperative visit, the continuation of the use of the volar splint is determined based upon the patient's unsupported finger alignment. If an ulnar drift posture is present, splinting is continued for the next 6 to 9 months. If the fingers are in neutral alignment, splinting is discontinued.[98]

Physical Agents and Mechanical Modalities

Thermotherapy, in the form of paraffin, fluidotherapy, or hot packs may be used to increase muscle/tendon extensibility of the small muscles of the hand and increase blood flow to promote healing.[102] Paraffin is the modality of choice since it has a mineral oil base to help soften the scar.[102] Thermotherapy in the form of cold packs or contrast baths may also be used. Cold packs are used after the exercise session to reduce edema, and pain, if necessary.[102] Contrast baths are beneficial to reduce edema, reduce discomfort, and improve blood flow to promote healing.[103,104]

COORDINATION, COMMUNICATION, AND DOCUMENTATION

Communication will occur with Mrs. Solomon and her family. A plan of care will be discussed with the patient. All elements of her management will be documented. Discharge planning will be provided.

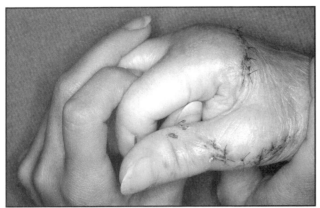

Figure 8-8. Therapist performing passive flexion of the MCP joint.

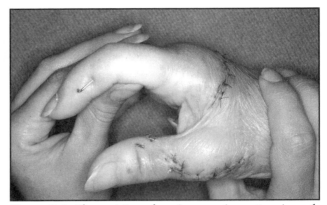

Figure 8-9. Therapist performing passive extension of the MCP joint.

PATIENT/CLIENT-RELATED INSTRUCTION

Instruction for this patient ideally begins preoperatively. There are two main objectives of the preoperative session: 1) to fabricate a custom-made dorsally based outrigger splint with a radial bar attachment, and 2) to facilitate patient understanding of the need for active participation in the postoperative therapy process. This includes the importance and rationale of initially attending physical therapy sessions three times a week and compliance with a daily home exercise program. This session also answers questions the patient might have about the surgery, the postoperative recovery, and anticipated functional outcomes.

Postoperatively, Mrs. Solomon will be provided instruction regarding her home exercise program, donning and doffing the outrigger splint, splint usage, time frames for progression of her program, and precautions.

THERAPEUTIC EXERCISE

- ◆ Fragile or inflammatory stage (PO 1 to 5 days)
  - AAROM and AROM exercises to improve the mobility of the MCP joints of the right hand
  - Assisted MCP joint extension guided by the slings on the outrigger splint
  - Active flexion of the MCP joints guided by the slings on the outrigger
  - AROM of the forearm/wrist: Supination and pronation, flexion, extension, ulnar and radial deviation, with fingers supported in neutral, using the other hand
  - Thumb
    - Opposition, thumb tip to each finger tip, and blocked IP joint flexion and extension
  - AROM of the MCP joints in flexion, guided in the supported slings of the outrigger
  - Blocked AROM of the IP joint of the thumb
    - By limiting motion of the CMC and MP joints

of the thumb with the left hand, the forces acting at the CMC and MP joints will be redirected to the IP joint of the thumb and allow for increased motion
  - The radial walk: Finger AROM in radial deviation is initiated on a powder board or tabletop and is the only exercise or activity performed out of the splint at this time
  - No unsupported AROM of the fingers or wrist is permitted
  - AROM of the elbow is permitted and full AROM of the elbow is encouraged
- ◆ Early fibroplastic or remolding stage (PO 5 to 10 days)
  - Finger exercises are continued within the confines of the dorsal outrigger splint (guided MCP joint flexion and assisted extension) except for the radial walk, in which the fingers are supported on a tabletop
  - Wrist and elbow AROM exercises are continued as outlined above
  - PROM of the MCP joints in flexion and extension is initiated if the therapist determines that there is tightness developing in the dorsal capsule (Figures 8-8 and 8-9)
    - This is performed only by the therapist and is not given to the patient as a home exercise
    - Refer to the different range requirements for each finger (Table 8-16)[98]
    - Late fibroplastic stage (PO 3 to 4 weeks)
  - All exercises are continued in the outrigger splint
  - Exercises that can now be performed out of the splint
    - K-wires are removed
    - The radial walk supported on a table top or a powder board
    - Active flexion/extension of the MCP joints, using finger cylinders to block PIP and DIP joint motion. This directs all forces to the MCP joint

level, allowing for increased motion at the MCP joint

- Wrist AROM in all directions
- Extensor digitorum communis glides (composite fist: MCP, PIP, and DIP joints in flexion) to intrinsic plus position (claw: MCP joints in neutral, PIP and DIP joints in flexion) and back to composite fist position

♦ Transitional stage (PO 4 to 6 weeks)

- Mrs. Solomon may perform light ADL while out of the splint, such as bathing, eating, and most self-dressing tasks, still avoiding forceful pinch
- Avoid strong key pinch activities, such as tying shoelaces and using a key, due to the ulnar deviating forces of the thumb on the index and middle fingers
- Active flexion exercise of the MCP joints

♦ End of transitional stage (PO 6 weeks)

- Gross grip strength on the right hand was below normal at 13 lbs (average of three trials); normal is 57 lbs for a right-hand dominant 56-year-old woman[96]
- Pinch strength, three-jaw chuck, index and middle fingers to thumb was also below normal at 3 lbs (average of three trials); normal is 12 lbs[96]
- Key pinch was not assessed because of the high degree of ulnar deviating forces placed on the index and middle fingers during this pinch pattern
- Gentle resistive exercises are begun using light resistance putty for grip strengthening
  - The putty is placed below the distal palmar crease and a fist is tightly sustained for 5 seconds
- The outrigger is used periodically during the day for exercise

♦ Early scar maturation stage (PO 6 weeks to 6 months)

- Progress resistance in all exercises to patient's tolerance
  - For example, putty resistance may be incrementally increased for grip strengthening
  - The thumb may be strengthened against the resistance of the putty as long as there is no pain at the MP joint (arthrodesis site)
- Focus is on functional power and endurance
- Low weight PREs are used to improve wrist strength in both flexion and extension
  - Starting with an 8-oz weight held in the hand, slowly perform 10 reps in wrist flexion and extension
  - The reps may be increased by five every week or according to the patient's tolerance

♦ Late scar maturation stage (6 months to 1 year postoperative)

- Progress resistive exercise program of putty exercises

Table 8-16
AROM GOALS FOR THE MCP JOINT FOLLOWING ARTHROPLASTY[98]

	Extension	Flexion
Index finger	Full 0 degrees	45 degrees
Middle finger	Full 0 degrees	60 degrees
Ring finger	Full 0 degrees	70 degrees
Small finger	Full 0 degrees	70 degrees

to improve grip and pinch strength

- PREs are progressed by increasing repetitions and weight to improve strength and endurance

FUNCTIONAL TRAINING IN SELF-CARE AND HOME MANAGEMENT

♦ Self-care

- Dressing: Adaptive equipment includes the use of Velcro closure shoes in place of shoe laces and a built-up handled button hook and zipper pull
- Eating: Adaptive equipment includes built-up handles for eating utensils (fork and spoon), a rocking T knife, built-up handles for serving utensils, and a double-handled mug and glass
- Grooming: Adaptive equipment includes built-up handles for comb and brush and a wash cloth mitt for the bath
- Toileting: A built-up handle bar was installed on the right side of her toilet

♦ Home management

- Activities that involve the thumb creating a strong key pinch and forceful ulnar deviation of the index and middle fingers should be avoided during household chores, cooking, cleaning, and shopping (Figure 8-10)
- Adaptive equipment includes: Rubber doorknob extensions, EZ key turner, built-up handle pens and grips for pencils, lamp switch enlargers, and sink knob covers with built-in levers

FUNCTIONAL TRAINING IN WORK, COMMUNITY, AND LEISURE INTEGRATION OR REINTEGRATION

♦ Community and leisure

- Mrs. Solomon uses a cardholder at her weekly bridge games

MANUAL THERAPY TECHNIQUES

♦ Massage[101]

- Retrograde massage

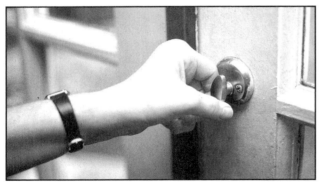

Figure 8-10. Forceful pressure of the index and middle fingers into ulnar deviation.

■ Begin at the first postoperative visit
■ Fluid flushing massage to reduce postoperative edema
■ Starting from the tips of each finger, working proximally to in between the MC heads (implant level), into the hand and up the arm
● Cross friction massage
■ Begin during the early part of the late fibroplastic phase about 1 week following suture removal when the wound margins can tolerate the pressure of the stroke
■ During the end of the late fibroplastic stage and the early part of the transitional stage (PO 3 to 4 weeks)
▸ Progress to deep circular friction massage when wound margins can tolerate
▸ Using pure lanolin or cocoa butter will reduce friction on the incision and soften the skin
▸ Adherence of the incision to the extensor digitorum communis tendon will limit extensor digitorum communis glide resulting in an extension lag at the MCP joint level and/ or limiting composite flexion
▸ Performing extensor digitorum communis gliding exercises while massaging the incision will address adhesions (claw, fist, claw)
♦ Passive range of motion
● Gentle passive flexion of the MCP joint (MCP joint in flexion with the PIP and DIP joints in full extension) and composite flexion stretching exercises (full MCP, PIP, and DIP joint flexion fist)

PRESCRIPTION, APPLICATION, AND, AS APPROPRIATE, FABRICATION OF DEVICES AND EQUIPMENT

♦ Fragile or inflammatory stage (PO 1 to 5 days)
● The base of the outrigger splint needs to be adjusted to accommodate the bulky surgical dressing
● The base was reformed to the contour of the dressing and without pressure on the surgical site
● The underside of the splint was padded using adhesive-backed foam to prevent shearing forces on the incision
● The slings on the dorsal outrigger bar were applied to each proximal phalanx at a 90-degree angle of pull
● Slings from the radial bar were placed on the index and middle fingers at the middle phalanx level
● The force couple created by the dorsal sling and the radial sling positioned the index and middle fingers in supination to allow for pad-to-pad pinch with the thumb
● The tension on the rubber bands is tight enough to support the MCP joints in zero degrees extension (neutral) but allow for 70 to 75 degrees of active MCP joint flexion
● The outrigger is worn full-time, except for wound care and the radial walk
♦ Early fibroplastic or remolding stage (PO 5 to 10 days)
● Continued use of the outrigger splint on a full-time basis
♦ Late fibroplastic stage (PO 10 days to 3 to 4 weeks)
● Begin weaning from full-time use of the outrigger, starting with half-hour increments
● Since Mrs. Solomon has limited PROM (0 to 40 degrees) at the MCP joints of the index, middle, ring, and small fingers, a dynamic flexion cuff splint is utilized to elongate the newly forming dorsal capsule and improve passive MCP flexion
■ Volar slings that originate from the flexion cuff are applied to the ring and small fingers
■ The flexion cuff sling is rarely used on the index finger because it requires stability over mobility
■ These slings are worn in 30-minute intervals, followed by active flexion exercises of the MCP joints
♦ Transitional stage (PO 4 to 6 weeks)
● A custom fabricated volar resting splint that is used to position the fingers in neutral alignment replaces the outrigger for nighttime use
● The volar resting splint is only worn during the day with severe joint instability
● The outrigger is used periodically during the day for rest and exercise

♦ Early scar maturation stage (PO 6 weeks to 6 months)
  • Most patients will be out of the outrigger splint all day

♦ Late scar maturation stage (PO 6 months to 1 year)
  • Continue nighttime splinting until the 1-year assessment
  • Splinting is continued if a recurrent ulnar drift pattern of the fingers is noted

INTEGUMENTARY REPAIR AND PROTECTION TECHNIQUES

♦ Mrs. Solomon is instructed in appropriate daily wound care and dressing changes while the sutures are in situ

♦ She is instructed to rinse the suture area using hydrogen peroxide, pat dry, then let air dry, and then cover with sterile gauze

♦ During wound care the hand and fingers are supported in neutral on the table

PHYSICAL AGENTS AND MECHANICAL MODALITIES

The following modalities may be used after complete wound closure:

♦ Thermotherapy parameters[102]
  • Paraffin baths
    ▪ Use "glove" application method
    ▪ Immerse hand into paraffin unit 6 to 12 times
    ▪ Cover hand using plastic bag or wax paper and than cover this using terry cloth mitt or towel
    ▪ Duration of treatment is 20 minutes
  • Fluidotherapy
    ▪ Treatments are delivered at 105° to 125°F
    ▪ Duration of treatment is 20 to 30 minutes

♦ Cold packs
  • Using commercial packs treatments are delivered at 0° to 10°F
  • Duration of treatment is 15 to 20 minutes, depending upon amount of discomfort

♦ Contrast baths
  • Use two basins, one filled with cold water (55° to 65°F) and the other filled with warm water (100° to 110°F)
  • Immerse hand for 15 seconds into the basin filled with the cold water, remove, and immediately immerse into the warm water basin for 15 seconds
  • Alternating between the warm and cold water
  • Duration of treatment is 15 minutes.
  • Always start and end in the cold-water basin[103,104]

ANTICIPATED GOALS AND EXPECTED OUTCOMES

♦ Impact on pathology/pathophysiology
  • Edema, lymphedema, or effusion is reduced.
  • Joint swelling, inflammation, or restriction is reduced.
  • Nutrient delivery to tissue is increased.
  • Pain is decreased.
  • Soft tissue inflammation, edema, and restriction are reduced.

♦ Impact on impairments
  • Endurance is improved.
  • Integumentary integrity is improved.
  • Joint integrity and mobility are improved.
  • Motor function is improved.
  • Muscle performance is increased.
  • Quality and quantity of movement between and across body segments are improved.
  • Relaxation is increased.
  • ROM is improved: Full MCP joint extension of all fingers, index finger=0 to 45 degrees, middle finger=0 to 60 degrees, and ring and small fingers=0 to 70 degrees.

♦ Impact on functional limitations
  • Ability to assume or resume required self-care, home management, work, community, and leisure roles is improved.
  • Ability to independently perform physical actions, tasks, and activities related to ADL/IADL in self-care, home management, work, community, and leisure with or without assistive devices and equipment is increased.

♦ Risk reduction/prevention
  • Postoperative complications are reduced.
  • Risk factors are reduced.
  • Risk of secondary impairments is reduced.
  • Self-management of symptoms is improved.

♦ Impact on health, wellness, and fitness
  • Behaviors that foster healthy habits, wellness, and prevention are acquired.
  • Decision making is enhanced regarding health, wellness, and fitness needs.
  • Health status and physical function are improved.

♦ Impact on societal resources
  • Available resources are maximally utilized.
  • Documentation occurs throughout patient management and across all settings and follows APTA's *Guidelines for Physical Therapy Documentation.*[80]
  • Utilization of physical therapy services is optimized.
  • Utilization of physical therapy services results in efficient use of health care dollars.

♦ Patient/client satisfaction
  ● Access, availability, and services provided are acceptable to patient/client.
  ● Case is managed throughout the episode of care.
  ● Clinical proficiency and interpersonal skills of the physical therapist are acceptable to patient.
  ● Coordination of care is acceptable to patient.
  ● Patient and family knowledge and awareness of the diagnosis, prognosis, interventions, and understanding of anticipated goals and expected outcomes are increased.
  ● Sense of well-being is improved.

REEXAMINATION

Reexamination is performed throughout the episode of care, particularly as the setting of care changes and as the stages change.

DISCHARGE

Mrs. Solomon is discharged from physical therapy after a total of 30 physical therapy sessions and attainment of her goals and expectations. These sessions have covered her entire episode of care except for her 1-year follow-up assessment visit which is used to determine whether splinting should be continued. She is discharged because she has achieved her goals and expected outcomes.

Case Study #5: Carpometacarpal Joint Osteoarthritis With Ligament Reconstruction Tendon Interpositional Arthroplasty

Mrs. Laura Norton is a 55-year-old female with bilateral basal joint osteoarthritis and bilateral de Quervain's stenosing tenosynovitis who has undergone a right ligament reconstruction tendon interpositional arthroplasty.

PHYSICAL THERAPIST EXAMINATION

HISTORY

♦ General demographics: Laura Norton is a 55-year-old, right-hand dominant female. She is a college graduate and her primary language is English.
♦ Social history: Mrs. Norton is married and has one daughter, 35 years old, and a 1-year-old granddaughter.
♦ Employment/work: Mrs. Norton worked as a dental hygienist for 30 years. She retired 5 years ago because of bilateral hand pain, localized to the base of her thumbs (R>L) that was exacerbated while working.
♦ Living environment: Mrs. Norton lives with her husband in a one family, two-story home in the suburbs.
♦ General health status
  ● General health perception: Mrs. Norton reports being in excellent health.
  ● Physical function: Prior to the surgery, Mrs. Norton was independent in all ADL. However, she did have increased pain while performing activities that required prolonged pinch, such as zippering, writing, and needlepoint.
  ● Psychological function: Normal.
  ● Role function: Wife, mother, grandmother.
  ● Social function: Mrs. Norton enjoys doing handcrafts and likes to take classes to perfect her skills. Crocheting, knitting, and needlepoint are her favorite crafts.
♦ Social/health habits: She reports being a non-smoker and social drinker.
♦ Family history: Noncontributory.
♦ Medical/surgical history: She is in generally good health except for a history of OA, especially in both hands.
♦ Prior hospitalizations: Bilateral carpal tunnel releases 10 years ago.
♦ Preexisting medical and other health-related conditions: She has bilateral de Quervain's stenosing tenosynovitis.
♦ Current condition(s)/chief complaint(s): She had pain in both thumbs prior to surgery. Mrs. Norton attended 6 weeks of physical therapy for conservative management of bilateral basal joint pain and de Quervain's stenosing tenosynovitis. Her preoperative treatment consisted of paraffin and phonophoresis with a topical ibuprofen. Two forearm based thumb spica splints were custom fabricated, one for each hand (Figure 8-11). Her overall pain on the left was reduced at rest to 1/10 and with attempted motion 3/10, but pain on the right persisted at 6/10 at rest and 8/10 with motion. At the end of 6 weeks of therapy, Mrs. Norton still had a positive grind test on the right hand. Radiographs confirmed Stage III involvement on the left and Stage IV involvement on the right.[65] Mrs. Norton had a right LRTI arthroplasty with complete trapezium excision, an MP joint arthrodesis, and a local decompression tenosynovectomy of the first dorsal extensor tendon compartment 4 1/2 weeks ago.
♦ Functional status and activity level: She had been independent in all ADL, although she had thumb pain. She avoided activities that required prolonged pinch due to pain.
♦ Medications: She had been taking two 200 mg ibupro-

fen tablets daily to control hand pain.

♦ Other clinical tests: Preoperative radiographs confirmed Stage III[105] involvement in the left and Stage IV in the right.

SYSTEMS REVIEW

♦ Cardiovascular/pulmonary
  • BP: 120/80 mmHg
  • Edema: Moderate dorsal edema of the right hand
  • HR: 73 bpm
  • RR: 12 bpm
♦ Integumentary
  • Presence of scar formation
    ▪ A vertical incision was noted on the dorsal radial aspect of the right hand extending distally from the radial styloid process to the base of the first MC
    ▪ Moderate edema localized to the region of the surgical site was present
  • Skin color: Mild ecchymosis is present and localized to the region of the surgical site
  • Skin integrity: Well-healed, mature scar was present on the palm at the carpal tunnel
♦ Musculoskeletal
  • Gross range of motion
    ▪ Right forearm, wrist, and thumb limited
    ▪ Left thumb limited
  • Gross strength
    ▪ BLE and the LUE were WFL
    ▪ No strength testing was performed on the RUE at this time
  • Gross symmetry: Symmetrical
  • Height: 5'5" (1.65 m)
  • Weight: 150 lbs (55.98 kg)
♦ Neuromuscular
  • Gross coordinated movements (balance, locomotion, transfers, and transitions) are all WFL
♦ Communication, affect, cognition, language, and learning style
  • Mrs. Norton is oriented to person, place, and time
  • She is able to express herself and make her needs known to others
  • Mrs. Norton stated she is an auditory learner
  • No barriers to learning are noted nor expected

TESTS AND MEASURES

♦ Aerobic capacity/endurance during functional activities was not tested at this time
♦ Anthropometric characteristics
  • BMI=705 x (body weight [in pounds] divided by

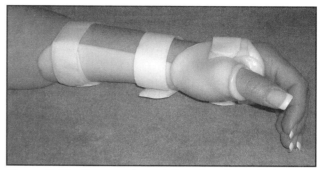

Figure 8-11. Forearm-based thumb spica splint.

height² [in inches])
    ▪ Mrs. Norton's BMI=25.02
    ▪ BMI values between 25 and 30 are considered to be overweight[93]
  • Circumferential measurements around the right MCP joint level was 25 cm as compared to the left MCP joint level which was 15 cm
  • Edema
    ▪ Volumetric measurements were used so that the edema of the hand was measured by the amount of water displaced, and a comparison was made between the right and left hands
      ‣ The procedure followed the technique described by Brand[105]
      ‣ Preoperative measurements revealed:
        ○ Right hand: 15 mL of water displacement
        ○ Left hand: 8 mL of water displacement
      ‣ Postoperative measurements (4 1/2 weeks) revealed:
        ○ Right hand: 25 mL of water displacement
        ○ Left hand: 8 mL of water displacement
♦ Assistive and adaptive devices
  • Two forearm based thumb spica splints were custom fabricated
  • Following the initial 6 weeks postoperative, the splint is to be used only for protection and rest
♦ Cranial and peripheral nerve integrity
  • Cranial nerves are intact
  • Peripheral nerve tests included were light touch, deep touch, moving touch, and two-point static touch
  • All tests are WNL except for diminished sensation distal to the incision on the dorsal aspect of the right thumb
  • Sensory testing on the left hand was normal
♦ Environmental, home, and work barriers
  • There are no barriers at home
  • Mrs. Norton is retired so there are no work barriers
♦ Ergonomics and body mechanics

- Dexterity and coordination during leisure activities are restricted at this time
♦ Gait, locomotion, and balance
  - No assistive devices are required
  - Balance is intact
  - Arm swing diminished during gait
♦ Integumentary integrity
  - Associated skin
    ▪ Skin over surgical site was slightly warm to the touch and mildly eccymotic
  - Wound
    ▪ No signs of infection were noted
    ▪ The incision was closed and healing well
    ▪ Sutures were removed at 14 days post surgery
♦ Motor function
  - Dexterity, coordination, and agility
    ▪ Fine motor dexterity not tested at this time, will be tested at 7 weeks postoperatively
    ▪ Hand function remains limited and protected until 8 weeks following surgery
♦ Muscle performance
  - MMT: Not performed at this time
  - Grip and pinch strength of the left hand were tested using a Jamar dynamometer and a Jamar pinch gauge, respectively according to the recommendations of the American Society of Hand Therapists[95]
    ▪ These instruments are commonly used to assess grip and pinch strength, however, their reliability is based on the condition that they are calibrated annually[94]
    ▪ Testing position
      ▸ Shoulder adducted, next to side of body, elbow flexed to 90 degrees, forearm in neutral rotation, wrist between 0 to 30 degrees of extension and in slight ulnar deviation
      ▸ The dynamometer was on the "second" handle position
      ▸ The test is performed three times with a short rest period allowed between readings so that the results are not affected by fatigue[95]
    ▪ Left hand grip strength recordings were 20 lbs, 15 lbs, and 10 lbs for an average of 15 lbs over three trials
      ▸ Normal grip strength is 57.3 lbs on the non-dominant hand of a 55-year-old woman[96]
    ▪ Left key pinch strength recordings were 10 lbs, 10 lbs, and 8 lbs for an average of 9.3 lbs over three trials
      ▸ Normal key pinch is 14.7 lbs[96] on the non-dominant hand of a 55-year-old woman

- Her limiting factor is discomfort at the basal joint with sustained force
- Grip and pinch strength on the right hand were not tested until 8 weeks postoperatively using a Jamar dynamometer and a Jamar pinch gauge as indicated above
  ▪ Right hand grip strength recordings were 7 lbs, 5 lbs, and 5 lbs for an average of 5.6 lbs over three trials
    ▸ Normal grip strength for the dominant hand of a 55-year-old woman is 57.3 lbs[96]
  ▪ Right hand pinch strength (key pinch) recordings were 1 lb, 1lb, and 1lb for an average of 1 lb over three trials
    ▸ Normal pinch strength for the dominant hand of a 55-year-old woman is 15.7 lbs[96]
  ▪ Left hand grip strength recordings at 8 weeks postoperatively were now 20 lbs, 20 lbs, and 15 lb for an average of 18.3 lbs
  ▪ Left hand pinch strength (key pinch) recordings were now 10 lbs, 10 lbs, and 10 lbs for an average of 10 lbs over three trials
- MMT for the right forearm, wrist, and fingers=4/5
- Thumb was not tested at this time due to arthrodesis
♦ Orthotic, protective, and supportive devices
  - A supported, protective orthotic, forearm based, thumb spica splint with the IP joint free was custom fabricated during the preoperative/conservative management phase of therapy
    ▪ The purpose of the splint was to support the weakened and painful basal joint and thumb during conservative management
  - Postoperatively, the same splint was used to support, protect, and rest the newly constructed joint, the decompressed first extensor tendon compartment, and the MP joint arthrodesis
  - The thumb spica splint was worn from immediately following cast removal at 4 1/2 weeks until 12 weeks postoperatively
    ▪ From 4 1/2 to 6 weeks, the splint is worn full-time including during sleeping
      ▸ During this period, the splint is only removed for controlled AROM exercise for the thumb and wrist, wound care at the surgical and pin sites, and retrograde massage for edema reduction
    ▪ At 8 weeks postoperative, the splint is to be worn during the day for protection and at night for rest
    ▪ At 12 weeks, the splint is to be worn only for rest if needed

♦ Pain
  • Pain at rest was 6/10 on the right and 2/10 on the left on the NPS with 0=no pain and 10=the worst pain possible[97]
  • Pain with motion was 8/10 on the right localized at the surgical site and 4/10 on the left on the NPS
♦ Posture
  • The patient has a FHP, mild kyphosis, and slightly protracted shoulders
♦ Range of motion
  • AROM and PROM tested with a goniometer revealed:
    ▪ Cervical spine: WNL
    ▪ Bilateral shoulders and elbows: WNL
    ▪ Right forearm: Supination=0 to 60 degrees, pronation=0 to 60 degrees
    ▪ Left forearm: Supination and pronation were WNL
    ▪ Right wrist: Extension=0 to 40 degrees, flexion=0 to 40 degrees
    ▪ Left wrist: WNL
    ▪ Bilateral terminal finger: Flexion and extension were WNL
    ▪ Right thumb
      ▸ Opposition limited to the radial side of the index finger tip
      ▸ MP joint arthrodesed in 30 degrees of flexion
      ▸ IP joint: Extension=+5 degrees, flexion=0 to 40 degrees
    ▪ Left thumb
      ▸ Opposition limited to the PIP joint crease of the small finger
      ▸ MP joint postured in 10 degrees of hyperextension
      ▸ IP joint postured in 10 degrees of flexion
      ▸ Zigzag deformity pattern of the thumb is present
    ▪ Limiting factor on right hand reported to be pain
  • PROM
    ▪ Wrist and forearm PROM: Not tested at this time
    ▪ Thumb PROM: Not tested at this time
♦ Reflex integrity
  • Deep reflexes: WNL
  • Superficial reflexes: WNL
♦ Self-care and home management
  • An interview concerning the ability to safely manage self-care and home management actions, tasks, and activities revealed that bilateral tasks in these areas required minimal to moderate assistance

  • Minimal assistance was required for most bilateral self-care tasks
♦ Work, community, and leisure integration or reintegration
  • An interview concerning the ability to safely manage community and leisure actions, tasks, and activities revealed the need for minimal assistance if the task was bilateral and required use of the thumb

EVALUATION

Laura Norton's history indicated that she is a 55-year-old, right-hand dominant female who retired early from her position as a dental hygienist at the age of 50 because of bilateral hand (thumb) discomfort. Ten years ago, she underwent bilateral carpal tunnel releases after which she reported full restoration of sensation and full functional use of both hands. Prior to this current surgery, Mrs. Norton attended 6 weeks of physical therapy for conservative management of bilateral thumb pain. At that time, she presented with a prominent shoulder sign at the right basal joint, a positive grind test, Stage IV CMC OA on the right, based on the Eaton radiographic grading system,[65] and right de Quervain's stenosing tenosynovitis.

The patient is now 4 1/2 weeks post a right CMC, LRTI arthroplasty, MP joint arthrodesis, and local decompression of the first dorsal extensor tendon compartment. She has limited AROM of the right UE: supination/pronation 0 to 60 degrees and wrist extension/flexion 0 to 40 degrees. Opposition of the thumb is limited to the radial side of the index finger tip. The MP joint of the thumb is fused. The IP joint is limited in extension 0/+5, and flexion is 0 to 40 degrees. She reports pain of 6/10 at the surgical site at rest and 8/10 with attempted thumb motion. Moderate edema, localized to the dorsum of the hand, is noted.

DIAGNOSIS

Mrs. Norton has undergone a right CMC, LRTI right arthroplasty, MP joint arthrodesis, and a de Quervain's release and she has pain. She has impaired: anthropometric characteristics; ergonomics and body mechanics; motor function; muscle performance; posture; and range of motion. She is functionally limited in self-care and home management and in work, community, and leisure actions, tasks, and activities. She will be using an orthotic device. These impairments and functional limitations will be addressed in determining the prognosis and the plan of care.

PROGNOSIS AND PLAN OF CARE

Over the course of the visits, the following mutually established outcomes have been determined:

- Ability to perform 95% of all ADL independently is achieved
- Ability to perform home management, community, and leisure actions, tasks, and activities independently is achieved
- AROM is improved
- Coordination is improved
- Deformity is lessened
- Endurance during fine motor activities is improved
- Gross grip strength is improved
- Joint edema and inflammation are reduced
- Joint mobility is improved
- Pain is reduced, both at rest and during pinch activities
- Pinch strength is improved

To achieve these outcomes the appropriate interventions for this patient are determined. These will include: coordination, communication, and documentation; patient/client-related instruction; therapeutic exercise; functional training in self-care and home management; functional training in work, community, and leisure integration or reintegration; manual therapy techniques; prescription, application, and, as appropriate, fabrication of devices and equipment; electrotherapeutic modalities; and physical agents and mechanical modalities.

Based on the diagnosis and prognosis, Mrs. Norton is expected to require between 20 to 30 visits over a 14- to 15-week period of time. Mrs. Norton has good family support and motivation, and there were no postoperative complications.

INTERVENTIONS

RATIONALE FOR SELECTED INTERVENTIONS

The rationale of the specific postoperative exercise program that Mrs. Norton will follow is based on the different stages of wound healing.[43] These stages have already been detailed in the MCP joint implant arthroplasty. Their importance necessitates their repetition here. The wound healing stages are:

- Fragile or inflammatory stage (PO 1 to 5 days)
- Early fibroplastic or remolding stage (PO 5 to 10 days)
- Late fibroplastic stage (PO 10 days to 3 to 4 weeks)
- Transitional stage (PO 4 to 6 weeks)
- Early scar maturation stage (PO 6 weeks to 6 months)
- Late scar maturation stage (PO 6 months to 1 year)

Poole and Pellegrini recommend immediate referral to physical therapy following surgery, while the patient is still in the plaster thumb spica cast, during the inflammatory and early fibroplastic stages of wound healing. The patient is instructed in AROM exercises of the shoulder, elbow, and fingers in order to reduce joint stiffness. Elevation instructions are also given to minimize postoperative edema.[7] All aspects of care should facilitate the encapsulation process. Swanson and his associates[98] address this process by the following statement:

> The greatest challenge in postoperative rehabilitation is to maintain a proper balance between good healing of the surrounding scar tissue and at the same time, application of proper amounts of tension across the scar to maintain the desired ROM. Controlled motion during this period will train the new capsule to have sufficient looseness for mobility and sufficient tightness for stability.

Therapeutic Exercise

The postoperative exercise program is guided by the progressive increase in the tensile strength of the forming pseudocapsule. Following cast removal, the focus of the therapy is to reduce postoperative edema, scar management, protecting the MP joint arthrodesis, and improving thumb mobility while maintaining CMC stability. Mobility of the thumb is achieved only by AROM exercises. PROM is not used at the CMC joint following arthroplasty. By using AROM exercises without passive force, mobility at this joint is increased, while simultaneously reinforcing it's stability. Mobility of the thumb enhances function. However, stability at the base of the thumb is necessary for pain-free motion.[28]

Exercises for the patient with this diagnosis will be progressed to include resistance for strengthening according to the different stages of wound healing and radiographic confirmation of healing.[98]

Manual Therapy Techniques

The patient is instructed in massage techniques, including fluid flushing, gentle cross friction, and deep circular massage. These techniques are incorporated into the home program at different stages. The fluid flushing massage is used to reduce the postoperative edema of the fingers, hand, and wrist.[101] The second massage technique, cross friction massage, is introduced about 1 week following suture removal, when the wound margins can tolerate the pressure.

A deep circular massage is used after the third postoperative week. The cross friction and deep circular massages are used to reduce the propensity of the incision to adhere to the underlying extensor tendons of the thumb.[101]

Prescription, Application, and, as Appropriate, Fabrication of Devices and Equipment

Following cast removal, at 4 1/2 weeks (in between the late fibroplastic and the transitional stages) a thermoplastic thumb spica splint is fabricated. The schedule for wearing the splint changes as the collagen of the pseudocapsule matures.

Refer to the rationale for Prescription, Application, and,

as Appropriate, Fabrication of Devices and Equipment in Case Study #4.

Electrotherapeutic Modalities

Electrotherapeutic modalities are not routinely used when treating a patient following arthroplasty surgery. However, they may be instrumental in treating secondary problems, such as pain and edema that may be the result of the surgery. For example, high-volt pulsed current (HVPC) may be used to promote healing and reduce postoperative edema. Edema may be curbed or reduced using the polar effects of HVPC. Following acute injury or surgery, proteins escape from the microvasculature. Cathodal stimulation expels these proteins from the area, taking excess fluid with them.[106] Pain following surgery may also be reduced through the use of TENS.[102] Conventional mode TENS relieves pain through a proposed spinal gate theory mechanism.[107]

Physical Agents and Mechanical Modalities

A variety of primary modalities may be used following cast removal. Thermotherapy may be in the form of heat or cold. Thermotherapy, in the form of heat, may include paraffin, hot packs, and fluidotherapy. Heat will increase muscle/tendon extensibility of the small muscles of the hand and increase blood flow needed to promote the healing process.[104] Paraffin is often the modality of choice. Its mineral oil base helps soften the scar in addition to providing the benefits of thermotherapy.[102]

Thermotherapy, in the form of cold, may include cold packs or contrast baths. If necessary, cold packs may be used following the exercise session to reduce discomfort and edema. Contrast baths utilize immersion of the hand in alternating hot and cold water to increase blood flow to promote healing and decrease joint stiffness. Contrast baths may alleviate pain, stiffness, and edema by externally inducing vasodilatation and vasoconstriction that is usually produced by normally contracting muscles.[103] The alternating water temperature increases the blood flow to the affected area and induces a "vascular pumping" effect resulting in vasoconstriction, edema reduction, and increased mobility. Contrast baths reduce discomfort, edema, and subsequent discomfort and improve blood flow to promote healing.[104] Contrast baths are an excellent modality that may be used in the clinic or at home.

COORDINATION, COMMUNICATION, AND DOCUMENTATION

Communication will occur with Mrs. Norton. A plan of care will be discussed with her, and all elements of her management will be documented. Discharge planning will be provided.

PATIENT/CLIENT-RELATED INSTRUCTION

Preoperatively, Mrs. Norton was custom fitted with a forearm based thumb spica splint as part of her conservative management. On her last preoperative visit, she was instructed in AROM exercises for the unaffected joints of the entire UE in order to prevent joint stiffness due to non-use. She was also instructed to elevate of the entire arm following surgery (day and night) to reduce post-surgical edema. The rationale for both of these instructions were explained to Mrs. Norton.

Postoperatively, Mrs. Norton was provided instruction regarding her home exercise program. She will also be provided instructions in joint protection and in ways to modify the pinch pattern to protect the arthroplasty.

THERAPEUTIC EXERCISE

- ◆ First postoperative week: Fragile or inflammatory stage (PO 1 to 5 days)
  - • With the below elbow thumb spica cast on, elevation of the arm above the heart level for edema control.
  - • Shoulder, elbow, and finger AROM (within the confines of the cast), to prevent stiffness of unaffected joints.
- ◆ Early fibroplastic or remolding stage (PO 5 to 10 days)
  - • Continued AROM of all unaffected joints of the UE
- ◆ Late fibroplastic stage (PO 10 days to 3 to 4 weeks)
  - • Early referral of the patient may be made to the therapist for initial assessment if the surgeon notices excessive postoperative edema and/or joint stiffness of the unaffected joints, especially the shoulder and fingers
- ◆ Transition stage (PO 4 to 6 weeks)
  - • At 4 1/2 to 5 weeks, the cast is removed, and the arthroplasty pin is taken out
  - • The patient is referred to therapy for her initial postoperative assessment, if not previously referred with the cast on
  - • Exercises include:
    - ▪ AROM for fingers, wrist, and elbow
    - ▪ Continue with shoulder exercise if indicated
    - ▪ AROM of the thumb IP joint, while supporting the thumb MP joint fusion with the other hand
    - ▪ Opposition to the index finger only
    - ▪ Stability over mobility is stressed
- ◆ End of transition stage into early scar maturation stage (PO 5 to 8 weeks)
  - • Active opposition of the thumb to all fingertips, and slide down of small finger to the distal palmar crease
  - • Isometric thenar exercises

- Light functional activities initiated
- ◆ Early scar maturation stage (PO 6 weeks to 6 months)
  - 8 to 12 weeks
    - Progressive grip strengthening
      - ▸ Grip strengthening using light resistant putty
      - ▸ Place putty below the distal palmar crease of the palm and tightly sustain a fist around the putty for 5 seconds
      - ▸ Initially repeat five times and slowly progress to 10 times during this 4-week period
      - ▸ The difficulty of this exercise may be progressed by using a heavy grade putty
      - ▸ Progressions are based on each individual patient's needs
    - Progressive pinch strengthening
      - ▸ Pinch strengthening using a light resistant sponge
        - ○ Place the sponge between the pulp of the thumb and the side tip of the index finger and pinch
        - ○ Pinch around the perimeter of the sponge two to three times depending upon patient tolerance
      - ▸ Pinch strengthening is progressed to light resistance putty
        - ○ Place a high cylinder of putty on the radial side/tip of the index finger
        - ○ Press into the top of the cylinder using the pulp of the thumb
        - ○ Continue to press into the putty until the pulp of the thumb is touching the side/tip of the index finger
        - ○ Initially repeat five times and progress very slowly to 10 times during this 4-week period
        - ○ The difficulty of this pinch exercise should be progressed according to the patient's tolerance and needs
        - ○ This can be done by gradually increasing the resistance of the putty
  - End of early scar maturation stage (PO 3 to 6 months)
    - Unrestricted functional activities
- ◆ Late scar maturation stage (PO 6 months to 1 year)
  - Unrestricted work and activities

FUNCTIONAL TRAINING IN SELF-CARE AND HOME MANAGEMENT

- ◆ Self-care
  - Dressing: Adaptive equipment includes a built-up handle button hook and zipper pull

- Eating: Adaptive equipment includes a built-up handle fork, knife, and spoon and selective serving utensils, such as spatula, wooden spoon, and ladle
- Grooming: Adaptive equipment includes built-up handles for brush and comb, toothbrush, and toothpaste squeeze
- ◆ Home management
  - Forceful prolonged pinch or grip should be avoided for 12 weeks following surgery during household chores, cooking, shopping, and cleaning
  - Adaptive equipment included an EZ key turner and a rubber doorknob extension
  - Built-up handle pens and grips for pencils

FUNCTIONAL TRAINING IN WORK, COMMUNITY, AND LEISURE INTEGRATION OR REINTEGRATION

- ◆ Community and leisure
  - Mrs. Norton's personal goal was to return to her knitting and needlepoint following surgery
  - At 5 months, she did resume knitting using built-up "needles"
  - She resumed needlepoint at 6 months post surgery, however limiting her time spent performing this task to 15 minutes, four times per day
  - She increased the time spent working on her needlepoint weekly
  - 4 to 6 months postoperative return to unrestricted leisure actions, tasks, and activities

MANUAL THERAPY TECHNIQUES

- ◆ Massage[101]
  - Transitional stage (PO 4 to 6 weeks)
    - Retrograde massage
      - ▸ Begun 4 1/2 to 5 weeks immediately following cast removal
      - ▸ Fluid flushing massage to reduce postoperative edema
      - ▸ Massage distal to proximal on each finger and thumb in a "milking" fashion
      - ▸ Continue into the hand and work proximally towards the wrist
    - Friction massage using a deep circular stroke
      - ▸ Initiate when the wound margins can tolerate the pressure[101]
      - ▸ Lanolin or cocoa butter will reduce friction on the incision and also help to soften the skin
    - Cross friction massage
      - ▸ Begin 5 to 8 weeks when the wound margins can tolerate the pressure

♦ Passive range of motion
  ● PROM of all fingers, in composite flexion (full fist) to improve joint mobility and muscle flexibility

PRESCRIPTION, APPLICATION, AND, AS APPROPRIATE, FABRICATION OF DEVICES AND EQUIPMENT

♦ Immediately postoperative to 12 weeks
  ● Adaptive devices and equipment
    ▪ Built-up handle fork, knife, and spoon
    ▪ Built-up serving utensils (spatula, wooden spoon, and ladle)
    ▪ Built-up handle brush and comb
    ▪ Built-up toothbrush and toothpaste squeeze
    ▪ EZ key turner
    ▪ Rubber doorknob extensions
    ▪ Built-up pens and pencils
  ● Orthotic device
    ▪ A thumb spica splint is used for protection/support and rest
♦ 4 1/2 to 5 weeks
  ● Orthotic device: When the cast is removed and the arthroplasty pin is taken out, a custom forearm based thumb spica splint is fabricated if it was not previously done as part of conservative management preoperatively
♦ 8 to 12 weeks
  ● Orthotic device: Start weaning from using the splint in protected situations (start weaning at home and progress to outside activities)
♦ 3 to 6 months
  ● Adaptive device
    ▪ Built-up knitting needles
  ● Orthotic device
    ▪ Discontinue protective splinting
    ▪ Splint will be worn only for rest, if needed

ELECTROTHERAPEUTIC MODALITIES

♦ HVPC to promote healing and reduce edema
♦ TENS to reduce pain

PHYSICAL AGENTS AND MECHANICAL MODALITIES

♦ Thermotherapy[102] can be used following cast removal
  ● Paraffin baths
    ▪ Use "glove" application method
    ▪ Immerse hand into paraffin unit 6 to 12 times
    ▪ Cover hand using plastic bag or wax paper and then cover with a terry cloth mitt or towel

    ▪ Duration of treatment is 20 minutes
  ● Fluidotherapy
    ▪ Treatments are delivered at 105° to 125°F
    ▪ Duration of treatment is 20 to 30 minutes
♦ Cold packs
  ● Using commercial packs treatments are delivered at 0° to 10°F
  ● Duration of treatment is 15 to 20 minutes, depending upon amount of discomfort
♦ Contrast baths
  ● Use two basins, one filled with cold water (55° to 65°F) and the other filled with warm water (100° to 110°F)
  ● Immerse hand for 15 seconds into the basin filled with the cold water, remove, and immediately immerse in to the warm water basin for 15 seconds
  ● Alternating between the warm and cold water
  ● Duration of treatment is 15 minutes.
  ● Always start and end in the cold-water basin[103,104]

ANTICIPATED GOALS AND EXPECTED OUTCOMES

♦ Impact on pathology/pathophysiology
  ● Edema, lymphedema, or effusion is reduced.
  ● Joint swelling, inflammation, or restriction is reduced.
  ● Nutrient delivery to tissue is increased.
  ● Pain is decreased.
  ● Soft tissue inflammation, edema, and restriction are reduced.
  ● Tissue perfusion and oxygenation are increased.
♦ Impact on impairments
  ● Endurance in using hand is increased.
  ● Integumentary integrity is improved.
  ● Motor function is improved.
  ● Muscle performance is increased.
  ● Quality of movement between and across body segments is improved.
  ● Relaxation is increased.
  ● ROM is maintained.
♦ Impact on functional limitations
  ● Ability to assume or resume required self-care, home management, work, community, and leisure roles is improved.
  ● Ability to independently perform physical actions, tasks, and activities related to ADL/IADL in self-care, home management, work, community, and leisure with or without assistive devices and equipment is increased.
  ● Level of supervision required for task performance is

decreased.

- Tolerance of actions, tasks, and activities is increased.
♦ Risk reduction/prevention
- Postoperative complications are reduced.
- Risk factors are reduced.
- Risk of recurrence of condition is reduced.
- Risk of secondary impairments is reduced.
- Safety is improved.
- Self management of symptoms is improved.
♦ Impact on health, wellness, and fitness
- Behaviors that foster healthy habits, wellness, and prevention are acquired.
- Decision making is enhanced regarding health, wellness, and fitness needs.
- Physical function is improved.
♦ Impact on societal resources
- Available resources are maximally utilized.
- Documentation occurs throughout patient management and across all settings and follows APTA's *Guidelines for Physical Therapy Documentation.*[80]
- Utilization of physical therapy services is optimized
♦ Patient/client satisfaction
- Access, availability, and services provided are acceptable to patient/client.
- Case is managed throughout the episode of care.
- Clinical proficiency and interpersonal skills of the physical therapist are acceptable to patient/client.
- Coordination of care is acceptable to patient/client.
- Intensity of care is decreased.
- Patient and family knowledge and awareness of the diagnosis, prognosis, interventions, and understanding of anticipated goals and expected outcomes are increased.
- Sense of well-being is improved.
- Stresses are decreased.

REEXAMINATION

Reexamination is performed throughout the episode of care, particularly as the setting of care changes and as the stages change.

DISCHARGE

Mrs. Norton is discharged from physical therapy after a total of 25 physical therapy sessions and attainment of her goals and expectations. These sessions have covered her entire episode of care. She is discharged because she has achieved her goals and expected outcomes.

REFERENCES

1. Moore KL. In: Gardner JN, ed. *Clinically Oriented Anatomy.* 2nd ed. Baltimore, Md: Williams & Wilkins; 1985.
2. Pansky B. *Review of Gross Anatomy.* 5th ed. New York, NY: Macmillan Publishing Co; 1984.
3. Harkness JW. Arthroplasty of hip. In: Canale ST, ed. *Campbell's Operative Orthopaedics.* St. Louis, Mo: Mosby; 1998:296-471.
4. Norkin CC, Levangie PK. *Joint Structure and Function.* 2nd ed. Philadelphia, Pa: FA Davis Co; 1992.
5. Moore KL, Dalley AF. *Clinically Oriented Anatomy.* 4th ed. Philadelphia, Pa: Lippincott Williams & Wilkins; 1999.
6. Beasley RW. *Hand Injuries.* Philadelphia, Pa: WB Saunders Co; 1981.
7. Poole JU, Pellegrini VD Jr. Arthritis of the thumb basal joint complex. *J Hand Ther.* 2000;13(2):91-107.
8. Glickel SZ, Horne LJ. *Current Opinion in Orthopedics.* Philadelphia, Pa: Lippincott Williams & Wilkins; 2001:290-294.
9. Tomaino M. *Hand Clinics: Thumb Arthritis.* Vol 17. Philadelphia, Pa: WB Saunders Co; 2001.
10. Eaton R, Littler JW. Ligament reconstruction for the painful thumb carpometacarpal joint. *J Bone Joint Surg.* 1973;55A:1655-1666.
11. Nordin M, Frankel VH. *Basic Biomechanics of the Musculoskeletal System.* 2nd ed. Philadelphia, Pa: Lea and Febiger; 1989.
12. Bergmann G. Loads acting at the hip joint. In: Sedel L, Cabanela ME, eds. *Hip Surgery; Materials and Developments.* London, England: Martin Dunitz Ltd; 1998:1-8.
13. Johnston RC, Smidt GL. Hip motion measurements for selected activities of daily living. *Clinical Orthop.* 1970;72:205-215.
14. Kettelkamp DB, Johnson RJ, Smidt GL. An electrogoniometric study of knee motion in normal gait. *J Bone Joint Surg (Am).* 1970;52a:775-790.
15. Norkin CC, Levangie PK. *Joint Structure and Function: A Comprehensive Analysis.* Philadelphia, Pa: FA Davis Co; 1983.
16. Bejjani F, Landsmeer J. Biomechanics of the hand. In: Nordin M, Frankel V, eds. *Basic Biomechanics of the Musculoskeletal System.* 2nd ed. Philadelphia, Pa: Lea and Febiger; 1989:275-301.
17. Lehmkuhl LD, Smith L. *Brunnstrom's Clinical Kinesiology.* 4th ed. Philadelphia, Pa: FA Davis Co; 1983.
18. Cooney W, Lucca M, Chao E, Linscheid,R. The kinesiology of the thumb trapeziometacarpal joint. *J Bone Joint Surg.* 1981;63A:1371.
19. Brander V, Mullarkey CF, Stulberg SD. Rehabilitation after total joint replacement for osteoarthritis: an evidence based approach. *Physical Medicine and Rehabilitation: State of the Art Reviews.* 2001;15(1):175-197.
20. Hochberg MC, Altman RD, Brandt KD, et al. Guidelines for the medical management of osteoarthritis of the knee. *Arthritis Rheum.* 1995;38:1541-1546.
21. Berman AT, Quinn RH, Zarro VJ. Quantitative analysis in unilateral and bilateral total hip replacements. *Arch Phys Med Rehabil.* 1991;72:190-194.
22. Azar FM, Wright PE. Arthroplasty of shoulder and elbow. In: Canale ST, ed. *Campbell's Operative Orthopaedics.* St. Louis,

Mo: Mosby; 1998:473-496.

23. Craig EV. Total shoulder replacement for primary osteoarthritis and osteonecrosis. In: Craig EV, ed. *Master Techniques in Orthopaedic Surgery. The Shoulder.* New York, NY: Raven Press, Ltd; 1995:311-342.

24. Fenlin JM, Frieman BG. Indications, technique and results of total shoulder arthroplasty in osteoarthritis. *Orthop Clin North Am.* 1998;29(3):423-434.

25. Stirrat CR. Metacarpophalangeal joint in rheumatoid arthritis of the hand. *Hand Clin.* 1996;12:515-529.

26. Biese J, Goudzwaard P. Postoperative management of metacarpal implant resection arthroplasty. *Orthopaedic Physical Therapy Clinics of North America.* 2001;10(4):595-615.

27. Flatt AE. Restoration of rheumatoid finger joint function: interim report on trial of prosthetic replacement. *J Bone Joint Surg (Am).* 1961;43:753-774.

28. Melone CM Jr, Gilbert DH, Bos M. Thumb basal joint arthroplasty: trapezium excision and abductor pollicis longus stabilization technique and results in 200 cases. Presented at AAOS annual meeting, February 1996, Atlanta, Ga.

29. Tomaino M, Pellegrini V, Burton R. Arthroplasty of the basal joint of the thumb. Long term follow-up after ligament reconstruction with tendon interposition. *J Bone Joint Surg.* 1995;77-A(3):346-355.

30. Melvin J. Therapist's management of osteoarthritis in the hand. In: Mackin EJ, Callahan A. Skirven T, et al, eds. *Rehabilitation of the Hand and Upper Extremity.* Vol 2. 5th ed. St. Louis, Mo: Mosby; 1995:1646-1676.

31. American Academy of Orthopaedic Surgeons. Available at: http//www.AAOS.org. Accessed August 31, 2003.

32. Total hip replacement. NIH Consensus Statement Online 1994 September 12-14;12(5):1-31. Available at: www.consensus.nih.gov/cons/098/098_into.htm. Accessed July 10, 2004.

33. Bannister GC. The hip, complications of total hip replacement. In: *Clinical Challenges in Orthopaedics.* London, England: Martin Dunitz Ltd; 2002:81-89.

34. Li E, Meding JB, Ritter MA, et al. The natural history of a posteriorly dislocated total hip replacement. *J Arthroplasty.* 1999;14:964-968.

35. Bullock DP, Sprorer SM, Shirreffs TG. Comparison of simultaneous bilateral with unilateral total knee arthroplasty in terms of perioperative complications. *J Bone Joint Surg.* 2003;85-A(10):1981-1986.

36. Lombardi AV, Mallory, TH, Fada RA, et al. Simultaneous bilateral total knee arthroplasties: who decides? *Clin Orthop.* 2001;1(392):319-329.

37. Hennigan SP, Iannotti JP. Instability after prosthetic arthroplasty of the shoulder. *Orthop Clin North Am.* 2001;32(4):649-659.

38. Wirth MA, Rockwood CA Jr. Complications of shoulder arthroplasty. *Clinical Orthop.* 1994;307:47-69.

39. Brannon EW, Klein G. Experiences with a finger joint prosthesis. *J Bone Joint Surg (Am).* 1959;41:87-102.

40. Swanson AB. Silicone rubber replacements of arthritic or destroyed joints in the hand. *Surg Clin North Am.* 1968;48.

41. Swanson AB, deGroot Swanson G, Ishikawa H. Use of grommets for flexible implant resection arthroplasty of metacarpophalangeal joint. *Clinical Orthop.* 1997;342:22-33.

42. Bass RL, Stern PJ, Nairus JG. High implant fracture incidence with sutter silicone metacarpophalangeal joint arthroplasty. *J Hand Surg (Am).* 1996;1:813-818.

43. Swanson AB. Finger joint replacement by silicone rubber implants and the concept of implant fixation by encapsulation. *Ann Rheum Dis.* 1969;28(Suppl):47-55.

44. Swanson A. Disabling arthritis at the base of the thumb: treatment by resection of the trapezium and flexible (silicone) implant arthroplasty. *J Bone Joint Surg (Am).* 1972;54:45.

45. Niebauer J, Shaw J, Doren W. The silicon-dacron hinge prosthesis: design, evaluation and application. *J Bone Joint Surg (Am).* 1968;50:634.

46. Swanson AB, deGroot Swanson G, Watermeier JJ. Trapezium implant arthroplasty: long term evaluation of 150 cases. *J Hand Surg.* 1981;6:125-141.

47. Khoo CTK. Silicone synovitis: the current role of silicone elastomer implants in joint reconstruction. *J Hand Surg (Br).* 1993;18(6):679-686.

48. Peimer CA, Medige J, Eckert B, Wright JR, Howard CS. Reactive synovitis after silicone arthroplasty. *J Hand Surg (Am).* 1986;11(5):624-638.

49. Gervis WH. Excision for the trapezium for osteoarthritis of the trapeziometacarpal joint. *J Bone Joint Surg.* 1949;31B:537-539.

50. Gervis WH, Wells T. A review of excision of the trapezium for osteoarthritis of the trapezio-metacarpal joint after twenty-five years. *J Bone Joint Surg.* 1973;55B:56-57.

51. Dhar S, Gray ICM, Jones WA, Beddow FM. Simple excision of the trapezium for osteoarthritis of the carpometacarpal joint of the thumb. *J Hand Surg.* 1994;19B:485-488.

52. Froimson AI. Tendon arthroplasty of the trapeziometacarpal joint. *Clinical Orthop.* 1970;70:191-199.

53. Carroll RE. Fascial arthroplasty for the carpometacarpal joint of the thumb. *Orthopedic Transactions.* 1977;1:15.

54. Amadio PC, Millender LH, Smith RJ. Silicone spacer or tendon spacer for trapezium resection arthroplasty—comparison of results. *J Hand Surg.* 1984;7A:237-244.

55. Menon J, Schoene HR, Hohl JC. Trapeziometacarpal arthritis-results of tendon interpositional arthroplasty. *J Hand Surg.* 1981;6:442-446.

56. Eaton RG, Glickel SZ, Littler JW. Tendon interposition arthroplasty for degenerative arthritis of the trapeziometacarpal joint of the thumb. *J Hand Surg.* 1985;10A:645-654.

57. Burton RI, Pellegrini VD. Surgical management of basal joint arthritis of the thumb. Part II: ligament reconstruction with tendon interposition arthroplasty. *J Hand Surg.* 1986;11A:324-332.

58. Robinson D, Aghasi M, Halperin N. Abductor pollicis longus tendon arthroplasty of the trapeziometacarpal joint: surgical technique and results. *J Hand Surg.* 1991;16A:504-509.

59. Smith RJ, Atkinson RE, Jupiter J. Silicone synovitis of the wrist. *J Hand Surg.* 1985;10A:47-60.

60. Thompson JS. "Suspensioplasty" a trapeziometacarpal reconstruction. *Orthopedic Transactions.* 1991;26:355-356.

61. Weilby A. Tendon interposition arthroplasty of the first carpometacarpal joint. *J Hand Surg.* 1988;13B:421-425.

62. Melone CP Jr, Beavers B, Isani A. The basal joint pain syndrome. *Clinical Orthop.* 1987;200:58-67.

63. Swanson AB, deGroot Swanson G, Watermeier JJ. Trapezium implant arthroplasty: long term evaluation of 150 cases. *J Hand Surg.* 1981;6:125-141.

64. Carter PR, Benton LJ, Dysert PA. Silicon rubber carpal implants: study of the incident of late osseous complications.

J Hand Surg. 1986;11A:639-644.

65. Eaton RG, Glickel SZ. Trapeziometacarpal osteoarthritis: staging as a rationale for treatment. *Hand Clin.* 1987;3(4):455-471.

66. Alter S, Feldon P, Terrono AL. Pathomechanics of deformities in the arthritic hand and wrist. In: Mackin EJ, Callahan AD, Skirven TM, et al. *Rehabilitation of the Hand and Upper Extremity.* 5th ed. Vol 2. St. Louis, Mo: Mosby; 2002.

67. Gajraj NM. Cyclooxygenase-2 inhibitors. *Anesth Analg.* 2003;96(6):1720-1738.

68. Malan TP, Marsh G, Hakki SI, Grossman E, Traylor L, Hubbard RC. Parecoxib sodium a parenteral cyclooxygenase 2 selective inhibitor, improves morphine analgesia and is opiod-sparing following total hip arthroplasty. *Anesthesiology.* 2003;98(4):950-956.

69. DeWeese FT, Akbari Z, Carline E. Pain control after knee arthroplasty: intraarticular versus epidural anesthesia. *Clin Orthop.* 2001;1(392):226-231.

70. Harada N, Chiu V, Stewart AL. Mobility-related function in older adults: assessment with a 6-minute walk test. *Arch Phys Med Rehabil.* 1999;80:837-841.

71. Newton R. Balance screening of an inner city older adult population. *Arch Phys Med Rehabil.* 1997;78:587-591.

72. Finch E, Brooks D, Stratford P, Mayo N. *Physical Rehabilitation Outcomes Measures: A Guide to Enhanced Clinical Decision Making.* 2nd ed. Baltimore, Md: Lippincott Williams & Wilkins; 2002.

73. Heitmann DK, Gossman MR, Shaddeau SA, Jackson JR. Balance performance and step width in noninstitutionalized, elderly, female faller and nonfallers. *Phys Ther.* 1989;69(11):923-931.

74. Gilbey HJ, Ackland TR, Wang AW, Morton AR, Trouchet T, Tapper J. Exercise improves early functional recovery after total hip arthroplasty. *Clinical Orthop.* 2003;408:193-200.

75. Roos E. Effectiveness and practice variation of rehabilitation after joint replacement. *Curr Opin Rheumatol.* 2003;15(2):160-162.

76. Freburger J. An analysis of the relationship between the utilization of physical therapy services and outcomes of care for patients after total hip arthroplasty. *Phys Ther.* 2000;80(5):448-458.

77. Boardman ND, Cofield RH, Bengtson KA, Little R, Jones MC, Rowland CM. Rehabilitation after total shoulder arthroplasty. *J Arthroplasty.* 2001;16(4):483-486.

78. van den Bogert AJ, et al. An analysis of hip joint loading during walking, running, and skiing. *Med Sci Sports Exerc.* 1999;10(3):131-141.

79. Healy WL, Iorio R, Lemos MJ. Athletic activity after joint replacement. *Am J Sports Med.* 2001;29(3):377-388.

80. American Physical Therapy Association. Guide to Physical Therapist Practice. 2nd ed. *Phys Ther.* 2001;81:9-744.

81. Lorentzen JS, Petersen MM, Brot C, et al. Early changes in muscle strength after total knee arthroplasty. *Acta Orthop Scand.* 1999;70:176-179.

82. Stevens JE, Mizner RL, Snyder-Mackler L. Quadriceps strength and volitional activation before and after total knee arthroplasty for osteoarthritis. *J Orthop Res.* 2003;21(5):775-779.

83. Avramidis K, Strike PW, Taylor PN, Swain ID. Effectiveness of electric stimulation of the vastus medialis muscle in the rehabilitation of patients after total knee arthroplasty. *Arch Phys Med Rehabil.* 2003;84:1850-1853.

84. Gotlin RS, Hershkowitz S, Juris PM, Gonzalez EG, Scott WN, Insall JN. Electrical stimulation effect on extensor lag and length of hospital stay after total knee arthroplasty. *Arch Phys Med Rehabil.* 1994;75:957-959.

85. Kumar P, McPherson E, Dorr L, Wan Z, Baldwin K. Rehabilitation after total knee arthroplasty: a comparison of 2 rehabilitation techniques. *Clin Orthop.* 1996;331:93-101.

86. Worland R, Arredondo J, Angles F, Lopez-Jimenez F, Jessup D. Home continuous passive motion machine versus professional physical therapy following total knee replacement. *J Arthroplasty.* 1998;13(7):784-787.

87. Chen B, Zimmerman JR, Soulen L, DeLisa JA. Continuous passive motion after total knee arthroplasty: a prospective study. *Am J Phys Med Rehabil.* 2000;79:421-426.

88. Brems JJ. Rehabilitation following total shoulder arthroplasty. *Clinical Orthop.* 1994;307:70-85.

89. Brown DD, Friedman RJ. Postoperative rehabilitation following total shoulder arthroplasty. *Orthop Clin North Am.* 1998;29(3):535-547.

90. Foley A, Halbert J, Hewitt T, Crotty M. Does hydrotherapy improve strength and physical function in patients with osteoarthritis—a randomized controlled trial comparing a gym based and a hydrotherapy based strengthening program. *Ann Rheum Dis.* 2003;62:1162-1167.

91. Speer KP, Warren RF, Horowitz L. The efficacy of cryotherapy in the postoperative shoulder. *J Shoulder Elbow Surg.* 1996;5(1):62-68.

92. Craig EV. Continuous passive motion in the rehabilitation of the surgically reconstructed shoulder: a preliminary report. *Orthopaedic Transactions.* 1986;10:219.

93. USDA Center for Nutrition Policy and Promotion. Body mass index and health. *Nutrition Insight.* 2000;March.

94. Bechtol CO. Grip test: use of a dynamometer with adjustable handle spacing. *J Bone Joint Surg (Am).* 1954;36A:820-824.

95. Fess EE. The effects of Jamar dynamometer handle position and test protocol on normal grip strength: procedures of the American Society of Hand Therapists. *J Hand Surg.* 1982;7:308.

96. Mathiowetz B, Kashman N, Volland G, et al. Grip and pinch strength, normative data for adults. *Arch Phys Med Rehabil.* 1995;66:71-72.

97. Downie W, Leatham PA, Rhind VM, et al. Studies with pain rating scales. *Ann Rheum Dis.* 1978;37.

98. Swanson AB, deGroot Swanson G, Leonard J, et al. Postoperative rehabilitation programs in flexible implant arthroplasty of the digits. In: Hunter JM, Schneider LH, Mackin EJ et al, eds. *Rehabilitation of the Hand.* 3rd ed. St. Louis, Mo: CV Mosby; 1990.

99. Madden MD, Devore G, Arem MD. A rational postoperative management program for metacarpophalangeal joint implant arthroplasty. *J Hand Surg.* 1977;2:385-386.

100. Cannon N, et al. *MP Implant Arthroplasties: Postoperative Management (for Rheumatoid Arthritis), Diagnosis and Treatment Manual for Physicians and Therapists.* 3rd ed. Indianapolis, Ind: Hand Rehabilitation Center of Indiana; 1991.

101. Beard G, Wood E. *Massage Principles and Techniques.* Philadelphia, Pa: WB Saunders Co; 1964.

102. Hayes K. *Manual for Physical Agent.* 5th ed. Upper Saddle River, NJ: Prentice Hall Health; 1999.

103. Engel JP, Wakim KG, Erickson DJ, Krusen FH. The effects of contrast baths on the peripheral circulation in patients with rheumatoid arthritis. *Arch Phys Med Rehabil.* 1950;31:135-144.

104. Breger-Stanton D, Bear-Lehman J, Graziano M, Ryan C. Contrast baths: what do we know about their use? *J Hand Ther.* 2003;16(4):343-345.

105. Brand PW, Hollister A. *Clinical Mechanics of the Hand.* 2nd ed. St. Louis, Mo: Mosby Year Book; 1993.

106. Reed BV. Effects of high voltage pulsed electrical stimulation on microvascular permeability to plasma proteins: a possible mechanism in minimizing edema. *Phys Ther.* 1988;68:491-495.

107. Melzack R, Wall P. Pain mechanisms: a new theory. *Science.* 1965;150:971-979.

Impaired Joint Mobility, Motor Function, Muscle Performance, and Range of Motion Associated With Bony or Soft Tissue Surgery (Pattern I)

Joshua A. Cleland, PT, DPT, PhD, OCS
Matthew B. Garber, PT, DSc, OCS, FAAOMPT
Marc Campolo, PT, PhD, SCS, ATC, CSCS

ANATOMY

BONY ANATOMY

The microscopic and macroscopic anatomy and physiology of bone has been described in detail in the chapters on Pattern A: Primary Prevention/Risk Reduction for Skeletal Demineralization and Pattern G: Impaired Joint Mobility, Muscle Performance, and Range of Motion Associated With Fracture and will not be reiterated. This chapter will focus on the pathophysiology associated with bony surgery, the method of bone healing associated with surgical fixation, with case studies in the format of the *Guide to Physical Therapist Practice, Second Edition.*[1]

In general, bony surgery may consist of a variety of surgical procedures, including osteotomies, bone lengthening procedures, and fixation of fractures. Osteotomies can be performed for the purpose of transferring a bony landmark to improve the mechanical advantage of muscles, as in the case of the tibial tubercle transfer.[2] Osteotomies are also performed in an attempt to relieve pain, alter the varus or valgus producing forces, and redistribute weightbearing forces in order to facilitate increased function of an osteoarthritic joint.[3] Limb lengthening procedures are occasionally utilized to obtain leg length equality, with the goal of improving

skeletal alignment and function.[4] More often bony surgery will be performed for the purpose of fixating a malaligned, displaced, or nonunion fracture.[5] Based upon clinical experience, the anticipated exposure of physical therapists to bony surgery is most likely to occur following surgical fixation of a fracture.

SOFT TISSUE ANATOMY

The anatomy and physiology of muscle and connective tissue are further detailed in Pattern C: Impaired Muscle Performance and Pattern D: Impaired Joint Mobility, Motor Function, Muscle Performance, and Range of Motion Associated With Connective Tissue Dysfunction. This chapter will also focus on the pathophysiology associated with soft tissue surgery, especially that related to rotator cuff tear and ACL repair, with two case studies in the format of the *Guide.*[1]

Soft tissue is described as all neuromusculoskeletal tissues except bone and articular cartilage.[6] Muscles are dynamic tissues that produce contractions that move body parts, including the extremities, internal organs, and the skin. The energy of their contractions is made mechanically effective by means of tendons, aponeuroses, and fascia. These structures secure the ends of muscles to the skeleton and control the direction of their pull.[7] Muscles account for approximately 40% of body weight in humans and vary greatly in size. Muscle is a resilient tissue that is capable of generating large forces. It has the ability to adapt to the demands of daily life and has the potential to regenerate should it become damaged. Muscles also give form to the body and provide it with heat. There are three types of muscle: skeletal, cardiac, and smooth. Skeletal muscle moves bones and other structures, such as the eyes and tongue. Cardiac muscle forms most of the walls of the heart and adjacent parts of the great vessels, such as the aorta. Smooth muscle lines the walls of most vessels and hollow organs, moves substances through viscera such as the intestine, and controls movement through blood vessels.[8]

The name of a muscle may be derived from its shape, size, location, attachments, or function. Shape is used to describe such muscles as the trapezius (shaped like a trapezoid), deltoid (triangular or delta-shaped), or gracilis (slender). Size is used in the description of such muscles as the gluteus maximus (largest) and the gluteus minimus (smallest) muscles. Location accounts for the name of such muscles as the supraspinatus and infraspinatus, ie, above (supra) and below (infra) the spine of the scapula. Muscles may also be named according to their attachments (eg, sternohyoid), their function (eg, levator scapulae), or the direction of their fibers (eg, transversus abdominis).[9]

There are more than 600 skeletal muscles in the body that are responsible for producing movement. These are sometimes referred to as voluntary muscles because they can be controlled at will. However, there are times when they function involuntarily (eg, the diaphragm). Skeletal muscles that produce movement by shortening are also referred to as striated muscle because of the striped appearance of their cells under microscopy. When a muscle contracts and shortens, one of its attachments usually remains fixed while the other one moves. The origin is usually located at the proximal end and remains fixed during muscular contraction. The insertion is usually located at the distal end of the muscle and moves. However, some muscles can move in both directions under certain circumstances. Most skeletal muscles are attached to bones. Some exceptions include the muscles of facial expression that are attached to the skin and the lumbrical muscles of the hand that are attached to tendons of other muscles. In some parts of the body (eg, abdominal wall) the muscle tendon spreads out in a broad, flat sheet called an aponeurosis. This sheet-like attachment is directly or indirectly connected with the various muscle sheaths and in some cases with the periosteum covering a bone.

Skeletal muscles develop by differentiation of cells from the mesoderm, the middle layer of the embryo. The structural unit of the muscle is the muscle cell. Muscle cells are often called muscle fibers because they are long and narrow when relaxed. A number of noncontractile connective tissue elements are necessary for the organization of the contractile muscle fibers into effective instruments of movement.

Individual muscle cells are surrounded by a fine connective tissue sheath called the endomysium. An additional layer of connective tissue, the perimysium, surrounds a bundle of up to 150 fibers, called a fasciculus. Depending on the muscle, varying numbers of fasciculi are organized into the gross muscle that is surrounded by a strong sheath called the epimysium. The epimysium is continuous with the muscle tendon that connects both ends of the muscle to the periosteum, the outermost covering of the bone.

Microscopically, skeletal muscle is comprised of 75% water, 20% protein, and the remaining 5% consists of salts and other substances. These include: the high-energy phosphates, urea, and lactate; the minerals calcium, potassium, and phosphorus; various enzymes including sodium, potassium, and chloride ions; as well as amino acids, fats, and carbohydrates. The most abundant muscle proteins are myosin, actin, and tropomyosin. Additionally, each 100 gm of muscle tissue contains approximately 700 mg of myoglobin, the molecular relative of hemoglobin.[10]

Skeletal muscles have a rich vascular supply. Arteries and veins that are oriented parallel to individual muscle fibers divide into numerous arterioles, capillaries, and venules to form a vast network in and around the endomysium. This ensures that each muscle fiber has adequate blood supply.

A single muscle fiber contains smaller functional units known as myofibrils that lie parallel to the muscle fiber's long axis. Each myofibril contains even smaller subunits named myofilaments that similarly lie parallel to the long axis of the myofibril. Myofilaments mainly consist of a serial arrangement of two proteins, actin and myosin, that make up the majority of the myofibrilar complex. Myofibrils are composed of a sequential arrangement of sarcomeres that are the muscle fiber's basic functional unit of shortening and force generation. Sarcomeres consist of a recurring parallel arrangement of actin (thin filaments) and myosin (thick filaments) that result in an interdigitating overlap of the two filaments. This arrangement contributes to the mechanical process of muscle contraction.

Microscopically, a muscle fiber presents with alternating light and dark bands providing the characteristic striated appearance. The lighter area is known as the I-band and the darker area is the A-band. The I-band corresponds to the area of thin filaments that is not overlapped by thick filaments. The Z-line consists of a connective tissue network that bisects the I-band, anchors the thin filaments, and provides structural integrity to the sarcomere. The A-band corresponds to the zone of thick filaments. The H zone is located in the middle of the A-band and is the region of thick filaments not overlapped by thin filaments. The M-band bisects the H-zone and represents the middle of the sarcomere. The M-band consists of protein structures that support the arrangement of the myosin filaments.

The sliding filament theory of muscle contraction in its simplest form proposes that actin filaments at each end of the sarcomere slide inward on myosin filaments, passing each other without changing length. The myosin cross bridges cyclically attach, rotate, flex, and detach from actin filaments using energy from ATP hydrolysis. This results in the movement of the actin filaments, causing fiber shortening and a change in relative size within the sarcomere's zones and bands (the I-band and H-zone decrease in length while the length of the A-band remains constant) and produces a force at the Z-band. Due to the fact that only a very small amount of displacement of the actin filament occurs with each flexion of the myosin cross-bridge, very rapid, repeated flexions must occur in many cross-bridges throughout the entire muscle for measurable movement to occur.[11]

The number of myosin cross-bridges that are attached to actin filaments at any one time dictates how much force is being produced in that particular muscle. The number of myosin cross-bridges that can attach to actin is affected by the relative length of the sarcomere. When a sarcomere is in a shortened state, the actin attachment sites are diminished because the actin and myosin are overlapped, reducing the number of active attachment sites. Similarly, when a sarcomere is in a lengthened state, the number of active actin sites is reduced because they are out of reach of the myosin cross-bridges. At resting length, however, the optimal number of myosin cross-bridge heads is able to align with active actin sites creating maximal force potential.

Morphologically, skeletal muscles are roughly divided into two types: fusiform and pennate. Fusiform fiber muscles have their muscle cells aligned almost parallel to the line of the action of the muscle that allows for rapid muscle shortening. Pennate muscles have fibers that insert into the tendon at an angle. This allows for more sarcomeres per unit area, resulting in greater force production, but sacrificing contractile velocity.[10-12]

Tendons are bands of strong, fibrous tissue that attach muscle to bone. They are responsible for transmitting the force created in the muscle to the bone, making joint movement possible. Tendons vary in size and shape and may be cylindrical, flat, ribbon, or fan shaped. Healthy tendons are white, glistening, fibroelastic tissues that are an extension of the deep fascia and/or the epimysium surrounding the muscle. They possess considerable strength, demonstrate great resistance to mechanical loads, and are important in reducing the strain on muscles. Each muscle has two tendons: one proximal and one distal. The site of the muscle and tendon union is referred to as the myotendinous junction. The site of the bone and tendon union is referred to as the osseotendinous junction. The gross morphology of each tendon reflects the function of its muscle.[13-15]

Kannus[13] describes five categories of structures that surround tendons. Retinacula are canals composed of fibrous sheaths through which the long tendons glide. The retinacula help to reduce friction as tendons glide through bony grooves and notches. Reflection pulleys consist of anatomic reinforcements of the retinacula in locations where there are curves along the course of the tendon. They are responsible for keeping the tendon inside its sliding bed. Synovial sheaths are essentially fibrous tunnels that contain peritendinous fluid for lubrication located at bony or other anatomic surfaces that might cause friction. A paratenon is a peritendinous sheath composed of loose fibrillar tissue that functions as an elastic sleeve, permitting free movement of the tendon against surrounding tissues. Tendon bursae are fluid-filled sacs located at the site where a tendon may course over a bony prominence. Their role is to reduce friction and wear of the gliding tendon.

Tendons are comprised of 65% to 80% collagen and 2% elastin fibers that are embedded in a PG water-based matrix. Ninety-five percent of the collagen in adult tendons is Type I. It has tremendous tensile strength and can withstand great amounts of force without being broken. The fiber arrangement is mainly longitudinal. However, approximately 10% of the collagen fibers are orientated transversely and horizontally.[13-15] This arrangement allows the tendon to handle high uniaxial tensile loading as well as transverse and rotational forces during activity.

Ligaments are short bands of tough, but flexible, dense regular fibrous connective tissue that attach bone to bone and act to stabilize joints. They also provide passive support and guidance to joints, resist the forces of elongation to restrict joint mobility, and have a role in joint proprioception. They are pliant enough to allow precise freedom of movement, but are also strong and inextensible enough to prevent them from readily yielding to applied force. Ligaments provide initial and increasing resistance to tensile loading. This allows movement of the joint to occur within its normal limits, but offering increased resistance to movement outside the joints normal range. There are several hundred ligaments in the human body, and they are named according to structural and functional features. They may be named according to their position in the body (eg, collateral), bony attachments (eg, AC), shape (eg, deltoid), or relationship to each other (eg, cruciates).[14,16]

Microscopically, ligaments are composed of water, collagen, PGs, elastin, and other glycoproteins. The main component is water, which constitutes 60% to 70% of the ligament's net weight. Collagen is the most abundant dry substance found in ligaments and constitutes about 25% of their overall makeup. Whether found in ligaments, tendons, or skin, collagen is all similar and is composed of densely packed collagen fibers, of which approximately 90% are Type I collagen and less than 10% are Type III. Collagen fibers in ligaments, however, are arranged in a less regular manner in the direction of functional need. An important structural feature of ligaments is that there is a periodic wave of collagen throughout the ligament known as crimps. This crimp pattern is believed to contribute to the non-linear mechanical properties of the ligament. This allows for a certain degree of elasticity that enables ligaments to accommodate for large internal stresses that occur during normal joint motion. Elastin makes up less than 5% of most skeletal ligaments. It is arranged in a complex, coiled manner that can be straightened out when stress is applied and recoils when the stress is removed. This supplies a small part of the ligament's tensile resistance and some of its elastic recoverability. Ligament PGs make up less than 1% of the ligament's dry weight. However, they play a key role in function by assisting in the formation of the ligament's gel-like extracellular matrix.[14,16]

The pertinent soft tissue anatomy and physiology for this pattern relates to the rotator cuff muscles and the anterior cruciate ligament because they are the most common soft tissue structures that are surgically repaired.

ANATOMY OF THE ROTATOR CUFF

The rotator cuff has been described as a group of muscles consisting of the supraspinatus, infraspinatus, teres minor, and subscapularis (SITS muscles). They are referred to as the rotator cuff muscles because they form a musculotendinous rotator cuff around the GH joint. These muscles act as a dynamic steering mechanism for the humeral head.[17] A unique feature of the rotator cuff muscles is that they blend with the articular capsule of the GH joint, thus reinforcing it.

The subscapularis represents the anterior portion while the supraspinatus, infraspinatus, and teres minor represent the superior and posterior aspect of the cuff. The supraspinatus originates from the supraspinous fossa of the scapula and inserts on the superior facet of the greater tubercle, located on the superior/posterior aspect of the humeral head. The infraspinatus originates from the infraspinous fossa, extends laterally, and inserts on the middle facet of the greater tubercle. The teres minor originates from the dorsal surface of the axillary border of the scapula, extends laterally and superiorly, and inserts on the most inferior facet of the greater tubercle. The subscapularis originates from the subscapular fossa located on the anterior portion of the scapula and extends laterally to its insertion on the lesser tubercle of the humerus. All the rotator cuff muscles with the exception of the supraspinatus are rotators of the humerus.

The current view of the function of the rotator cuff is that it plays a major role in directing the humeral head and helps to maintain a normal arthrokinematic pattern of the shoulder.[18] This is accomplished by the rotator cuff's role in providing stability and balancing force couples about the GH joint.[19,20] A force couple is defined as two equal forces acting in opposite directions to rotate a part about its axis of motion.[21] In the coronal plane it is generally accepted that the supraspinatus and the deltoid are prime movers of GH abduction.[22] The angle of pull of the deltoid muscle results in an upward translation of the humeral head. This can lead to contact with the coracoacromial arch and restriction of abduction if

unchecked. This motion is opposed by the inferior rotator cuff (the infraspinatus, teres minor, and the subscapularis) that applies a downward translatory compressive force allowing abduction to occur. The force couple in the transverse plane is the result of a balance of the anterior moments of the subscapularis and posterior moments of the infraspinatus and teres minor. Blasier and associates[20] describe four ways in which the rotator cuff musculature stabilizes the shoulder joint: 1) by its passive bulk, 2) by developing muscle tensions that compress the joint surfaces together, 3) by moving the humerus with respect to the glenoid and thereby tightening static restraints, and 4) by limiting the arc of motion of the GH joint by muscle tensions. An intact rotator cuff will maintain the head of the humerus in equilibrium in the glenoid fossa in the coronal plane. Tears of the subscapularis or posterior cuff muscle insufficiency will result in anterior translation of the humeral head, disrupting the GH equilibrium.

ANATOMY OF THE KNEE AND ANTERIOR CRUCIATE LIGAMENT

The knee joint is the largest joint of the body. It is a ginglymoid, or a modified hinge joint, and consists of three bones and two articulations. The tibiofemoral joint is the articulation between the distal femur and the proximal tibia. The patellofemoral joint is the articulation between the patella and the femur. These joints are contained within one joint capsule. The knee joint allows for six degrees of freedom that includes: 1) three translations—anterior-posterior, medial-lateral, and proximal-distal, and 2) three rotations—internal-external, varus-valgus, and flexion-extension.[23] It also allows for sliding of the patella on the femur.

The knee joint is inherently unstable due to its architecture and the fact that it is located at the ends of two long lever arms, the femur and the tibia. As a result, it depends on muscular and ligamentous structures for its stability.

The integrity of the knee joint is maintained by a fibrous capsule that is lined with synovium. The capsule is strengthened by the surrounding ligaments: the patellar ligament, tibial collateral ligament, fibular collateral ligament, POL, APL, posterior cruciate ligament (PCL), and ACL. These ligaments prevent or control excessive knee extension, varus/valgus stresses, anterior/posterior displacement of the tibia, medial/lateral rotation of the tibia, and combinations of anterior/posterior displacement and rotations of the tibia.

The patellar ligament is the central portion of the common tendon of the quadriceps femoris. It is a strong, flat ligamentous band that is attached proximally to the apex of the patella and distally to the tubercle of the tibia. The function of the patellar ligament is to provide anterior reinforcement to the joint capsule.

The tibial (medial) collateral ligament is a broad, flat membranous band that originates at the adductor tubercle on the medial femoral condyle and is attached to the medial surface of the body of the tibia distally, approximately 3 to 4 inches below the joint line. It consists of two separate layers: superficial and deep. The deep layer attaches to the medial meniscus and serves to stabilize and secure it. The tibial collateral ligament resists valgus stresses and checks ER of the tibia.

The fibular (lateral) collateral ligament is a strong, rounded, fibrous cord that originates from the lateral femoral condyle, passing distally and posteriorly over the popliteus tendon and inserting onto the lateral proximal fibular head. The fibular collateral ligament is not attached to the lateral meniscus. It resists varus stresses.

The oblique popliteal (or posterior oblique) ligament extends obliquely from the inferomedial aspect of the posterior knee at the site of the semimembranosus insertion on the tibia and travels superolaterally to insert into the capsule posterior to the lateral femoral condyle. The oblique popliteal ligament forms part of the floor of the popliteal fossa and resists ER.

The arcuate popliteal ligament arches distally from the lateral condyle of the femur and merges into the posterior capsular ligament. It is attached to the styloid process of the head of the fibula by two converging bands. It reinforces the lateral side of the knee, the posterior capsule, and is a secondary restraint to posterior tibial translation.

The cruciate ligaments are located within the articular capsule, but outside the synovial cavity. They have considerable strength and are located in the middle of the joint, situated more posterior than anterior. They are called the cruciate ligaments because they cross each other as in the letter "X." The cruciates have been named anterior and posterior based on the position of their attachments to the tibia.

The ACL originates from the posterior aspect of the medial surface of the lateral femoral condyle. It travels anteriorly, medially, and distally and inserts onto the tibial plateau anterolateral to the anterior tibial spine. The ACL is divided into two separate bands. The anteromedial and posterolateral bands are named according to their relationship at the tibial attachment. The anteromedial band is taut in flexion and lax in extension while the posterolateral band is taut in extension and lax in flexion. Additionally, between the two bands, there is an intermediate region that allows for some portion of the ACL to remain taut throughout the ROM of the knee. The primary function of the ACL is to prevent anterior translation of the tibia on the femur. However, it also checks ER of the tibia, hyperextension, and assists in controlling the normal rolling and gliding motions of the knee.

The PCL is stronger, shorter, and less oblique than the ACL. It arises from the posterior aspect of the tibial intercondylar region and travels anteriorly and medially passing behind the ACL to attach to the lateral surface of the medial femoral condyle. The PCL also consists of two bundles, the anterolateral and the posteromedial. The anterolateral band is taut in flexion while the posteromedial band is taut in extension. The primary function of the PCL is to prevent posterior translation of the tibia on the femur. It also serves to prevent hyperextension, maintain rotary stability, and acts as the knee's central axis of rotation.

The menisci are two asymmetric, crescent-shaped fibrocartilage plates located on the articular surface of the tibia. They are wedge shaped with the peripheral border being thicker, convex, and attached to the inner capsule of the joint. The superior surface is concave to accept the femoral condyles, while the inferior surface is flat and attached to the tibia. They serve to deepen the articular surfaces of the tibia and function as shock absorbers by distributing the weightbearing forces across the joint. The internal edges of the menisci are poorly vascularized and therefore do not heal well.

The muscle that provides the most stability to the knee joint is the quadriceps femoris. Table 9-1 lists the muscles surrounding the knee joint and their function.[7,8,23]

PATHOPHYSIOLOGY

BONY PATHOPHYSIOLOGY

It is reported that 90% to 95% of the estimated 5.6 million fractures sustained annually in the United States heal

Table 9-1			
KNEE JOINT MUSCLES AND THEIR FUNCTION			
Flexion	*Extension*	*Internal Rotation*	*External Rotation*
Semimembranosus	Quadriceps femoris	Popliteus	Biceps femoris
Semitendinosus	Tensor fascia latae	Semimembranosus	
Biceps femoris		Semitendinosus	
Sartorius		Sartorius	
Gracilis		Gracilis	
Popliteus			
Gastrocnemius			
Plantaris			

without complications; the remaining go on to delayed union or nonunion.[24,25] Management of uncomplicated fractures has been discussed in detail in Pattern G: Impaired Joint Mobility, Muscle Performance, and Range of Motion Associated With Fracture. However, with a complicated fracture the consequences may include delayed or nonunion, both of which may require surgical intervention to achieve adequate reduction and healing. Operative treatment of fractures is also warranted if closed reduction cannot be obtained or articular surfaces are disrupted to the extent that function may be disturbed.[26] The goals of surgical fixation include reduction, immobilization or stabilization, realignment, and preservation of function.[27]

Fracture union is the process whereby the strength of a healing bone is restored by the process of bone regeneration and is typically complete within 4 to 6 months.[28] However, if complete healing is not accomplished during this time frame then the fracture is classified as delayed.[29] Delayed union is typically attributed to lack of blood supply, excessive motion at the fracture site, excessively wide gap between bony fragments, presence of comorbidites that result in poor tissue healing (diabetes), nerve damage, infection, or the nature of the inciting event.[30,31] If delayed union persists it is likely that endosteal and periosteal osteogenesis will cease and be outweighed by bone resorption. The fibrocartilage will begin to seal off the medullary canals, obliterating blood flow to the fracture site and resulting in a nonunion.[28,29]

If open reduction is indicated, the surgeon has a choice of four methods to stabilize the segments. These methods of fixation include: rigid with plates or screws, dynamically with wires or lag screws, intramedullary nails, and external fixators.[31-33] In addition, bone grafts are occasionally utilized in instances where a significant amount of bone loss exists and results in nonunion of a fracture. Bone grafts are osteoconductive and provide a structural framework for angiogenesis, chondrogenesis, and a site for osteoprogenitor cells to deposit newly formed bone.[34] Three different types of bone grafts exist including autografts, with a common donor site being the iliac crest, allografts, and synthetic bone supplements, the most common being bone morphogenic proteins.[34]

FRACTURE HEALING

As discussed in the Fracture section of Pattern G: Impaired Joint Mobility, Muscle Performance, and Range of Motion Associated With Fracture, bone is the only tissue that is regenerated rather than repaired by poorly organized scar tissue.[35,36] Fracture healing may occur through two biological mechanisms: primary and secondary. Rigid surgical fixation of a fracture provides conditions conducive to primary bone formation.[37] Primary bone healing requires intimate contact and stability of the bony fragment to establish mechanical continuity of the fracture.[32,35] Stability of a fracture occurs when rigid fixation is utilized to compress the fracture fragments to the extent that no displacement will

occur.[38] Under these conditions, direct osteonal migration occurs across the fracture gap and osteoclastic cells undergo a tunneling response resulting in the establishment of new haversian systems, providing pathways for angiogenesis. Accompanying the blood vessels are mesenchymal cells that become osteoprogenitor cells, later developing into osteoblasts.[35] However, internal fixation can disrupt the continuity of the periosteal blood supply and therefore potentially reduce cortical blood flow in the short term by up to 70%.[28] Primary healing response does not result in the formation of an external callus.[32] Secondary healing requires a minute degree of movement at the fracture sites and therefore is more likely to occur in circumstances where rigid fixation has not been performed. Pattern G: Impaired Joint Mobility, Muscle Performance, and Range of Motion Associated With Fracture provides further details on secondary healing.

SOFT TISSUE PATHOPHYSIOLOGY

Injury to muscles and tendons are referred to as strains, while injuries to ligaments are referred to as sprains. Muscle strain is damage to some part of the contractile unit from overuse or overstress and is classified in three grades: Grade I (mild), Grade II (moderate), and Grade III (severe). Grade I strains involve only a small amount of mechanical injury (a few fibers) to the tissue and are accompanied by mild local pain, local tenderness, mild swelling, and ecchymosis without a loss of function. Grade II strains involve up to half of the contractile unit and are accompanied by more severe pain and tenderness, moderate swelling, and ecchymosis with some weakness and loss of function. Grade III strains involve complete rupture of the contractile unit, and as a result the signs and symptoms are severe and with a complete loss of function of the involved muscle.[39]

Ligament injuries may be partial or complete and are also classified in three grades. In a Grade I injury there is mild stretching with no gross disruption of fibers and no significant laxity (<5 mm distraction with stress test). The signs and symptoms are mild, and there may be a minor loss of function of the joint involved. In a Grade II there is a partial tear (approximately half the fibers are involved), some laxity (5 to 10 mm), more moderate symptoms and loss of function. In Grade III there is a complete tear, major instability (>10 mm of distraction), severe symptoms, and loss of function.[39]

PATHOPHYSIOLOGY OF THE ROTATOR CUFF

Rotator cuff pathologies are common and are usually the result of subacromial impingement.[40,41] They may be categorized as tendinitis, partial-thickness tears, or full-thickness tears. They occur most frequently in inactive patients over the age of 40 or in the athletic population that participates in overhead activities. Fukuda[42] classified the pathogenesis of rotator cuff tears as intrinsic, extrinsic, or traumatic. Intrinsic factors include factors such as changes in vascularity of the rotator cuff or other metabolic changes associated with aging, leading to degeneration. Extrinsic factors involve impingement of the rotator cuff tendon as a result of narrowing of the supraspinatus outlet by abnormalities of the coracoacromial arch. Traumatic factors involve excessive tensile loading of the tendon from either a single event or repetitive microtrauma. Other etiological factors of rotator cuff tears may include GH ligament laxity, contracture of the posterior capsule, poor scapular mechanics, and rotator cuff muscle insufficiency.[41,43] All of these factors may lead to impingement resulting in rotator cuff pathology.

Management of rotator cuff pathology includes both nonoperative and surgical techniques. The method of treatment is based on the exact cause, severity of the lesion, and the individual's functional requirements.

In most instances, rotator cuff injuries may be managed conservatively and may include the use of: NSAIDs; local rest; modification of activities; anti-inflammatory modalities such as phonophoresis, iontophoresis, and ice; mobilization; and therapeutic exercise as indicated.

Surgical management is considered when conservative treatment fails. Surgical techniques include debridement of the partial tear, acromioplasty, acromioplasty and debridement, or rotator cuff repair in combination with acromioplasty. These procedures may be performed using open, arthroscopic, or arthroscopically assisted (mini-open) techniques. The decision to use either open or arthroscopic techniques is influenced by the patient's age, occupation, underlying pathology, extent of the tear, other medical conditions, and the surgeon's preference, skill, and experience.[41,42]

Arthroscopic evaluation is necessary to determine the extent of the lesion. If a lesion involves less than 50% of cuff thickness, acromioplasty and debridement should be sufficient to manage the injury. If the tendon edge becomes frayed, careful debridement is accomplished by a motorized shaver. In addition, if there is degeneration of the humerus, glenoid, or glenoid labrum, these surfaces may also be debrided. The coracoacromial arch is formed by the inferior aspect of the acromion and the coracoid process of the scapula with the coracoacromial ligament spanning between them. The coracoacromial ligament is usually composed of anterolateral and posteriomedial bands. To ensure clinical success of arthroscopic acromioplasty, it is necessary to release this ligament. In the older patient, a complete excision of this ligament may be performed, while in the young overhead athlete, only the anterolateral band is excised. After soft tissue debridement, removal of spurs and any bony prominence of the anterior acromial margins is performed.

If the tear is thicker then 50%, then surgical repair of the rotator cuff tendon may be necessary.[41,42] For small to medium-sized tears of the rotator cuff without significant retraction, the mini-open rotator cuff repair is used. This involves using a 3-cm incision on the anterolateral aspect of the shoulder with a small split in the deltoid, minimizing soft tissue damage resulting from the surgery. Stay sutures are placed in the tendon's edge, and the tear is mobilized until it reaches the greater tubercle. The tendon edge may be secured to the bone by sutures using bone (transosseous) tunnels or bone anchors.

In larger, less mobile tears an open repair may be preferred. The technique is similar to the mini-open except that a larger incision is made in the skin and the deltoid. This allows for better access, resulting in more precise and accurate rotator cuff mobilization, suture passing, knot tying, and anchor placement. The drawback is that the open technique is more invasive and associated with greater subacromial and deltoid trauma necessitating a more conservative rehabilitation approach.

PATHOPHYSIOLOGY OF THE ANTERIOR CRUCIATE LIGAMENT

The ACL is the most commonly injured knee ligament.[44] Injury to the anterior cruciate ligament is one of the most common injuries in sports, although relatively uncommon in the general population.[45] High risk sports for ACL injury include: basketball, football, soccer, volleyball, gymnastics, and skiing. The classic history of an ACL injury includes a noncontact deceleration injury. The main mechanism of the noncontact injury occurs when the foot is planted on the ground with the knee flexed and a sudden change in direction occurs. This creates a valgus force applied to the knee while the leg is in ER, resulting in an immediate disruption of the ligament. A similar mechanism occurs in contact sports when a player's foot is planted on the ground and a force is directed at the posterolateral aspect of the knee. Less frequently, an ACL tear may result from hyperextending the knee with the leg internally rotated. A patient typically describes hearing or feeling a pop. An individual who has sustained an ACL tear will normally not be able to continue in the activity. He or she will have a lack of knee extension and ambulate with a bent-knee gait. A moderate to severe hemarthrosis may develop within 6 to 12 hours.

The treatment approach for an ACL tear varies depending on the goals of the patient. Individuals wishing to continue to participate in high risk sports that involve cutting and jumping need to have surgical reconstruction of the ACL. Those individuals who are willing to modify their lifestyle and restrict themselves to sports that do not involve high-risk activities, such as running, bicycling, or swimming, may do well with a conservative approach.

ACL reconstruction is the treatment of choice for those who elect to have surgery. Various structures have been used for ACL substitutes and have been classified as autografts that are the patient's own tissue, allografts that are tissue from another human donor, or synthetic tissue. Autograft tissue is the most commonly used graft material, because it has the advantages of low risk adverse inflammatory reaction and virtually no risk of disease transmission. Currently, bone-patellar tendon-bone (BPTB) and hamstring autografts are the standard procedures and are used equally as often for ACL reconstruction.[46]

The surgical technique for using the BPTB graft involves harvesting a 10-mm autogenous patellar tendon graft with 25-mm bone plugs from both the patella and tibial ends through a 4- to 6-cm incision made medial to the tibial tubercle. The graft is placed in a bony tunnel drilled through both the tibia and femur, reproducing the anatomy and function of an intact anterior cruciate ligament. There are many methods of fixating a replacement graft that include interference screws, staples, washers, crosspins, and suture-post. Each technique has advantages and disadvantages. The most common fixation technique for the BPTB graft is the interference screw that is placed parallel to both the bone plug of the graft and the tunnel.[46-49]

The use of hamstring tendon grafts for ACL reconstruction has gained popularity as a response to the post-surgical complications associated with the BPTB technique. Complications include a high incidence of anterior knee pain, extensor mechanism weakness and atrophy, and patellofemoral pathology.[48]

Initially, the semitendinosus and gracilis tendon were used together as two single strands. It was reported that their combined strength exceeded that of the ACL. More recently surgeons have chosen to fold the semitendinosus and gracilis tendons upon themselves, creating a quadruple hamstring graft, increasing its strength. The graft is placed in the bony tunnel in a similar fashion to that of the BPTB graft and fixated most commonly by using a crosspin device.[49]

It has been reported that quadruple hamstring tendon grafts have the size, stiffness, and ultimate strength equivalent to or greater than BPTB grafts.[46] However, the BPTB provides a more stable knee in the long term,[48,50] while the semitendinosus tendon graft presents fewer short-term complications.[47] There appears to be no significant difference between subjective and functional long-term outcomes between the two techniques.[50]

Rehabilitation considerations differ postoperatively between the two grafts. Harvesting the BPTB graft disrupts the extensor mechanism, resulting in pain and edema. These may create reflex inhibitory effects on the activation of the quadriceps mechanism, limiting the strength of the quadriceps.[46,51] Additionally, there may be secondary patellar tendinitis, contracture, and resulting patellofemoral dysfunction. In the early postoperative rehabilitation phases, immediate management of pain and swelling and a conservative progression will avoid irritating the weakened patellar tendon. When rehabilitating patients with a hamstring graft in the early stages, a slower progression of hamstring exercises is used.[46,52]

IMAGING

BONY IMAGING

Imaging procedures utilized to detect fractures have been described in detail in Pattern G: Impaired Joint Mobility, Muscle Performance, and Range of Motion Associated With Fracture. Plain radiographs are usually adequate to detect fractures that will require surgical fixation.[27] Following surgical intervention, plain film radiography is also used to determine appropriate reduction of the fracture.[27] Fracture healing is indicated by callus formations, and healing is considered complete when the fracture line is no longer visible.[32]

SOFT TISSUE IMAGING

The following diagnostic imaging techniques have been proven successful in diagnosing rotator cuff and ACL pathology.[41,53,54]

Although plain films are surpassed by other diagnostic techniques used for soft tissue diagnosis, there may be pertinent findings associated with chronic tears of the rotator cuff that can be identified by radiography. These include: anterior acromial spurs, irregularity of the greater tuberosity, narrowing of the subacromial space, erosion of the inferior aspect of the acromion, and Hill-Sachs defects (that are indicative of recurrent anterior subluxation). Plain film radiographic assessment of ACL injuries may be able to identify an avulsed portion of bone at the attachment site of the collateral ligament or some other associated bony pathology such as fractures or dislocations.

The use of contrast media with radiography permits visualization of anatomic structures of the shoulder that are not normally seen. An intact rotator cuff will confine the contrast medium within the joint capsule. Rotator cuff pathology may be identified by a collection of contrast medium at the site of the tear.

MRI is the technique of choice in the evaluation of rotator cuff and ACL injuries.[53] The MRI is able to obtain exquisite images of soft tissue and to provide complementary information regarding the surrounding joint. It is noninvasive, so it holds an advantage over contrast arthrography.

PHARMACOLOGY

BONY PHARMACOLOGY

Depending on the severity of the fracture, patients may be placed on medications to control pain. These may range from NSAIDs in mild cases to opioid analgesics in the case of severe pain. If the fracture is compound or is at risk for infection, the patient may be given antibiotics to combat or prevent infection.

If the fracture was a result of insufficient bone strength, the patient may be placed on a variety of other medications in an attempt to maximize bone density and strength. For a detailed description of these medications the readers are referred to Pattern A: Primary Prevention/Risk Reduction for Skeletal Demineralization. The reader is also referred to *Pharmacology in Rehabilitation*[55] for further information regarding the use of pharmacological management of this patient population.

SOFT TISSUE PHARMACOLOGY

The following pharmacological agents are utilized in both conservative and surgical management of patients who have rotator cuff and ACL pathology.[56,57]

Opioid analgesics act by depressing pain impulse transmission at the spinal cord level by interacting with opioid receptors. Products are divided into opiates and nonopiates. Most products are used to control moderate to severe pain and are used before and after surgery. Representative drugs include codeine, hydrocodone, oxycodone, and propoxyphene.

NSAIDs work by reducing inflammation (pain, swelling, redness, heat) and by inhibiting chemicals in the body that produce tissue irritation and cause inflammation. NSAIDs are used to treat mild to moderate pain and inflammation. Representative drugs include ibuprofen, naproxen, nabumtone, and meloxicam.

Case Study #1: Femoral Fracture

Mrs. Emmons is a 78-year-old female who experienced a fractured left femoral shaft and subsequently underwent open reduction internal fixation to stabilize the fracture segment (Figure 9-1).

PHYSICAL THERAPIST EXAMINATION

HISTORY

♦ General demographics: Mrs. Emmons is a 78-year-old white female whose primary language is English. She is a high school graduate.

♦ Social history: Mrs. Emmons has been married for 45 years. She has two adult children who live out of the state. She has six adult grandchildren and 14 great grandchildren.

♦ Employment/work: She is a retired bookkeeper and still does some part-time bookkeeping.

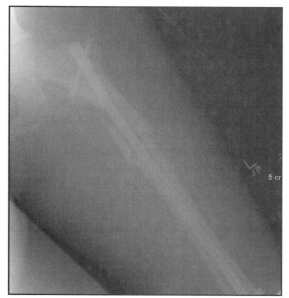

Figure 9-1. Radiograph of Mrs. Emmon's left comminuted femoral shaft fracture stabilized with intramedullary nailing.

♦ Living environment: She lives in a single-family home with her husband who is in good physical condition.

♦ General health status
  ● General health perception: Mrs. Emmons reports that her health was fair, for her age, prior to the fall.
  ● Physical function: Normal for her age prior to fall.
  ● Psychological function: Her husband reports that she has small bouts of dementia.
  ● Role function: Wife, mother, grandmother, great-grandmother.
  ● Social function: Mrs. Emmons participates in card tournaments with her friends on a weekly basis and is also an avid bird watcher.

♦ Social/health habits: Mrs. Emmons is a non-smoker and social drinker (one to two drinks per week).

♦ Family history: Her mother died of natural causes at 91, and her father died of lung cancer at 69.

♦ Medical/surgical history: She underwent a carotid endarterectomy 6 years ago. She also had an inguinal hernia repaired 3 years ago.

♦ Preexisting medical and other health-related conditions: She has a history of hyperlipidemia.

♦ Current condition(s)/chief complaint(s): Mrs. Emmons reports that she slipped on the ice approximately 2 weeks ago and landed on her left side on a curb resulting in a left femoral shaft fracture. After undergoing ORIF, she remained in the hospital for 1 week and then was transferred to a rehabilitation facility for 6 weeks. Current physician orders are for weightbearing as tolerated. She is now complaining of mild discomfort, general weakness, and fatigue.

◆ Functional status and activity level: Prior to the injury Mrs. Emmons was independent in all ADL and IADL. She has recently relinquished her driver's license, as she reports that she is too nervous.

◆ Medications: Currently taking 20 mg of Zocor per day for hyperlipidemia and 325 mg of aspirin every 4 hours for pain control.

◆ Other clinical tests: Radiographs taken 6 weeks post-injury revealed an ORIF (intramedullary nailing) and moderate healing of the fracture site. Radiographs of the pelvis taken at the time of the injury were negative.

SYSTEMS REVIEW

◆ Cardiovascular/pulmonary
  ● BP: 142/86 mmHg
  ● Edema: Noted left distal LE
  ● HR: 77 bpm
  ● RR: 16 bpm
◆ Integumentary
  ● Presence of scar formation: 32-cm long scar along the left lateral thigh
  ● Skin color: WNL
  ● Skin integrity: WNL
◆ Musculoskeletal
  ● Gross range of motion: BUE and RLE WNL, LLE moderately limited
  ● Gross strength: Moderate weakness demonstrated in LLE
  ● Gross symmetry: Disuse atrophy and poor quadriceps tone on left
  ● Height: 5'3" (1.6 m)
  ● Weight: 134 lbs (60.8 kg)
◆ Neuromuscular
  ● Balance: Unsteady with UE support on walker
  ● Locomotion, transfers, and transitions
    ■ Ambulates with wheeled walker
      ■ Demonstrates difficulty with sit to stand
    ■ Requires minimal assistance
    ■ Impaired bed mobility
◆ Communication, affect, cognition, language, and learning style
  ● Communication, affect, and cognition: WNL
  ● Learning preferences: Visual learner

TESTS AND MEASURES

◆ Aerobic capacity/endurance
  ● Fatigues easily when ambulating short distances (25 feet)
◆ Anthropometric characteristics

● BMI=23.75, WNL (weight [in kg] divided by height² [in meters])
  ● Mild pitting edema noted left distal extremity
◆ Assistive and adaptive devices
  ● Utilizes a wheeled walker for balance during gait and is currently weightbearing as tolerated
  ● She is only able to climb three stairs with moderate assistance and requires verbal cues for proper technique
◆ Cranial and peripheral nerve integrity
  ● Mild decrease in sensation para-incision
◆ Environmental, home, and work barriers
  ● Potential barriers include five steps to get into her single-level home
◆ Ergonomics and body mechanics
  ● Analysis of body mechanics during transfers revealed Mrs. Emmons utilized her UEs for considerable assist during sit-to-stand transfers and required minimal assistance, which raised some safety concerns
◆ Gait, locomotion, and balance
  ● Ambulates slowly with a wheeled walker
  ● Unable to maintain a static standing position without assistance secondary to immediate balance loss
◆ Integumentary integrity
  ● 32-cm long scar left lateral thigh
  ● Banding of scar noted
  ● No signs of infection
◆ Motor function
  ● Dexterity of UEs and RLE: WNL
  ● Lack of coordination during proprioceptive and kinesthetic assessment of her LLE, which included touching her left heel to her right toes and then to her right knee
◆ Muscle performance
  ● MMT revealed the following deviations from normal in her left hip and knee
    ■ Hip flexion=3/5
    ■ Hip abduction=3-/5
    ■ Hip extension=3+/5
    ■ Hip adduction=4/5
    ■ Hip ER=3+/5
    ■ Hip IR=4-/5
    ■ Knee flexion=4-/5
    ■ Knee extension=4/5
◆ Orthotic, protective, and supportive devices
  ● Mrs. Emmons is wearing bilateral elastic stockings
◆ Pain
  ● Patient reported pain of 1 to 2/10 on the NPS in the left hip and groin during ambulation and transfers
◆ Posture
  ● Observation of postural alignment and position

(static and dynamic) revealed:
- Standing with UE support
- FHP
- Increased thoracic kyphosis
- Elevated left ilium

♦ Range of motion
  • Left hip (goniometry)
    - Flexion=0 to 87 degrees
    - Extension=0 to 6 degrees
    - Abduction=0 to 12 degrees
  • Left knee (goniometry)
    - Flexion=0 to 112 degrees

♦ Self-care and home management
  • Interview with the patient reveals that the husband has been assisting with all basic ADL, including hygiene and grooming
  • Prior to the fracture she was independent in all self-care actions, tasks, and activities
  • Mr. Emmons is currently tending to all home management duties, whereas prior to the injury this was Mrs. Emmons responsibility

♦ Sensory integrity
  • Difficulty identifying passive positioning of the left great toe and ankle

♦ Work, community, and leisure integration or reintegration
  • Since the fracture, Mrs. Emmons has been unable to attend her weekly card games

EVALUATION

Her history indicated that she is an elderly white female who sustained a fracture during a fall and subsequently underwent ORIF. She lives in a one-story home with her husband, who is healthy and able to assist Mrs. Emmons with ADL and home management duties. Mrs. Emmons has decreased motor and muscle performance, altered posture, and decreased ROM of the LLE. In addition, she has mild edema in the distal LLE and pain in the left hip and groin. She has difficulty with transfers, balance, and gait.

DIAGNOSIS

Mrs. Emmons is a patient with mild dementia who sustained a fracture and underwent ORIF and who has pain and edema in the LLE. She has impaired: aerobic capacity/endurance; cranial and peripheral nerve integrity; ergonomics and body mechanics; gait, locomotion, and balance; integumentary integrity; motor function; muscle performance; posture; range of motion; and sensory integrity. She is functionally limited in self-care, home management, work, community, and leisure actions, tasks, and activities. She also has a poten-

tial home barrier. These findings are consistent with placement in Pattern I: Impaired Joint Mobility, Motor Function, Muscle Performance, and Range of Motion Associated With Bony or Soft Tissue Surgery. These impairments, functional limitations, and barriers will be addressed in determining the prognosis and the plan of care.

PROGNOSIS AND PLAN OF CARE

Over the course of the visits, the following mutually established outcomes have been determined:
- Ability to perform home management actions, tasks, and activities is improved
- Ability to perform physical actions, tasks, and activities including ADL is improved
- Aerobic capacity and endurance is increased
- Balance is improved
- Edema is improved
- Functional independence in ADL and IADL is increased
- Gait is improved
- Motor function is improved
- Muscle performance is increased
- Pain is decreased
- Physical function is improved
- Postural control is improved
- ROM is improved
- Self-management of symptoms is improved

To achieve these outcomes, the interventions will include: coordination, communication, and documentation; patient/client-related instruction; therapeutic exercise; functional training in self-care and home management; and functional training in work, community, and leisure integration or reintegration.

Based on the diagnosis and prognosis, Mrs. Emmons is expected to require between 6 and 24 visits over a 24-week period of time. Mrs. Emmons has good social support, is motivated, and will follow through with her home exercise program. She is not severely impaired and is generally healthy.

INTERVENTIONS

RATIONALE FOR SELECTED INTERVENTIONS

Therapeutic Exercise

The benefits of physical therapy in the management of geriatric patients who have undergone open reduction of the femur after sustaining a fracture is well documented.[58-62] Jones and associates[60] demonstrated that significant improvements in function had occurred at discharge and at a 6-week follow-up in patients receiving inpatient rehabilitation following ORIF of the femur. In addition, Guccione and associates[63] demonstrated that following ORIF for a femoral fracture, patients who had more than one physical therapy treatment per day had greater performance in transfers and gait with a walker prior to discharge. Also, those patients who received more than one physical therapy session per day in the acute phase were more likely to go directly home after discharge from the hospital. A randomized controlled trial by Mitchell and Stott[64] revealed that those patients receiving additional quadriceps training significantly increased leg extensor power and decreased disability at a 16-week follow-up. In addition, Lamb and associates[65] demonstrated the effectiveness of a regimen of quadriceps muscle training along with neuromuscular stimulation and suggested it might be effective in speeding the recovery after surgical fixation of hip fractures.

Numerous prospective studies[62,63,66] have demonstrated that physical therapy programs that incorporate balance and coordination training into the treatment plan following a hip fracture in the geriatric population result in significant improvements in strength, balance, gait, and functional independence. However, it must be noted that balance and coordination activities were not performed independently in these studies but incorporated with other interventions commonly used by physical therapists including strengthening/endurance exercises, mobility training, and functional training. In addition, a multi-modal physical therapy regimen including balance training has been demonstrated to significantly enhance strength, walking speed, and functional performance and reduce fall-related emotional states.[67]

COORDINATION, COMMUNICATION, AND DOCUMENTATION

Communication will occur with Mrs. Emmons and her husband regarding all components of her care and to engender support for her program. This began in the hospital and continued at home through her return to leisure activities. All elements of the patient's management, including examination, evaluation, diagnosis, prognosis, and interventions, will be documented.

PATIENT/CLIENT-RELATED INSTRUCTION

The patient will be instructed about her current condition, impairments, and functional limitations. The patient and family will be educated about the risk factors in the home and ways to address them to preclude further falls. The patient and family will understand the importance of her home exercise program and the outcomes that can be expected. Mrs. Emmons will receive ongoing instruction/modification of her exercise programs. Education regarding abnormal wound healing will include knowledge of the signs

of infection, including fever, chills, redness, swelling, drainage, and pain.

Instruction in enhancement of performance, health, wellness, and fitness programs will occur. She will also be informed of the plan of care that will include transitioning back into her hobbies of playing cards and bird watching.

THERAPEUTIC EXERCISE

- ◆ Phase I: Inpatient hospital, week 1
  - Aerobic capacity/endurance conditioning
    - Progressive ambulation with wheeled walker
    - Upper body ergometer starting with short durations (eg, starting with 2 minutes) considering the poor endurance exhibited by the patient and progress length of time according to patient tolerance with close monitoring of vital signs
  - Balance, coordination, and agility training
    - Bilateral stance in parallel bars
    - Tandem stance in parallel bars
    - Weight shifts standing in parallel bars
  - Body mechanics and postural stabilization
    - Supine, actively push shoulders into mat
    - Patient will maintain stance in front of a mirror to provide visual cues for postural correction
    - Postural cues during ambulation activities and all exercises
    - Seated scapula retractions
  - Flexibility exercises
    - Stretching exercises should be done after warming up, using a slow and steady stretch accompanied by deep breathing, and building hold up to 30 to 60 seconds
    - Supine left leg raise
    - Supine left knee to chest
  - Gait and locomotion training
    - Ambulate with wheeled walker focusing on eliminating deviations and progressing weightbearing status
    - Ambulation with wheeled walker focusing on proper heel strike and toe push off
    - Progress ambulation distance using wheeled walker
  - Strength, power, and endurance training
    - Bridging
    - Straight leg raising progression
    - Sidelying abduction
    - Short-arc quadriceps exercises
- ◆ Phase II: Inpatient rehabilitation, weeks 2 through 6
  - Aerobic capacity/endurance conditioning
    - Stationary bicycle, progress slowly

- Consider recumbent bike secondary to patient's age
- Balance, coordination, and agility training
  - Progress balance activities to external perturbations as appropriate
  - Ambulation with wheeled walker around obstacles
  - Bilateral stance in parallel bars on dynamic surface (foam pad)
- Body mechanics and postural stabilization
  - Standing with back to wall performing head and shoulder retractions
  - One arm stretch, hand on wall with elbow extended, shoulder horizontally abducted
- Flexibility exercises
  - Supine, flexed left knee and hip, perform horizontal adduction
  - Supine, flexed left knee and hip, perform horizontal abduction
  - Supine, use towel to pull left leg into abduction
- Gait and locomotion training
  - Progress from a wheeled walker to ambulation with a cane as appropriate
  - Progression of stair climbing with wheeled walker to a cane, as indicated
  - Ambulation activities with a cane are progressed for greater distances
  - Ambulation with cane through obstacles that require directional changes
- Strength, power, and endurance training
  - Single leg bridging when appropriate
  - Sidelying abduction
  - Short-arc quadriceps exercises
  - Long arc quadriceps exercises
  - Seated hip ER exercises
  - Progress the above exercises to include light weights (starting at 1 lb) as appropriate
  - Repeated sit to stand from varying chair heights
  - Standing hip abduction, flexion, and extension with progression to using light weights (1 lb)
  - Standing knee flexion, progressing to using light weights (1 lb)
- Phase III: Outpatient rehabilitation, weeks 7 through 24
  - Aerobic capacity/endurance conditioning
    - Progressive walking program: Wean from cane to no assistive device provided normal gait pattern and no pain
  - Balance, coordination, and agility training
    - Tandem stance in parallel bars on dynamic surface

- Ambulation with cane as appropriate
- Body mechanics and postural stabilization
  - One arm stretch, hand on wall with elbow extended, shoulder horizontally abducted
- Flexibility exercises
  - Seated in chair, walk hands down left leg, knee extended
  - Seated in chair, pull left leg toward chest
  - Right sidelying, extended left hip with flexed left knee (use towel for assistance)
- Gait and locomotion training
  - Ambulation with cane on uneven terrain
  - Progression of stair climbing with cane and railing (use railing that simulates home environment)
  - Progression of stair climbing with hand railing only
- Strength, power, and endurance training
  - 2-inch step-ups with UE support and progressing by increasing step height and reducing use of UEs as appropriate
  - Mini wall squats
  - Heel raises in standing with UE support (progress to reduced UE support as appropriate)

Maintenance of a regular exercise program must be instilled in this patient.

FUNCTIONAL TRAINING IN SELF-CARE AND HOME MANAGEMENT

- ◆ Self-care and home management
  - She will receive bed mobility and transfer training to be independent in these activities at home
  - Assistive devices for ambulation will include a walker and cane
  - Dressing will be assisted by the use of reacher, long-handled shoe horn, and sock aid
  - Bathing will be assisted by the use of a long-handled sponge
  - Review all actions, tasks, and activities and postural alignment for self-care and home management
- ◆ IADL training
  - Mrs. Emmons will slowly resume household chores that she performed prior to her fracture
- ◆ Injury prevention or reduction
  - Mrs. Emmons will receive education on principles to prevent falls and to improve her safety awareness
  - Barrier accommodations or modifications may be made to prevent or reduce risk of injury

FUNCTIONAL TRAINING IN WORK, COMMUNITY, AND LEISURE INTEGRATION OR REINTEGRATION

- ◆ Device and equipment use and training
  - Mrs. Emmons will use a walker and then a straight cane in her home
- ◆ IADL training
  - See functional training interventions in self-care and home management and IADL training above
- ◆ Leisure
  - Mr. Emmons will gradually return to her card playing
  - For return to her bird watching Mrs. Emmons must demonstrate the following:
    - Adequate ROM in all joints for specific activity
    - Adequate muscle strength
    - Adequate aerobic capacity

ANTICIPATED GOALS AND EXPECTED OUTCOMES

- ◆ Impact on pathology/pathophysiology
  - Pain is decreased from a 1-2/10 to a 1/10 during Phase I and a 0/10 during Phase II.
- ◆ Impact on impairments
  - Balance, endurance, motor function, muscle performance, postural control, and weightbearing status will improve and patient will be able to ambulate 100 feet with wheeled walker in Phase I, ambulate with a cane for distances of up to 200 feet in Phase II, and ambulate 300 feet with no assistive device and with minimal fatigue and no loss of balance in Phase III.
  - ROM improves to the following during Phase I: left hip flexion 90 degrees, extension 10 degrees, abduction 20 degrees, and knee flexion 120 degrees.
- ◆ Impact on functional limitations
  - During Phase I patient will demonstrate an understanding of the precautions associated with surgical pinning of the femur as well as modification of risk factors associated with cardiovascular disease.
  - Patient is able to ambulate at normal speed with wheeled walker during Phase I, ambulate with a straight cane and up two flights of stairs using hand railing during Phase II, and with no assistive devices and up three flights of stairs with no railings during Phase III.
  - Patient is able to use bathroom and bath with moderate assistance from husband during Phase I and will be able to perform all these activities independently during Phase II. During Phase II the patient will be

able to return to her part-time job of bookkeeping. During Phase III patient will achieve the ability to perform social activities including attending weekly card games and grocery shopping independently.

- Patient will achieve the ability to don/doff clothing with assistive devices during Phase I. Patient will achieve the ability to perform basic ADL including cooking, washing dishes, and proper hygiene and grooming of LEs during Phase II. During Phase III patient will achieve the ability to perform IADL including vacuuming and cleaning.
- ◆ Impact on health, wellness, and fitness
  - During Phase II the patient will begin practicing behaviors to modify risk factors associated with cardiovascular disease including maintaining a healthy diet.
  - Physical therapy services will be utilized optimally and result in the efficient use of health care dollars while assuring that patient makes optimal improvement toward both clinical and functional goals during the rehabilitation process.
  - Utilization and cost of health care services are decreased.
- ◆ Impact on societal resources
  - Documentation occurs throughout patient management and follows APTA's *Guidelines for Physical Therapy Documentation.*[1]
- ◆ Patient/client satisfaction
  - During Phase I the patient's husband will develop an understanding of precautions associated with surgical pinning of the femur as well as proper safety skills, including assistance with transfers and gait, as necessary.
  - Patient and family are satisfied with the access, availability, and quality of services provided and the clinical proficiency and interpersonal skills of the physical therapist during all three phases of rehabilitation.
  - Patient and family will develop understanding and knowledge of the diagnosis, prognosis, interventions, anticipated goals, and expected outcomes for all phases of rehabilitation.

REEXAMINATION

Reexamination is performed throughout the episode of care, particularly as the setting of care changes.

DISCHARGE

Mrs. Emmons is discharged from physical therapy after a total of 16 outpatient physical therapy sessions and attainment of her goals and expected outcomes.

Case Study #2: Distal Tibia and Fibula Fracture

Mr. John Palmer is a 20-year-old male who sustained a compound fracture of his distal left tibia and fibula that required open reduction internal fixation (Figure 9-2).

PHYSICAL THERAPIST EXAMINATION

HISTORY

- General demographics: Mr. Palmer is a 20-year-old black American male whose primary language in English. He is left-leg dominant.
- Social history: Mr. Palmer is single. He lives with his girlfriend of 2 years.
- Employment/work: He is currently a full-time student in his junior year of college majoring in business administration. He works part-time on the weekends landscaping for the university at which he attends classes.
- Living environment: He lives in a one-bedroom walk-up apartment on the third floor.
- General health status
  - General health perception: Mr. Palmer reports being in good health.
  - Physical function: His reported function is normal for his age.
  - Psychological function: Normal.
  - Role function: Student.
  - Social function: He has been involved in rugby and intramural basketball and soccer. He works out at a local health club three times weekly.
- Social/health habits: John is a non-smoker and heavy drinker (25+ drinks per week).
- Family history: His parents and four grandparents are alive and healthy to the best of his recollection.
- Medical/surgical history: Mr. Palmer reports that his medical and surgical history is nonsignificant.
- Prior hospitalizations: None reported.
- Preexisting medical and other health-related conditions: Noncontributory.
- Current condition(s)/chief complaint(s): John fractured his left tibia and fibula while playing rugby for the university. Subsequently he underwent ORIF to repair the fracture 6 weeks ago. He has been partial weightbearing since the time of surgery and has just been given clearance from the surgeon to begin weightbearing as tolerated. He is anxious to return to all functional activities,

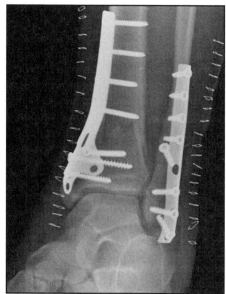

Figure 9-2. Radiograph of Mr. Palmer's left distal tibia and fibular fracture stabilized with compression plates and screws.

including athletics, at full capacity.

- Functional status and activity level: He is totally independent in all basic ADL. John has some difficulty with IADL because he has trouble carrying objects while using his crutches. He has to spend a great deal of time walking between classes on campus and has managed with assistance from friends up to this point.
- Medications: None currently besides an occasional Advil after a day on his feet.
- Other clinical tests: Radiographs taken 6 weeks postoperative revealed that the fractures were well healed.

SYSTEMS REVIEW

- Cardiovascular/pulmonary
  - BP: 118/74 mmHg
  - Edema: Visual inspection reveals mild edema left ankle and foot
  - HR: 58 bpm
  - RR: 10 bpm
- Integumentary
  - Presence of scar formation: 14-cm scar on medial aspect and 11-cm scar on lateral aspect of left ankle that are confined to the borders of the incision
  - Skin color: WNL
  - Skin integrity: WNL
- Musculoskeletal
  - Gross range of motion: WNL except for the left ankle that visually demonstrated decreased plan-

tarflexion, dorsiflexion, inversion, and eversion
- Gross strength: WNL except for left ankle that demonstrates weakness of the invertors, evertors, dorsiflexors, and plantarflexors
- Gross symmetry: Atrophy noted in left calf and thigh
- Height: 5'11" (1.8 m)
- Weight: 170 lbs (77.1 kg)
- Neuromuscular
  - Balance: Appears to be good with partial weightbearing and two crutches
  - Locomotion, transfers, and transitions
    - Ambulates with two crutches using a step-through gait with partial weightbearing of LLE
    - Transfers and transitions easily with crutches
- Communication, affect, cognition, language, and learning style
  - Communication, affect, and cognition: WNL
  - Learning preferences: Visual learner

TESTS AND MEASURES

- Aerobic capacity/endurance
  - Diminished, secondary to crutch ambulation and immobilization
- Anthropometric characteristics
  - BMI=23.79, WNL (weight [in kg] divided by height^2 [in meters])
  - Mild edema noted left distal extremity
- Assistive and adaptive devices
  - Uses two crutches that are fit appropriately to patient's specifications[68]
- Cranial and peripheral nerve integrity
  - Mild decrease in sensation para-incisions
- Environmental, home, and work barriers
  - Potential barriers include three flights of stairs to enter apartment and walking distance between classes (up to 30 minutes)
- Ergonomics and body mechanics
  - Analysis of body mechanics during transfers revealed that Mr. Palmer frequently hops on the RLE when transferring
- Gait, locomotion, and balance
  - Ambulates quickly with two crutches using a step-through gait pattern with partial weightbearing on the LLE
  - Exhibits decreased toe push off on the LLE
  - No recognized loss of balance
- Integumentary integrity
  - 14-cm scar on medial aspect of left ankle and 11-cm scar on lateral aspect of left ankle
  - Mild binding of scar noted

- No signs of infection
- Joint integrity and mobility
  - Joint mobility assessment revealed:
    - Moderate decrease in mobility of the talocrural joint
    - Moderate decrease of posterior mobility of both the proximal and distal tibiofibular joints
    - Decrease in intertarsal mobility on the left
- Motor function
  - Dexterity of UEs and RLE: WNL
  - Lack of coordination during proprioceptive and kinesthetic assessment of the left ankle
- Muscle performance
  - MMT of the LLE revealed the following deviations from normal:
    - Left hip abduction=4-/5
    - Left hip extension=4+/5
    - Left knee flexion=4/5
    - Left knee extension=4+/5
    - Left ankle dorsiflexion=4/5
    - Left ankle plantarflexion=4-/5
    - Left ankle inversion=4-/5
    - Left ankle eversion=3+/5
- Pain
  - Patient reported pain of 1-2/10 on the NPS in the left ankle when "putting too much weight" on the LLE
- Posture
  - Standing with UE support of two axillary crutches
  - Mild FHP
  - Left knee held in slight flexion
  - Left pelvis elevated
- Range of motion
  - AROM of left ankle revealed:
    - Plantarflexion=0 to 22 degrees
    - Dorsiflexion=0 to 2 degrees
    - Inversion=0 to 8 degrees
    - Eversion=0 to 14 degrees
  - PROM of left ankle revealed:
    - Goniometric measurements of ankle ROM for plantarflexion and dorsiflexion have demonstrated good intratester reliability (ICC=0.86 to 0.09), yet the intratester reliability for inversion and eversion measurements is poor (ICC=0.22 to 0.30)[69]
    - Plantarflexion=0 to 28 degrees
    - Dorsiflexion=0 to 5 degrees
    - Inversion=0 to 12 degrees
    - Eversion=0 to 21 degrees
  - Passive muscle flexibility testing revealed decreased extensibility of the left hamstrings, quadriceps, ankle

plantarflexors, and toe extensors
- ◆ Self-care and home management
  - ● Interview with the patient revealed:
    - ■ He is independent with all basic ADL
    - ■ John is limited in IADL that require any lifting and home management duties (taking out the trash)
    - ■ His live-in girlfriend has been assisting with IADL and home management actions, tasks, and activities
- ◆ Work, community, and leisure integration or reintegration
  - ● Mr. Palmer has continued to attend all courses but reports that he has had considerable assistance from friends with traveling to and from various class buildings and to and from school

EVALUATION

His history indicated that he is a young black American male who sustained a fracture of his left tibia and fibula during a rugby match and subsequently underwent ORIF. He lives in a one-bedroom apartment on the third floor with his girlfriend who assists him with IADL and home management duties. Mr. Palmer has postural deviations and decreased LLE motor and muscle performance, ROM, and scar tissue mobility. He is currently ambulating with two crutches using a step-through gait with partial weightbearing on the LLE. His physician has approved gait progression as tolerated.

DIAGNOSIS

Mr. Palmer is a patient who has sustained distal tibia and fibula fractures with ORIF. He has impaired: aerobic capacity/endurance; cranial and peripheral nerve integrity; gait, locomotion, and balance; joint integrity and mobility; motor function; muscle performance; posture; and range of motion. He is functionally limited in self-care and home management and in work, community, and leisure actions, tasks, and activities. These findings are consistent with placement in Pattern I: Impaired Joint Mobility, Motor Function, Muscle Performance, and Range of Motion Associated With Bony or Soft Tissue Surgery. These impairments and functional limitations will be addressed in determining the prognosis and the plan of care.

PROGNOSIS AND PLAN OF CARE

Over the course of the visits, the following mutually established outcomes have been determined:
- ◆ Ability to perform physical actions, tasks, and activities related to self-care, home management, work, commu-

nity, and leisure is improved
- ◆ Functional independence in ADL and IADL is increased
- ◆ Gait is improved
- ◆ Joint mobility is improved
- ◆ Motor function is improved
- ◆ Muscle performance is increased
- ◆ Pain is decreased
- ◆ Passive muscle flexibility is improved
- ◆ Physical function is improved
- ◆ Postural control is improved
- ◆ ROM is improved
- ◆ Self-management of symptoms is improved

To achieve these outcomes, the appropriate interventions for this patient are determined. These will include: coordination, communication, and documentation; patient/client-related instruction; therapeutic exercise; functional training in self-care and home management, functional training in work, community, and leisure integration or reintegration; and manual therapy techniques.

Based on the diagnosis and prognosis, Mr. Palmer is expected to require between 6 and 20 visits, over a 16-week period of time. Mr. Palmer is a young, healthy, motivated individual with good social support and will follow through with his home exercise program.

INTERVENTIONS

RATIONALE FOR SELECTED INTERVENTIONS

Therapeutic Exercise

The effects of immobilization on strength and torque of the triceps surae muscle group, ROM, and function have been well documented in the literature.[70-74] Duchateau[71] demonstrated that when subjected to 5 weeks of bed rest the triceps surae muscle group exhibited a 46% decrease in maximum voluntary contraction with 33% being attributed to central activation and 13% attributed to a decrease in muscle force generating capacities. However, it should be noted that the Duchateau[71] study was carried out on an individual who had not sustained an injury to the ankle joint. Conversely, Geboers and associates[72] demonstrated that 4 to 6 weeks after immobilization for an ankle fracture, there was a 28% decrease in dorsiflexion torque as compared to the unaffected side.

Vandenborne and associates[75] demonstrated that after 8 weeks of cast immobilization following ORIF for a tibia fracture, a 22-year-old male exhibited a 50% deficit in plantarflexion strength and significant reductions in cross sectional area of the lateral gastrocnemius, medial gastrocnemius, and soleus of 32.4%, 22.9%, and 20.1%, respectively. These physical impairments were associated with considerable functional deficits. However, following 8 weeks of rehabilitation that included strength and endurance training, significant improvements in all impairments were noted and subsequently translated into functional improvements. Rozzi and associates[76] demonstrated that a 4-week balance, coordination, and agility training program significantly improved ankle stability and joint proprioception.

Perhaps of greater clinical relevance, Shaffer and associates[73] investigated the effects of plantarflexion torque, fatigue resistance, and functional ability following an ORIF and 8 weeks of immobilization as a result of an ankle fracture. Their findings demonstrated that following immobilization plantarflexion torque was significantly decreased, fatigue resistance was significantly lower, and function was significantly less than in an age- and sex-matched control group. However, following a 10-week rehabilitation program consisting of strengthening exercises, tibiotalar joint mobilizations, passive stretching, and proprioceptive training, the patients exhibited significant improvement with all the aforementioned impairments. Following the course of rehabilitation, the plantarflexion torque surpassed the initial torque of the contralateral limb. Functional improvements were noted throughout the entire 10 weeks with the largest improvements occurring during the first 4 weeks. A strong relationship between plantarflexor peak torque and function was demonstrated through regression analysis.

Early mobilization and the initiation of exercise following surgical reduction is essential for optimal rehabilitation.[31] A randomized clinical trial[70] investigating the effects of early mobilization (within 24 hours following ORIF for an ankle fracture) demonstrated there was no significant improvement in pain or ROM when compared to a group who remained immobilized for 2 weeks. However, and perhaps of greater relevance, was the significant improvements in function exhibited by the group receiving immediate non-weightbearing exercises at the 12 week follow-up.[70]

Manual Therapy Techniques

As previously discussed, patients who underwent a rehabilitation program consisting of ambulation, strengthening, proprioceptive retraining, and joint mobilization made significant improvements in functional performance and through the course of treatment returned to control levels.[73] A pilot study by Wilson and associates[77] demonstrated exercise plus manual therapy (joint mobilization and traction to hypomobile joints) was superior to exercise therapy alone in increasing ROM and function in a group of patients who had been immobilized for 6 weeks following an ankle fracture.

Tropp and Norlin[74] found that patients who were immobilized for 6 weeks in a plaster cast following ORIF of an ankle fracture demonstrated considerable reductions in ankle dorsiflexion, as compared to a group that was placed in a hinged brace, following ORIF. The hinged brace allowed dorsiflexion and plantarflexion movements, and the results suggested that early ROM might decrease impairments associated with dorsiflexion. Immobilization may have considerable consequences on the capsular structures of a joint and may result in disorganization of the collagenous weave patterns.[78] Threlkeld[79] purported that joint mobilizations may be beneficial in breaking some of the links between connective tissue fibers. It has been advocated that once the fracture site is sufficiently healed, mobilization of the affected joints should be initiated to ensure optimal return of motion.[80]

COORDINATION, COMMUNICATION, AND DOCUMENTATION

Communication will occur with Mr. Palmer regarding all components of his care. This began in the hospital and continued at home through his return to leisure activities. All elements of the patient's management, including examination, evaluation, diagnosis, prognosis, and interventions, will be documented.

PATIENT/CLIENT-RELATED INSTRUCTION

The patient will be instructed about his current condition, impairments, and functional limitations. He will be instructed in enhancement of performance, health, wellness, and fitness programs. John will also be informed of the plan of care and transition across settings.

THERAPEUTIC EXERCISE

- ◆ Phase I: Non-weightbearing, weeks 1 through 6
  - ● Aerobic capacity/endurance conditioning
    - ■ Upper body ergometer
    - ■ Crutch walking, non-weightbearing
  - ● Flexibility exercises
    - ■ Hamstring, quadriceps, and hip flexor stretching
  - ● Strength, power, and endurance training
    - ■ Long-arc quadriceps and hamstring curls
    - ■ Hip straight leg raising for flexion, extension, abduction, and adduction
- ◆ Phase II: Weightbearing as tolerated, weeks 6 through 16
  - ● Aerobic capacity/endurance conditioning
    - ■ Start with stationary bicycle and progress to walking as weightbearing increases
    - ■ Begin with small duration of exercise until patient's physiological responses to exercise can be monitored and adjusted to reach THR and progress accordingly
    - ■ Intensity will be 60% to 80% of THR with

appropriate perceived exertion according to Borg scale[81]

- Frequency will be three to four times per week
- Progress to walking on treadmill including inclines
- Progress to light jogging as appropriate

● Balance, coordination, and agility training
  - Gait progression forward and backward with eyes open and closed
  - Carioca
  - Single leg balance activities, first on static surface progressing to dynamic surface
  - Single leg stance, while catching and throwing a ball
  - Single leg stance, while catching and throwing a ball on a dynamic surface
  - Controlled single leg dorsiflexion and plantarflexion on wobble board
  - Controlled single leg inversion and eversion on wobble board
  - Lunges with front foot on half roller
  - Single leg hops when appropriate
  - Single leg hops over short hurdles, forward, backward, side to side

● Flexibility exercises
  - Stretching exercises should be done after warming up, using a slow and steady stretch accompanied by deep breathing, and building hold up to 30 to 60 seconds
  - Gastrocnemius and soleus stretching in long sitting with assistance from towel wrapped around foot, with 30-second holds
  - Gastrocnemius and soleus stretching leaning against a wall in tandem stance, with 30-second holds
  - Gastrocnemius and soleus stretching, on slant board, with 30-second holds
  - Sitting and doorway stretch for hamstring muscle on the left, with 30-second holds
  - Sidelying quadriceps stretch, with assistance from towel wrapped around foot, with 30-second holds
  - Standing quadriceps stretch, with assistance from towel wrapped around foot, with 30-second holds
  - Standing hamstring stretch, with left leg on low table, with 30-second holds
  - Supine hamstring stretch, with knee extended, with 30-second holds
  - Seated with knee to chest, pull foot into plantarflexion and toes into flexion, with 30-second holds

● Gait and locomotion training
  - Gait in front of mirror for visual cues
  - Forward and backward walking with eyes open and closed
  - Gait on treadmill
  - Gait on uneven terrain
  - Stair walking with various stair heights
  - Gait around obstacles at progressive speeds

● Strength, power, and endurance training
  - Ankle AROM, all planes, with elastic band resistance
  - Standing hip abduction, with elastic band at ankle for resistance
  - Sidelying hip abduction, with elastic band or progressive ankle weights
  - Toe raises, with UE support progressing from bilateral to unilateral
  - Heel raises, with UE support progressing from bilateral to unilateral
  - Bridging on static surface
  - Bridging on therapeutic ball
  - Supine leg curls with therapeutic ball under ankles
  - Mini squats
  - One-legged squats
  - Lunges
  - One-legged step ups on platform with progressive step heights
  - Controlled ankle inversion and eversion on a wobble board

FUNCTIONAL TRAINING IN SELF-CARE AND HOME MANAGEMENT

◆ Self-care and home management
  ● Review and simulation of all actions, tasks, and activities and postural alignment for self-care and home management
  ● Stair climbing
  ● Review of energy conservation techniques

FUNCTIONAL TRAINING IN WORK, COMMUNITY, AND LEISURE INTEGRATION OR REINTEGRATION

◆ School and work
  ● Simulated ambulation activities on uneven terrain similar to that of the college campus
  ● Simulation of activities required for part-time work
◆ Leisure
  ● Training for return to sport activities when appropriate

MANUAL THERAPY TECHNIQUES

♦ Massage
  ● Connective tissue massage
  ● Scar tissue massage, to both the medial and lateral ankle incisions, to promote proper scar formation
♦ Mobilization/manipulation
  ● Joint mobilization to the left talocrural joint, emphasizing posterior glide of talus, starting with Grades I and II mobilizations and quickly progressing to Grades III and IV
  ● Joint mobilization/manipulation of the left intertarsal joints in both a dorsal and volar direction, starting with Grades III and IV and progressing to Grade V, if necessary
  ● Joint mobilizations of the proximal tibiofibular joints in a posterior direction, beginning with Grade III and progressing to Grades IV and V if necessary
♦ Passive range of motion
  ● PROM of the left ankle in the directions of plantarflexion, dorsiflexion, inversion, and eversion, maintaining a low load prolonged stretch at end range of all planes
  ● PROM to promote elongation of the hamstrings using both the SLR and supine knee extension with the hip flexed to 90 degrees
  ● Prone knee flexion to facilitate elongation of the quadriceps muscles
  ● PROM to facilitate flexibility of the quadriceps muscles
  ● PROM to promote maximum excursion of the toe extensors with the ankle in a plantarflexed position

ANTICIPATED GOALS AND EXPECTED OUTCOMES

♦ Impact on pathology/pathophysiology
  ● Pain is decreased from a 1 to 2/10 with weightbearing activities to a 0/10 in 4 weeks.
♦ Impact on impairments
  ● Patient will achieve improvements in active mobility of the ankle to the following: plantarflexion 40 degrees, dorsiflexion 15 degrees, inversion 25 degrees, and eversion 20 degrees in 3 to 4 weeks.
  ● Patient will achieve improvements in muscle strength to the following: left hip abduction 4+/5, left hip extension 4/5, left knee flexion 5/5, left knee extension 5/5, left ankle dorsiflexion 4+/5, left ankle plantarflexion, 4+/5, left ankle inversion 4+/5, and left ankle eversion 4/5 in 4 weeks.
  ● Patient will ambulate up to one-quarter mile without an assistive device and up seven flights of stairs with minimal fatigue in 4 to 6 weeks.

● Patient will ambulate without assistive devices in a busy university setting with no loss of balance in 4 to 6 weeks.
● Patient will be able to weightbear on LLE with no assistive devices and no pain in 4 to 6 weeks.
● Patient will exhibit improved coordination and kinesthetic awareness of the left ankle, allowing him to ambulate on uneven terrain for distances up to 100 feet without assistive devices in 2 weeks.
● Patient will walk to and from class, carrying a backpack, with minimal fatigue in 4 to 6 weeks.
♦ Impact on functional limitations
  ● Patient will ambulate for periods up to 30 minutes, while commuting between classes, with normal gait and climb up and down seven flights of stairs without an assistive device in 4 to 6 weeks.
  ● Patient will perform all ADLs independently, as well as all physical actions required for reintegration into school, community, and leisure actions, tasks, and activities (with the exception of rugby) in 6 weeks.
♦ Impact on health, wellness, and fitness
  ● Patient will develop an understanding of the consequences associated with large amounts of alcohol consumption and will begin to modify this activity in 2 weeks.
♦ Impact on societal resources
  ● Documentation occurs throughout the patient management and follows APTA's *Guidelines for Physical Therapy Documentation.*[1]
  ● Patient will develop a knowledge, awareness, and understanding of the diagnosis, prognosis, interventions, and anticipated goals and expected outcomes.
  ● The rehabilitation process will focus on maximizing both clinical and functional outcomes, while ensuring that the number of visits utilized is managed in both a clinically effective and cost-effective manner.
  ● Through coordination, communication, and documentation there is expected to be a smooth transition from the hospital to home and school and to full independence.

REEXAMINATION

Reexamination is performed throughout the episode of care.

DISCHARGE

Mr. Palmer is discharged from physical therapy after a total of 12 physical therapy sessions and attainment of his goals and expected outcomes.

Case Study #3:
Rotator Cuff Tear

Mrs. Marge Spevak is a 67-year-old female who underwent a right rotator cuff repair 6 weeks ago.

PHYSICAL THERAPIST EXAMINATION

HISTORY

♦ General demographics: Mrs. Spevak is a 67-year-old white female whose primary language is English. She is right-hand dominant, and she graduated from community college with an associate's degree in bookkeeping.

♦ Social history: Mrs. Spevak is married, lives with her husband and has four children, three daughters and one son, all of whom are adults and live on their own.

♦ Employment/work: Mrs. Spevak is a retired bookkeeper who relies on her and her husband's Social Security income for financial support.

♦ Living environment: Mrs. Spevak lives in a two-story private house.

♦ General health status
  - General health perception: Mrs. Spevak reports that she is in good health.
  - Physical function: She reports that her physical function is normal for her age, and she was completely independent in all aspects of her life prior to her surgery.
  - Psychological function: Normal.
  - Role function: Wife, mother, grandmother.
  - Social function: Mrs. Spevak is active in many social activities, including tennis, biking, working out at the local health club, wine tasting, and other group events for retired individuals. She also enjoys spending time with her grandchildren.

♦ Social/health habits: She is a non-smoker and drinks alcohol socially.

♦ Family history: Her mother had a history of breast cancer, and her father had a history of coronary heart disease. Both are deceased.

♦ Medical/surgical history: Mrs. Spevak has been diagnosed with high cholesterol, which she manages with diet and medication. She denies any other significant past medical history.

♦ Prior hospitalizations: She was hospitalized for the birth of each of her children.

♦ Preexisting medical and other health-related conditions: Unremarkable.

♦ Current condition(s)/chief complaint(s): Mrs. Spevak sustained a full-thickness rotator cuff tear as a result of falling off a bicycle on an outstretched arm. She went to her physician 2 weeks after her accident due to her inability to move her arm and pain that wakened her at night. X-ray and MRI studies revealed a full-thickness tear in her right rotator cuff, and her physician elected to perform corrective surgery using an open procedure. Mrs. Spevak has been using a sling for her RUE and was recently instructed to discontinue its use and to begin physical therapy. She complains of pain, stiffness, lack of ROM, and weakness in her right shoulder. She also complains of her lack of independence in various self-care and home management activities as a result of the surgery.

♦ Functional status and activity level: Prior to her surgery, Mrs. Spevak was completely independent in all self-care and home management activities, including all ADL. She currently requires assistance for certain self-care and home management activities such as dressing, cooking, and cleaning her house. She is not able to participate in her leisure activities at this time.

♦ Medications: Percocet 5 mg by mouth for pain every 4 to 6 hours as needed, Zocor 5 mg/day by mouth for high cholesterol.

♦ Other clinical tests: Radiograph was negative for bony lesions, and MRI was positive for a full-thickness tear of the right supraspinatus tendon.

SYSTEMS REVIEW

♦ Cardiovascular/pulmonary
  - BP: 128/72 mmHg
  - Edema: Unremarkable
  - HR: 72 bpm
  - RR: 12 bpm

♦ Integumentary
  - Presence of scar formation: Scar well healed, thin, and pink, approximately 5 inches in length and extends from anterior/lateral aspect of shoulder to the posterior/superior aspect in a crescent-like shape
  - Skin color: WNL
  - Skin integrity: WNL

♦ Musculoskeletal
  - Gross range of motion
    - Right shoulder motion grossly decreased in all directions
    - Right scapula moderately hypomobile
    - Right elbow, wrist, and hand: WNL
    - LUE and both LEs: WFL
  - Gross strength
    - Gross strength WNL for age except for right shoulder girdle musculature, which was grossly limited
  - Gross symmetry: Atrophy noted in right shoul-

der girdle in the area of the supraspinatus and infraspinatus when compared to left
- Height: 5'1" (1.55 m)
- Weight: 140 lbs (63.50 kg)

♦ Neuromuscular
- Balance: Normal
- Locomotion, transfers, and transitions: WNL

♦ Communication, affect, cognition, language, and learning style
- Communication, affect, and cognition: WNL
- Learning preferences: Learns by demonstration and practice

TESTS AND MEASURES

♦ Aerobic capacity/endurance
- The 1-Mile Walk test revealed that Mrs. Spevak had a predicted VO$_{2max}$ of 11.9 ml/kg^1/min^1
- This is an indication that the patient requires improvement in cardiorespiratory fitness (CRF)[46]

♦ Anthropometric characteristics
- BMI=26.46, which indicates that the patient is overweight with a slightly elevated risk of developing obesity-related conditions[82] (weight [in kg] divided by height^2 [in meters])

♦ Assistive and adaptive devices: None required

♦ Cranial and peripheral nerve integrity
- Sensation to light touch of the RUE: WNL

♦ Ergonomics and body mechanics
- Analysis of body mechanics during self-care, home management, work, community, and leisure actions, tasks, and activities revealed difficulty with overhead activities, dressing, and various home management skills, such as putting groceries in upper cabinets and cleaning chores

♦ Gait, locomotion, and balance
- Patient exhibited decreased arm swing on the right during gait
- Otherwise, gait and balance were WNL

♦ Integumentary integrity
- Skin color, temperature, texture, and turgor: WNL
- Wound is well-healed, pliable, and exhibits normal texture and sensation

♦ Joint integrity and mobility
- Passive joint mobility assessment revealed moderate hypomobility of the inferior and posterior glide of the right GH joint
- Lateral scapula glide test was positive on the right indicating scapula dyskinesia
- Right AC and SC joint mobility: WNL
- Right elbow, wrist, and hand joints: WNL

♦ Motor function

- Dexterity, coordination, and agility: WNL except for the right shoulder
- Right shoulder displayed altered SH rhythm and GH joint function
- Mrs. Spevak scored poorly (11/25) on the UCLA Shoulder Scale
  - The self-report section of the UCLA Shoulder Scale includes three single-item subscales to evaluate pain, functional level, and satisfaction
  - The items are Likert scale type and are scored from 1 to 10 for pain and function and 0 to 5 for satisfaction
  - The score ranges from 0 to 25, with higher scores indicating less pain, greater function, and higher satisfaction
  - The UCLA Shoulder Scale has been described as having good internal consistency[83]

♦ Muscle performance
- MMT was not performed at this time to prevent disruption of the surgical repair
- Right shoulder flexion, abduction, IR and ER, and gross scapular motion appear to be at least in the fair range (3/5) within the available ROM

♦ Pain
- Using the NPS, the patient described her pain to be a 3/10 at rest escalating to a 5/10 with overhead movement and when she rolls over onto that side while sleeping
  - The NPS is the simplest subjective rating scale
  - The patient is asked to quantify her pain with rest and certain activities using a scale from 0 (no pain) to 10 (worst pain ever imagined)
  - The NPS enables the examiner to place an objective value on the patient's symptoms and allows for comparison on reexaminations

♦ Posture
- Mrs. Spevak is holding her UE in a protective pain posture of shoulder adduction and IR with her elbow flexed to 90 degrees and held on her abdomen
- Observation reveals poor slumped posture with a forward head and protracted shoulders

♦ Range of motion
- Shoulder (goniometer)
  - Flexion=R 0 to 80 degrees, L 0 to 170 degrees
  - Extension=R 0 to 30 degrees, L 0 to 40 degrees
  - Abduction=R 0 to 85 degrees, L 0 to 170 degrees
  - ER=R 0 to 40 degrees, L 0 to 85 degrees
  - IR=R 0 to 30 degrees, L 0 to 60 degrees
- Scapular
  - Posterior tilt, retraction, and depression are all moderately decreased

- Elbow, wrist, and hand (goniometry): WNL
◆ Reflex integrity: WNL
◆ Self-care and home management
  - Mrs. Spevak has difficulty performing dressing and grooming activities when they involve reaching behind her back or overhead movements
  - She expresses that she has difficulty with various home management skills, such as putting groceries in upper cabinets and cleaning chores that involve overhead movements or heavy lifting
◆ Work, community, and leisure integration or reintegration
  - She has not been able to resume leisure activities that she had been involved with prior to her surgery because she is fearful about reinjuring her shoulder

EVALUATION

Her history indicated that she is a 67-year-old female who sustained a rotator cuff tear as a result of a fall from a bicycle accident. She underwent an open repair of her rotator cuff 6 weeks prior and has been maintained in a sling since that time. As a result of the immobilization, she has developed impaired ROM and accessory motions of the right GH joint, altered SH rhythm, and altered muscle performance. She also has difficulty performing any task requiring reaching behind her back, overhead movements, or lifting. Additionally, she is a socially active non-smoker who occasionally drinks alcohol, is slightly overweight, and needs improvement in her level of CRF.

DIAGNOSIS

Mrs. Spevak is a patient who has undergone surgical repair of a right rotator cuff tear and has pain in that shoulder. She has impaired aerobic capacity/endurance; anthropometric characteristics; ergonomics and body mechanics; gait, locomotion, and balance; joint integrity and mobility; motor function; muscle performance; posture; and range of motion. She is functionally limited in self-care and home management and in work, community, and leisure actions, tasks, and activities. These findings are consistent with placement in Pattern I: Impaired Joint Mobility, Motor Function, Muscle Performance, and Range of Motion Associated With Bony or Soft Tissue Surgery. These impairments and functional limitations will be addressed in determining the prognosis and the plan of care.

PROGNOSIS AND PLAN OF CARE

Over the course of the visits, the following mutually established outcomes have been determined:
◆ Ability to perform physical actions, tasks, and activities

related to self-care, home management, work, community, and leisure is improved
◆ Ability to resume community and leisure actions, tasks, and activities is improved
◆ Aerobic capacity is increased
◆ Gait is improved
◆ Joint integrity and mobility are improved
◆ Motor function and muscle performance are improved
◆ Pain is decreased
◆ Physical capacity is improved
◆ Physical function is improved
◆ Posture is improved
◆ ROM is improved

To achieve these outcomes, the appropriate interventions for this patient are determined. These will include coordination, communication, and documentation; patient/client-related instruction; therapeutic exercise; functional training in self-care and home management; functional training in work, community, and leisure integration or reintegration; manual therapy techniques; prescription, application, and, as appropriate, fabrication of devices and equipment; electrotherapeutic modalities; and physical agents and mechanical modalities.

Based on the diagnosis and prognosis, Mrs. Spevak is expected to require between 16 and 24 visits. Mrs. Spevak has good social support, is motivated, and follows through with her home exercise program. She is not severely impaired and is generally healthy.

INTERVENTIONS

RATIONALE FOR SELECTED INTERVENTIONS

Successful rehabilitation of the shoulder involves addressing all the impairments discovered during examination, including posture, scapula position, scapular dyskinesia, ROM, mobility, and strength deficits of the entire shoulder girdle.[84]

Therapeutic Exercise

Posture and Scapula Position

Focus on the scapula in shoulder rehabilitation has increased considerably in recent years because of increased understanding of its role in normal shoulder mechanics. Culham and Peat[22] described the resting position of the scapula as follows: with the arm dependent, the superior angle of the scapula lies at the level of the second thoracic vertebra; the root of the scapula spine is at the level of the third thoracic SP; and the inferior angle is at the level of the seventh or eighth thoracic vertebra. The vertebral border lies 5 to 6 cm from midline, with the scapula itself being orientated 30 to 45 degrees anterior to the coronal plane and having a slight forward tilt (approximately 10 degrees) in the sagittal plane. It has been postulated that alterations of this resting position may lead to shoulder dysfunction. Most individuals with shoulder pathology have poor posture. This slouched position results in protracted shoulders and an increase of the anterior tilt of the scapula, causing increased activity of the levator scapulae and pectoralis minor muscles and relative weakness of the rhomboids.[85] MRI studies reveal that as the shoulder moves from a retracted to a protracted position, the subacromial space becomes narrowed predisposing an individual to impingement and associated rotator cuff tears.[85] Therefore, shoulder protraction must be addressed during shoulder rehabilitation.

Scapular Dyskinesia

Ludewig and associates[86] demonstrated that during shoulder elevation the scapula not only upwardly rotates, it moves from an anterior to a posterior tipped position. In another study, Ludewig and Cook[87] found that individuals with shoulder impingement demonstrated decreased scapula upward rotation and increased anterior tipping of the scapula during UE elevation. As a result of these studies, it is apparent that anterior tilt of the scapula must also be considered in shoulder rehabilitation.

Strengthening Exercises

In normal UE motion, the scapula provides a stable base for GH mobility. The scapula muscles are responsible for positioning the glenoid to allow for efficient GH movement. When the muscles are weak or fatigued, the scapulohumeral rhythm is compromised and shoulder dysfunction may occur.[88,89] It is important to stress scapula rehabilitation prior to emphasizing rotator cuff strengthening in the rehabilitation sequence. Kibler[90] stated that the most physiologic way to reestablish normal motor firing patterns for the scapula is with CKC activities. CKC exercises have been associated with greater compressive forces, joint congruity, decreased shear, stimulation of proprioceptors, and enhanced dynamic stabilization.[91]

Incorporation of four core exercises to target the scapula stabilizers will enhance the exercise program in the early rehabilitation phase. These include: scaption, rowing, push-ups plus (adding protraction to the end of a push-up), and press-ups.[84,92] Once scapula stabilization has been addressed, OKC exercises, including typical rotator cuff exercises such as IR and ER, PNF patterns, and plyometric activities may be added.[84,93,94]

Manual Therapy Techniques

Posterior capsule hypomobilty is common in patients with shoulder dysfunction and results in decreased GH IR.[84] Lack of GH IR may cause compensatory elevation and protraction of the medial border of the scapula from the thorax, resulting in altered scapula mechanics and associated

shoulder dysfunction.[41] It has been reported that manual physical therapy combined with supervised exercise is better than exercise alone for increasing strength, decreasing pain, and improving function with shoulder impingement syndrome.[95] As a result, it is important to include manual therapy techniques to address posterior capsule dysfunction in shoulder rehabilitation.

COORDINATION, COMMUNICATION, AND DOCUMENTATION

Communication will occur with Mrs. Spevak and her husband regarding all components of her care and to engender support for her program. This will continue at home through her return to leisure activities. All elements of the patient's management will be documented.

PATIENT/CLIENT-RELATED INSTRUCTION

The patient will be instructed in appropriate activity modification to avoid placing stress on soft tissue structures that are currently impaired. Mrs. Spevak will be instructed in proper postural habits and body mechanics during home management and leisure activities. She will be provided information on the impairments identified during the examination, plan of care, and prognosis and how they will be addressed. She will also be educated on the stages of tissue healing that will include advice about avoiding any painful activities.

THERAPEUTIC EXERCISE

Post-surgical management of rotator cuff repairs are separated into the Maximum Protective Phase, the Moderate Protective Phase, and the Minimum Protective Phase.[96]

- Maximum Protective Phase (1 to 8 weeks): The primary objectives of the Maximum Protective Phase are to protect the repaired tissue and prevent the adverse effects of immobilization. The immobilizer is removed for therapy sessions
  - Body mechanics and postural stabilization
    - Use of mirror for visual input of appropriate postural alignment
    - Head retractions to improve FHP
    - Shoulder retraction and depression
    - Chicken wing position (hands behind head, horizontal abduction of shoulders)
    - Bridging
    - Pelvic tilts
    - Dead bug (reciprocal movement of arms and legs while maintaining pelvis in neutral position in supine)
    - Ball exercises for postural control
    - Maintenance of good posture during positional changes

- Maintenance of good posture while performing functional and leisure activities
- Flexibility exercises
  - AAROM of elbow to maintain ROM
  - AROM of wrist and hand to maintain ROM
  - PROM of the shoulder joint within safe pain-free range, progress to AAROM when appropriate
  - Pendulum exercises
- Gait and locomotion training
  - Use of mirror for visual input of proper gait
  - Verbal instruction and cueing of proper gait
- Strength, power, and endurance training
  - Submaximal isometrics to scapula muscles
- Moderate Protection Phase (can begin as early as 4 weeks or as late as 6 to 12 weeks depending on the surgery): The objectives of the Moderate Protection Phase are to achieve normal ROM and progress the patient to active and resistive motion, so that the extremity can be used for functional activities
  - Aerobic capacity/endurance conditioning
    - Mode: Walking or stationary bicycle program
    - Duration: Work up to 20 to 30 minutes
    - Intensity: 60% to 70% predicted MHR
    - Frequency: Two to three times a week
  - Body mechanics and postural stabilization
    - Continue as in Maximum Protective Phase
    - Active exercise to increase retraction of the cervical spine
  - Flexibility exercises
    - General cervical spine ROM exercises
    - AROM of the shoulder joint through increasing ranges progressing to full ROM
  - Strength, power, and endurance training
    - Strengthening of the scapula stabilizers using PNF techniques, such as, alternating isometrics and rhythmic stabilization, and dynamic exercises, such as, rowing, prone horizontal abduction, protraction, and retraction
    - CKC scapular stabilization activities, such as, press-ups, push-ups, and push-up plus, progressing from minimum to maximum weightbearing (ie, weightbearing on wall initially, progressing to quadruped position, and then to a full push-up position if the patient is able to tolerate)
    - Rotator cuff PRE including scaption, sidelying ER, and prone IR
    - PNF for the scapula and UE including:
      - Rhythmic initiation to promote the ability to initiate a movement pattern by moving the patient's limb passively through the available range of the desired movement pattern, in order for the patient to become familiar with the movement pattern
      - Reversal of antagonists, which involves a weak movement pattern by first resisting the antagonist pattern
      - Rhythmic stabilization, which uses a progression of alternating isometrics around the joint in order to promote stability through co-contraction of the shoulder girdle muscles
    - Upper body ergometer for muscle endurance, progressing from 1 minute to 20 minutes as tolerated in both forward and reverse directions
- Minimum Protective Phase (begins as early as 3 months or as late as 5 months depending on the surgery and state of the repair): The objective of the Minimum Protective Phase is to gradually return the patient to unrestricted activity
  - Aerobic capacity/endurance conditioning
    - Continue walking or stationary bicycle program, 30 minutes, at 60% to 70% predicted MHR, two to three times a week
  - Body mechanics and postural stabilization
    - Continue to stress good postural alignment during all activities
  - Flexibility exercises
    - Maintain full ROM of shoulders
  - Strength, power, and endurance training
    - Use of isokinetic dynamometers
    - Plyometric activities, such as throwing and catching weighted balls
    - For younger patients Marine style push-ups (the patient propels up off the floor during the up phase and lands on the floor with his or her hands during the down phase) may be used
    - Functional exercises such as overhead lifting, pushing, and pulling while incorporating proper shoulder and body mechanics
    - For younger patients functional overhead lifting, pushing, and pulling may use weighted carts or lifting and stacking weighted objects

FUNCTIONAL TRAINING IN SELF-CARE AND HOME MANAGEMENT

- Moderate and Minimum Protective Phases
  - Self-care and home management
    - Review all actions, tasks, and activities and postural alignment for self-care and home management
      - Practice dressing and grooming activities involving reaching behind her back or overhead movements

▶ Practice putting groceries in upper cabinets and cleaning chores that involve overhead movements or heavy lifting

FUNCTIONAL TRAINING IN WORK, COMMUNITY, AND LEISURE INTEGRATION OR REINTEGRATION

◆ Moderate and Minimum Protective Phases
  ● Leisure
    ■ Review all actions, tasks, and activities and postural alignment for leisure

MANUAL THERAPY TECHNIQUES

◆ Maximum Protective Phase
  ● PROM
    ■ PROM of GH and ST joints
◆ Moderate and Minimum Protective Phases
  ● Mobilization/manipulation techniques
    ■ Posterior, inferior, and anterior glides (Grades III and IV) to the GH joint to increase UE elevation, IR, and ER
    ■ Scapula mobilization including superior, inferior, medial, lateral, and diagonal glides to improve general scapula mobility
    ■ STM to improve scapula mobility and restore posterior tilt
      ▶ Techniques include having the patient sidelying and performing medial and posterior glides of the scapula to decrease protraction
      ▶ Techniques for pectoralis minor stretching to decrease anterior tilt
    ■ Cervical joint mobilization to increase mobility of the cervical spine, including gentle manual traction

PRESCRIPTION, APPLICATION, AND, AS APPROPRIATE, FABRICATION OF DEVICES AND EQUIPMENT

◆ Maximum Protective Phase
  ● The UE is typically immobilized in a sling or abduction splint from 1 to 8 weeks, depending on the surgery

ELECTROTHERAPEUTIC MODALITIES

◆ Maximum Protective Phase
  ● Electrical stimulation
    ■ HVPC to right shoulder to decrease pain, joint swelling, and inflammation
    ■ The acute pain protocol will be used and consists

of the following parameters:
  ▶ Frequency: 100 pps
  ▶ Amplitude: Sensory stimulation
  ▶ Polarity: Negative
  ▶ Pulse duration: Fixed in HVPC
  ▶ Pad placement: Over injury site[97]

PHYSICAL AGENTS AND MECHANICAL MODALITIES

◆ Maximum Protective Phase
  ● Physical agents
    ■ Thermotherapy: Moist heat to enhance tissue perfusion and oxygenation[92]
    ■ Cryotherapy: Ice or cold packs to decrease pain, joint swelling, and inflammation[92]
  ● Mechanical modalities
    ■ CPM of the shoulder joint 0 to 90 degrees for first 48 hours

ANTICIPATED GOALS AND EXPECTED OUTCOMES

◆ Impact on pathology/pathophysiology
  ● No edema is present in the RUE within 2 to 3 weeks
  ● Nutrient delivery to tissue is increased.
  ● Pain is decreased from 3/10 to 0/10 at rest and 5/10 to 2/10 at its worst with overhead activity over 4 to 6 weeks.
  ● Soft tissue healing is enhanced.
  ● Soft tissue swelling and inflammation are decreased.
  ● Tissue perfusion and oxygenation are enhanced.
◆ Impact on impairments
  ● Aerobic capacity is increased during the Moderate and Minimum Protective Phases as evidenced by ability to work at 60% to 70% of max predicted HR for 30 minutes.
  ● Gait is improved as evidenced by normal reciprocal arm swing within 6 to 8 weeks.
  ● Joint mobility is improved to minimum hypomobility of inferior and posterior glide of the right GH joint.
  ● Joint stability is improved.
  ● Motor function is improved.
  ● Muscle performance is improved as evidenced by increased control of scapula movement during the Moderate and Minimum Protective Phases.
  ● Muscle strength and endurance are restored during the Moderate and Minimum Protective Phases.
  ● Postural alignment is achieved during the Maximum and Moderate Protective Phases as evidenced by decreased forward head and forward shoulder.

- Protective pain posture of the shoulder is eliminated.
- ROM is improved through the Maximum Protective Phase and pain-free ROM is achieved during the Moderate Protective Phase as evidenced by 150 degrees of shoulder elevation and 75 degrees of ER.
- Scapula dyskinesia is normalized within 6 to 8 weeks.

- ◆ Impact on functional limitations
  - Ability to resume and perform independently required physical actions, tasks, and activities related to ADL and IADL of self-care (including personal hygiene, dressing, and washing her hair), home management (including reaching items in kitchen cabinets, putting groceries on shelves, removing items from the refrigerator), community, and leisure is achieved by the Minimum Protective Phase.
  - Self-management of symptoms is improved.
  - Tolerance of positions and actions, tasks, and activities is increased.

- ◆ Risk reduction/prevention
  - Mrs. Spevak will learn behaviors that will foster prevention.
  - Postoperative complications are reduced.
  - Pressure on body tissues is reduced.
  - Protection of body parts is increased.
  - Risk factors are reduced.
  - Risk of secondary impairment is reduced.
  - Safety is improved.
  - Stresses precipitating injury are decreased.

- ◆ Impact on health, wellness, and fitness
  - Fitness and health status are improved.
  - Physical capacity and physical function are increased.
  - Mrs. Spevak will learn behaviors that will foster healthy habits and wellness.

- ◆ Impact on societal resources
  - Resources available to the Spevaks will be maximally utilized.

- ◆ Patient/client satisfaction
  - Documentation occurs throughout patient management and follows APTA's *Guidelines for Physical Therapy Documentation* located in *Guide to Physical Therapist Practice.*[1]
  - Patient and family knowledge and awareness regarding her diagnosis, prognosis, and interventions and their understanding of anticipated goals and expected outcomes are increased.

REEXAMINATION

Reexamination is performed throughout the episode of care, particularly as the phase of protection changes.

DISCHARGE

Mrs. Spevak is discharged from physical therapy after a total of 18 physical therapy sessions and attainment of her goals and expectations. These sessions have covered her entire episode of care. She is discharged because she has achieved her goals and expected outcomes.

Case Study #4: Anterior Cruciate Ligament Repair

Mr. Al Langert is a 16-year-old healthy male who underwent a right anterior cruciate ligament reconstruction 8 days ago.

PHYSICAL THERAPIST EXAMINATION

HISTORY

- ◆ General demographics: Al is a 16-year-old white male whose primary language is English. He is right-hand dominant and is presently attending high school.
- ◆ Social history: He is the oldest of four children and currently lives with both of his parents.
- ◆ Employment/work: Al works part-time at a video game store; he is not dependent on this income, however, as he receives full financial support from his parents.
- ◆ Living environment: Al lives in a two-story private house.
- ◆ General health status:
  - General health perception: Al reports that he is in excellent health.
  - Physical function: He reports that his physical function had been excellent as he excelled in athletics.
  - Psychological function: Normal.
  - Role function: Son, brother, student.
  - Social function: Al is involved with several high school sports and after school activities.
- ◆ Social/health habits: He is a non-smoker and non-drinker who prides himself on eating healthily and working out in order to keep himself physically fit.
- ◆ Family history: Unremarkable.
- ◆ Medical/surgical history: Unremarkable.

◆ Prior hospitalizations: None.

◆ Preexisting medical and other health-related conditions: Unremarkable.

◆ Current condition(s)/chief complaint(s): He sustained an ACL rupture when he attempted to decelerate and pivot while playing football. The patient was sent to the emergency room for immediate care and x-ray evaluation. Following his emergency room visit, Al was referred to an orthopedic surgeon who diagnosed his condition as a Grade III ACL tear because of his clinical and MRI evaluation. Al received 3 weeks of preoperative physical therapy prior to his scheduled reconstructive surgery that involved an intra-articular ACL reconstruction using a patellar tendon graft. Al currently complains of pain, lack of ROM, and decreased strength in his right knee. He also reports he has low endurance and is frustrated that he cannot ambulate without crutches.

◆ Functional status and activity level: Prior to his injury, Al was completely independent in all ADL and IADL. He is not able to participate in his sport or after school activities at this time.

◆ Medications: Percocet 5 mg PO for pain q 4 to 6 hr as needed.

◆ Other clinical tests: X-ray negative for bony lesions, MRI positive for Grade III ACL tear.

SYSTEMS REVIEW

◆ Cardiovascular/pulmonary
  ● BP: 120/70 mmHg
  ● Edema: Moderate right knee edema noted
  ● HR: 60 bpm
  ● RR: 12 bpm
◆ Integumentary
  ● Presence of scar formation
    ▪ A 6-cm well-healing scar, without signs and symptoms of infection, is noted on the central aspect of right knee
    ▪ A small scar is located at the drain site and is also healing well
  ● Skin color: Grossly WNL in area of the knee, with some redness noted over scar
  ● Skin integrity: WNL
◆ Musculoskeletal
  ● Gross range of motion
    ▪ Right knee flexion proportionately decreased greater than extension
    ▪ All other ROM: WFL
  ● Gross strength
    ▪ RLE grossly limited
    ▪ All other gross strength: WNL
  ● Gross symmetry: Atrophy noted in right quadriceps

muscle when compared to left
  ● Height: 5'8" (1.73 m)
  ● Weight: 175 lbs (79.38 kg)
◆ Neuromuscular
  ● Balance: Patient exhibited poor static and dynamic balance
  ● Locomotion, transfers, and transitions: Patient requires minimal assistance with transfers from chair to treatment table because of his poor balance
◆ Communication, affect, cognition, language, and learning style
  ● Communication, affect, and cognition: WNL
  ● Learning preferences: Learns by demonstration and practice.

TESTS AND MEASURES

◆ Aerobic capacity/endurance: Not evaluated at this time.
◆ Anthropometric characteristics
  ● Body composition was determined by use of a Lange skin fold caliper
    ▪ Skin fold measurement provides fairly consistent and meaningful information about body fat[10]
    ▪ An age-appropriate formula was utilized as fat deposition patterns varies with age
    ▪ The following formula was developed for young men:
      ‣ % body fat=0.43A + 0.58B + 1.47, where A=triceps skin fold (mm), and B=subscapular skin fold (mm)
    ▪ The patient's body fat percentage was calculated to be 15%, which is average for his age
  ● Girth measurements revealed approximately a 1-inch increase in the suprapatella region as a result of edema and approximately 1.5-inch decrease of the quadriceps indicating atrophy
◆ Assistive and adaptive devices
  ● He requires use of axillary crutches to ambulate
◆ Cranial and peripheral nerve integrity
  ● Sensation to light touch of the RLE: WNL, except a small area of decreased sensation over area of the scar
◆ Ergonomics and body mechanics
  ● Analysis of body mechanics during self-care, home management, work, community, and leisure, actions, tasks, and activities revealed difficulty with transfer activities and various ADL that involve the lower body
◆ Gait, locomotion, and balance
  ● Patient ambulates partial weightbearing on right with knee immobilizer, requiring supervision and

verbal cueing as he exhibits decreased dynamic balance

♦ Integumentary integrity
  ● Skin color, temperature, texture, and turgor all appear WNL in area of knee, except over scar, where slight redness noted
  ● Wounds are healing well, are pliable, and exhibit normal texture

♦ Joint integrity and mobility
  ● Passive joint mobility assessment revealed moderately hypomobile posterior and anterior glide of the right knee capsule, and superior glide of the patella
  ● In Phase I (preoperatively), the Lachman test, which is a one-plane anterior instability test used to assess the integrity of the ACL, was positive
    ■ The Lachman test has been reported to be the best test for assessing the integrity of the posterolateral band of the ACL and is the most practical test for assessing the integrity of the ACL in an acutely injured knee because of the position utilized with testing[23]
    ■ The Lachman is performed by having the patient lie in supine with the knee flexed to 25 to 30 degrees, a position that may be accomplished by placing a 6-inch firm bolster under the patient's knee
    ■ The examiner places the proximal hand over the patient's thigh while simultaneously palpating the knee joint line
    ■ The distal hand is used to grasp the posterior aspect of the leg and apply an anteriorly directed force
    ■ If there is greater than a 3-mm difference in anterior translation between the injured and uninjured leg, the test is positive for an ACL tear
  ● In Phase I (preoperatively), Al had a positive result on the KT 1000
    ■ The KT 1000 knee ligament arthrometer is an instrumented stress device used to measure tibial displacement and verifies suspected ACL and PCL tears
    ■ It objectively quantifies ligamentous laxity in millimeters, with a 3-mm displacement being indicative of a ligament tear
    ■ Knee ligament arthrometers may assist in the initial diagnosis but are more effective in evaluating patients with chronic ACL ligament disruptions and documenting post-surgical results[23]

♦ Motor function
  ● Dexterity, coordination, and agility all appeared WNL except in the RLE, where altered joint biomechanics were noted

  ● The patient maintained the knee in a guarded position of slight flexion during ambulation and transfers

♦ Muscle performance
  ● Patient was unable to perform a quad set or SLR on the right due to pain and weakness
  ● Knee flexion appeared to be 3/5 in the available ROM
  ● Otherwise, strength appeared to be normal throughout

♦ Orthotic, protective, and supportive devices
  ● Patient required the use of a knee immobilizer on his right knee

♦ Pain
  ● Patient reported his pain was 5/10 on the NPS at rest escalating to a 8/10 with movement

♦ Posture
  ● Upper body posture: WNL
  ● RLE maintained in a protective pain posture of slight knee flexion

♦ Range of motion
  ● WNL throughout except in the right knee
  ● AROM and PROM for the R knee were the same and were as follows:
    ■ Extension=L 0 degrees, R -5 degrees
    ■ Flexion=L 150 degrees, R 45 degrees

♦ Reflex integrity: WNL

♦ Self-care and home management
  ● Patient has some difficulty dressing his lower body, transferring, and showering at this time.

♦ Work, community, and leisure integration or reintegration
  ● Patient unable to participate in sports activities or after school activities at this time

EVALUATION

Al's previously outlined history indicated that he is a 16-year-old male who sustained an ACL tear as a result of a football injury. He underwent an ACL reconstruction using a BPTB graft 8 days ago. He is currently ambulating partial weightbearing and is using a knee immobilizer. He exhibits decreased balance during gait and requires minimal assistance when transferring. Also noted are decreased right knee ROM, decreased quadriceps and hamstring function, and right knee edema. He has not been able to attend school or function socially since his surgery.

DIAGNOSIS

Al is a patient who has undergone ACL reconstruction as a result of a tear and has pain in his right knee. He has impaired:

anthropometric characteristics; ergonomics and body mechanics; gait, locomotion, and balance; joint integrity and mobility; motor function; muscle performance; posture; and range of motion. He is functionally limited in self-care and home management and in work, community, and leisure actions, tasks, and activities. These findings are consistent with placement in Pattern I: Impaired Joint Mobility, Motor Function, Muscle Performance, and Range of Motion Associated With Bony or Soft Tissue Surgery. These impairments and functional limitations will be addressed in determining the prognosis and the plan of care.

PROGNOSIS AND PLAN OF CARE

Over the course of the visits, the following mutually established outcomes have been determined:

♦ Ability to perform physical actions, tasks, and activities related to self-care, home management, work, community, and leisure is improved

♦ Ability to resume community and leisure actions, tasks, and activities is improved

♦ Edema is decreased

♦ Gait and transfers are improved

♦ Joint integrity and mobility are improved

♦ Motor function and muscle performance are improved

♦ Pain is decreased

♦ ROM is improved

To achieve these outcomes, the appropriate interventions for this patient are determined. These will include coordination, communication, and documentation; patient/client-related instruction; therapeutic exercise; functional training in self-care and home management; functional training in work, community, and leisure integration or reintegration; manual therapy techniques; electrotherapeutic modalities; and physical agents and mechanical modalities.

Based on the diagnosis and prognosis, Al is expected to require between 16 and 24 visits. Al has good social support, is motivated, and follows through with his home exercise program. He is not severely impaired and is young and healthy.

INTERVENTIONS

RATIONALE FOR SELECTED INTERVENTIONS

Early emphasis on the quadriceps muscle group is critical for successful return to functional activity. It has been noted that a combination of both OKC non-weightbearing and CKC weightbearing exercises performed in the correct manner should be incorporated for successful and safe quadriceps rehabilitation.[98] However, it is important to know when and how to incorporate each activity as well as its possible effect on the ACL.

Therapeutic Exercise

Prior to instituting a therapeutic exercise program with a patient who has an injured ACL or a healing ACL graft, one must understand the effect the exercises have on the graft. Early work by Paulos and associates[99] revealed that strain on the ACL dramatically increased during the last 30 degrees of OKC knee extension. Similarly, it was reported by Arms and associates[100] that quadriceps activity did not strain the normal or reconstructed ACL when the knee was flexed beyond 60 degrees; however, the activity significantly strained the ACL from 0 to 45 degrees. Beynnon[101] reported that isotonic quadriceps contraction consistently produced positive strain values between 10 and 48 degrees of flexion and an unstrained region between 48 and 110 degrees of flexion. Additionally, isometric contraction of the hamstring muscles at 15, 30, 60, and 90 degrees of flexion did not strain the ACL. Taken together, these findings suggest that AROM and OKC extension exercises may be safe from 100 to 50 degrees of flexion and that OKC flexion exercises do not pose a risk early in rehabilitation. Beynnon also reported that passive motion of the knee between 110 degrees and full extension produced little strain in the range between 11.5 and 110 degrees, indicating that CPM in this range should be safe for the ACL graft immediately post-surgery.

Closed-Kinetic-Chain Exercises

The value of CKC over OKC exercises in quadriceps rehabilitation post ACL surgery has also been promoted. In a classic study by Henning and associates,[102] it was reported that isometric knee extension at 0 and 22 degrees produced five to 17 times more strain on the ACL than weightbearing exercises. This finding supported the benefit of strengthening the quadriceps using CKC exercises. In a separate study, Yack and associates[103] compared OKC knee extension to the CKC parallel squats in subjects with anterior cruciate deficient knees. Their results revealed that the anterior cruciate deficient knee had significantly greater anterior tibial displacement during extension from 64 to 10 degrees in the OKC knee extension exercise, as compared to the CKC parallel squat exercise. The authors concluded that stress on the ACL is minimized by using CKC exercises.

Palmitier and associates[104] proposed a biomechanical model to explain the benefits of CKC exercise that included reduced anterior shear forces and tibial translation, both of which result in increased strain on the ACL. The authors hypothesized that these effects were due to tibial-femoral joint compression, co-contraction of the hamstrings providing a posterior force on the tibia decreasing the anterior shear, and changing the angles of applied forces. Other researchers have also demonstrated decreased anterior translation with CKC exercises.[105]

More recent studies[101,106] indicated that ACL strain does not differ with either OKC and CKC exercises. These studies did note that increasing loads with CKC exercises did not increase the strain on the ACL. This may be a benefit when performing CKC exercises.

Rehabilitation Phases

Current rehabilitation of ACL reconstruction is divided into four phases: Phase I, preoperative phase (3 to 5 weeks); Phase II, immediate or acute postoperative phase (week 1); Phase III, intermediate postoperative phase (2 to 4 weeks); and Phase IV, advanced rehabilitation/functional training (5 weeks to 4 to 5 months). The phases were developed to coincide with the healing of the ACL graft. Timelines given may vary depending on the surgeon and the ability to meet the goals of one phase prior to advancing to the next. The rationale for incorporating the preoperative phase is that it has been noted that if a patient undergoes surgery with pain, edema, lack of ROM, and poor quad function the post surgical outcome will be poor.[23]

COORDINATION, COMMUNICATION, AND DOCUMENTATION

Communication will occur with Al and his parents. This began in the preoperative period and continued through his return to school, part-time work, and leisure activities. All elements of the patient's management will be documented.

PATIENT/CLIENT-RELATED INSTRUCTION

Instruction began for Al preoperatively, when the patient had the postoperative procedures explained to him. Postoperatively, the patient was instructed in appropriate activity modification to avoid placing stress on soft tissue structures that were currently impaired. Al was instructed in proper postural habits and body mechanics during home management and school activities. The impairments identified during the examination, prognosis, and plan of care were all reviewed with Al. He was provided instruction on the stages of tissue healing, which included advice about avoiding any painful activities or activities that may disrupt the graft.

THERAPEUTIC EXERCISE

Management of ACL reconstruction is divided into four phases: Phase I, preoperative phase (3 to 5 weeks); Phase II, immediate or acute postoperative phase (week 1); Phase III, intermediate postoperative phase (2 to 4 weeks); and Phase IV, advanced rehabilitation/functional training (5 weeks to 4 to 5 months).

- ◆ Phase I: Preoperative phase
  - Aerobic capacity/endurance conditioning
    - Stationary bicycle
    - Stairmaster
  - Body mechanics and postural stabilization
    - Maintain a neutral aligned position with the natural cervical lordosis, thoracic kyphosis, and lumbar lordosis
    - Achieve pelvic neutral position (midposition between anterior and posterior pelvis tilt) in order to attain and maintain a neutral spine
    - Instruct and correct standing and sitting postures using a mirror, verbal cueing, and a plumb line
    - Instruct in proper sit-to stand, lifting, and pushing techniques incorporating a neutral pelvis and spine
  - Flexibility exercises
    - Prone hangs with lower leg hanging off the edge of a table in a gravity-assisted position for extension of the knee
      - ‣ A light weight may be placed over the ankle to assist in achieving full knee extension
    - Heel slides sitting in long sitting and sliding the heel toward the buttocks for flexion of the knee
  - Gait and locomotion training
    - Gait training with crutches
  - Strength, power, and endurance training
    - Quad-sets and SLR for quad control
    - CKC strengthening, such as leg press, one-quarter squats, step-downs, stationary bicycle, and the Stairmaster
- ◆ Phase II: Immediate or acute postoperative phase
  - Body mechanics and postural stabilization
    - Same activities as Phase I
    - Physioball activities while sitting to improve trunk stabilization including single arm lateral reach, bilateral arm reach, side foot reach (sitting with arms crossed extend foot to one side), lateral pelvic glide (patient sits in pelvic neutral and rolls pelvis from side to side returning to neutral), and bounce (patient sits in pelvic neutral and maintains this position while he bounces on ball, may then incorporate alternating arms)
    - Begin weight shifting in parallel bars: Anterior to posterior, side to side, and obliquely
    - Progress to single leg stance
    - Perform single leg stance while moving arms in various planes, frontal, sagittal, and transverse
  - Flexibility exercises
    - Bicycle to gain ROM, first by peddling forward and backward in the available range until such time that enough range is gained in order to complete a full revolution
    - Pillow extensions: Patient supine with heel propped on a pillow to allow gravity to assist in

gaining full knee extension
- Wall slides: Supine with hip and knee flexed to 90 degrees with foot placed on a wall, slide foot toward the floor to gain flexion
- General flexibility for all major LE muscle groups
- Gait and locomotion training
  - Ambulation training with weightbearing as tolerated, partial to full weightbearing without crutches
- Strength, power, and endurance training
  - Active-assisted knee flexion
  - Quad-sets, hamstring sets, and adductor sets
  - SLRs

♦ Phase III: Intermediate postoperative phase
- Aerobic capacity/endurance conditioning
  - Aerobic activities, such as bicycling, Stairmaster, and swimming, progressing up to 20 minutes a session at least three times a week
- Balance, coordination, and agility training
  - Balance and proprioceptive activities using the mini trampoline, foam rubber mats, low balance beam, BAPS board, and like apparatus
    - ‣ These activities are used to improve balance by challenging the patient's center of gravity and making the patient aware of his knee position in space by performing activities first with eyes open then eyes closed
    - ‣ Activities may be progressed by providing manual resistance or having the patient catch a Physioball while balancing on a particular apparatus
- Body mechanics and postural training
  - Isometric resistance to pelvis in standing in all planes while the patient maintains his standing balance
  - Rhythmic stabilization in standing achieved by applying alternating force to shoulders and pelvis in varying planes while the patient maintains his standing balance
  - Perform above first in double leg stance then in single leg stance
- Flexibility exercises
  - Continue as in Phase II
- Gait and locomotion training
  - Ambulation training full weightbearing, correcting any gait deviations
- Strength, power, and endurance training
  - Quad sets
  - Four-way SLRs, perform SLRs in hip flexion, abduction, adduction, and extension

- PREs to hamstrings
- Initiate OKC knee extension 90 to 40 degrees
- CKC activities when sufficient control is available including:
  - ‣ Unilateral leg press
  - ‣ One-quarter squats
  - ‣ Reverse lunge
  - ‣ Step-ups and step-downs
  - ‣ Stairmaster

♦ Phase IV: Advanced rehabilitation/functional training
- Aerobic capacity/endurance conditioning
  - Running activities progressed to full speed
  - Between 4 to 6 weeks if all the goals from the previous phases are met and strength is approximately 60% to 70% of the uninvolved side, may begin a running program
  - After a 3- to 5-minute warm-up consisting of biking or a slow jog, the following functional running progression is performed:
    - ‣ Running on level surface at 50% maximum speed, 1/4 mile
    - ‣ Running on level surface at 75% maximum speed, 1/4 mile
    - ‣ Running on level surface at 100% maximum speed, 1/4 mile
    - ‣ Running on level surface at 100% maximum speed, 1/2 mile
    - ‣ Running on level surface at 100% maximum speed, 3/4 mile
    - ‣ Running on level surface at 100% maximum speed, 1 mile
    - ‣ The distance is progressively increased by 1/4 mile increments until desired distance is achieved, then running on incline surfaces may be incorporated using a similar progression
    - ‣ Once achieved, the speed of the running may be increased as long as there are no adverse effects
- Balance, coordination, and agility training
  - Agility training, such as jump rope, single-leg hop, shuttle run, carioca (alternately crossing legs while side running)
- Body mechanics and postural stabilization
  - Continue with activities in Phase III
  - Resisted walking activities by applying manual resistance or use of an elastic band while having the patient walk correctly
  - Isometric resistance and rhythmic stabilization applied to trunk while patient on an unstable surface such as mini trampoline, rocker board, or BAPS board

- Flexibility exercises
  - Achieve full ROM of knee
  - Lunges and full squats as tolerated
- Gait and locomotion training
  - Running activities (see aerobic capacity/endurance training) progressed to full speed
- Strength, power, and endurance training
  - OKC knee flexion and extension in appropriate ROM (see Rationale for Therapeutic Exercise)
  - All CKC activities in Phase III plus lunges and full squats as tolerated
  - Sport-specific activities, such as shooting baskets, dribbling soccer ball, and football blocking drill
  - Isokinetic evaluation may be performed, typically at faster speeds (180 degrees/sec) with an extension block initially at around 4 to 6 weeks

FUNCTIONAL TRAINING IN SELF-CARE AND HOME MANAGEMENT

- ◆ Self-care and home management
  - Review and simulation of all actions, tasks, and activities for self-care and home management
  - Review of energy conservation techniques
  - Stair climbing

FUNCTIONAL TRAINING IN WORK, COMMUNITY, AND LEISURE INTEGRATION OR REINTEGRATION

- ◆ School and work
  - Simulated ambulation activities similar to those required at school
  - Simulation of activities required for part-time work
- ◆ Leisure
  - Training for return to sport activities when appropriate

MANUAL THERAPY TECHNIQUES

- ◆ Phases I and II
  - Anterior-posterior and medial-lateral glides (Grades III and IV) of the tibia to increase extension and flexion of the tibiofemoral joint
  - Patella mobilization using superior and medial glides (Grades III and IV) to prevent retraction of patella tendon
  - PROM of tibiofemoral joint to increase extension and flexion

ELECTROTHERAPEUTIC MODALITIES

- ◆ Phases I and II

- HVPC to right knee to decrease pain, joint swelling, and inflammation
  - Acute pain protocol incorporated using the following parameters
    - ▸ Frequency: 100 pps
    - ▸ Amplitude: Sensory stimulation
    - ▸ Polarity: Negative
    - ▸ Pulse duration: Fixed in HVPC
    - ▸ Pad placement: Over injury site[97]
- Variable muscle stimulation (VMS) for muscle reeducation
  - Parameters are as follows
    - ▸ Amplitude: Motor level stimulation
    - ▸ Frequency: 35 pps
    - ▸ Polarity: NA
    - ▸ Pulse duration: 300 usec
    - ▸ Pad placement: Vastus medialis oblique/vastus lateralis motor points[97]

PHYSICAL AGENTS AND MECHANICAL MODALITIES

- ◆ Physical agents
  - Phases I, II, and III as necessary
    - Cryotherapy to decrease pain, joint swelling, and inflammation post-treatment[97]
    - Compression and/or combination cold/compression unit to decrease edema[97]
- ◆ Mechanical modality
  - Phase II
    - CPM is set at 5-0-40 degrees for the first 24 hours and is left on at all times except to perform exercises and use the restroom
    - It is then used 8 hours a day over the next 2 weeks progressively increasing the ROM approximately 5 degrees per day until 110 degrees flexion is achieved (CPM protocol is physician dependent)

ANTICIPATED GOALS AND EXPECTED OUTCOMES

- ◆ Impact on pathology/pathophysiology
  - No effusion in right knee in 2 to 4 weeks.
  - Pain is decreased to 1 to 2/10 with ambulation in 2 to 3 weeks and 0/10 with ambulation x 4 to 6 weeks.
- ◆ Impact on impairments
  - Full AROM to allow for stairclimbing and normal gait without assistive device in 6 weeks.
  - Increase strength in right quadriceps to allow for active SLR without lag in 7 to 10 days.
  - Normal quadriceps and hamstring strength via

MMT in 3 to 4 months and 75% to 80% of the uninvolved side via isokinetic testing in 6 to 9 months.

- Patient will exhibit improved coordination and kinesthetic awareness of the RLE, allowing him to ambulate on uneven terrain for distances up to ½ mile in 2 to 3 months.

♦ Impact on functional limitations

- Patient will achieve the ability to ambulate for a period of up to 60 minutes with normal gait and to climb up and down eight flights of stairs without an assistive device in 4 to 6 months.
- Patient will achieve the ability to perform all ADL independently as well as all physical actions, tasks, and activities required for reintegration into school, community, and leisure/sports activities in 6 to 9 months.

♦ Risk reduction/prevention

- Patient will be able to verbalize signs and symptoms of infection when asked by attending providers.

♦ Impact on health, wellness, and fitness

- Patient will develop an understanding of the healing times for his condition, relative to returning to sports, and the risks of reinjury.

♦ Impact on societal resources

- The rehabilitation process will focus on maximizing both clinical and functional outcomes, while ensuring that the number of visits utilized is managed in both a clinically effective and cost-effective manner.
- Documentation occurs throughout the patient management and follows APTA's *Guidelines for Physical Therapy Documentation.*[1]
- Patient will develop a knowledge, awareness, and understanding of the diagnosis, prognosis, interventions, and anticipated goals and expected outcomes.

REEXAMINATION

Reexamination is performed throughout the episode of care, particularly as the setting of care changes and as the protection phases change.

DISCHARGE

Al is discharged from physical therapy after a total of 21 physical therapy sessions and attainment of his goals and expectations. These sessions have covered his entire episode of care, beginning in the acute care hospital, to his transfer home with home care, and after 4 weeks of outpatient physical therapy. He is discharged because he has achieved his goals and expected outcomes.

ACKNOWLEDGMENTS

The authors of the Bony Surgery portion of this chapter would like to thank the following individuals who have contributed to the completion of this project including: Jessica Palmer, SPT; the library staff at the Franklin Pierce College, Rindge, New Hampshire; the Physical Therapy Staff at Brooke Army Medical Center, Ft. Sam Houston, Texas; and Dr. Liem Mansfield, Department of Radiology, Brooke Army Medical Center, Ft. Sam Houston, Texas.

REFERENCES

1. American Physical Therapy Association. Guide to physical therapist practice. 2nd ed. *Phys Ther*. 2001;81:9-744.
2. Stetson WB, Friedman MJ, Fulkerson JP, Cheng M, Buck D. Fracture of the proximal tibia with immediate weightbearing after a Fulkerson osteotomy. *Am J Sports Med*. 1997;25:570-573.
3. Marti RK, Verhagen RAW, Kerkhoffs GMMJ, Moojen TM. Proximal tibial varus osteotomy. *J Bone Joint Surg*. 2001;83A:164-170.
4. McCarthy JJ, MacEwen GD. Management of leg length inequality. *J South Orthop Assoc*. 2001;10:73-85.
5. Delforge G. Therapeutic implications: fracture healing. In: Delforge G, ed. *Musculoskeletal Trauma: Implications for Sports Injury*. Champaign, Ill: Human Kinetics; 2002:133-154.
6. Bottomley JM. *Quick Reference Dictionary for Physical Therapy*. 2nd ed. Thorofare, NJ: SLACK Incorporated; 2003.
7. Gray FRSH. *Gray's Anatomy*. New York, NY: Barnes & Noble Books; 1995.
8. Moore KL, Dalley AF. *Clinically Oriented Anatomy*. 4th ed. Philadelphia, Pa: Lippincott Williams & Wilkins; 1999.
9. Smith PE. *Bailey's Text-Book of Histology*. 9th ed. Baltimore, Md: William Wood & Co; 1936.
10. McArdle WD, Katch FI, Katch VL. *Exercise Physiology: Energy, Nutrition, and Human Performance*. 5th ed. Philadelphia, Pa: Lippincott Williams & Wilkins; 2001.
11. Baechle TR, Earle RW. *Essentials of Strength Training and Conditioning*. 2nd ed. Champaign, Ill: Human Kinetics; 2000.
12. Fukunaga T, Kawakami Y, Kuno S, Funato K, Fukashiro S. Muscle architecture and function in humans. *J Biomechanics*. 1997;30(5):457-463.
13. Kannus P. Structure of the tendon connective tissue. *Scandinavian Journal of Medicine & Science in Sports*. 2000;10:312-320.
14. Lundon K. *Orthopedic Rehabilitation Science: Principles for Clinical Management of Nonmineralized Connective Tissue*. Boston, Mass: Butterworth-Heinemann; 2003.
15. Jozsa L, Kannus P. *Human Tendons: Anatomy, Physiology, and Pathology*. Champaign, Ill: Human Kinetics; 1997.
16. Woo S, Buckwalter A, eds. *Injury and Repair of the Musculoskeletal Soft Tissues*. Park Ridge, Ill: American Academy of Orthopaedic Surgeons; 1988.
17. Terry GC, Chopp TM. Functional anatomy of the shoulder. *Journal of Athletic Training*. 2000;35(3):248-255.

18. Tovin BJ, Greenfield BH. *Evaluation and Treatment of the Shoulder: An Integration of the Guide to Physical Therapist Practice.* Philadelphia, Pa: FA Davis Co; 2001.

19. Lo IKY, Burkhart SS. Current concepts in arthoscopic rotator cuff repair. *Am J Sports Med.* 2003;31(2):308-324.

20. Blasier RB, Guldberg RE, Rothman ED. Anterior shoulder stability: contributions of rotator cuff forces and the capsular ligaments in a cadaver model. *J Shoulder Elbow Surg.* 1992;140-150.

21. Schenkman M, Rugo de Cartaya V. Kinesiology of the shoulder complex. *J Orthop Sports Phys Ther.* 1987;8(9):439-449.

22. Culham E, Peat M. Functional anatomy of the shoulder complex. *J Orthop Sports Phys Ther.* 1993;18(1):342-350.

23. Ellenbecker TS. *Knee Ligament Rehabilitation.* 1st ed. Philadelphia, Pa: Churchill Livingstone; 2000.

24. Slade JF, Chou KH. Bony tissue repair. *J Hand Ther.* 1998;April-June:118-124.

25. Stern PJ. Fractures of the metacarpals and phalanges. In: Green DP, ed. *Operative Hand Surgery.* 3rd ed. New York, NY: Churchill-Livingstone; 1993:695-758.

26. Roberts JM. Operative treatment of fractures about the knee. *Orthop Clin North Am.* 1990;21:365-379.

27. Furlow B. Bone fracture fixation. *Radiol Technol.* 2000;71:543-561.

28. Marsh D, Einhorn TA, Lane JM. Concepts of fracture union, delayed union, and nonunion. *Clin Orthop.* 1998;355(Suppl): S22-S30.

29. Rosen H. Fracture nonunion in the elderly: principles of management. *Journal of Musculoskeletal Medicine.* 1999;16:364-376.

30. Roman HA, Brighton CT, Esterhai JL, Einhorn TA, Lane JM. Pathophysiology of delayed healing. *Clin Orthop.* 1998;355(Suppl):S31-S40.

31. Sarmiento A, Waddell J, Latta LL. Diaphyseal humeral fractures: treatment options. *J Bone Joint Surg.* 2001;83A:1566-1579.

32. Hoppenfeld S, Murthy VL. *Treatment and Rehabilitation of Fractures.* Philadelphia, Pa: Lipincott Williams & Wilkins; 2000.

33. Perry CR, Elstrom JA. *Handbook of Fractures.* 2nd ed. New York, NY: McGraw-Hill Inc; 2000.

34. Allen GJ. Bone grafting in fracture management. *Surgical Technology.* 1994;26(8):8-13.

35. Einhorn TA. The cell and molecular biology of fracture healing. *Clin Orthop.* 1998;355(Suppl):S7-S21.

36. Engles M. Tissue response. In: Donatelli RA, Wooden MJ, eds. *Orthopaedic Physical Therapy.* 3rd ed. New York, NY: Churchill Livingstone; 2001:1-24.

37. Slatis Par, Paavolainen P, Karaharju E, Holmstrom T. Structural and biomechanical changes in bone after rigid fixation. *Can J Surg.* 1980;23:247-249.

38. Stephan PM. Evolution of the internal fixation of long bone fractures: the scientific basis of biological internal fixation: choosing a new balance between stability and biology. *J Bone Joint Surg (Br).* 2002;84B:1093-1110.

39. Schenck RC. *Athletic Training and Sports Medicine.* 3rd ed. Rosemont, Ill: American Academy of Orthopaedic Surgeons; 1999.

40. Thompson WO, Debski RE, Boardman ND, Taskiran, et al. A biomechanical analysis of rotator cuff deficiency in a cadav-

eric model. *Am J Sports Med.* 1996;24(3):286-289.

41. Williams GR, Kelley M. Management of rotator cuff and impingement injuries in the athlete. *Journal of Athletic Training.* 2000;35(3):300-315.

42. Fukuda H. Review article: the management of partial-thickness tears of the rotator cuff. *J Bone Joint Surg.* 2003;85(1):3-12.

43. Jobe CM, Coen MJ, Screnar P. Evaluation of impingement syndromes in the overhead-throwing athlete. *Journal of Athletic Training.* 2000;35(3):293-299.

44. Houglum PA. *Therapeutic Exercise for Athletic Injuries.* Champaign, Ill: Human Kinetics; 2001.

45. Brandsson S, et al. A prospective four-to seven-year follow-up after arthroscopic anterior cruciate ligament reconstruction. *Scand J Med Sci Sports.* 2001;11:23-27.

46. Grant JA, Mohtadi NG. ACL reconstruction with autografts weighing performance considerations and postoperative care. *The Physician and Sports Medicine.* 2003;31(4):27-34.

47. Fu FH, Bennett CH, Latterman C, Benjamin CM. Current trends in anterior cruciate ligament reconstruction: part 1: biology and biomechanics of reconstruction. *Am J Sports Med.* 1999;27(6):821-832.

48. Starch DW, et al. Multistranded hamstring tendon graft fixation with a central four-quadrant or a standard tibial interference screw for anterior cruciate ligament reconstruction. *Am J Sports Med.* 2003;31(3):338-345.

49. Canale ST, Cambell WC. *Campbell's Operative Orthopaedics.* 10th ed. St. Louis. Mo: Elsevier; 2002.

50. Anderson AF, Synder RB, Lipscomb AB Jr. Anterior cruciate ligament reconstruction: a prospective study of three surgical methods. *Am J Sports Med.* 2001;29(3):272-279.

51. Faherer H, Rentsch HU, Gerber NJ, Beyellar C, Hess CW, Grunig B. Knee effusion and reflex inhibition of the quadriceps. *J Bone Joint Surg.* 1988;70(4):635-638.

52. Eriksson K, Anderberg P, Hamgreg P, Olerud P, Wredmark T. There are differences in early morbidity after ACL reconstruction when comparing patellar tendon and semitendinosus tendon graft. *Scand J Med Sci Sports.* 2001;11:170-177.

53. McKinnis LN. *Fundamentals of Orthopedic Radiology.* Philadelphia, Pa: FA Davis Co; 1997.

54. Mettler FA. *Essentials of Radiology.* Philadelphia, Pa: WB Saunders Co; 1996.

55. Ciccone CD. *Pharmacology in Rehabilitation.* 2nd ed. Philadelphia, Pa: FA Davis Co; 1996.

56. Kizior RJ, Hodgson BB. *Saunders Drug Handbook for Health Professions.* 2nd ed. Philadelphia, Pa: WB Saunders Co; 2002.

57. Karch AM. *Lippincott's Nursing Drug Guide.* Philadelphia, Pa: Lippincott Williams & Wilkins; 2004.

58. Crotty M, Whitehead CH, Gray S, Finucane PM. Early rehabilitation after hip fracture achieves functional improvements: a randomized controlled trial. *Clin Rehabil.* 2002;16:406-413.

59. Huusko TM, Karappi P, Avikanien V, Kautiainen H, Sulkuva R. Randomised, clinically controlled trial of intensive geriatric rehabilitation in patient with hip fracture: subgroup analysis of patients with dementia. *BMJ.* 2000;321:1107-1111.

60. Jones GR, Miller T, Petrella RJ. Evaluation of rehabilitation outcomes in older patients with hip fractures. *Am J Phys Med Rehabil.* 2002;7:489-497.

61. Ruchlin HS, Elkin EB, Allegrante JP. The economic impact

of a multifactorial intervention to improve postoperative rehabilitation of hip fractures. *Arthritis Care and Research.* 2001;45:446-452.

62. Tinetti ME, Baker DL, Gottschalk M, et al. Systematic home-based physical and functional therapy for older persons after hip fracture. *Arch Phys Med Rehabil.* 1997;78:1237-1247.

63. Guccione AA, Fagerson TL, Anderson JJ. Regaining functional independence in the acute care setting following hip fracture. *Phys Ther.* 1996;76:818-826.

64. Mitchell SL, Stott DJ. Randomized controlled trial of quadriceps training after proximal femoral fracture. *Clin Rehabil.* 2001;15:282-290.

65. Lamb SE, Oldham JA, Morse RE, Evans JG. Neuromuscular stimulation of the quadriceps muscle after hip fractures: a randomized controlled trial. *Arch Phys Med Rehabil.* 2002;83:1087-1092.

66. Sherrington C, Stephen LR, Herbert RD. A randomized trial of weight-bearing versus non-weight-bearing exercise for improving physical ability in inpatients after hip fracture. *Aust J Physiother.* 2003;49:15-22.

67. Hauer K, Specht N, Schuler M, Bartsch P, Oster P. Intensive physical training in geriatric patients after severe falls and hip surgery. *Age Ageing.* 2002;31:49-57.

68. Deuesterhaus Minor MA, Deuesterhaus Minor S. *Patient Care Skills.* Norwalk, Conn: Appleton and Lange; 1995:340-399.

69. Eleveru RA, Rothstein JM, Lamb RL. Goniometric reliability in a clinical setting: subtalar and ankle joint measurements. *Phys Ther.* 1988;68:672-677.

70. Dogra AS, Rangan A. Early mobilisation versus immobilization of surgically treated ankle fractures. Prospective randomized control trial. *Injury.* 1999;30:417-419.

71. Duchateau J. Bed rest induces neural and contractile adaptations in triceps surae. *Med Sci Sports Exerc.* 1995;27:1581-1589.

72. Geboers JFM, van Tuijl, Seelen HAM, Drost MR. Effect of immobilization on ankle dorsiflexion strength. *Scand J Rehabil Med.* 2000;32:66-71.

73. Shaffer MA, Okereke E, Esterhai J, et al. Effects of immobilization on plantar-flexion torque, fatigue, resistance, and functional ability following an ankle fracture. *Phys Ther.* 2000;80:769-780.

74. Tropp H, Norlin R. Ankle performance after ankle fracture: a randomized study of early mobilization. *Foot Ankle Int.* 1995;16:7-83.

75. Vandenborne K, Elliott MA, Walter GA, et al. Longitudinal study of skeletal muscle adaptations during immobilization and rehabilitation. *Muscle Nerve.* 1998;21:1006-1012.

76. Rozzi SL, Lephart SM, Sterner R, Kuligowski L. Balance training for persons with functionally unstable ankles. *J Orthop and Sports Phys Ther.* 1999;29:478-486.

77. Wilson FM. Manual therapy versus traditional exercises in mobilization of the ankle post-ankle fracture. *New Zealand Journal of Physiotherapy.* 1991;12:11-16.

78. Olson VL. *Connective Tissue Response to Injury, Immobilization, and Mobilization.* Orthopaedic Section, American Physical Therapy Association, La Crosse, Wisc, 2001.

79. Threlkeld JA. The effects of manual therapy on connective tissue. *Phys Ther.* 1992;72:893-902.

80. Uhl RL, Hartshorn T. Mobilization after fractures of the hand. *Operative Techniques in Orthopaedics.* 1997;7:145-151.

81. Scherer S, Cassady SL. Rating of perceived exertion: development and clinical applications for physical therapy exercise testing and prescription. *Cardiopulmonary Physical Therapy Journal.* 1999;10:143-147.

82. Howley ET, Franks BD. *Health Fitness Instructor's Handbook.* 3rd ed. Champaign, Ill: Human Kinetics; 1997.

83. Cook KF, et al. Reliability by surgical status of self-reported outcomes in patients who have shoulder pathologies. *J Orthop Sports Phys Ther.* 2002;32(7):336-346.

84. DePalma MJ, Johnson EW. Detecting and treating shoulder impingement sydrome: the role of scapulothoracic. *The Physician and Sports Medicine.* 2003;31(7):25.

85. Solem-Bertoft E, Thuomas K, Westerberg C. The influence of scapular retraction and protraction on the width of the subacromial space. *Clinical Orthop.* 1993;Nov(296):99-103.

86. Ludewig PM, Cook TM, Nawoczenski DA. Three-dimensional scapular orientation and muscle activity at selected positions of humeral elevation. *J Orthop Sports Phys Ther.* 1996;24(2):57-65.

87. Ludewig PM, Cook TM. Alterations in shoulder kinematics and associated muscle activity in people with symptoms of shoulder impingement. *Physical Therapy.* 2000;80(3):276-289.

88. Voight ML, Thomson BC. The role of the scapula in the rehabilitation of shoulder injuries. *Journal of Athletic Training.* 2000;35(3):364-372.

89. Chen S, Simonian PT, Wickiewicz TL, Otis JC, Warren RF. Radiograftic evaluation of glenohumeral kinematics: a muscle fatigue model. *J Shoulder Elbow Surg.* 1999;8(1):49-52.

90. Kibler WB. The role of the scapula in athletic shoulder function. *Am J Sports Med.* 1998;26(2):325-337.

91. Lephart SM, Henry TJ. The physiological basis for open and closed kinetic chain rehabilitation for the upper extremity. *Journal of Sport Rehabilitation.* 1996;5:71-87.

92. Moseley JB Jr, Jobe FW, Pink M, et al. EMG analysis of the scapular muscles during a shoulder rehabilitation program. *Am J Sports Med.* 1992;20(2):128-134.

93. Takeda Y, Kashiwaguchi S, Endo K, Matsuura T, Sasa T. The most effective exercise for strengthening the supraspinatus muscle: evaluation by magnetic resonance imaging. *Am J Sports Med.* 2002;30(3):374-382.

94. Ballantyne BT, O'Hare SJ, Paschall JL, et al. Electromyograftic activity of selected shoulder muscles in commonly used therapeutic exercises. *Phys Ther.* 1993;73(10):668-682.

95. Bang MD, Deyle GD. Comparison of supervised exercise with and without manual physical therapy for patients with shoulder impingement syndrome. *J Orthop Sports Phys Ther.* 2000;30(3):126-137.

96. Kisner C, Colby L. *Therapeutic Exercise: Foundations and Techniques.* 4th ed. Philadelphia, Pa: FA Davis Co; 2002.

97. Belanger A. *Evidenced-Based Guide to Therapeutic Physical Agents.* 1st ed. Baltimore, Md: Lippinocott Williams & Wilkins; 2002.

98. Snyder-Mackler L, Delitto A, Stralka SW. Strength of the quadriceps femoris muscle and functional recovery after reconstruction of the anterior cruciate ligament. *J Bone Joint Surg.* 1995;77(8):1166-1173.

99. Paulos L, Noyes FR, Grood E, Butler DL. Knee rehabilitation after anterior cruciate ligament reconstruction and repair. *Am J Sports Med.* 1981;9(3):140-149.

100. Arms SW, Pope MH, Johnson RJ, et al. The biomechanics of anterior cruciate rehabilitation and reconstruction. *Am J Sports Med.* 1984;12(1):8-18.

101. Beynnon BD. Anatomy and biomechanics of the knee. In: Garrett WE, Speer KP, Kirkendall DT, eds. *Principles & Practice of Orthopaedic Sports Medicine.* 1st ed. Philadelpha, Pa: Lippincott Williams & Wilkins; 2000:623-643.

102. Henning CE, Lynch MA, Glick JR. An in vivo strain gauge study: study of elongation of the anterior cruciate ligament. *Am J Sports Med.* 1985;13(1):22-26.

103. Yack JH, Collins CE, Whieldon TJ. Comparison of closed and open kinetic chain exercise in the anterior cruciate ligament-deficient knee. *Am J Sports Med.* 1993;21(1):49-54.

104. Palmitier RA, An K, Scoot SG, Chao E. Kinetic chain exercise in knee rehabilitation. *Sports Med.* 1991;11(6):402-413.

105. Voight M, Bell S, Rhoades D. Instrumented testing of anterior tibial translation in open vs closed chain activity. *Phys Ther.* 1991;71(Suppl):S98.

106. Fleming BC, Ohlen G, Renstrom PA, et al. The effects of compressive load and knee joint torque on peak anterior cruciate ligament strains. *Am J Sports Med.* 2003;31(5):701-711.

CHAPTER TEN

Impaired Motor Function, Muscle Performance, Range of Motion, Gait, Locomotion, and Balance Associated With Amputation (Pattern J)

Bella J. May, PT, EdD, FAPTA
with contributions from Tom Holland, PT, PhD

ANATOMY

Anatomically, the structures that are missing affect patient function and the physical therapy approach to management. In both the UEs and LEs and for all amputation levels, there is loss of sensation and sensory input from the part that has been amputated. This impacts LE function where sensory input assists with balance and adjustment to different terrains and surfaces. Amputation has a major impact on UE activity where the sense of touch is critical to function.

The most commonly seen levels of amputation of the LEs may range from the toe to the hip. The majority of LE amputations are at the transtibial or transfemoral levels. The levels include:

- Toe amputation is the removal of a single toe through the phalanx or through the base of the proximal phalanx.
- Complete ray amputation is the removal of a toe plus the MT.
- Transmetatarsal amputation is the removal of all the toes and distal portion of the MTs. A shoe with a filler and rocker bottom is indicated for individuals with this level of amputation.
- Ankle disarticulation or Syme's amputation is a disarticulation through the ankle maintaining the heel flap to allow weightbearing.

- Transtibial or below the knee amputation includes all levels of amputations from the knee to the ankle.
- Knee disarticulation occurs through the knee joint. In some instances the patella is attached to the bottom of the femur. This level provides a long lever arm for good prosthetic control. This level is usually used with traumatic amputations or malignancies.
- Transfemoral or above the knee amputation includes all levels of amputations from the hip to the knee.
- Hip disarticulation is the resection of the entire femur.
- Hemipelvectomy occurs at the pelvis with resection of part of the pelvis and the entire LE.

Levels of amputation of the UE may range from the fingers to the shoulder. These levels include:

- Finger (digit) amputation is the removal of any of the phalangeal joints.
- Wrist disarticulation is an amputation that occurs at the level of the wrist.
- Transradial/ulnar or below elbow amputation is any amputation that occurs between the elbow and the wrist.
- Elbow disarticulation is an amputation that occurs at the level of the elbow.
- Transhumeral or above elbow amputation is any amputation that occurs between the shoulder and the elbow.
- Total shoulder complex or four quarter amputation is a

type of amputation that requires removal of the shoulder girdle including the scapula and the clavicle and the entire UE. Functional status is poor.

PHYSIOLOGY

Since circulatory compromise is often implicated as a cause of amputation, the physiology of circulation is important in this pattern. This has been detailed in Integumentary Pattern C: Impaired Integumentary Integrity Associated With Partial-Thickness Skin Involvement and Scar Formation and Cardiovascular/Pulmonary Pattern D: Impaired Aerobic Capacity/Endurance Associated With Cardiovascular Pump Dysfunction or Failure. The physiology of bone is detailed in Pattern A: Primary Prevention/Risk Reduction for Skeletal Demineralization and Pattern G: Impaired Joint Mobility, Muscle Performance, and Range of Motion Associated With Fracture since pathological fractures due to cancer of the bone may also lead to amputation.

PATHOPHYSIOLOGY

The three major causes of amputations in the LE are peripheral arterial occlusive disease (PAOD), trauma, and cancer. Additionally, children may be born without part or all of a limb or limbs or with deformities that require amputation. In the UE, trauma is the leading cause of amputation followed by cancer.[1,2]

In addition to the major causes of amputations, phantom pain and phantom sensation are pathophysiological factors with which individuals who have undergone an amputation may experience.

PERIPHERAL OCCLUSIVE DISEASE

The leading cause of amputation in the LE is vascular disease, usually PAOD. There are a number of terms used to refer to variations in PAOD. Some may be used interchangeably in the literature, such as arteriosclerosis and atherosclerosis (ASO). Either term refers to a thickening, hardening, and narrowing of the arterial walls. Generally, fibrous plaques narrow the vessels, eventually leading to ischemia of the tissue distally. The distal segment of the superficial femoral artery is a common site of involvement. Other frequently involved sites include the common femoral artery, the midportion of the popliteal artery, and the origins of the tibial arteries. In some situations an embolus in the popliteal artery may lead to amputation by blocking blood flow to the lower limb leading to tissue necrosis. Tissue necrosis may often be prevented by early diagnosis and treatment. There are other forms of PAOD, but the basic pathophysiology is a slow gradual occlusion of one or more major arteries leading to distal tissue ischemia. Generally, large arteries are involved in individuals without diabetes, while medium and small arteries are more generally involved in individuals with diabetes.[2]

PAOD occurs in about 5% of men over the age of 50 and women over the age of 60. It is estimated that approximately 25% of individuals with ASO eventually have reconstructive surgery, and 5% of these individual have one or more LE amputations.[3] The incidence of PAOD and amputations increases when ASO is associated with diabetes. Individuals with diabetes account for more than 50% of the amputations performed in the United States today.[4]

Diabetes is a systemic metabolic disease related to insulin deficiency and impaired glucose tolerance. The American Diabetes Association[5] estimates that approximately 6.2% of the population have diabetes including: 13% of black Americans, 10% of Latino Americans, and 15% of Native Americans. There are two major types of diabetes, but only Type 2 is related to amputations. PAOD associated with diabetes generally affects both microvascular and macrovascular tissues. The broad spectrum of vascular tissue affected by diabetes may lead to other complications, such as nephropathy and end stage renal disease, retinopathy with deteriorating vision and possible blindness, loss of sensation distally often leading to foot ulcers that fail to heal secondary to lack of adequate vascularization, and neuropathy with loss of function particularly in the intrinsic muscles of the hands and feet.

Amputation secondary to vascular disease is usually performed after attempts at revascularization surgically. There are numerous revascularization procedures that are employed initially with many factors affecting the rate of success. Generally, revascularization procedures are more successful in individuals without diabetes than with diabetes with a reported 20.7 amputations per 100,000 revascularization procedures as found in a longitudinal study.[6] It is also estimated by the National Commission on Diabetes[5] that 5% to 15% of all individuals with diabetes will require one or more amputations in their lifetime. As people are living longer with vascular disease, the rate of amputation has increased slightly over time. In a study in Minnesota, the authors reported that, although amputation rates had declined in the past 20 years, the total number of amputations had increased. They predicted that the number of amputations would double by the year 2030.[7] Recent studies also indicated that the rate of amputation for vascular disease among black Americans is considerably higher than that for other races and seems to be increasing.[8]

TRAUMA

From a pathophysiological perspective, a traumatic amputation may result in major loss of bone, muscle, vascular supply, and nerve tissue. It may also result in infection secondary to the trauma, blood loss leading to loss of tissue viability below the site of injury, or actual limb ablation.

There are no national statistics on the rate of amputation for trauma. Outside of war-related limb loss in the LE, vehicular accidents are the major cause, followed by gunshot wounds, and other types of explosions. Farm and industrial accidents are the leading cause of amputation in the UE.[1]

CANCER

The rate of amputation for soft tissue and bone malignancies is decreasing as improved detection and management procedures are developed. When the tumor is well encapsulated, it may be excised; limb salvage procedures are used to replace lost tissue and long-term survival is not statistically different between amputation and tumor excision.

PHANTOM PAIN AND PHANTOM SENSATION

It is estimated that approximately 70% of patients experience phantom limb pain after amputation, and 50% still experience phantom pain 5 years after surgery.[9] Patients describe burning, stabbing, twisting, cramping, or throbbing pains in the missing part. There is thought to be a relationship between pre-amputation pain and phantom pain.[9] Phantom pain is generally not disabling and does not, in and of itself, counter the successful use of a prosthesis. However, phantom pain may become chronic and may be disabling, interfering with prosthetic use and reintegration into a normal life.

Phantom sensation, as differentiated from phantom pain, is described as the sensation of the absent limb. It may be the whole limb but more frequently is a part of the limb.

PATHOKINESIOLOGY

UNILATERAL LOWER EXTREMITY AMPUTATIONS

Unique considerations exist for individuals with amputations as they relate to kinesiology. Amputation of a toe or a complete ray will affect balance and the pressures generated in the foot from weightbearing. Depending on which digit is involved, the change in pressure could lead to callous formation or ulceration. In some instances, an individually molded shoe insert is helpful for individuals who have had one or more toes amputated.

Partial foot or transmetatarsal amputation leads to the loss of terminal stance support and push off. Prosthetic replacement is not required for bipedal function, but a shoe insert greatly enhances terminal stance and may reduce the possibility of secondary complications.

Ankle disarticulation or Syme's amputation is a very functional level of amputation. An individual with a Syme's amputation is capable of independent ambulation without a prosthetic device, although a significant leg length discrepancy exists. Function is improved with a prosthesis that has an ankle foot assembly that simulates normal ankle foot movements observed during ambulation.

Patients with unilateral transtibial amputations regardless of age are quite likely to become functional prosthetic users. These individuals should be community ambulators provided the intact LE has sufficient strength, mobility, and tolerance for weightbearing.

The presence or absence of the knee joint has a major impact on function. The residual limb in a knee disarticulation with its intact femoral condyles requires some adaptation of the prosthetic socket, but with the development of multiaxis knee mechanisms, individuals with a knee disarticulation can become quite functional. The longer lever arm makes ambulation easier and less energy demanding.

Older adults with unilateral transfemoral amputations have more difficulty becoming prosthetically independent.[10,11]

BILATERAL LOWER EXTREMITY AMPUTATIONS

Individuals who lose both lower limbs above the partial foot level will not be able to ambulate without prosthetic replacement. Depending on the presence of co-morbidities, individuals with bilateral transtibial (below the knee) amputations will generally be able to ambulate with prostheses. The higher the levels of amputation the greater the physiological demands of prosthetic ambulation. Whether the individual with one transtibial and one transfemoral amputation or with two transfemoral amputations will be able to functionally use prostheses depends on a great many factors including strength, balance, coordination, motivation, cardiopulmonary status, and the presence of other pathological problems. Most patients with bilateral transfemoral amputations do not become functional prosthetic users.[10,11]

New computerized prosthetic components have improved the functional capabilities of individuals with bilateral transfemoral amputations while reducing the energy demands for ambulation.

Patients who have undergone a hemipelvectomy require a special prosthesis that is stable throughout the stance phase. The individual sits in a plastic socket that encircles the pelvis and may stabilize on the lower ribs. The gait pattern, initiated by pelvic tilting and momentum, is slow with little variation in speed or stride length. Many individuals with this level of amputation may choose to use a wheelchair.

UNILATERAL UPPER EXTREMITY AMPUTATIONS

All UE amputations reduce manual dexterity and may reduce or eliminate bimanual function. Although prosthetic replacements have become quite sophisticated, many individuals prefer to function primarily with one hand. These individuals perform many bimanual functions using other body parts for stabilization or using adapted devices for one hand.

Most individuals who have lost a digit or partial hand do not use any prosthetic replacement.

Individuals with a wrist disarticulation amputation may use a prosthesis with a terminal device to replace the lost hand or may function without a prosthesis as they use the residual limb for stabilization purposes.

Many individuals with amputations at the transradial/ulnar (below the elbow) level use the remaining hand as the dominant hand and may prefer to use the residual limb as an assistive entity mainly for stabilization.

Individuals who have had an elbow disarticulation benefit from this type of amputation since the length of the residual limb is preserved and the remaining humeral condyles allow for a better prosthetic fit.

Individuals with a transhumeral amputation may use a prosthesis that has both a terminal device and mechanical elbow joint.

Individuals who have undergone a total shoulder complex or four quarter amputation usually have a poor prognosis functionally.

BILATERAL UPPER EXTREMITY AMPUTATIONS

Individuals who lose two UEs at any level are dependent on prostheses to perform ADL. Children who are born with congenital loss of the UEs or part thereof are fitted in relation to normal development and usually integrate the prostheses into daily life.

PHARMACOLOGY

There are no specific medications used in the management of patients with amputations per se. However, people with amputations may have a variety of conditions requiring the use of medications. Individuals with vascular disease, diabetes, cardiovascular conditions, among others, may use medications. These pharmacological agents are detailed in Integumentary Pattern C: Impaired Integumentary Integrity Associated With Partial-Thickness Skin Involvement and Scar Formation and Cardiovascular/Pulmonary Pattern D: Impaired Aerobic Capacity/Endurance Associated With Cardiovascular Pump Dysfunction or Failure.

Generally control of pain associated with phantom sensation is usually achieved with OTC medications. Over the years a great variety of pharmacological agents have been tried in the treatment of chronic, disabling phantom pain including pre-amputation analgesic drips and narcotic medications. While some treatments have been successful with some individuals, no consistent successful treatment for chronic phantom pain exists.

PROSTHETIC DEVICES

The field of prosthetics is quite complex today with numerous options for all components depending on the level of amputation, level of activity, finances, leisure activities, and age. There are some components that are not made for very small children.

A prosthetic device must meet three major criteria: 1) it must be comfortable or the person will not wear it, 2) it must be functional and thus enable the wearer to meet all the demands of daily life, and 3) it must be cosmetically pleasing. The importance of cosmesis varies from individual to individual. Many people with amputations value function over cosmesis and the wearing of a prosthesis without cosmetic cover occurs most frequently among young athletic individuals. Components for toddlers and young children must be concerned with both function and safety.

PROSTHETIC COMPONENTS—LOWER EXTREMITY

Transtibial Prosthesis

The transtibial prosthesis includes a foot, a pylon or connecting rod, a socket, and a means of suspending the prosthesis. The transtibial socket is designed for patellar tendon weightbearing with stabilization forces on the flares of the tibia and the soft tissue around the residual limb. Increasingly, socket designs are fabricated for total surface bearing with weightbearing throughout the residual limb avoiding bony prominences, such as the crest of the tibia or sensitive areas, such as the peroneal nerve as it wraps around the head of the fibula. Most transtibial sockets are made of lightweight hard plastic with a gel liner acting as an interface between the residual limb and socket.

The transtibial socket may be suspended by means of a supracondylar cuff, suction, a shuttle lock system, or a neoprene sleeve that pulls up over the distal part of the thigh. There are variations on all these methods.

The foot is connected to the end of the socket by a light aluminum pipe called a pylon. In some cases a telescoping shock absorbing pylon is used, particularly for individuals who will participate in sports or other high-energy activities. The purpose is to protect the residual limb from the stress of running, jumping, and other such activities.

Most prosthetic feet provide some degree of energy response. Some provide only minimal energy return (>20%), while others are constructed for very high energy return (<60%).[12] Feet may also be either single axis (primarily substitute for anterior/posterior movements) or multiaxis (substitute for medial/lateral and anterior/posterior movements). Foot movements, naturally, are reactive not proactive. Technology and advanced materials and the addition of hydraulics increasingly provide a smoother transition through the weightbearing cycle.

Transfemoral Prosthesis

The transfemoral prosthesis includes all the above components and in addition, a knee mechanism. There are currently three different designs for the transfemoral prosthetic socket. The quadrilateral socket is the traditional socket design that is used primarily for individuals who have worn this design for many years and do not want to change to newer design technologies. The patient literally "sits" on top of the posterior wall of the socket with major weightbearing through the ischial tuberosity. The quadrilateral socket has a larger medial/lateral dimension than anterior/posterior.

The ischial containment (IC) socket reflects a different design. It is closer to the transtibial socket with some weightbearing on the ischial tuberosity that is contained within the socket and some on the soft tissue throughout the socket. It has a narrow medial/lateral dimension to provide improved stability on stance by exerting controlling pressure against the femur.

The third design is a variation on the IC design currently called the Hanger Comfort Flex Socket. Many IC sockets are made of flexible plastic materials encased in a rigid frame often constructed of carbon graphite. Most individuals with new amputations are fitted with the IC socket design. The Hanger Comfort Flex Socket is best suited for more active individuals.

As with the transtibial prosthesis, the transfemoral system may be suspended by suction, a webbing strap around the pelvis called a Silesian band or a neoprene elastic band that fits around the hips.

There are a large number of prosthetic knee mechanisms on the market. Knees may be single or multiaxis; may function primarily through a friction mechanism, alignment, and patient control; may incorporate a hydraulic or pneumatic mechanism; or may be computer driven. Knee mechanisms may provide swing phase control that will vary the swing speed of the shank in relation to the person's speed of gait. The degree to which each knee responds to changes in speed varies with the knee mechanism. Generally, hydraulic knee mechanisms are more responsive than friction mechanisms, and computer driven are the most responsive. A knee mechanism may also provide stance phase control that slows the rate of knee flexion on weightbearing if the knee is not totally straight at initial contact. Some hydraulic and computer driven knees provide both stance and swing phase control. Stance phase control is best for those individuals who do not have a strong step over step gait pattern and who do not greatly vary their speed. More active individuals function best with swing and stance phase control knee mechanisms.

Feet have been previously described and may be used with any LE prosthesis.

PROSTHETIC COMPONENTS—UPPER EXTREMITY

The prosthetic rehabilitation of an individual with an UE amputation requires specialized post professional training for physical therapists. Early fitting is desirable and possible as soon as the incision has healed.

Components

A large variety of possible components exist for an UE prosthesis. While no prosthetic component can substitute for the complex capabilities of the human hand, and no prosthetic component to date provides sensory input, devices operated myoelectrically can be quite functional for those requiring bilateral hand function. Skin electrodes are embedded in the socket on top of functioning muscles. When the patient contracts the muscle, an electrical signal is sent that opens or closes the terminal device, usually a hand. It is beyond the scope of this chapter to present and discuss these many components and the reader is referred to other sources.[13-15]

The UE prosthesis consists of a socket, a method of suspension, an elbow unit if transhumeral, a wrist unit, and one or more terminal devices. The terminal device may be a hook or a hand. There are a great variety of hooks depending on the individual's required activities and prehensile needs. The hook is more durable and functional than the hand; the hand is more cosmetic. The prosthetist must be actively involved in component selection. There are also many specialized components to help the person with special needs including individuals with higher-level amputations or with bilateral amputations.

The UE prosthesis may be body powered using the shoulder muscles or may be powered by myoelectric controls imbedded in the socket and stimulated by contraction of selected residual limb muscles. If myoelectric fitting is anticipated, the program focuses on functional activities and development of the musculature in potential myoelectric sites.

Training

Training an individual to use an UE prosthesis is a specialized activity and physical therapists involved with UE prosthetic rehabilitation, especially with individuals using myoelectric devices, should complete specialized training in that area. Selection and training of muscles for myoelectric use requires an understanding of the functions of myoelectric devices and is beyond the scope of this chapter. Generally, the individual must first develop skill in the basic operations of the prosthesis. If transhumeral, that will include locking and unlocking the elbow mechanisms in synchrony with terminal device operation. The range of terminal device operation must also be learned whether it is voluntary opening or voluntary closing. A voluntary opening device is preferred since there is no need for active muscle contractions in the residual limb while maintaining terminal device grasp on an object. The individual then learns to control prehension power by picking up and moving objects of all sizes and densities. Finally, use is incorporated in bilateral activities appropriate to the individual's particular vocation and leisure activities.

PROSTHETIC CHECK OUT

Prior to the initiation of mobility training the prosthesis is evaluated for fit. The checkout varies to some extent depending on the specific components. During this initial training period, the prosthetist and physical therapist need to maintain close communication. If prosthetic problems are identified, the prosthetist must be notified promptly and further training delayed until the problems have been remedied to avoid possible injury to the residual limb. Today, most prosthetic sockets are fabricated from computer-generated replicas of the residual limb from detailed information provided by the prosthetist. Actual socket construction problems are rare. The more common socket fit problems are related to a patient's weight gain or to not properly wrapping the residual limb for edema control between the time measurements are taken and the time the socket is delivered.

During check out and any time during prosthetic training, the patient may complain of pain. Residual limb pain and pain related to the prosthesis itself must be differentiated from phantom limb pain through careful evaluation and interview. Residual limb pain may be the result of a poorly fitting prosthesis, neuroma development, or overuse from excess activity or stress caused by changes in mobility.

If the person indicates that the pain only occurs when wearing the prosthesis and can point to a specific area on the residual limb, a prosthetic fit problem or a neuroma must be considered. Neuroma pain, as most nerve pain, is a tingling sensation that may move up the residual limb. It may often be replicated by tapping with a fingertip over the designated area. On occasion, the neuroma may be moved back into the soft tissue through gentle massage, which the patient can be taught to do. On occasion the prosthetic socket can be relieved in an area. Severe neuroma pain requires referral back to the physician for further treatment. Prosthetic fit problems need to be referred back to the prosthetist for adjustment. If the pain is general, non-specific, and occurs with and without the prosthesis on, phantom limb pain must be considered.

In addition, a proper fitting socket and good skin tolerance should be included in the prosthetic checkout of the individual with an UE amputation. An initial evaluation of the proper cosmetic design and function of prosthetic components should be performed prior to prosthetic application. ADL and other functional activity performance with the prosthesis on should be evaluated during UE prosthetic checkout.

REHABILITATION PROGRAM

The rehabilitation of individuals following UE or LE amputation usually occurs in three distinct phases. Ideally, the patient is referred to physical therapy immediately after the amputation; and Phase 1, the post-surgical phase, is initiated while the patient is still in the hospital. Barring complications, patients are only kept in the hospital for a few days following surgery, and the initial post-surgical program focuses on discharge planning, functional activities to enhance discharge, prevention of contractures in the residual limb, and education for proper residual limb care.

Phase 2 is the time between discharge from the acute care hospital and the decision to fit or not to fit the patient with a prosthesis. This period varies in length depending on the cause of amputation, the presence of co-morbidities, the availability of rehabilitation facilities or a local clinic for persons with amputations, and the surgeon's preference. During this phase, the goals are to increase muscle strength, endurance, functional abilities, and prepare the residual limb for the prosthesis. Patients may be fitted with a prosthesis as early as 10 to 12 weeks following surgery or fitting may be delayed for many months due to complications. The length of time between amputation and prosthetic fitting may affect outcomes. If individuals are not referred for continued post-surgical care following discharge from the hospital and/or are not referred for prosthetic evaluation and fitting for many months, they may become weaker and may develop joint contractures. Individuals with a LE amputation may become habituated to a wheelchair existence.

Older individuals with a LE amputation, who are often limited in ambulation using the intact leg, are particularly susceptible to complications from poor follow-up and delayed fitting. It is important for the physical therapist to initiate discharge planning early in the hospitalization period. Not all individuals with a LE amputation are candidates for prosthetic fitting. A high amputation level, limited or absent ambulatory and general mobility status prior to amputation, and the presence of co-morbid conditions, such as cardiovascular/pulmonary disease, may preclude the decision for a prosthesis. The Amputee Mobility Predictor[16] is a simple validated instrument that provides information on balance and mobility capabilities and is a helpful tool in decision making when the potential for successful prosthetic rehabilitation is a concern.

Phase 3 is prosthetic fitting and rehabilitation. The clinic team working with patients with amputations is usually composed of physicians, physical therapists, prosthetists, and occupational therapists. These individuals evaluate the patient's status at each stage and establish goals and recommend treatment.[10] The patient's status is monitored as healing takes place. If a clinic is not easily available, it is important that the patient be referred to a prosthetist as soon as feasible. Any delay may cause complications, such as residual limb weakness and decreased general conditioning that mitigate against a successful outcome.[11] During this phase, it is also important that physical therapists understand the regulations and work with the payer communities to maximize the prosthetic potential of the patient.

Case Study #1: Below-Knee Amputation

Mrs. Natalie Hooper is a 63-year-old female who underwent a right transtibial (below the knee, 14-inch bone length) amputation yesterday secondary to diabetic gangrene.

PHASE 1: IN-HOSPITAL PHASE

PHYSICAL THERAPIST EXAMINATION: PHASE 1

HISTORY: PHASES 1, 2, AND 3

- ◆ General demographics: Mrs. Natalie Hooper is a 63-year-old black American female who lives in a middle-sized Southern city. Mrs. Hooper is left-hand dominant.
- ◆ Social history: Mrs. Hooper is married to a high school teacher and has two grown children and a 2-year-old granddaughter.
- ◆ Employment/work: She was employed as a sales person in a large chain department store until 3 months ago when the increasing development of a plantar ulcer made it impossible for her to be on her feet. She is on unpaid medical leave but continues to be covered by the store's health plan.
- ◆ Living environment: Mr. and Mrs. Hooper live in their own home. There are four entry-level steps with a railing on the right.
- ◆ General health status
  - • General health perception: Ms. Hooper reports the status of her health to be fair.
  - • Physical function: Prior to the onset of the current problem, Ms. Hooper was independent in all functional activities, worked, and took care of the home. She was an active individual prior to this episode.
  - • Psychological function: Ms Hooper had no known psychological problems prior to the amputation. While she is now accepting of the amputation, she is apprehensive about future prosthetic use. She is also

afraid of losing the other limb and is concerned with her ability to return to her previous lifestyle.
  - • Role function: Salesperson, wife, mother, grandmother.
  - • Social function: She was involved in church activities.
- ◆ Social/health habits: Mrs. Hooper is a non-smoker and drinks wine socially on occasion.
- ◆ Family history: Her mother had diabetes and died of CAD. Her father had OA and peripheral vascular disease (PVD).
- ◆ Medical/surgical history: Mrs. Hooper was diagnosed with adult onset diabetes approximately 15 years ago. The diabetes has been controlled with diet and oral medication. Mrs. Hooper also has high BP controlled by medication and ASO as a result of the diabetes. She had lost protective sensation in both feet several years ago. She had a history of several small ulcers on the right foot that healed with foot care and shoe inserts. Mrs. Hooper underwent a femoral-popliteal bypass 6 months ago to try to increase the circulation in her right foot. The ulcer on the plantar surface of the right foot began approximately 3 months ago. It was treated with reduced weightbearing and off loading shoe wear, wet to dry dressings, and antibiotics, but the ulcer did not heal. A ray amputation was performed 3 weeks ago but did not heal and transtibial amputation was performed yesterday secondary to diabetic gangrene from the plantar ulcer.
- ◆ Prior hospitalizations: She was hospitalized for the birth of her children and for the femoral-popliteal bypass and the ray amputation.
- ◆ Preexisting medical and other health-related conditions: Mrs. Hooper has diabetes, ASO, and high BP.
- ◆ Current condition(s)/chief complaint(s): Mrs. Hooper complains of pain at the incision site, 3/10 with medication and 6/10 without medication on the NPS.
- ◆ Functional status and activity level: To be determined during tests and measures.
- ◆ Medications: Mrs. Hooper is taking Orinase, Darvocet (q 4 hrs prn), and Capoten.
- ◆ Other clinical tests: Her most recent blood sugar was 98. Abnormal arterial sounds were heard during Doppler examination. She has a decreased left ankle brachial index (0.65).

SYSTEMS REVIEW: PHASE 1

- ◆ Cardiovascular/pulmonary
  - • BP: 128/78 mmHg
  - • Edema: Residual limb cannot be determined at this time, slight edema in left ankle
  - • HR: 66 bpm

- RR: 15 bpm
- Integumentary (Note: In the early postoperative period in the hospital, the physical therapist may not have the opportunity to inspect the residual limb suture line. The dressing is a soft gauze dressing with an elastic wrap to mid thigh covering the gauze.)
  - Presence of scar formation
    - Patient has a long posterior flap sutured by means of an anterior closure according to the operative report
    - This type of closure is advantageous as the posterior tissues are well vascularized
    - However, the scar on the anterior distal end of the residual limb may sometimes lead to pressure problems in the prosthesis
  - Skin color: WNL
  - Skin integrity: From the nursing notes
    - A drain is in place with minimal drainage at the surgical site (drain usually removed 24 to 48 hours after surgery)
    - No apparent signs of infection
    - Skin of intact LLE is dry but warm to touch
- Musculoskeletal
  - Gross range of motion
    - LLE: WFL
    - Right hip extension: Limited
  - Gross strength
    - Both UEs and LLE: WFL
    - Gross strength R hip: At least in 3/5 range
  - Gross symmetry: Leans to the left
  - Height: 5'4" (1.62 m)
  - Weight: 162 lbs (73.48 kg)
- Neuromuscular
  - Balance
    - Static sitting independent
    - Dynamic sitting required close supervision
  - Locomotion, transfers, and transitions
    - Bed mobility: Apprehensive about moving residual limb in bed requiring minimal assistance
    - Bed to chair transfer: Able to transfer with minimal assist of one person
    - Standing by bed with walker: Able to stand for a few seconds before tiring requiring contact guarding
- Communication, affect, cognition, language, and learning style
  - Communication and affect: WNL
  - Cognition: Alert and aware of her situation
  - Learning preferences: Visual leaner

TESTS AND MEASURES: PHASE 1

- Aerobic capacity/endurance
  - Poor aerobic capacity with increased energy expenditure per unit of work
- Anthropometric characteristics
  - BMI=27.8 (this is considered overweight based on Centers for Disease Control and Prevention)[17]
  - Edema: Observed at distal end of residual limb around incision site during dressing changes and slight edema left ankle
- Arousal, attention, and cognition
  - Patient alert and oriented x 3
  - Mrs. Hooper is motivated to improve
- Assistive and adaptive devices
  - Mrs. Hooper is using a standard walker to assist ambulation
  - Mrs. Hooper uses a wheelchair when she is tired and for longer distances
- Circulation
  - Left popliteal pulse: 3+
  - Left tibial pulse: 3+
  - Temperature LLE: Warm to palpation
- Cranial and peripheral nerve integrity
  - Peripheral nerves intact
  - Mild sensory neuropathy in distal LLE
  - Loss of protective sensation on plantar surface of L foot
- Environmental, home, and work barriers
  - Mrs. Hooper lives with her husband in their own home
  - There are four entry-level steps with a railing on the right
  - The department store in which she worked is handicap accessible
- Ergonomics and body mechanics
  - Cannot be tested at this time
- Gait, locomotion, and balance
  - Stands with walker at bedside for 10 seconds requiring contact guarding
- Integumentary integrity
  - No evidence of sores or pressure areas
  - Trophic changes in L foot included shiny skin, edema, thick discolored nails
- Joint integrity and mobility
  - Patient displays some rigidity in the L foot due to diabetic neuropathy
  - Other joints: WNL
- Motor function
  - Performs functional activities in a coordinated manner
- Muscle performance

- MMT revealed strength to be WFL for her UEs and LLE
- Her RLE was not tested at this time, but decreased strength expected as a result of the surgical incision and pain
♦ Orthotic, protective, and supportive devices
  - Soft dressing with elastic wrap to mid thigh in place
♦ Pain
  - NPS (0=no pain and 10=worst possible pain) revealed 3/10 with medications and 6/10 without medications
♦ Posture
  - Forward head and thoracic kyphosis noted in sitting
  - Lateral trunk lean to the right detected during standing activities
♦ Prosthetic requirements
  - Transtibial prosthesis with appropriate ankle foot assembly, shank, socket, and suspension will be required
♦ Range of motion
  - Goniometric measurements revealed:
    - All UE joints: WNL
    - All LLE joints: WNL except dorsiflexion=0 to 5 degrees
    - R hip flexion=10 to 120 degrees with tightness noted
    - R hip extension=-10 degrees
    - R knee flexion=5 to 105 degrees with tightness noted
♦ Self-care and home management
  - Requires minimal assistance with bed mobility
  - Independent in upper body grooming and dressing
  - Requires assistance in lower body grooming and dressing
♦ Ventilation and respiration/gas exchange
  - Patient has strong, nonproductive cough
  - Patient is using an incentive spirometer
  - No abnormal breath sounds noted during auscultation
♦ Work, community, and leisure integration or reintegration
  - Presently on leave of absence from work
  - Extremely supportive family and friends

EVALUATION: PHASE 1

Her history previously outlined indicated that she is a 63-year old black American female salesperson, non-smoker, and overweight. She has high BP, ASO, and adult onset diabetes. She has just undergone a transtibial amputation of her RLE. Mrs. Hooper is alert and aware and was active prior to the onset of the most recent problem. Her potential for eventual prosthetic rehabilitation appears good. It is critically important that plans for continued therapy and post-surgical rehabilitation be initiated as soon as possible so the patient makes a smooth transition from inpatient hospital care to either home health care or outpatient physical therapy.

DIAGNOSIS: PHASE 1

Mrs. Hooper is a patient who has diabetes and ASO and has undergone a transtibial amputation of her RLE. She has pain in the residual LE. She has impaired: aerobic capacity/endurance; anthropometric characteristics; circulation; peripheral nerve integrity; gait, locomotion, and balance; integumentary integrity; joint integrity and mobility; muscle performance; posture; and range of motion. She is functionally limited in self-care and home management and in work, community, and leisure actions, tasks, and activities. She requires assistive, adaptive, protective, supportive, and prosthetic devices and equipment. These findings are consistent with placement in Pattern J: Impaired Motor Function, Muscle Performance, Range of Motion, Gait, Locomotion, and Balance Associated With Amputation. These impairments, functional limitations, and device and equipment requirements will be addressed in determining the prognosis and the plan of care.

PROGNOSIS AND PLAN OF CARE: PHASE 1

Over the course of the visits, the following mutually established outcomes have been determined:
♦ Ability to perform physical actions, tasks, and activities related to self-care is improved
♦ Care is coordinated with patient, family, and other professionals
♦ Case is managed throughout episode of care
♦ Decrease dependence for stand pivot transfers
♦ Dynamic sitting balance is improved
♦ Edema is decreased
♦ Integumentary integrity is improved
♦ Knowledge of behaviors that foster healthy habits is gained
♦ Muscle strength is increased
♦ Pain is decreased
♦ Placement needs are determined
♦ Risk factors are reduced
♦ Risk of secondary impairments is reduced
♦ ROM is increased
♦ Standing balance is improved
♦ Standing tolerance is increased
♦ Stress is decreased

To achieve these outcomes, the appropriate interventions for this patient are determined. These will include: coordination, communication, and documentation; patient/client-related instruction; therapeutic exercise; functional training in self-care and home management; and airway clearance techniques.

Based on the diagnosis and prognosis, Mrs. Hooper is expected to require between two to eight visits over a 5-day period of time depending on the length of hospitalization. In this example, the physical therapist must consider that Mrs. Hooper has multiple system involvement and has limited endurance. While in the hospital, Mrs. Hooper will be seen twice a day. Upon discharge she may be referred to home health or to a rehabilitation agency. Continued therapy after discharge is required, and the physical therapist has the responsibility to ensure that an appropriate referral is made.

INTERVENTIONS: PHASE 1

RATIONALE FOR SELECTED INTERVENTIONS

Therapeutic Exercise

The initial interventions are directed toward preparing the patient for discharge from the hospital. Independent mobility, care of the residual limb and the other extremity, and a home exercise program are important. The therapeutic exercises are directed toward decreasing contractures or contracture prevention in order to prepare the residual limb for eventual prosthetic use. Positioning and active exercises are used to maintain joint ROM and muscle flexibility in the residual limb following amputation.[1,18] The prone and supine positions are recommended to avoid joint contractures at the hip and the knee. Functional training should include bed mobility to promote frequent position changes following surgery. Poor bed mobility is a major risk factor for the development of pressure sores due to prolonged unrelieved pressure.[19] Transfer training and sitting balance exercises are progressed as tolerated by the patient to promote increased functional independence. Exercises may be initiated after surgery as long as stress is avoided to the incision and underlying tissue. Therapeutic exercises will help to prevent muscle atrophy and deconditioning. Strengthening exercises for the UEs, LLE, and the trunk are implemented to improve transfer, standing, and ambulation activities. Shoulder girdle depressor and elbow extensor strength are important for transfer and ambulation activities.[20]

Airway Clearance Techniques

Physical therapy airway clearance techniques should be used if the patient exhibits abnormal breathing indicative of excessive pulmonary secretions. Clearance of excessive pulmonary secretions is assisted by the techniques of percussion, vibration, and deep breathing exercises.[21]

Other Techniques

Treatment of chronic phantom pain includes pre-amputation analgesic drip, TENS, regional nerve blocks, epidural injections, narcotic medications, biofeedback, and even hypnosis. While success has been reported with some treatments in some instances, there has been no consistent successful approach to chronic phantom pain.[22-24]

COORDINATION, COMMUNICATION, AND DOCUMENTATION

Communication will occur with Mrs. Hooper. Education regarding her current condition, impairments, and functional limitations will be discussed. A plan of care will be developed and discussed with the patient. All elements of the patient's management will be documented. Early communication with the physician is necessary for post hospital planning and referral to either outpatient therapy, a rehabilitation center, or home health. Collaboration with a rehabilitation center will occur. The patient and family need to be involved in discharge planning for the best placement. Discharge planning will be provided.

PATIENT/CLIENT-RELATED INSTRUCTION

The patient will be instructed in bed mobility; proper bed and chair positioning of the RLE, including keeping right hip and knee straight in bed and keeping right knee straight on a board or pillow when sitting in any chair; wound care; proper residual limb wrapping; and care of LLE, including diabetic foot care. Instruction will be given in proper footwear, shoe fitting, and foot care. Risk factors will be discussed including a discussion concerning weight management. A nutritional referral will be made. The patient will receive education concerning the need for a prosthetic rehabilitation program that is to begin in a timely manner.

THERAPEUTIC EXERCISE

- ◆ Aerobic capacity/endurance conditioning
  - Increase ambulation distance and decrease time
  - Increase standing endurance with walker
- ◆ Balance, coordination, and agility training
  - Balance on LLE at bedside using walker
  - Balance two hand support, then one hand support
- ◆ Body mechanics and postural stabilization
  - If mirror available, work on postural alignment with altered center of mass
  - Maintain right hip and knee in neutral
  - Core strengthening exercises to strengthen and improve endurance in trunk and pelvic musculature

♦ Flexibility exercises
  ● Stretching exercises should be done after warming up, using a slow and steady stretch accompanied by deep breathing, and building hold up to 30 to 60 seconds
  ● Stretch R hip flexors using Thomas test position and active hip extension sidelying
  ● Stretch hamstrings in long sit position or supine with SLR
  ● Stretch left ankle plantar flexors
♦ Gait and locomotion training
  ● Standing endurance with walker
  ● Gait training with walker or crutches
♦ Strength, power, and endurance training
  ● Active exercises for right hip extensors, abductors, and internal rotators
  ● Active hip extension sidelying on left
  ● Ankle pump LLE
  ● Gentle active knee flexion and extension without stretching or pain at incision site
  ● Isometric exercises for gluts, quads, and hamstrings
  ● Resistive exercises, as tolerated, for LLE and UEs
  ● Core strengthening

FUNCTIONAL TRAINING IN SELF-CARE AND HOME MANAGEMENT

♦ Self-care
  ● Bed mobility
  ● Learn to move safely in and out of bed
  ● Independent mobility with assistive device
  ● Instruction in dressing and toilet activities
  ● Skin inspection of residual limb
  ● Skin care of residual limb and LLE
  ● Learn proper residual limb wrapping
♦ Injury prevention or reduction
  ● Awareness of safety precautions involved with self-care
  ● Injury protection while using walker
♦ Safety awareness training during self-care

AIRWAY CLEARANCE TECHNIQUES

♦ Breathing strategies
  ● Active cycles of breathing (forced expiratory techniques)
  ● Assisted cough/huff techniques
  ● Autogenic drainage
  ● Paced breathing
  ● Pursed lip breathing
♦ Manual/mechanical techniques
  ● Chest percussion, vibration, and shaking

♦ Positioning
  ● Positioning to maximize ventilation and perfusion

ANTICIPATED GOALS AND EXPECTED OUTCOMES

♦ Impact on pathology/pathophysiology
  ● Pain is decreased to 2/10 with medication and 3/10 without medication.
  ● Physiological response to increased oxygen demand is improved.
  ● Soft tissue inflammation, edema, and restriction are reduced.
  ● Tissue perfusion and oxygenation are enhanced.
  ● Ventilation and respiration/gas exchange are improved.
♦ Impact on impairments
  ● Airway clearance is improved so lungs are clear.
  ● Balance is improved in dynamic sitting balance requiring standby supervision.
  ● Cough is eliminated.
  ● Endurance is increased and can stand for 30 seconds with walker.
  ● Energy expenditure per unit of work is decreased.
  ● Exercise tolerance is improved to tolerating 20 minutes of exercise.
  ● Gait and locomotion are improved and can ambulate 10 feet with walker with contact guarding.
  ● Muscle performance, including strength, power, and endurance, is increased; UEs and LLE are WFL; and RLE hip strength is 3+/5 and knee strength is 4-/5.
  ● Postural awareness is improved.
  ● ROM is increased to point where LLE is WFL and right hip and knee are limited at end ranges.
  ● Sensory awareness is increased.
  ● Work of breathing is decreased.
♦ Impact on functional limitations
  ● Ability to perform physical actions, tasks, and activities related to self-care is improved.
  ● Ability to resume self-care is improved.
  ● Functional independence in ADL is improved so that the patient is independent in UE dressing and requires minimal assistance for LE dressing.
  ● Level of supervision required for task performance is decreased.
  ● Patient is independent in wheelchair mobility and requires contact guarding for bed to wheelchair transfers.
  ● Performance level of self-care is improved.
  ● Performance of ADL with devices is increased.
♦ Risk reduction/prevention
  ● Risk factors and risk of secondary impairments are

reduced.
- Safety is improved.
- Self-management of symptoms is improved.
♦ Impact on health, wellness, and fitness
  - Behaviors that promote healthy nutrition, physical activity, and wellness are promoted.
  - Physical capacity is increased.
  - Physical function is improved.
♦ Impact on societal resources
  - Documentation will occur throughout the patient management and across all settings and follows APTA's *Guidelines for Physical Therapy Documentation.*[25]
♦ Patient/client satisfaction
  - Care is coordinated with patient, family, and other professionals.
  - Case is managed throughout the episode of care.
  - Collaboration and coordination occurs with the rehabilitation center.
  - Decision making is enhanced regarding patient health and use of health care resources by patient and family.
  - Interdisciplinary collaboration occurs through case conferences.
  - Patient and family knowledge and awareness of the diagnosis, prognosis, interventions, and anticipated goals and expected outcomes are increased.
  - Placement needs are determined.

PHASE 2: POST-HOSPITAL PHASE

PHYSICAL THERAPIST EXAMINATION: PHASE 2

Mrs. Hooper has been referred to a local rehabilitation center for continued therapy and care 5 days post amputation.

SYSTEMS REVIEW: PHASE 2

♦ Cardiovascular/pulmonary
  - BP: 130/76 mmHg
  - Edema: Noted in the residual limb and left ankle
  - HR: 70 bpm
  - RR: 15 bpm
♦ Integumentary
  - Presence of scar formation: Long posterior flap sutured anteriorly
  - Skin color: WNL
  - Skin integrity: Incision healing well, no apparent signs of infection, wire sutures in place
♦ Musculoskeletal

- Gross range of motion
  - Both UEs and LLE: WFL, except for limited left ankle dorsiflexion
  - R hip and knee limited at end ranges
- Gross strength
  - Both UEs and LLE: WFL
  - RLE: Decreased
- Gross symmetry: Slight lean to the left
- Height: 5'4" (1.62 m)
- Weight: 162 lbs (73.48 kg)
♦ Neuromuscular
  - Balance: Independent in static and dynamic sitting
  - Locomotion, transfers, and transitions
    - Bed mobility: Independent
    - Bed to chair transfer: Independent in standing pivot transfer
    - Standing by bed with walker
    - Gait: Ambulating with a walker
♦ Communication, affect, cognition, language, and learning style
  - Communication and affect: WNL
  - Cognition: Alert and aware of her situation
  - Learning preferences: Visual learner

TESTS AND MEASURES: PHASE 2

♦ Aerobic capacity/endurance
  - Poor aerobic capacity with increased energy expenditure per unit of work
  - Increased cardiovascular response to low level work loads
  - Increased perceived exertion with functional activities
♦ Anthropometric characteristics
  - BMI=27.8 (this is considered overweight based on Centers for Disease Control and Prevention)[17]
  - Edema: Circumferential measurements taken the length of the residual limb.
  - Shape of residual limb: Cylindrical
♦ Arousal, attention, and cognition
  - Patient alert and oriented x 3
  - Mrs. Hooper is motivated to improve
♦ Assistive and adaptive devices
  - Mrs. Hooper is using a standard walker to assist ambulation
  - Mrs. Hooper uses a wheelchair when she is tired and for longer distances
♦ Circulation
  - Right popliteal pulse=3+
  - Left PT pulse=2+
  - Residual limb skin in normal condition

- Temperature: Warm to palpation
- Edema in residual limb and slight edema in left ankle
♦ Cranial and peripheral nerve integrity
  - PNs intact
  - Mild sensory neuropathy in distal LLE
  - Semmes-Weinstein monofilaments used for quantitative assessment of touch, and 1 g, 10 g, and 75 g are the most common sizes
    - Normal sensation is the perception of 1 g, and protective sensation is perception of 10 g
    - Individuals who require a higher force for perception are at risk of ulceration[26]
    - Mrs. Hooper is unable to perceive 1 g but easily perceives 10 g
♦ Environmental, home, and work barriers
  - Mr. and Mrs. Hooper live in their own home in a middle class area of town
  - There are four entry level steps with a railing on the right
  - Employment/work
    - She was employed as a sales person in a large chain department store until 3 months ago
    - The department store is handicap accessible
♦ Ergonomics and body mechanics
  - Patient able to perform functional activities in a safe and efficient manner
♦ Gait, locomotion, and balance
  - Could stand with walker at bedside independently for 30 seconds
  - Ambulating with walker 10 feet with contact guarding
  - Sitting balance independent both static and dynamic
♦ Integumentary integrity
  - No evidence of sores or pressure areas
  - Trophic changes remain in foot
  - Long posterior flap sutured anteriorly
  - Incision healing well
  - No apparent signs of infection noted
  - Wire sutures in place
♦ Joint integrity and mobility
  - Patient displays some rigidity in the left foot due to diabetic neuropathy
  - Other joints: WNL
♦ Motor function
  - Performs functional activities in a coordinated manner
♦ Muscle performance
  - MMT revealed:
    - Both UEs and LLE: WFL

- RLE
  - Hip flexion=4/5
  - Hip extension=3+/5
  - Hip abduction=4/5
  - Hip adduction=4/5
  - Hip IR=3+/5
  - Hip ER=3+/5
  - Knee flexion=3+/5
  - Knee extension=3+/5
♦ Orthotic, protective, and supportive devices
  - Limb wrapped in elastic bandage
  - Mrs. Hopper is wearing an extra depth shoe with inserts on L foot
♦ Pain
  - NPS (0=no pain and 10=worst possible pain) revealed 1/10 with medications and 3/10 without medications
  - Reports occasional phantom burning and itching to right foot
♦ Posture
  - Forward head and thoracic kyphosis noted in sitting.
  - Lateral trunk lean to the right detected during standing activities
♦ Prosthetic requirements
  - Transtibial prosthesis with appropriate ankle foot assembly, shank, socket, and suspension
♦ Range of motion
  - Goniometric measurements revealed:
    - All UE joints: WNL
    - All LLE joints: WNL except dorsiflexion which was 0 to 5 degrees
  - Bilateral hip extension=0 degrees
  - Right knee flexion=3 to 130 degrees
♦ Self-care and home management
  - Ambulating short distances with walker requiring contact guarding
  - Independent in upper body grooming and dressing
  - Requires minimal assistance with lower body grooming and dressing
♦ Ventilation and respiration/gas exchange
  - WFL
♦ Work, community, and leisure integration or reintegration
  - Presently on leave of absence from work
  - Extremely supportive family and friends

EVALUATION: PHASE 2

Her history previously outlined indicated that she is a 63-year old black American female salesperson, non-smoker, and overweight. She has high BP, ASO, and adult onset diabetes. She is status post a transtibial amputation of her RLE 5 days ago. Mrs. Hooper is alert and aware and was active prior to the onset of the most recent problem. Her potential for eventual prosthetic rehabilitation appears good. It is critically important that plans for continued therapy and prosthetic placement be initiated as soon as possible so the patient makes a smooth transition from the rehabilitation center to prosthetic placement.

DIAGNOSIS: PHASE 2

Mrs. Hooper has undergone a transtibial amputation of her RLE and has pain in her right residual limb, as well as phantom burning and itching. She has impaired: aerobic capacity/endurance; anthropometric characteristics; circulation, peripheral nerve integrity; gait, locomotion, and balance; integumentary integrity; joint integrity and mobility; muscle performance; posture; and range of motion. She is functionally limited in self-care and home management and in work, community, and leisure actions, tasks, and activities. Mrs. Hooper will need a transtibial prosthesis with appropriate ankle foot assembly, shank, socket, and suspension. She will also need assistive, adaptive, protective, and supportive devices and equipment. These findings are consistent with placement in Pattern J: Impaired Motor Function, Muscle Performance, Range of Motion, Gait, Locomotion, and Balance Associated With Amputation. These impairments, functional limitations, and device and equipment requirements will be addressed in determining the prognosis and the plan of care.

PROGNOSIS AND PLAN OF CARE: PHASE 2

Over the course of the visits, the following mutually established outcomes have been determined:
- Ability to perform physical actions, tasks, and activities related to self-care is improved
- Care is coordinated with patient, family, and other professionals
- Case is managed throughout episode of care
- Integumentary integrity is improved
- Knowledge of behaviors that foster healthy habits is gained
- Pain is decreased
- Placement needs are determined
- Residual limb edema is decreased
- Risk factors are reduced
- Risk of secondary impairments is reduced
- ROM is increased
- Standing balance is improved
- Stress is decreased

To achieve these outcomes, the appropriate interventions for this patient are determined. These will include: coordination, communication, and documentation; patient/client-related instruction; therapeutic exercise; and functional training in self-care and home management.

Based on the diagnosis and prognosis, Mrs. Hooper is expected to be in the rehabilitation center 7 to 10 days until she has achieved independence in ambulation, residual limb care, and ADL training. She will be discharged with a home program and be ready for prosthetic fitting approximately 3 to 4 months after surgery. She may be referred to a local amputee clinic by the vascular surgeon or be referred directly to a prosthetist. Mrs. Hooper has multiple system involvement and has limited endurance.

INTERVENTIONS: PHASE 2

RATIONALE FOR SELECTED INTERVENTIONS

Therapeutic Exercise

Residual limb strengthening exercises are important to prepare for prosthetic ambulation. One recent study regarding the relationship of muscle strength and weightbearing of the residual limb demonstrated a positive correlation between increased hip abductor strength and prosthetic gait stability.[27,28] The therapeutic exercise program should place an emphasis on the muscles needed for prosthetic ambulation. Sitting and standing balance activities are essential for prosthetic ambulation. Once the patient is independent in self-care and mobility activities and competent in a home program of exercises and residual limb care, physical therapy may be temporarily discontinued with a definite date for return to the amputee clinic for prosthetic prescription. Depending on the healing status, the patient may be ready for fitting in approximately 10 to 12 weeks. However, more often patients with diabetes and vascular problems are not fitted for 3 to 4 months. Early prosthetic fitting is important to maintain strength and balance and to assure a positive transition to prosthetic use.[29] Temporary fitting cannot be considered until the residual limb is well healed and nontender.

Manual Therapy Techniques

Active stretching techniques and joint mobilization may be used to prevent residual limb contractures. PNF hold-relax technique has been effectively used in reducing knee flexion contracture.[30] Massage may be used to help reduce swelling, muscles spasms, and pain in certain traumatic amputations where adherence may be an issue.[31] Soft tissue mobilization may assist in maintaining adequate circulation and muscle flexibility for improved functional use. If necessary, soft tissue mobilization may be applied above and below the scar and to the surrounding tissues as appropriate to improve tissue mobility and prevent adhesions. When the incision is well healed, gentle mobilization may be directed to the scar itself.[32]

Prescription, Application, and, as Appropriate, Fabrication of Devices and Equipment

Residual limb edema control is important in this phase of rehabilitation. Edema increases pain and interferes with suture line healing in the residual limb.[33] The application of a residual limb shrinker or ace wraps is indicated to promote reabsorption of postoperative edema and to begin shaping the residual limb.[34] In addition, the application of a dressing protects the residual limb from infection and trauma and helps to desensitize the residual limb in preparation for prosthetic fitting.[34]

COORDINATION, COMMUNICATION, AND DOCUMENTATION

Communication will occur with Mrs. Hooper. Education regarding her current condition, impairments, and functional limitations will be discussed. A plan of care will be developed and discussed with the patient. All elements of the patient's management will be documented. Early communication with the physician is necessary for post rehabilitation planning and referral for prosthetic placement. Collaboration with a prosthetic center will occur. The patient and family need to be involved in discharge planning for the best placement. Discharge planning will be provided.

PATIENT/CLIENT-RELATED INSTRUCTION

The patient will be instructed in wound care, prevention of skin problems, and proper wrapping of the residual limb. Instruction will be given in proper footwear, shoe fitting, and foot care for the LLE. Risk factors will be discussed including a discussion concerning weight management. A nutritional referral will be made because of her diabetes. The patient will receive education concerning the need for a prosthetic rehabilitation program that is to begin in a timely manner. Preparation for prosthetic fitting may include demonstration or pictures shown of different prostheses and components explaining uses and limitations. Discussion of the role of an amputee clinic and the importance of acting proactively for early prosthetic fitting shall occur.

THERAPEUTIC EXERCISE

- ♦ Aerobic capacity/endurance conditioning
  - • Increased workload over time
  - • Progressive wheelchair propulsion program
- ♦ Balance, coordination, and agility training
  - • Balance on left leg using walker
  - • Balance two hand support, then one hand support

- • Ball throwing in short sit and or long sit position
- • Progress to ball throwing in standing as tolerated
- • Closed kinematic exercises in the parallel bars
- • Coordination activities with residual limb
  - ▪ Making figure eights
  - ▪ Drawing numbers
- ♦ Body mechanics and postural stabilization
  - • Using a mirror, work on postural alignment with altered center of mass
  - • Maintain right hip and knee in neutral
- ♦ Flexibility exercises
  - • Stretching exercises should be done after warming up, using a slow and steady stretch accompanied by deep breathing, and building hold up to 30 to 60 seconds
  - • ROM for L ankle dorsiflexion
  - • ROM for R knee flexion and extension
  - • ROM for R hip flexion and extension
- ♦ Gait and locomotion training
  - • Gait training with assistive device on level surfaces
  - • Gait training with assistive device on stairs, curbs, and ramps
- ♦ Strength, power, and endurance training
  - • Active exercises for right hip extensors, abductors, and internal and external rotators, and for knee flexors and extensors
  - • Active to resistive hip extension prone
  - • Active to resistive exercises for gluts, quads, and hamstrings
  - • Dynamic residual limb exercises emphasizing hip adduction, hip extension, and knee flexion and extension.
  - • Progress to resistive exercises as tolerated for RLE using elastic bands or weights
  - • Combination residual limb exercises, such as modified bridging over a bolster or roll for combined hip extension/knee extension
  - • Weightbearing exercises as tolerated through the residual limb by kneeling on a cushion on a chair/stool of appropriate height
  - • Resistive exercises for LLE and UEs using elastic bands or weights
  - • Seated push-ups
  - • Core strengthening

FUNCTIONAL TRAINING IN SELF-CARE AND HOME MANAGEMENT

- ♦ Self-care
  - • Independent mobility with assistive device
  - • Instruction in dressing and grooming activities
  - • Skin inspection of residual limb and LLE

- Independent skin care of residual limb and LLE
- Ensure proper residual limb bandaging until sutures are removed then fit with a shrinker
- Injury prevention or reduction
  - Awareness of safety precautions involved with self-care
  - Injury protection while using walker or other assistive devices
  - Wound prevention for the intact LE
  - Protection of residual limb
- Safety awareness training during self-care

ANTICIPATED GOALS AND EXPECTED OUTCOMES

- Impact on pathology/pathophysiology
  - Pain is decreased to 0/10 with medication and 2/10 without medication.
  - Phantom sensation is present but tolerated.
  - Soft tissue inflammation, edema, and restrictions are reduced to allow for prosthetic fitting.
- Impact on impairments
  - Balance is independent static and dynamic standing with walker.
  - Endurance is increased and can stand for 60 seconds with walker.
  - Energy expenditure per unit of work is decreased.
  - Exercise tolerance is improved to 30 minutes.
  - Gait and locomotion are improved and can independently ambulate 100 feet and contact guarding required for elevation activities.
  - Muscle performance, including strength, power, and endurance, is increased so that UEs and LLE are WFL and RLE is 4-4+/5.
  - Postural awareness is improved with less lateral trunk lean in standing.
  - ROM and flexibility increased to point where LLE and R knee are WFL and R hip extension is +5 degrees.
- Impact on functional limitations
  - Ability to perform physical actions, tasks, and activities related to self-care is independent in personal hygiene and dressing.
  - Ability to resume self-care is independent.
  - Performance level of self-care is improved and can perform independent self-care of residual limb and LLE.
  - Performance of ADL with devices is independent.
- Risk reduction/prevention
  - Demonstrate proper care of remaining LE and foot.
  - Risk factors and risk of secondary impairments are reduced: Residual limb is properly bandaged and protected during all activities.
  - Safety is demonstrated in all activities on level surfaces.
  - Self-management of symptoms is improved.
- Impact on health, wellness, and fitness
  - Behaviors that promote healthy nutrition, physical activity, and wellness are promoted.
  - Physical capacity is increased.
  - Physical function is improved.
- Impact on societal resources
  - Documentation will occur throughout the patient management and across all settings and follows APTA's *Guidelines for Physical Therapy Documentation.*[25]
- Patient/client satisfaction
  - Care is coordinated with patient, family, and other professionals.
  - Case is managed throughout the episode of care.
  - Collaboration and coordination occurs with the rehabilitation center.
  - Decision making is enhanced regarding patient health and use of health care resources by patient and family.
  - Interdisciplinary collaboration occurs through case conferences.
  - Patient and family knowledge and awareness of the diagnosis, prognosis, interventions, and anticipated goals and expected outcomes are increased.
  - Placement needs are determined.

PHASE 3: PROSTHETIC EVALUATION AND TRAINING

PHYSICAL THERAPIST EXAMINATION: PHASE 3

Mrs. Hooper has been referred to a local amputee clinic for evaluation for prosthetic fitting approximately 3 months after amputation.

SYSTEMS REVIEW: PHASE 3

- Cardiovascular/pulmonary
  - BP: 131/76 mmHg
  - Edema: Slight in left ankle
  - HR: 72 bpm
  - RR: 15 bpm
- Integumentary
  - Presence of scar formation: Long posterior flap with anterior suture line closure
  - Skin color: WNL

- Skin integrity: Incision well healed, scar mobile and non tender
- ◆ Musculoskeletal
  - Gross range of motion
    - Both UEs and LLE: WFL
    - R hip extension: Limited end range
    - R knee: WFL
  - Gross strength
    - Both UEs and LLE: WFL
    - Gross strength of RLE: Minimally decreased
  - Gross symmetry: Symmetrical while sitting and slight left lean while standing
  - Height: 5'4" (1.62 m)
  - Weight: 162 lbs (73.48 kg)
- ◆ Neuromuscular
  - Balance: Independent sitting and standing with a standard walker
  - Locomotion, transfers, and transitions
    - Stand pivot transfers independent
    - Able to stand with walker for at least 60 seconds
    - Independent ambulation with a walker for 100 feet
    - Requires contact guarding with elevation activities
- ◆ Communication, affect, cognition, language, and learning style
  - Communication and affect: WNL
  - Cognition: Alert and aware of her situation
  - Learning preferences: Visual learner

TESTS AND MEASURES: PHASE 3

- ◆ Aerobic capacity/endurance training
  - Fair aerobic capacity with increased energy expenditure per unit of work
- ◆ Anthropometric characteristics
  - BMI=27.8 (this is considered overweight based on Centers for Disease Control and Prevention)[17]
  - Edema: Slightly edematous L ankle
  - Shape of residual limb: Cylindrical
- ◆ Arousal, attention, and cognition
  - Patient alert and oriented x 3
  - Patient is motivated to improve
- ◆ Assistive and adaptive devices
  - Mrs. Hooper is using a standard walker to ambulate
  - Mrs. Hooper uses a wheelchair when she is tired or needs to go long distances
- ◆ Circulation
  - Right popliteal pulse=3+
  - Left PT pulse=2+
  - LLE is hairless and slightly edematous at the ankle and tropic changes in foot

- Temperature: Warm to palpation
- ◆ Cranial and peripheral nerve integrity
  - Peripheral nerves intact
  - Mild sensory neuropathy in distal LLE
  - Sensation in the left foot is diminished with a 1 g monofilament but has good response with a 10 g monofilament
- ◆ Environmental, home, and work barriers
  - Mr. and Mrs. Hooper live in their own home. There are four entry-level steps with a railing on the right
  - She was employed as a sales person in a large chain department store until 6 months ago. The department store is handicap accessible
- ◆ Ergonomics and body mechanics
  - Patient able to perform functional activities in a safe and efficient manner
- ◆ Gait, locomotion, and balance
  - Stands with walker for at least 60 seconds
  - Ambulating with walker independently 100 feet
  - Gait evaluation while walking in her transtibial prosthesis includes observations noted in Table 10-1
- ◆ Integumentary integrity
  - No evidence of sores or pressure areas
  - Long posterior flap with anterior suture line closure
  - Incision well healed, scar mobile and nontender
- ◆ Joint integrity and mobility
  - Patient displays some rigidity in the left foot due to diabetic neuropathy, other joints WNL
- ◆ Motor function
  - Performs functional activities in a coordinated manner
- ◆ Muscle performance
  - MMT revealed:
    - UEs and LLE: WFL
    - RLE:
      - Hip flexion=4+/5
      - Hip extension=4/5
      - Hip abduction=4+/5
      - Hip adduction=4+/5
      - Hip IR=4/5
      - Hip ER=4/5
      - Knee flexion=4/5
      - Knee extension=4/5
- ◆ Orthotic, protective, and supportive devices
  - Limb is encased in a shrinker
  - Ms. Hooper is wearing an extra depth shoe on the left
- ◆ Pain
  - NPS (0=no pain and 10=worst possible pain) revealed 1/10 without medications
- ◆ Posture

	Table 10-1		
TRANSTIBIAL GAIT DEVIATIONS			
Problem	*Characteristics*	*Prosthetic Causes*	*Client Causes*
Knee extension through stance	Knee is extended from heel contact to foot flat	Too long toe lever arm too soft heel cushion (varies with type of foot)	Wearing lower heel shoes Weak quadriceps Bad habit
Knee instability	Tendency for the knee to buckle at initial or terminal stance	Initial stance=heel cushion too hard Terminal stance=short toe lever arm If client tries to extend knee against buckling force it will lead to anterior distal pressure and abrasions	Wearing higher heel shoes than on initial checkout
Hip rises on stance	Hip on prosthetic side raises on stance; may also have lateral trunk lean	Prosthesis too long	If client puts on too many socks or residual limb is edematous, it may simulate long prosthesis
Hip drops on stance	Hip on prosthetic side drops on stance; may also have lateral trunk lean	Prosthesis too short	If the residual limb has shrunk and client does not have enough socks, it may simulate a short prosthesis
Wide-based gait	Walks with leg further than 2 inches away from midline	Outset foot Medial leaning pylon (from floor up)	Client afraid to shift weight onto prosthesis at stance Bad habit
Narrow-based gait (excessive lateral thrust of prosthesis)	Malleoli pass close to each other on gait (top of socket may be seen to move away from knee on stance)	Inset foot Lateral leaning pylon (from the floor up)	This deviation is usually caused by improper socket alignment
Pistoning on swing	Socket drops away from limb on swing	Inadequate suspension	Client not pulling suspension sleeve over socks to skin level
Uneven steps	Long prosthetic step and short step with other leg	Pain on weightbearing from poorly fitting socket Sensitive residual limb	Client is afraid of putting weight on the prosthesis
Circumduction	Prosthesis swings out to the side on swing returning to the midline on stance	Prosthesis too long Inadequate suspension	Client has difficulty bending knee and hip

Copyright BJM Enterprises.

- Patient displays a FHP and an increased thoracic kyphosis
♦ Prosthetic requirements
  - Ms. Hooper's prosthesis will include the following components:
    ■ Socket: Patellar tendon bearing with a gel liner
    ■ Suspension: Over-the-knee sleeve
    ■ Pylon: Standard lightweight connecting pylon
    ■ Foot: Lightweight single axis dynamic response foot
  - Static evaluation of the fit of the transtibial prosthesis was initially performed (Table 10-2)

♦ Range of motion (goniometry)
  • All UE joints: WNL
  • All LLE joints: WNL except dorsiflexion=0 to 10 degrees
  • Bilateral hip extension=0 to 5 degrees
  • Right knee ROM=0 to 135 degrees
♦ Self-care and home management
  • Independent in upper and lower body grooming and dressing
  • Transfers independently to the shower using a shower chair
  • Requires help with home management
♦ Work, community, and leisure integration or reintegration
  • Presently on leave of absence from work
  • Has returned to community work at her church

EVALUATION: PHASE 3

Her history previously outlined indicated that she is a 63-year old black American female salesperson, non-smoker, and overweight. She has high BP, ASO, and adult onset diabetes. She is status post a transtibial amputation of her RLE 3 months ago. She has a well-healed scar and a cylindrical residual limb. She has circulatory changes, decreased muscle strength in her RLE, decreased ROM, and decreased endurance. Mrs. Hooper is alert and aware and was active prior to the onset of the most recent problem. Her potential for prosthetic fitting appears good.

DIAGNOSIS: PHASE 3

Mrs. Hooper is a patient who underwent a transtibial amputation of her RLE 3 months ago and still has pain in the limb. She has impaired: aerobic capacity; anthropometric characteristics; circulation; peripheral nerve integrity; gait, locomotion, and balance; joint integrity and mobility; muscle performance; posture; and range of motion. She is functionally limited in self-care and home management and in work, community, and leisure actions, tasks, and activities. Mrs. Hooper's prosthetic requirements will include a patellar tendon bearing prosthesis with a gel liner, an over the knee sleeve, a standard lightweight connecting pylon, and a lightweight single axis dynamic response foot. These findings are consistent with placement in Pattern J: Impaired Motor Function, Muscle Performance, Range of Motion, Gait, Locomotion, and Balance Associated With Amputation. These impairments, functional limitations, and prosthetic requirements will be addressed in determining the prognosis and the plan of care.

PROGNOSIS AND PLAN OF CARE: PHASE 3

Over the course of the visits, the following mutually established outcomes have been determined:
♦ Ability to perform physical actions, tasks, and activities related to self-care is improved
♦ Care is coordinated with patient, family, and other professionals
♦ Case is managed throughout episode of care
♦ Integumentary integrity is improved
♦ Knowledge of behaviors that foster healthy habits is gained
♦ Placement needs are determined
♦ Risk factors are reduced
♦ Risk of secondary impairments is reduced
♦ ROM is increased
♦ Standing balance is improved
♦ Stress is decreased

To achieve these outcomes, the appropriate interventions for this patient are determined. These will include: coordination, communication, and documentation; patient/client-related instruction; therapeutic exercise; functional training in self-care and home management; and functional training in work, community, and leisure integration or reintegration.

Based on the diagnosis and prognosis, Mrs. Hooper is expected to require 10 to 15 visits of daily prosthetic training followed by three to five visits over a 2-week period then long-term follow-up through the amputee clinic.

INTERVENTIONS: PHASE 3

RATIONALE FOR SELECTED INTERVENTIONS

Therapeutic Exercise

The prosthetic training program should start in a safe and controlled environment (parallel bars) and incorporate activities that require the person to integrate the prosthesis into functional activities.[35] The ability to accept weight on the prosthesis has been shown to be an important indicator for successful prosthetic ambulation.[36] Initial training is performed in the closed environment and emphasizes balance on the prosthesis. Once the patient has developed confidence, balance, and good prosthetic control, ambulation activities in an open environment is begun. Over dependence on an assistive device is discouraged to maximize prosthetic use and to promote community ambulation on all surfaces and elevations. Constant gait evaluation and interventions are done to minimize gait deviations. A high correlation exists between

Table 10-2

STATIC TRANSTIBIAL PROSTHETIC CHECKOUT

Checkout Item	What to Check	Possible Problems
Sitting:		
Is the person comfortable while sitting with the sole of the shoe flat on the floor?	Check for excessive pressure between residual limb and socket	Excessive pressure may lead to skin abrasions
Is there adequate flaring of the posterior trim line to accommodate the hamstring tendons?	Check for pressure on the hamstrings when sitting	Client will keep leg outstretched when sitting to reduce pressure
Are the tissue rolls in the popliteal area excessive?	Check the posterior wall of the socket	Too much tissue may indicate inadequate AP dimensions
Is the residual limb forced out of the socket excessively?	The stump will rise out of the socket a little when sitting	May indicate a socket that is too small The client is wearing too many socks The client has gained weight
Can the patient sit comfortably with knees flexed to at least 90 degrees without excessive pressure on knees?	The residual limb tends to move up a little when person sits Sleeve or liner need to stretch adequately to prevent excessive pressure	May push residual limb to bottom or front of socket excessively Client will keep leg outstretched to reduce pressure
Are the knees level?	The length of the shank should correspond to the other side	May lead to gait deviations
Are the color and contour of the prosthesis similar to the sound leg?	The finished prosthesis should match the other leg	Poor cosmesis may lead to non-wearing
Standing:		
Does the client have any pain or discomfort when bearing weight on the prosthesis?	Check limb/socket interface, particularly bony prominences	Excessive pressures may lead to skin problems
Is the knee stable? Does the patient have to resist to prevent the knee from being forced into flexion or extension?	PTB socket aligned in 5 to 8 degrees of flexion	Too much flexion will lead to counter knee extension and anterior distal pressure Too little flexion may lead to end bearing
Is the pelvis level when the patient bears his or her weight equally on both feet?	Palpate the iliac crests with client standing evenly on both feet	A long or short prosthesis will lead to gait deviations
Is the pylon vertical when weight is borne on the prosthesis?	On weightbearing, check the pylon connecting the socket and foot	May see medial and lateral leaning pylon on gait deviations
Does the sole of the shoe maintain even contact with the floor?	Check that the foot is fully on the floor on weightbearing	May lead to excessive knee pressures on gait
Are tissue rolls around the trim line of the socket or the cuff suspension minimal?	Check the edges of the residual limb at the socket line	Excessive rolls may indicate a socket that is too tight proximally
Is there gapping at the brim of the socket?	Check the edges of the residual limb at the socket line	Gapping may indicate a socket that is too large proximally

continued

Table 10-2 (continued)		
STATIC TRANSTIBIAL PROSTHETIC CHECKOUT		
Checkout Item	*What to Check*	*Possible Problems*
Is there evidence of total contact?	If the person has a Pelite liner, total contact may be checked by putting a little ball of playdough at the end of the socket; the client stands and bears weight; and the displacement of the playdough indicates the extent of total contact If the person is wearing a gel liner, palpate the distal residual limb after the gel liner has been donned and before inserting into the socket	Too little contact may cause distal end skin problems and a stretching pain Too much may cause excessive pressure at the end of the stump and pressure pain
If wearing a gel liner, does it fit properly and smoothly?	The liner should be smooth, free of wrinkles, worn areas, or holes	Gel liners have a limited life span Wrinkles, holes, or worn areas create skin abrasions
Is suspension maintained when patient lifts leg off the floor?	Check that there is not excessive movement of the prosthesis away from limb when weight is removed On weightbearing, make a small pencil mark at the anterior socket brim or, if sleeve or shuttle lock suspension, place a finger lightly at edge of socket	Too much movement between residual limb and socket creates abrasions and may lead to toe drag on swing
Does the sleeve extend over residual limb socks (if worn)?	The sleeve should be in direct contact with the skin for at least 2 inches above any socks	Failure to have skin to sleeve contact will lead to loss of suspension and pistoning

Adapted from May BJ. *Amputations and Prosthetics: A Case Study Approach.* 2nd ed. Philadelphia, Pa: FA Davis Co; 2002.

gait deviations and energy expenditure during prosthetic ambulation.[37]

An aerobic exercise program should be designed to help improve exercise tolerance and endurance and to prepare the patient for the energy demands of prosthetic ambulation.[32]

Functional Training in Self-Care and Home Management/Functional Training in Work, Community, and Leisure Integration or Reintegration

ADL training with the prosthesis on (ie, picking up objects from the floor, stepping over obstacles, descending and rising from the floor, curb negotiation, carrying objects) should be incorporated in the prosthetic training program to maximize independence. Ambulation and elevation training on all surfaces is required to prepare the patient for a return to her pre-amputation activities.

Prescription, Application, and, as Appropriate, Fabrication of Devices and Equipment

The patient will have a patellar tendon bearing prosthesis with a standard lightweight connecting pylon with a gel liner. The suspension will be an over-the-knee sleeve. The foot will be a lightweight single axis dynamic response foot allowing for anterior/posterior movements.

COORDINATION, COMMUNICATION, AND DOCUMENTATION

Communication will occur with Mrs. Hooper. Education regarding her current condition, impairments, and functional limitations will be discussed. A plan of care will be developed and discussed with the patient. All elements of the patient's management will be documented. Collaboration with the prosthetic center will occur. The patient and family need to be involved in decision making about the type of prosthesis and prosthetic training.

PATIENT/CLIENT-RELATED INSTRUCTION

In addition to all previous instruction, the patient will be instructed in the care of the prosthesis and will be made aware of warning signs for poor socket fit due to weight or residual limb size changes. In addition, the following will also be included in her instructional program:

- ♦ Techniques for inspection of the residual limb for sores or problems before and after wearing the prosthesis
- ♦ Instructions in donning the prosthesis
- ♦ Instructions in how to prevent wrinkles and creases in gel liner
- ♦ The techniques to clean the prosthetic socket and gel liner each night
- ♦ Ways to adjust the fit of the prosthesis with socks external to the gel liner as the residual limb shrinks
- ♦ The need to contact the prosthetist for regular prosthetic maintenance

THERAPEUTIC EXERCISE

- ♦ Aerobic capacity/endurance conditioning
  - Gait and locomotor endurance training
  - Increased workload over time
  - Progressive walking program
- ♦ Balance, coordination, and agility training
  - Weight shifting and balance activities with the prosthesis in a closed environment (eg, parallel bars)
    - Weight shift side to side
    - Weight shift forward and backward
    - Reaching for objects held in different positions
    - Kicking a softball, alternating feet
    - Sit to stand using hands, progressing to no support
    - Standing balance on prosthesis without hand support for a few seconds
    - Obstacle course
- ♦ Body mechanics and postural stabilization
  - Using a mirror, work on postural alignment with altered center of mass
- ♦ Flexibility exercises
  - Stretching exercises should be done after warming up, using a slow and steady stretch accompanied by deep breathing, and building hold up to 30 to 60 seconds
  - Increase flexibility of:
    - Left ankle dorsiflexors
    - Right hip and knee flexors
    - Right hip abductors, adductors, internal and external rotators
- ♦ Gait and locomotion training
  - Gait training with prosthesis in/out of parallel bars

- Forward walking
- Backward walking
- Side stepping both directions
- Gait training with cane
- Negotiating stairs and curbs
- Walking on different surfaces
- Picking objects up from floor
- Catching and throwing a ball
- ♦ Strength, power, and endurance training
  - Resistive exercises as tolerated for both LEs using elastic bands or weights as part of the home program.
  - Carrying objects of different weights
  - Core strengthening
  - Advanced activities
    - Pickup objects from floor
    - Getting up from the floor
    - Catching and throwing a ball
    - Stepping over obstacles

FUNCTIONAL TRAINING IN SELF-CARE AND HOME MANAGEMENT

- ♦ Self-care
  - Independent mobility with prosthesis
  - Independent in donning and doffing the prosthesis
  - Skin inspection of residual limb
  - Independent skin care
- ♦ Injury prevention or reduction
  - Awareness of safety precautions involved with self-care
  - Safety awareness training during self-care

FUNCTIONAL TRAINING IN WORK, COMMUNITY, AND LEISURE INTEGRATION OR REINTEGRATION

- ♦ Functional training programs
- ♦ Simulated environments and tasks
- ♦ Task adaptation
- ♦ Task training
- ♦ Work conditioning

PRESCRIPTION, APPLICATION, AND, AS APPOPRIATE, FABRICATION OF DEVICES AND EQUIPMENT

- ♦ Continue to monitor and check transtibial prosthesis and fit (see Table 10-2)

ANTICIPATED GOALS AND EXPECTED OUTCOMES

◆ Impact on pathology/pathophysiology
- Pain is eliminated.

◆ Impact on impairments
- Aerobic capacity is increased.
- Balance is independent in sitting and standing.
- Endurance is improved to standing with walker for 90 seconds.
- Energy expenditure per unit of work is decreased.
- Exercise tolerance is improved to 45 minutes.
- Gait and locomotion are improved with patient ambulating with walker for 200 feet.
- Improved weightbearing on the prosthetic leg.
- Muscle performance, including strength, power, and endurance, is 4+-5/5.
- Postural awareness is improved so that lateral lean is eliminated.

◆ Impact on functional limitations
- Ability to perform physical actions, tasks, and activities related to self-care and home management is improved.
- Ability to perform physical actions, tasks, and activities related to work, community, and leisure and leisure integration or reintegration is improved.
- Able to ambulate independently with prosthesis and walker outside the home including elevation activities.
- Performance of ADL with devices is increased including donning and caring for prosthesis.
- Performance of and independence in IADL with or without devices and equipment are increased.

◆ Risk reduction/prevention
- Risk factors and risk of secondary impairments are reduced.
- Safety is achieved in all activities.

◆ Impact on health, wellness, and fitness
- Behaviors that promote healthy nutrition, physical activity, and wellness are promoted.
- Resumes pre-amputation level of activity.

◆ Impact on societal resources
- Documentation will occur throughout the patient management and across all settings and follows APTA's *Guidelines for Physical Therapy Documentation.*[25]

◆ Patient/client satisfaction
- Care is coordinated with patient, family, and other professionals.
- Case is managed throughout the episode of care.
- Collaboration and coordination occurs with the prosthetic center.

- Decision making is enhanced regarding patient health and use of health care resources by patient and family.
- Interdisciplinary collaboration occurs through case conferences.
- Patient and family knowledge and awareness of the diagnosis, prognosis, interventions, and anticipated goals and expected outcomes are increased.

REEXAMINATION

Reexamination is performed throughout the episode of care.

DISCHARGE

Mrs. Hooper is discharged from physical therapy after completing phases 1 (5 days), 2 (10 days), and 3 (3 weeks) of physical therapy and attainment of her goals and expectations. These sessions have covered her entire episode of service. She is discharged because she has achieved her goals and expected outcomes.

Case Study #2: Above-Knee Amputation

Mr. Kenneth Jardin is a 20-year-old male who underwent a left transfemoral (above the knee, 14-inch bone length) amputation secondary to a motor vehicle accident.

PHASE 2: POST HOSPITAL PHASE

PHYSICAL THERAPIST EXAMINATION: PHASE 2

Mr. Jardin has been referred to an outpatient rehabilitation center 10 days post amputation. (Mr. Jardin was not seen for physical therapy during Phase 1, the inhospital, postoperative phase.)

HISTORY: PHASES 2 AND 3

◆ General demographics: Mr. Kenneth Jardin is a 20-year-old white male who attends a local university. He is a sophomore attending college on a baseball scholarship. Mr. Jardin is right-hand dominant.

◆ Social history: Mr. Jardin is single. He is the oldest of three children. His father is a senior vice president of a bank, and his mother is an attorney.

- Employment/work: Mr. Jardin is a college student who had been involved in college baseball and other sports.
- Living environment: Mr. Jardin shares an apartment with two other college students. His apartment is on the second floor and requires negotiation of 13 steps with railings on both sides. His family lives about 4 hours away.
- General health status
  - General health perception: Mr. Jardin reported that the status of his health prior to the accident was excellent.
  - Physical function: Prior to the onset of the current problem, Mr. Jardin was independent in all functional activities.
  - Psychological function: He was well-adjusted prior to amputation. He is now accepting of his amputation, but he is apprehensive of his prosthetic replacement. He is concerned about the effect that the amputation will have on his body image, his future, and about whether he will be able to return to his previous lifestyle.
  - Role function: Student, son.
  - Social function: He was involved in sports, especially baseball prior to the amputation. He was active in college social life.
- Social/health habits: Mr. Jardin is a non-smoker and drinks beer socially. He is active in fitness and sports activities.
- Family history: His mother has HTN, and his father has spinal stenosis.
- Medical/surgical history: Mr. Jardin reports only sports-related injuries, including chronic ankle and shoulder sprains.
- Prior hospitalizations: Mr. Jardin was never hospitalized.
- Preexisting medical and other health-related conditions: None.
- Current condition(s)/chief complaint(s): Mr. Jardin has undergone a transfemoral amputation of his LLE as a result of a motorcycle accident 10 days ago. Mr. Jardin reports that the accident occurred on the highway when he was returning from a weekend at home. He reports that he lost control of the motorcycle while trying to avoid an oncoming car and ran into a guard rail. Mr. Jardin complains of slight pain at the incision site. He also complains of feeling the absent limb.
- Functional status and activity level: Mr. Jardin is ambulating independently with crutches with the residual limb encased in a removable rigid dressing suspended by a Silesian band around the waist. He reports that he tires if he walks more than two blocks. Mr. Jardin is independent in his personal care.
- Medications: He had taken Darvocet as needed for pain but now uses only OTC pain medication. He is not taking any other medication.
- Other clinical tests: None.

SYSTEMS REVIEW: PHASE 2

- Cardiovascular/pulmonary
  - BP: 110/65 mmHg
  - Edema: No edema noted in residual limb secondary to rigid dressing
  - HR: 68 bpm
  - RR: 14 bpm
- Integumentary
  - Residual limb healing well; incision at anterior aspect of distal end of residual limb
  - Skin color: WNL
  - Skin integrity: No drainage; incision healing well
- Musculoskeletal
  - Gross range of motion
    - RLE and both UEs: WFL
    - Hip motion LLE slightly limited in extension
  - Gross strength
    - Both UEs and RLE: WFL
    - Slight limitation in L hip extension as compared to RLE; Hip flexion, abduction and adduction WNL
  - Gross symmetry: Slight asymmetry
  - Height: 6'2" (1.93 m)
  - Weight: 188 lbs (82.27 kg)
- Neuromuscular
  - Balance: Independent sitting and standing
  - Locomotion, transfers, and transitions
    - Stand pivot transfers: Independent
    - Gait: Independent with axillary crutches on all surfaces
- Communication, affect, cognition, language, and learning style
  - Communication and affect: WNL
  - Cognition: WNL
  - Learning preferences: Mixed style learner

TESTS AND MEASURES: PHASE 2

An individual wearing a removable rigid dressing must wear it 24 hours a day 7 days a week. It may be removed briefly for wound inspection and necessary measurements but must be reapplied quickly.

- Aerobic capacity/endurance
  - Increased energy expenditure noted per unit of work
- Anthropometric characteristics
  - BMI=24.1 (this is considered WNL based on Centers for Disease Control and Prevention)[17]

- Bone and tissue length measured from greater trochanter: 35 cm to bone; 37 cm to incision (65% of the intact leg)
- Edema
  - Edema develops if rigid dressing removed for longer than 20 to 30 minutes.
  - Circumferential measurements taken at regular intervals from proximal to distal
- Shape of residual limb: Cone shaped
- Arousal, attention, and cognition
  - Alert and oriented x 3
  - Extremely motivated
- Assistive and adaptive devices
  - Using axillary crutches to ambulate
- Cranial and peripheral nerve integrity
  - PNs intact
  - Sensation WNL
- Environmental, home, and work barriers
  - Lives on the second floor of an apartment with two other college students
  - Requires negotiation of 13 steps with railings on both sides
  - Family lives about 4 hours away
- Ergonomics and body mechanics
  - Performs functional activities in a safe and efficient manner
- Gait, locomotion, and balance
  - Ambulating independently with axillary crutches on all surfaces for at least two blocks
  - Standing balance good on RLE
- Integumentary integrity
  - Wire sutures in place
  - Incision closed, no drainage noted
  - Temperature: Warm to palpation
- Joint integrity and mobility
  - Slight hypermobility in the right ankle
- Motor function
  - Performs functional activities in a coordinated manner
  - Good dexterity and agility
- Muscle performance
  - MMT revealed:
    - UEs and RLE: WFL
    - LLE
      - Extension=4+/5
      - Flexion=4+/5
      - Abduction=4/5
      - Adduction=4/5
- Orthotic, protective, and supportive devices
  - Rigid dressing in place to residual limb

- Pain
  - NPS (0=no pain and 10=worst possible pain) revealed 1/10 with medications and 2/10 without medications
  - Intermittent sensation of burning/itching to left ankle and knee
- Posture
  - Slightly increased lumbar lordotic curve and anterior pelvic tilt
- Prosthetic requirements
  - Transfemoral prosthesis with appropriate ankle foot assembly, shank, knee unit, socket and suspension
- Range of motion
  - Goniometric measurements revealed:
    - All UE and RLE joints: WNL
    - LLE hip extension 0 to 5 degrees, all other LLE motions: WFL
- Self-care and home management
  - Independent with bed mobility
  - Independent in grooming and dressing
  - Ambulating two blocks independently with axillary crutches before tiring
- Work, community, and leisure integration or reintegration.
  - Sophomore in college planning to return to school on a part time basis with eventual return to full-time studies
  - To be referred for vocational counseling
  - To return to the gym and some form of sports activity
  - Patient's family and friends very supportive

EVALUATION: PHASE 2

His history previously outlined indicated that he is a 20-year-old white male college sophomore, non-smoker, and casual drinker who has just undergone a transfemoral amputation of his LLE as a result of a MVA. He has impaired integumentary integrity, muscle performance, pain, posture, and ROM in the residual limb. Mr. Jardin is alert and aware and was active prior to the onset of the most recent problem. His potential for eventual prosthetic rehabilitation appears good. It is critically important that plans for continued therapy and prosthetic evaluation be initiated as soon as Mr. Jardin's condition allows.

DIAGNOSIS: PHASE 2

Mr. Jardin has undergone a left transfemoral amputation secondary to a MVA, and he has slight pain in the residual limb. He has minimal impairment of aerobic capacity/endurance; anthropometric characteristics; gait, locomotion, and balance; joint integrity and mobility; muscle performance; posture; and range of motion. He is functionally limited in work, community, and leisure actions, tasks, and activities. He is in need of assistive, protective, and prosthetic devices and equipment. These impairments, functional limitations, and device and equipment requirements will then be addressed in determining the prognosis and the plan of care. These findings are consistent with placement in Pattern J: Impaired Motor Function, Muscle Performance, Range of Motion, Gait, Locomotion, and Balance Associated With Amputation. These impairments, functional limitations, and devices and equipment requirements will be addressed in determining the prognosis and the plan of care.

PROGNOSIS AND PLAN OF CARE: PHASE 2

Over the course of the visits, the following mutually established outcomes have been determined:
- Care is coordinated with patient, family, and other professionals
- Case is managed throughout episode of care
- Endurance is improved
- Integumentary integrity is improved
- Knowledge of behaviors that foster healthy habits is gained
- Muscle strength is improved
- Pain is decreased
- Risk factors are reduced
- Risk of secondary impairments is reduced
- ROM is increased
- Stress is decreased

To achieve these outcomes, the appropriate interventions for this patient are determined. These will include: coordination, communication, and documentation; patient/client-related instruction; therapeutic exercise; functional training in self-care and home management; and prescription, application, and, as appropriate, fabrication of devices and equipment.

Based on the diagnosis and prognosis, Mr. Jardin is expected to require between six to nine visits over a 7- to 10-day period for this phase. Mr. Jardin is in good physical health and highly motivated.

INTERVENTIONS: PHASE 2

RATIONALE FOR SELECTED INTERVENTIONS

Therapeutic Exercise

Normal residual limb hip ROM and strength are important for future prosthetic use. A major contributory factor to prosthetic gait deviations and increased energy expenditure is a residual limb with decreased mobility and strength.[38] Following suture removal and residual limb healing, resistive exercise including dynamic stump exercises are indicated. In addition, strengthening exercises for the trunk and RLE will further contribute to successful and efficient prosthetic function. Exercises that challenge postural control should also be included.[32] An aerobic exercise program is indicated to improve general endurance to help the patient resume his pre-amputation lifestyle. The aerobic exercise program should be designed to help improve exercise tolerance and endurance and to prepare the patient for the energy demands of prosthetic ambulation.[32] General fitness level has been highly correlated between endurance and LE prosthetic function.[39] Barring any complications, the patient should be ready for prosthetic fitting in 8 to 10 weeks post surgery. Patient education for residual limb hygiene, suture line mobilization, and shaping is essential during this time to assist in the preparation for prosthetic fitting.[1]

Prescription, Application, and, as Appropriate, Fabrication of Devices and Equipment

Residual limb edema control is important in this phase of rehabilitation. Edema increases pain and interferes with suture line healing in the residual limb.[33] This patient has been fitted with a removable rigid dressing that he will wear until fitted with a prosthesis. Rigid dressings may be fabricated of plaster of paris or some form of thermo plastics. Depending on the type of dressing, a new dressing may be fabricated as the residual limb shrinks or the dressing may incorporate straps that allow for changing residual limb size. Assistive devices needed for ambulation are provided to the patient.

COORDINATION, COMMUNICATION, AND DOCUMENTATION

Communication will occur with Mr. Jardin. Education regarding his current condition, impairments, functional limitations, and device and equipment requirements will be discussed. The plan of care will be discussed with the patient. All elements of the patient's management will be documented. Early communication with the physician and collaboration with the rehabilitation center will occur. The patient and family need to be involved in planning for prosthetic evaluation.

Finances and future plans will be discussed. As a college student, Mr. Jardin may be eligible for support from the Division of Vocational Rehabilitation and should be referred for evaluation. Depending on his preinjury college major, he may or may not need to reevaluate career goals. As an athlete, he needs to be made aware of the athletic program for persons with amputations of the American

Orthotic and Prosthetic Association (www.oandp.org) and of the International Paralympics Organization (www.paralympic.org).

PATIENT/CLIENT-RELATED INSTRUCTION

The patient will be instructed in care of the residual limb including the incision, care of the rigid dressing, and prevention of contractures. Risk factors will be discussed. A consult to a psychologist or other professional counselor will be made if needed to discuss changes in body image and concerns with sexuality. There are also amputee support groups that may provide emotional assistance. The Amputee Coalition of America (www.aca.org) provides many resources for individuals to adjust to life with an amputation. The patient will receive education concerning the need for a prosthetic rehabilitation program that is to begin in a timely manner.

THERAPEUTIC EXERCISE

- ◆ Balance, coordination, and agility training
  - Balance on right leg
  - Balance two hand support, then one hand support
  - Throwing/catching a ball in long sit and short sit
  - Progress to standing position as tolerated
- ◆ Body mechanics and postural stabilization
  - If mirror available, work on postural alignment with altered center of mass
  - Maintain right hip in neutral
- ◆ Flexibility exercises
  - Left hip flexors
- ◆ Gait and locomotion training
  - Gait training with crutches level surfaces increasing distance
  - Gait training on stairs and inclines
- ◆ Strength, power, and endurance training
  - Active exercises for left hip extensors, abductors, and internal rotators
  - Active hip extension sidelying on right
  - Isometric exercises for gluts
  - Isometric exercises for residual limb musculature using visualization of knee flexion and extension
  - Dynamic stump exercises
    - ▪ Hip adduction with patient sidelying with stool. Push down on stool (covered with towel) into adduction
    - ▪ Hip extension in supine with a small roll under the residual limb
  - Resistive exercises, as tolerated, for RLE and UEs using elastic bands or weights
  - Weightbearing exercises as tolerated through residual limb

- PNF exercises to UEs and intact LE
- Seated push ups
- Dip exercises
- Core strengthening

FUNCTIONAL TRAINING IN SELF-CARE AND HOME MANAGEMENT

- ◆ Self-care
  - Skin inspection of residual limb
  - Monitoring rigid dressing fit
  - Independent mobility with assistive device
  - Instruction in bathing and positioning
  - Instruction regarding removal and replacement of the rigid dressing for bathing
  - Instruction regarding the signs and symptoms associated with infection
- ◆ Injury prevention or reduction
  - Awareness of safety precautions involved with self-care
  - Injury protection while using crutches
  - Safety awareness training during self-care

PRESCRIPTION, APPLICATION, AND, AS APPROPRIATE, FABRICATION OF DEVICES AND EQUIPMENT

- ◆ Assistive devices: Crutches
- ◆ Supportive devices: Removable rigid dressing

ANTICIPATED GOALS AND EXPECTED OUTCOMES

- ◆ Impact on pathology/pathophysiology
  - Pain is decreased to 1/10 with medication and 2/10 without medication.
- ◆ Impact on impairments
  - Balance is independent in sitting and standing.
  - Gait and locomotion are improved so that he is independent with crutches for three to four blocks.
  - Muscle performance, including strength, power, and endurance, is increased so that L hip is WFL.
  - Postural awareness is improved with decreased lumbar lordosis and anterior pelvic tilt.
- ◆ Impact on functional limitations
  - Ability to perform physical actions, tasks, and activities related to self-care and home management is independent.
  - Ability to perform physical actions, tasks, and activities related to work, community, and leisure and leisure integration or reintegration is independent.
  - Functional independence in ADL.

- Level of supervision required for task performance is decreased so patient is independent.
- Performance of ADL with devices is independent.

◆ Risk reduction/prevention
- Risk factors and risk of secondary impairments are reduced.
- Safety is improved so patient is independent on level surfaces.
- Self-management of symptoms is improved.

◆ Impact on health, wellness, and fitness
- Behaviors that promote healthy nutrition, physical activity, and wellness are promoted.
- Physical capacity is increased.
- Physical function is improved.

◆ Impact on societal resources
- Documentation will occur throughout the patient management and across all settings and follows APTA's *Guidelines for Physical Therapy Documentation.*[25]

◆ Patient/client satisfaction
- Care is coordinated with patient, family, and other professionals.
- Case is managed throughout the episode of care.
- Collaboration and coordination will occur with the rehabilitation center.
- Decision making is enhanced regarding patient health and use of health care resources by patient and family.
- Interdisciplinary collaboration will occur through case conferences.
- Patient and family knowledge and awareness of the diagnosis, prognosis, interventions, and anticipated goals and expected outcomes are increased.
- Placement needs will be determined.

PHASE 3: PROSTHETIC EVALUATION AND TRAINING

PHYSICAL THERAPIST EXAMINATION: PHASE 3

Mr. Jardin has been referred to the prosthetist for evaluation for prosthetic fitting approximately 10 weeks after amputation.

SYSTEMS REVIEW: PHASE 3

◆ Cardiovascular/pulmonary
- BP: 110/65 mmHg
- Edema: None present
- HR: 68 bpm

- RR: 14 bpm
◆ Integumentary
- Presence of scar formation
  - Fishmouth incision with distal suture line
  - Incision well healed
  - Scar mobile and non tender
- Skin color: WNL
- Skin integrity: Good

◆ Musculoskeletal
- Gross range of motion
  - Both UEs and RLE: WFL
  - L hip: WFL
- Gross strength both UEs and RLE: WFL
- Gross symmetry: Slight asymmetry
- Height: 6'2" (1.93 m)
- Weight: 188 lbs (82.27 kg)

◆ Neuromuscular
- Balance: Independent sitting and standing
- Locomotion, transfers, and transitions
  - Transfers independent
  - Gait: Independent ambulation with crutches

◆ Communication, affect, cognition, language, and learning style
- Communication and affect: WNL
- Cognition: WNL
- Learning preferences: Mixed learning styles

TESTS AND MEASURES: PHASE 3

◆ Aerobic capacity/endurance
- Increased energy expenditure per unit of work

◆ Anthropometric characteristics
- BMI=24.1 (this is considered normal based on Centers for Disease Control and Prevention)[17]
- Edema: None observed
- Shape of residual limb: Cone shaped

◆ Arousal, attention, and cognition
- Alert and oriented x 3
- Extremely motivated

◆ Assistive and adaptive devices
- Using axillary crutches when ambulating

◆ Circulation
- All residual limb pulses WNL

◆ Cranial and peripheral nerve integrity
- PNs intact
- Sensation: WNL

◆ Environmental, home, and work barriers
- Lives on the second floor of an apartment with two other college students
- Requires negotiation of 13 steps with railings on both sides

- Family lives about 4 hours away
♦ Ergonomics and body mechanics
  - Performs functional activities in a safe and efficient manner
♦ Gait, locomotion, and balance
  - Ambulating independently with axillary crutches on level surfaces, stairs and inclines
  - Independent standing balance with axillary crutches
♦ Integumentary integrity
  - Scar well healed and mobile
  - Temperature: Warm to palpation
♦ Joint integrity and mobility
  - Slight hypermobility in the right ankle
♦ Motor function
  - Performs functional activities in a coordinated manner
  - Good dexterity and agility
♦ Muscle performance
  - MMT for both UEs and LEs: WNL
♦ Orthotic, protective, and supportive devices
  - Residual limb is encased in a rigid dressing
♦ Pain
  - NPS (0=no pain and 10=worst possible pain) revealed 0/10 without medications
♦ Posture
  - Slightly increased lumbar lordotic curve and anterior pelvic tilt
♦ Prosthetic requirements
  - The prosthesis probably will include:
    - Socket: IC socket with flexible inner socket and rigid frame.
    - Suspension: Suction (better for patients who will engage in sports activities)
    - Knee: Either a multiaxis standard knee or a hydraulic knee mechanism (computerized knee mechanisms are not always used with the first prosthesis)
    - Foot: Multiaxis dynamic response foot
♦ Range of motion (goniometry)
  - All UE and LE joints: WNL
♦ Self-care and home management
  - Ambulating independently with axillary crutches
  - Independent in upper and lower body grooming and dressing
  - Transfers independently to the shower using a shower chair
♦ Work, community, and leisure integration or reintegration
  - Sophomore in college planning to return to school on a part-time basis with eventual return to full-time studies

- To be referred to vocational counselor
- To return to the gym and sports on a modified level
- Independent in driving automatic transmission automobile
- Patient's family and friends very supportive

EVALUATION: PHASE 3

His history previously outlined indicated that he is a 20-year-old white male college sophomore, non-smoker, and casual drinker who has just undergone a transfemoral amputation of his LLE. He has minimal impairments at this time. Mr. Jardin is alert and aware and was active prior to the onset of the most recent problem. His potential for eventual prosthetic rehabilitation appears excellent. It is critically important that plans for therapy continue in order for Mr. Jardin to return to his activities as his condition allows.

DIAGNOSIS: PHASE 3

Mr. Jardin is a patient who has undergone a traumatic transfemoral amputation of his LLE. He has impaired: aerobic capacity/endurance; gait, locomotion, and balance; joint integrity; and posture. He is functionally limited in work, community, and leisure actions, tasks, and activities. He is in need of assistive and prosthetic devices and equipment. Mr. Jardin's prosthetic requirements will include an above-knee prosthesis with a suction suspension with either a multiaxis standard knee or a hydraulic knee and a multiaxis dynamic response foot. These findings are consistent with placement in Pattern J: Impaired Motor Function, Muscle Performance, Range of Motion, Gait, Locomotion, and Balance Associated With Amputation. These impairments, functional limitations, and assistive and prosthetic requirements will be addressed in determining the prognosis and the plan of care.

PROGNOSIS AND PLAN OF CARE: PHASE 3

Over the course of the visits, the following mutually established outcomes have been determined:
♦ Care is coordinated with patient, family, and other professionals
♦ Case is managed throughout episode of care
♦ Endurance is improved
♦ Knowledge of behaviors that foster healthy habits is gained
♦ Placement needs are determined
♦ Risk factors are reduced
♦ Risk of secondary impairments is reduced
♦ Stress is decreased

To achieve these outcomes, the appropriate interventions for this patient are determined. These will include: coordination, communication, and documentation; patient/client-related instruction; therapeutic exercise; functional training in work, community, and leisure integration or reintegration; and prescription, application, and, as appropriate, fabrication of devices and equipment.

Based on the diagnosis and prognosis, Mr. Jardin is expected to require between 10 to 15 visits over the course of 14 to 21 days. Mr. Jardin is in good physical health and highly motivated.

INTERVENTIONS: PHASE 3

RATIONALE FOR SELECTED INTERVENTIONS

Therapeutic Exercise

The prosthetic training program should start in a safe and controlled environment (parallel bars) and incorporate activities required for integration of the prosthesis into functional activities.[35] Pre-ambulation exercises to promote prosthetic knee control in the stance and swing phases of gait are used to improve safety and efficiency for prosthetic ambulation.[40] The ability to extend the residual limb hip and progress the pelvis and trunk over the prosthetic foot ensures prosthetic knee stability during the stance phase of gait. Ambulation progression in an open environment without an assistive device is indicated to improve overall function. Yigiter and associates[35] in a study of individuals with transfemoral amputations suggested that prosthetic training using PNF was more effective in improving weightbearing and gait than other traditional approaches. Treadmill walking at graded speeds has also been shown to improve ambulation function.[41] Constant evaluation and intervention for gait deviations is done to minimize habitual use of these deviations. There is a high correlation between gait deviations and energy expenditure during prosthetic ambulation.[37]

Functional Training in Work, Community, and Leisure Integration or Reintegration

ADL training with the prosthesis on (ie, picking up objects from the floor, stepping over obstacles, descending and rising from the floor, curb negotiation, carrying objects) should be incorporated in the prosthetic training program to maximize independence. Ambulation and elevation training on all surfaces is required to prepare the patient for a return to pre-amputation activities. Advanced activities such as running, jumping, and sports participation should be introduced as appropriate.

Prescription, Application, and, as Appropriate, Fabrication of Devices and Equipment

The patient has been fitted with an above-knee prosthesis with a Hangar Comfort Flex Socket, which is an ischial containment socket best suited for more active individuals. The suspension is suction. The knee is a computerized multiaxis knee providing both stance and swing phase control. The foot is a multiaxis dynamic response foot.

COORDINATION, COMMUNICATION, AND DOCUMENTATION

Communication will occur with Mr. Jardin. Education regarding his current condition, and functional limitations will be discussed. The plan of care will be discussed with the patient. All elements of the patient's management will be documented. Collaboration with prosthetist will occur. The patient and family need to be involved in decision making about type of prosthesis and prosthetic training.

Finances and future plans will be discussed. As a college student, Ken may be eligible for support from the Division of Vocational Rehabilitation and should be referred for evaluation. Depending on his pre injury college major, he may or may not need to reevaluate career goals. As an athlete, he needs to be made aware of the athletic program for persons with amputations of the American Orthotic and Prosthetic Association (www.oandp.org) and of the International Paralympics organization (www.paralympic.org).

PATIENT/CLIENT-RELATED INSTRUCTION

The patient will be instructed in proper residual limb wrapping and care of LLE. Instruction will be given in proper footwear, shoe fitting, and foot care. Risk factors will be discussed. The patient will receive education concerning types of prostheses and prosthetic training. Other instruction will include the need for:
- Inspecting the residual limb for sores or problems before and after wearing the prosthesis
- Contacting the prosthetist for regular prosthetic maintenance, especially as initial residual limb shrinkage occurs
- Cleaning the prosthetic socket each night

THERAPEUTIC EXERCISE
- Balance, coordination, and agility training
    - Weight shifting and balance activities with and without the prosthesis in a closed environment (eg, parallel bars)
        - Weight shift side to side in goal-oriented activities
        - Weight shift forward and backward in goal-oriented activities

- Flexing and extending prosthetic knee in standing to gain knee control
- Reaching for objects held in different positions to facilitate weight shifting
- Kicking a softball, alternating feet
- Balancing while turning head and trunk to one side and then to the other side
- Sit to stand using hands, progressing to no support
- Sit to stand from different heights and surfaces
- Standing balance on prosthesis without hand support for a few seconds
- Obstacle course
- Rhythmic stabilization standing
- Standing balance on dynamic surfaces: cushion, foam roller

♦ Body mechanics and postural stabilization
  - If mirror available, work on postural alignment with altered center of mass
♦ Flexibility exercises
  - Maintain ROM of:
    - Right hip abductors, adductors, and internal and external rotators
♦ Gait and locomotion training
  - Gait training with prosthesis in/out of parallel bars
    - Forward walking
    - Backward walking
    - Side stepping both directions
    - Ambulating on level ground without external support
    - Negotiating stairs and curbs
    - Walking on different surfaces
    - Catching and throwing a ball
    - Resisted ambulation
  - Continue to monitor and check for any gait deviations (Table 10-3)
  - Advanced activities
    - Pickup objects from floor
    - Carrying objects of different weights
    - Getting up from the floor
    - Clearing obstacles on the floor
    - Going downstairs step over step
    - Sports training activities
    - Running activities on different surfaces (eg, grass, treadmill with shock absorbing platforms)
    - Negotiating of all types of elevations
    - Jumping, hopping, and skipping activities to advance to the hop-skip running cycle

FUNCTIONAL TRAINING IN WORK, COMMUNITY, AND LEISURE INTEGRATION OR REINTEGRATION

♦ Work, community, and leisure
  - Independent mobility with prosthesis
  - Simulated environments and tasks
  - Task adaptation
  - Task training
  - Work conditioning
  - Functional training programs
♦ Injury prevention or reduction
  - Awareness of safety precautions involved in work, community, and leisure actions, tasks, and activities
  - Injury protection while ambulating without assistive devices
♦ Safety awareness training during work, community, and leisure actions, tasks, and activities

PRESCRIPTION, APPLICATION, AND, AS APPROPRIATE, FABRICATION OF DEVICES AND EQUIPMENT

♦ Continue to monitor and check transfemoral prosthesis and fit (Table 10-4)

ANTICIPATED GOALS AND EXPECTED OUTCOMES

♦ Impact on impairments
  - Balance is independent on all surfaces.
  - Endurance is WFL.
  - Gait and locomotion are improved so that patient can ambulate independently on all surfaces without an assistive device.
  - Muscle performance, including strength, power, and endurance, is WNL.
  - Postural awareness is improved with slight increase in lumbar lordosis.
  - Prosthetic fit is achieved.
  - Weightbearing status is improved so patient is able to bear full weight on prosthesis.
♦ Impact on functional limitations
  - Ability to perform physical actions, tasks, and activities related to self-care and home management is WNL.
  - Ability to perform physical actions, tasks, and activities related to work, community, and leisure integration or reintegration is WFL.
  - Independent in donning and doffing prosthesis.
  - Level of supervision required for task performance is decreased.

Table 10-3

TRANSFEMORAL GAIT DEVIATIONS

Problem	Characteristics	Prosthetic Causes	Patient Causes
Lateral bending of the trunk at mid stance	Excessive bending occurs laterally from the midline to the prosthetic side	Prosthesis may be too short Inadequate adduction forces in socket or alignment may fail to provide adequate support for the femur A high medial wall may cause the client to lean away to minimize discomfort	Patient may not have adequate balance Patient may have an abduction contracture The residual limb may be sensitive and painful A very short residual limb may fail to provide a sufficient lever arm for lateral control
Abducted gait	There is a wide-based gait with the prosthesis held away from the midline at all times	Prosthesis may be too long Inadequate adduction forces in socket or alignment may fail to provide adequate support for the femur A high medial wall may cause the patient to hold the prosthesis away to avoid ramus pressure Pelvic band (if worn) may be positioned too far away from the patient's body	May have abduction contracture Defect may be due to habit pattern if the patient is afraid to bend knee on swing
Circumducted gait	The prosthesis swings laterally in a wide area during swing phase	Prosthesis may be too long Prosthesis may have too much alignment stability or hydraulic knee flexion set too high, making it difficult to bend the knee in swing through	May not be coming over the toe of the prosthesis at terminal stance May have abduction contracture of the residual limb May be due to lack of confidence for flexing the prosthetic knee because of muscle weakness or fear of stubbing toe Defect may be due to habit pattern
Vaulting	Rising on the toe of the sound foot permits the patient to swing the prosthesis through with little knee flexion	Prosthesis may be too long There may be inadequate socket suspension Excessive stability in the alignment or some limitation of knee flexion, such as a knee lock, may cause this deficit	Vaulting is a fairly frequent habit pattern Fear of stubbing toe may cause this defect Residual limb discomfort may be a factor
Uneven arm swing	The arm on the prosthetic side is held close to the body during locomotion	None	Patient may not have developed good balance Fear and insecurity Bad habit pattern
Uneven timing	Taking steps of unequal duration and length with short stance phase on prosthesis	Improperly fitting socket may cause pain Unstable knee from poor alignment or mechanical problems	Weak hip extensors Poor training

continued

Table 10-3 (continued)

TRANSFEMORAL GAIT DEVIATIONS

Problem	*Characteristics*	*Prosthetic Causes*	*Patient Causes*
Uneven heel rise	The prosthetic heel rises quite markedly and rapidly when the knee is flexed at the beginning of swing phase	Knee joint may have too little extension resistance (rarely seen with hydraulic or computerized knees)	Patient may be using more power than necessary to force the knee into flexion
Terminal swing impact	Rapid forward movement of the shin piece allows the knee to reach maximum extension with too much force before heel strike	Knee friction is insufficient (rarely seen with hydraulic or computerized knees)	Patient may try to assure self that the knee is in full extension by deliberately and forcibly extending the residual limb
Medial or lateral whips	Whips are best observed when the patient walks away from the observer A medial whip is present when the heel travels medially on initial flexion at the beginning of swing phase A lateral whip exists when the heel moves laterally	Lateral whips may result from excessive IR of the prosthetic knee Medial whips may result from excessive ER of the knee Socket may fit too tightly, thus reflecting residual limb rotation Excessive valgus or "knock" in the prosthetic knee may contribute to this defect	Patient has donned prosthesis in IR or ER
Instability of the prosthetic knee	Knee buckles at any part of the weightbearing phase	Knee joint may be too far ahead of the trochanter-knee-ankle line Insufficient socket flexion alignment	Patient may have hip extensor weakness Severe hip flexion contracture may cause instability
Drop-off at the end of stance	There is a downward movement of the trunk as the body moves forward over the prosthesis	The socket may have been placed too far anterior in relation to the foot	None
Long prosthetic step	Patient takes a longer step with the prosthesis than with the normal	Initial flexion in the socket is insufficient when an irreducible flexion contracture is present	Poor training Bad habit
Extensive trunk extension	Patient creates an active lumbar lordosis during stance phase	Insufficient initial flexion may have been built into the socket A hip flexion contracture may exist that is not accommodated by socket alignment	Patient may have a flexion contracture that cannot be accommodated prosthetically Patient may have weak hip extensors and may be substituting with lumbar erector spinae muscle Abdominal muscles may be weak Defect may be due to habit pattern

Table 10-4		
STATIC TRANSFEMORAL PROSTHETIC CHECKOUT		
Checkout Item	What to Check	Possible Problem
Before Donning:		
Is the prosthesis as prescribed?	Compare to prescription and residual limb	Changes in prescribed components need to be justified
Is the inside of the socket smoothly finished?	Feel the inside of the socket	Skin abrasions
Do all joints move freely and smoothly?	Check the knee joint Check stance support knee by putting weight on it with the knee in slight flexion	Too stiff or loose joints may cause gait deviations Failure of stance support may lead to falls
Sitting:		
Is the socket securely on the residual limb?	Pull on the socket slightly	Suspension should be maintained in all positions
Does the length of the shin and thigh correspond to the shin and thigh of the intact leg?	Check to see that the knees are level when the client is sitting with the knees flexed to 90 degrees	A high prosthetic knee could indicate a misaligned knee joint and lead to poor swing through
Can the patient sit comfortably without burning or pinching?	Check the posterior wall particularly the pressure of the posterior brim against the seat and residual limb	A sharp posterior wall may cause sciatic nerve pressure
Is the patient able to lean forward and reach his or her shoes?	Check the anterior wall height when sitting	The anterior wall may impinge on the abdominal area
Standing:		
Does the socket fit properly and comfortably?	Ask the patient if he or she is comfortable	Areas of discomfort may cause gait deviations, non-wearing, and skin problems
Is the knee stable when weight is placed on the prosthesis?	The knee joint is initially aligned on or just behind a line dropped from the trochanter to the knee axis If the knee is in front of the line, it will be unstable	An unstable knee may lead to an insecure gait
Is the pelvis level when weight is borne evenly on both legs?	Palpate both iliac crests with the patient standing with weight equally distributed on both legs	Too long or short a prosthesis will lead to gait deviations
Does the socket maintain good contact with the residual limb on all sides as the patient shifts his or her weight?	Check the brim of the socket as the patient shifts his or her weight	Too loose or tight a socket may lead to skin abrasions and discomfort
Is there an adductor roll?	Check high in the groin for excessive tissue around the medial wall	An adductor roll may be pinched between the top of the medial wall and the pubic ramus leading to pain and an abducted gait
Is there pressure on the pubic ramus?	Ask the patient	Pain may lead to an abducted gait

Adapted from May BJ. *Amputations and Prosthetics: A Case Study Approach.* 2nd ed. Philadelphia, Pa: FA Davis Co; 2002.

- Patient is independent in community activities including driving.
- Performance of ADL and IADL with devices is independent. Able to return to gym and sports on a modified level.
- ♦ Risk reduction/prevention
  - Pressure on body tissues is reduced.
  - Residual limb is protected from trauma.
  - Risk factors and risk of secondary impairments are reduced.
  - Safety is improved.
  - Self-management of symptoms is improved.
- ♦ Impact on health, wellness, and fitness
  - Behaviors that promote healthy nutrition, physical activity, and wellness are promoted.
  - Physical capacity is increased.
  - Physical function is improved.
- ♦ Impact on societal resources
  - Documentation will occur throughout the patient management and across all settings and follows APTA's *Guidelines for Physical Therapy Documentation.*[25]
- ♦ Patient/client satisfaction
  - Care is coordinated with patient, family, and other professionals.
  - Case is managed throughout the episode of care.
  - Collaboration and coordination will occur with the prosthetic center.
  - Decision making is enhanced regarding patient health and use of health care resources by patient and family.
  - Interdisciplinary collaboration will occur through case conferences.
  - Patient and family knowledge and awareness of the diagnosis, prognosis, interventions, and anticipated goals and expected outcomes are increased.
  - Placement needs will be determined.
  - Sense of well-being is improved.

REEXAMINATION

Reexamination is performed throughout the episode of care.

DISCHARGE

Mr. Jardin is discharged from physical therapy after completing Phases 2 (7 to 10 days) and 3 (10 to 15 days) of the physical therapy sessions and attainment of his goals and expectations. These sessions have covered his entire episode of service. He is discharged because he has achieved his goals and expected outcomes.

Case Study #3: Above-Elbow Amputation

Mr. Anthony Needham is a 45-year-old wheat farmer who underwent a right transhumeral amputation 2 days ago secondary to a farming accident.

PHYSICAL THERAPIST EXAMINATION: PHASE 1

HISTORY: PHASES 1, 2, AND 3

- ♦ General demographics: Mr. Needham is a 45-year-old wheat farmer.
- ♦ Social history: Mr. Needham lives with his wife and three of his four children.
- ♦ Employment/work: Mr. Needham worked long hours as a wheat farmer on his ranch prior to the accident.
- ♦ Growth and development: Mr. Needham is right-hand dominant and displays normal motor function in his right residual limb and other extremities.
- ♦ Living environment: He lives on his ranch in Nebraska with his wife and his three children.
- ♦ General health status
  - General health perception: He reports his health status to be good prior to the accident.
  - Physical function: Mr. Needham was independent in all activities prior to the accident.
  - Psychological function: Normal.
  - Role function: Father, husband, farmer.
  - Social function: Mr. Needham is active in a men's club and at church.
- ♦ Social/health habits: He reports to be a social drinker and a non-smoker.
- ♦ Family history: His father has HTN and his mother has gallbladder disease.
- ♦ Medical/surgical history: Mr. Needham has OA in both knees and occasional lower back pain.
- ♦ Prior hospitalizations: Mr. Needham reports no prior hospitalizations.
- ♦ Preexisting medical and other health-related conditions: None.
- ♦ Current condition(s)/chief complaint(s): Mr. Needham underwent a right transhumeral amputation 2 days ago secondary to a farming accident. He reports that his arm got caught in the threshing machine while trying to clear a machine jam. Mr. Needham reports that he can feel his hand and that it "itches" and "cramps." His right arm is wrapped in a plaster cast to the axilla with a webbing strap over his chest and under the left axilla.

- Functional status and activity level: Mr. Needham is independent in ambulation. He is presently having difficulty with self-care activities.
- Medications: Mr. Needham is not taking any medications at this time.
- Other clinical tests
  - Blood tests reveal that the patient is slightly anemic.

SYSTEMS REVIEW: PHASE 1

- Cardiovascular/pulmonary
  - BP: 130/65 mmHg
  - Edema: Cannot be determined secondary to plaster cast
  - HR: 60 bpm
  - RR: 15 bpm
- Integumentary
  - Presence of scar formation: Cannot be determined
  - Skin color: Cannot be determined
  - Skin integrity: Cannot be determined
- Musculoskeletal
  - Gross range of motion
    - Limited motion noted to the right shoulder and cervical spine
    - ROM modified to avoid pain and stretching of the incisional site
    - LUE and both LEs: WNL
  - Gross strength
    - Gross strength testing delayed secondary to rigid dressing.
    - LUE and both LEs: WFL
  - Gross symmetry
    - Slightly FHP
    - Right shoulder mildly elevated
  - Height: 5'11" (1.80 m)
  - Weight: 195 lbs (88.45 kg)
- Neuromuscular
  - Balance: Sitting and standing balance good
  - Locomotion, transfers, and transitions: WNL
- Communication, affect, cognition, language, and learning style
  - Communication, affect, and cognition: WNL
  - Learning preferences: Visual and auditory

TESTS AND MEASURES: PHASE 1

- Aerobic capacity/endurance
  - Energy expenditure per unit of work is WNL
- Anthropometric characteristics
  - BMI=27.3 (this is considered overweight based on Centers for Disease Control and Prevention)[17]
  - Right arm is wrapped in a plaster cast to the axilla

with a webbing strap over his chest and under his left axilla

- Arousal, attention, and cognition
  - Alert and oriented x 3
- Assistive and adaptive devices
  - Adaptive equipment (eg, one-handed jar and can openers) to be provided to Mr. Needham to increase his ADL independence
- Circulation
  - Left UE peripheral pulses=WNL
  - Right axillary pulses cannot be tested at this time.
- Cranial and peripheral nerve integrity
  - Cranial and peripheral nerves intact in RUE, intact in LUE proximal to amputation site
  - Sensation: WNL, except RUE not tested at this time
- Environmental, home, and work barriers
  - Farm equipment that requires use of both UEs
- Ergonomics and body mechanics
  - Performs functional activities in a safe and efficient manner
- Gait, locomotion, and balance
  - Standing and sitting balance good
  - Ambulating independently
- Integumentary integrity
  - Skin integrity intact in the residual limb
- Joint integrity and mobility
  - Right shoulder joint with normal integrity and decreased mobility due to rigid dressing
- Motor function
  - RUE functional activities slow, labored, and with decreased coordination; LUE WNL
- Muscle performance
  - MMT revealed:
    - LUE and both LEs: WFL
    - Resistive testing not performed to R shoulder and neck at this time
- Orthotic, protective, and supportive devices
  - Plaster cast to the axilla with a webbing strap over his chest and under the left axilla in place to protect the residual limb
- Pain
  - Reports that he can still feel his hand and that it itches and occasionally cramps due to phantom sensation and pain
- Posture
  - FHP
  - R head tilt
- Prosthetic requirements
  - Transhumeral prosthesis with appropriate terminal device, elbow unit, socket, and suspension

- Range of motion
  - Goniometry revealed LUE and both LEs: WNL
  - R shoulder testing modified to avoid pain and stretching of the incision, but appears to be WFL
- Self-care and home management
  - Mr. Needham has just started to feed himself, brush his teeth, and wash his face with his left hand
  - He attempts other self-care activities with his L hand
  - Assistance required for bilateral self-care activities
- Work, community, and leisure integration or reintegration
  - Evaluate occupational demands as patient returns to his work as a farmer
  - Provide adaptive devices to compensate for limb loss
  - Refer patient and family to support services as patient returns to social and recreational activities

EVALUATION: PHASE 1

His history previously outlined indicated that he is a 45-year-old wheat farmer, non-smoker, and social drinker. He is status post a traumatic transhumeral amputation of his RUE 2 days ago. He is overweight, has decreased muscle performance, and FHP. Mr. Needham is alert and aware and was active prior to the onset of the most recent problem. His potential for eventual prosthetic rehabilitation appears good. It is critically important that plans for continued therapy and prosthetic placement be initiated as soon as possible so the patient makes a smooth transition from the hospital to a rehabilitation center for prosthetic placement.

DIAGNOSIS: PHASE 1

Mr. Needham has undergone a traumatic transhumeral amputation of his RUE with loss of BUE function and dominant hand function and with phantom pain. He has impaired: anthropometric characteristics; integumentary integrity; motor function; muscle performance; and posture. He is functionally limited in self-care and home management and in work, community, and leisure actions, tasks, and activities. He is in need of a prosthetic device. In addition, he has work barriers that will need to be addressed. These findings are consistent with placement in Pattern J: Impaired Motor Function, Muscle Performance, Range of Motion, Gait, Locomotion, and Balance Associated With Amputation. These impairments, functional limitations, device and equipment needs, and barriers will then be addressed in determining the prognosis and the plan of care.

PROGNOSIS AND PLAN OF CARE: PHASE 1

Over the course of the visits, the following mutually established outcomes have been determined:
- Ability to perform physical actions, tasks, and activities related to self-care is improved
- Care is coordinated with patient, family, and other professionals
- Case is managed throughout episode of care
- Integumentary integrity is improved
- Knowledge of behaviors that foster healthy habits is gained
- Placement needs are determined
- Risk factors are reduced
- Risk of secondary impairments is reduced
- Stress is decreased

To achieve these outcomes, the appropriate interventions for this patient are determined. These will include: coordination, communication, and documentation; patient/client-related instruction; therapeutic exercise; functional training in self-care and home management; and prescription, application, and, as appropriate, fabrication of devices and equipment.

Based on the diagnosis and prognosis, Mr. Needham is expected to require between two to four visits in the hospital. Mr. Needham is a wheat farmer whose occupation requires the use of his UEs.

INTERVENTIONS: PHASE 1

RATIONALE FOR SELECTED INTERVENTIONS

Therapeutic Exercise

Postoperatively, patients with an UE amputation tend to hold their residual limb in a flexed and protected position.[15] Flexibility and ROM exercises in the residual limb are essential to prevent residual limb contractures. Positioning and active and passive exercises are used to maintain joint ROM and muscle flexibility in the residual limb following amputation.[18] Bed mobility, transfer training, and ambulation/elevation activities should be integrated in treatment interventions as needed.[42] Therapeutic exercises will help prevent muscle atrophy and deconditioning. Strengthening exercises for the shoulder girdle and the residual limb musculature are needed in preparation for prosthetic use. Postural exercises should be an integral part of the therapeutic exercise program in order to maintain function and improve self-image. Exercises that challenge postural control should be included.[32] Core stabilization exercises facilitate strength and control of the UEs. Coordination and agility training are also necessary to facilitate movement control of the residual limb with and without a prosthesis.

Prescription, Application, and, as Appropriate, Fabrication of Devices and Equipment

Immediate postoperative goals are to reduce pain, edema, and promote tissue healing in the residual limb. Edema control facilitates suture line healing, decreases pain, and contributes to easier movement in the residual limb.[32] Fitted with a rigid dressing, Mr Needham will not have difficulty with edema or related pain. If not fitted with a rigid dressing, consistent use of a shrinker or compressive wraps has been shown to decrease the severity of phantom limb phenomena and pain and shortens the time required to begin prosthetic fitting.[32]

Assistive devices may be needed to facilitate self-care and one-handed activities.

Physical Agents and Mechanical Modalities

Compression bandaging or compression garments may be used to control postoperative edema and to help shape the residual limb. Controlling the edema helps to decrease the time between the amputation and the initial prosthetic fit.[32] Wearing a shrinker or an elastic wrap also tends to control postoperative pain, phantom sensation, and phantom pain.[32] However, this patient has been fitted with a rigid dressing that also helps control postoperative and phantom pain.

COORDINATION, COMMUNICATION, AND DOCUMENTATION

Communication will occur with Mr. Needham. Education regarding his current condition, impairments, and functional limitations will be discussed. The plan of care will be discussed with the patient. All elements of the patient's management will be documented. Early communication with the physician is necessary for rehabilitation planning and referral for prosthetic placement. Collaboration with prosthetic center will occur. The patient and family need to be involved in discharge planning for the best placement. Discharge planning will be provided.

PATIENT/CLIENT-RELATED INSTRUCTION

The patient will be instructed in bed mobility, proper residual limb positioning, and care of the rigid dressing. Risk factors will be discussed. The patient will receive education concerning the need for a prosthetic rehabilitation program that is to begin in a timely manner. Preparation for prosthetic fitting may include demonstration or pictures shown of different prostheses and components and an explanation of their uses and limitations. Discussion of the role of an amputee clinic and the importance of acting proactively for early prosthetic fitting shall occur.

THERAPEUTIC EXERCISE

♦ Balance, coordination, and agility training
  ● One-handed ADL activities as required
  ● Writing activities with L hand
♦ Body mechanics and postural stabilization
  ● If mirror available, work on postural alignment with altered center of mass with visual cuing
  ● Chin tucks to correct forward head
  ● Shoulder shrugs bilaterally
  ● Scapula retraction bilaterally
  ● Scapula adduction and depression bilaterally
  ● Scapula adduction and downward rotation bilaterally
  ● Scapula abduction and upward rotation bilaterally
♦ Flexibility exercises
  ● Stretching exercises should be done after warming up, using a slow and steady stretch accompanied by deep breathing, and building hold up to 30 to 60 seconds
  ● Pectoral minor stretch
  ● Pectoral major stretch
  ● Shoulder medial and lateral rotator stretch
  ● ROM exercises
    ■ Cervical spine in all directions
    ■ R shoulder in all directions
    ■ R scapula in all directions
♦ Gait and locomotion training
  ● Encourage arm swing during gait
♦ Strength, power, and endurance training
  ● Resistive exercises for R shoulder girdle
  ● Repetitive endurance exercises for both UEs as allowed by rigid dressing.
  ● Core strengthening

FUNCTIONAL TRAINING IN SELF-CARE AND HOME MANAGEMENT

♦ Self-care
  ● Instruction regarding signs and symptoms associated with infection
  ● Monitoring rigid dressing fit
  ● Instruction in one-handed activities
  ● Instruction in bathing and protection of rigid dressing
  ● Instruction regarding positioning of the residual limb
  ● Instruction in grooming activities
  ● Instruction in dressing activities

- Instruction in feeding activities
- Instruction in writing activities with the left hand
- Instruction in the use of adaptive equipment needed for self-care activities
- Instruction in the performance of bimanual activities

♦ Injury prevention or reduction
- Awareness of safety precautions involved with self-care

♦ Safety awareness training during self-care

PRESCRIPTION, APPLICATION, AND, AS APPROPRIATE, FABRICATION OF DEVICES AND EQUIPMENT

♦ Assistive devices may be needed to facilitate self-care and one-handed activities

ANTICIPATED GOALS AND EXPECTED OUTCOMES

♦ Impact on impairments
- Balance is good in sitting and standing.
- Muscle performance, including strength, power and endurance, is increased; scapular is 3/5.
- Postural awareness is improved with decreased R head tilt.
- ROM is increased so that R shoulder is WNL.

♦ Impact on functional limitations
- Ability to perform physical actions, tasks, and activities related to self-care requires minimal assistance.
- Functional independence in ADL requires minimal assistance.
- Level of supervision required for task performance is decreased.

♦ Risk reduction/prevention
- Residual limb is protected from trauma.
- Risk factors and risk of secondary impairments are reduced.
- Safety is independent.
- Self-management of symptoms is improved.

♦ Impact on health, wellness, and fitness
- Behaviors that promote healthy nutrition, physical activity, and wellness are promoted.
- Physical capacity is increased.
- Physical function is improved.

♦ Impact on societal resources
- Documentation will occur throughout the patient management and across all settings and follows APTA's *Guidelines for Physical Therapy Documentation.*[25]

♦ Patient/client satisfaction
- Care is coordinated with patient, family, and other professionals.
- Case is managed throughout the episode of care.
- Collaboration and coordination will occur with the prosthetic center.
- Decision making is enhanced regarding patient health and use of health care resources by patient and family.
- Interdisciplinary collaboration will occur through case conferences.
- Patient and family knowledge and awareness of the diagnosis, prognosis, interventions, and anticipated goals and expected outcomes are increased.
- Placement needs will be determined.

PHYSICAL THERAPIST EXAMINATION: PHASES 2 AND 3

SYSTEMS REVIEW: PHASES 2 AND 3

♦ Cardiovascular/pulmonary
- BP: 130/65 mmHg
- Edema: Minimal postoperative edema in the residual limb
- HR: 60 bpm
- RR: 15 bpm

♦ Integumentary
- Presence of scar formation: Scarring noted around the perimeter of the suture line
- Skin color: Suture line well healed
- Skin integrity: Intact in the residual limb

♦ Musculoskeletal
- Gross range of motion
  - Limited at end ranges of motion to the right shoulder
  - LUE and both LEs: WNL
- Gross strength
  - Decreased strength noted to all right shoulder musculature
  - LUE and both LEs: WFL
- Gross symmetry: Slight tilt of head
- Height: 5'11" (1.80 m)
- Weight: 195 lbs (88.45 kg)

♦ Neuromuscular
- Balance: Sitting and standing balance good
- Locomotion, transfers, and transitions: WNL

♦ Communication, affect, cognition, language, and learning style
- Communication, affect, and cognition: WNL
- Learning preferences: Auditory learner

TESTS AND MEASURES: PHASES 2 AND 3

- Aerobic capacity/endurance
  - Energy expenditure per unit of work: WNL
- Anthropometric characteristics
  - Edema: Minimal edema noted in distal portion of the residual limb
  - BMI=27.3 (this is considered overweight based on Centers for Disease Control and Prevention)[17]
- Arousal, attention, and cognition
  - Alert and oriented x 3
- Assistive and adaptive devices
  - Adaptive equipment (eg, one-handed jar and can openers) to be provided to Mr. Needham to increase his ADL independence
- Circulation
  - BUE peripheral pulses: WNL
- Cranial and peripheral nerve integrity
  - Cranial and peripheral nerves intact
  - Sensation: WNL
  - RUE may be hypersensitive
- Environmental, home, and work barriers
  - Farm equipment that requires use of both UEs
- Ergonomics and body mechanics
  - Performs functional activities in a safe and efficient manner
- Gait, locomotion, and balance
  - Standing and sitting balance good
  - Ambulating independently
- Integumentary integrity
  - Suture line well healed with no discharge
  - Skin color and temperature in the residual limb: WNL
- Joint integrity and mobility
  - Right shoulder joint with normal integrity
- Motor function
  - RUE functional activities slow, labored, and with decreased coordination; LUE WNL
- Muscle performance
  - MMT revealed:
    - LUE and both LEs: WFL
    - R scapula
      - Elevation/abduction=4+/5
      - Adduction/depression=4+/5
    - R shoulder
      - Flexion/abduction/extension=4/5
      - Scaption=4/5
- Orthotic, protective, and supportive devices
  - Once the sutures are removed a new removable rigid dressing will be applied
- Pain

- Reports that he can still feel his hand and that it itches and occasionally cramps due to phantom sensation and pain
- Posture
  - FHP
  - R head tilt
- Prosthetic requirements
  - Transhumeral prosthesis with appropriate terminal device, elbow unit, socket, and suspension to enable return to heavy farm work to include:
    - Body powered cable prosthetic device
      - Socket: Double walled plastic laminate socket
      - Suspension: Figure eight harness
      - Dual cable control
      - Friction wrist
      - Internal locking elbow unit
      - Voluntary opening cantilevered split hook
    - Cosmetic hand for social occasions
- Range of motion
  - Goniometry revealed LUE and both LEs: WNL
  - R shoulder testing appears to be WFL
- Self-care and home management
  - Mr. Needham continues to feed himself with his L hand
  - Minimal assistance now required for all other self-care activities
- Work, community, and leisure integration or reintegration
  - Evaluate occupational demands as patient returns to his work as a farmer
  - Provide adaptive devices to compensate for limb loss
  - Refer patient and family to support services as patient returns to social and recreational activities

EVALUATION: PHASES 2 AND 3

His history previously outlined indicated that he is a 45-year old wheat farmer, non-smoker, and social drinker. He is status post a traumatic transhumeral amputation of his RUE 21 days ago. He is overweight, has altered integumentary integrity, decreased ROM, and some difficulty with self-care. Mr. Needham is alert and aware and was active prior to the onset of the most recent problem. His potential for eventual prosthetic rehabilitation appears good. It is critically important that plans for continued therapy and prosthetic placement be initiated as soon as possible so the patient makes a smooth transition from the hospital to a rehabilitation center for prosthetic placement.

DIAGNOSIS: PHASES 2 AND 3

Mr. Needham has undergone a traumatic transhumeral amputation of his RUE with loss of BUE function and dominant hand function and with phantom pain. He has impaired: anthropometric characteristics; motor function; muscle performance; and posture. He is functionally limited in self-care and home management and in work, community, and leisure actions, tasks, and activities. He is in need of assistive, adaptive, protective, and supportive devices and equipment. Mr. Needham will need a transhumeral prosthesis with appropriate terminal device, elbow unit, socket, and suspension. In addition, he has work barriers that will need to be addressed. These findings are consistent with placement in Pattern J: Impaired Motor Function, Muscle Performance, Range of Motion, Gait, Locomotion, and Balance Associated With Amputation. These impairments, functional limitations, device and equipment needs, and barriers will be addressed in determining the prognosis and the plan of care.

PROGNOSIS AND PLAN OF CARE: PHASES 2 AND 3

Over the course of the visits, the following mutually established outcomes have been determined:
♦ Ability to perform physical actions, tasks, and activities related to self-care is improved
♦ Care is coordinated with patient, family, and other professionals
♦ Case is managed throughout episode of care
♦ Integumentary integrity is improved
♦ Knowledge of behaviors that foster healthy habits is gained
♦ Placement needs are determined
♦ Risk factors are reduced
♦ Risk of secondary impairments is reduced
♦ ROM is increased
♦ Stress is decreased

To achieve these outcomes, the appropriate interventions for this patient are determined. These will include: coordination, communication, and documentation; patient/client-related instruction; therapeutic exercise; functional training in self-care and home management; functional training in work, community, and leisure integration or reintegration; and prescription, application, and, as appropriate, fabrication of devices and equipment.

Based on the diagnosis and prognosis, Mr. Needham is expected to require between 5 to 10 visits over a 14-day period of time if treated in physical therapy. He will need further therapy usually rendered in occupational therapy. Mr. Needham is a wheat farmer whose occupation requires the use of his UEs.

INTERVENTIONS: PHASES 2 AND 3

RATIONALE FOR SELECTED INTERVENTIONS

Therapeutic Exercise

The rehabilitation program is directed toward improving function both with and without a prosthetic device. A home exercise program of postural exercises, residual limb strengthening, and stretching is essential for effective use of myoelectric and body powered prostheses.[13,43] If myoelectric fitting is anticipated, the program focuses on functional activities for the hand and development of the musculature in potential myoelectric sites. Early intervention and referral to appropriate services are critical determinants in the successful return to occupational, recreational, and social activities.[44]

Functional Training in Self-Care and Home Management/Functional Training in Work, Community, and Leisure Integration or Reintegration

Functional training in ADL and in occupational and recreational activities will help the return to their pre-amputation life style.[45] It is important for the patient to develop skills in one-handed activities due to the limitations of prosthetic replacement for the individual with a transhumeral amputation.[42,46] Prescription of adaptive equipment will also help promote an easier transition for functional performance in individuals with an UE amputation.[45,46]

Prescription, Application, and, as Appropriate, Fabrication of Devices and Equipment

The patient has been fitted with a transhumeral prosthesis with a double-walled plastic laminate socket with a figure-eight harness. It is a dual-cable prosthesis with an internal locking elbow unit and a friction wrist. The terminal device is a voluntary opening cantilevered split hook. He has also been provided with a cosmetic hand for social occasions.

COORDINATION, COMMUNICATION, AND DOCUMENTATION

Communication will occur with Mr. Needham. Education regarding his current condition, impairments, and functional limitations will be discussed. The plan of care will be discussed with the patient. All elements of the patient's management will be documented. Communication with the physician will continue. Collaboration with the prosthetic center will occur. Discharge planning will be provided.

PATIENT/CLIENT-RELATED INSTRUCTION

The patient will be instructed in ROM, muscle strengthening, and use of adaptive equipment to enhance ADL. Risk factors will be discussed. The patient will receive education concerning different prosthetic options. Preparation for prosthetic fitting will include a demonstration or pictures of different UE prostheses and their components and an explanation of the uses and limitations of each.

THERAPEUTIC EXERCISE

- ◆ Balance, coordination, and agility training
  - Playing soccer, ball, or other sports activities to assist with altered center of mass
  - One-handed ADL activities as required
  - Writing activities with L hand
  - Fine prehensile activities with L hand
  - Bimanual activities with prosthesis
    - Cutting meat with a knife and fork
    - Hammering nails
    - Putting on socks
    - Tying shoelaces
- ◆ Body mechanics and postural stabilization
  - Work on postural alignment with altered center of mass using a mirror for visual feedback
  - Chin tucks to correct forward head
  - Shoulder shrugs bilaterally
  - Scapula retraction bilaterally
  - Wall standing postural exercises
- ◆ Flexibility exercises
  - Stretching exercises should be done after warming up, using a slow and steady stretch accompanied by deep breathing, and building hold up to 30 to 60 seconds
  - Posterior neck stretch
  - Pectoral minor stretch
  - Pectoral major stretch
  - Shoulder medial and lateral rotator stretch
  - ROM exercises
    - Cervical spine in all directions
    - R shoulder in all directions
    - R scapula in all directions
- ◆ Strength, power, and endurance training
  - Resistive exercises for R shoulder girdle
  - Repetitive endurance exercises for both UEs
  - Core strengthening

FUNCTIONAL TRAINING IN SELF-CARE AND HOME MANAGEMENT

- ◆ Self-care
  - Independent mobility with prosthesis
  - Independent in donning prosthesis
  - Skin inspection of residual limb
  - Independent skin care
  - Independent writing
  - Independent in one-handed activities
  - Independent in bimanual activities
- ◆ Injury prevention or reduction
  - Awareness of safety precautions involved with self-care
- ◆ Safety awareness training during self-care

FUNCTIONAL TRAINING IN WORK, COMMUNITY, AND LEISURE INTEGRATION OR REINTEGRATION

- ◆ Driving with adaptive devices
- ◆ Functional training programs
- ◆ Simulated environments and tasks
- ◆ Task adaptation
- ◆ Task training
- ◆ Work conditioning

PRESCRIPTION, APPLICATION, AND, AS APPROPRIATE, FABRICATION OF DEVICES AND EQUIPMENT

- ◆ Continue to monitor and check transhumeral prosthesis and fit (Table 10-5)

ANTICIPATED GOALS AND EXPECTED OUTCOMES

- ◆ Impact on impairments
  - Balance is independent.
  - Muscle performance, including strength, power, and endurance, is increased; scapula is 5/5 and R shoulder is 4+/5.
  - Postural awareness is improved so that the head is in midline.
  - Prosthetic fit is achieved.
  - Weightbearing status is improved to WFL.
- ◆ Impact on functional limitations
  - Ability to perform physical actions, tasks, and activities related to self-care is independent.
  - Ability to perform physical actions, tasks, and activities related to work, community, and leisure integration or reintegration is independent.
  - Independent in donning and doffing prosthesis.
  - Level of supervision required for task performance is decreased.
  - Performance of ADL with devices is independent.
  - Performance of and independence in IADL with or

	Table 10-5	
UPPER EXTREMITY PROSTHETIC CHECKOUT		
Checkout Item	*What to Check*	*Possible Problems*
Is the prosthesis as prescribed?	Compare to prescription	Changes in prescribed components need to be justified
Is the inside of the socket smoothly finished?	Check the inside of the socket	Skin abrasions
Is the socket secured on the residual limb?	Pull gently on socket	Suspension should be maintained in all positions for better stabilization and rotational control
Does the socket fit properly and comfortably?	Ask the patient if he or she is comfortable	Areas of discomfort may cause non-wearing and skin problems Improper fit will cause lack of control of the prosthesis
Does the harness fit properly and comfortably?	Ask the patient if he or she is comfortable	Improper fit will cause lack of control and poor suspension of the prosthesis
Is the friction component appropriate?	Check to see if friction is too tight or too loose	Too much or too little friction will cause poor control of the prosthesis
Do all joints move freely and smoothly?	Check elbow, wrist, and hand	Too stiff or loose joints may cause difficulty with prosthetic use
Are the color and contour of the prosthesis similar to the sound arm?	The finished prosthesis should match the sound arm	Poor cosmesis may lead to non-wearing
Does the length of the prosthesis correspond to the sound arm?	Check to see that the arms are level	Poor cosmesis may lead to non-wearing

without devices and equipment.

♦ Risk reduction/prevention
  • Residual limb is protected from trauma.
  • Risk factors and risk of secondary impairments are reduced.
  • Safety is improved.
  • Self-management of symptoms is improved.
♦ Impact on health, wellness, and fitness
  • Behaviors that promote healthy nutrition, physical activity, and wellness are promoted.
  • Physical capacity is increased.
  • Physical function is improved.
♦ Impact on societal resources
  • Documentation will occur throughout the patient management and across all settings and follows APTA's *Guidelines for Physical Therapy Documentation.*[25]
♦ Patient/client satisfaction
  • Care is coordinated with patient, family, and other professionals.
  • Case is managed throughout the episode of care.
  • Collaboration and coordination will occur with the prosthetist.
  • Decision making is enhanced regarding patient

health and use of health care resources by patient and family.
  • Interdisciplinary collaboration will occur through case conferences.
  • Patient and family knowledge and awareness of the diagnosis, prognosis, interventions, and anticipated goals and expected outcomes are increased.
  • Placement needs will be determined.
  • Sense of well-being is improved.

REEXAMINATION

Reexamination is performed throughout the episode of care.

DISCHARGE

Mr. Needham is discharged from physical therapy after completing Phase 1 (5 to 10 days) and Phases 2 and 3 (10 days) of his physical therapy sessions and attainment of his physical therapy goals and expectations. These sessions have covered his physical therapy episode of service. He is discharged because he has achieved his goals and expected outcomes.

REFERENCES

1. May BJ. *Amputations and Prosthetics: A Case Study Approach.* 2nd ed. Philadelphia, Pa: FA Davis Co; 2002.

2. Krajewski LP, Olin JW. Atherosclerosis of the aorta and lower extremities arteries. In: Young JR, et al, eds. *Peripheral Vascular Diseases.* St. Louis, Mo: Mosby Year Book; 1991.

3. Steinberg FU, et al. Prosthetic rehabilitation of geriatric amputee patients: a follow-up study. *Arch Phys Med Rehabil.* 1985;66:742-745.

4. Reiber GE, et al, eds. Risk factors for amputation in patients with diabetes mellitus: a case-control study. *Ann Intern Med.* 1992;117:97-105.

5. American Diabetes Association Webpage. Available at: http://www.diabetes.org. Accessed June 15, 2003.

6. Feinglass J, et al. Peripheral bypass surgery and amputation. Northern Illinois demographics, 1993-1997. *Arch Surg.* 2000;135(1):75-80.

7. Fletcher DD, Andrews KL, Hallett JW Jr, Butters MA, Rowland CM, Jacobsen SJ. Trends in rehabilitation after amputation for geriatric patients with vascular disease: implications for future health resource allocation. *Arch Phys Med Rehabil.* 2002;83(10):1389-1393.

8. Dillingham TR, Pezzin LE, MacKenzie EJ. Racial differences in the incidence of limb loss secondary to peripheral vascular disease: a population-based study. *Arch Phys Med Rehabil.* 2002;83(9):1252-1257.

9. Bloomquist T. Amputation and phantom limb pain: a pain-prevention model. *AANA J.* 2001;69(3):211-217.

10. May BJ. A statewide amputee rehabilitation programme. *Prosthet Orthot Int.* 1978;2:24-26.

11. Meikle B, Devlin M, Garfinkel S. Interruptions to amputee rehabilitation. *Arch Phys Med Rehabil.* 2002;83(9):1222-1228.

12. Geil MD. Energy loss and stiffness properties of dynamic elastic response prosthetic feet. *Journal of Prosthetics and Orthotics.* 2001;13(3):70-73.

13. Edelstein J. Upper limb amputations. In: May BJ, ed. *Amputations and Prosthetics: A Case Study Approach.* 2nd ed. Philadelphia, Pa: FA Davis Co; 2002:236-254.

14. Bowker JH, Michael JW, eds. *Atlas of Limb Prosthetics: Surgical, Prosthetic and Rehabilitation Principles.* St. Louis, Mo: Mosby Year Book; 1992.

15. Lipschutz RD. Upper extremity amputations and prosthetic management. In: Lusardi MM, Nielsen CC, eds. *Orthotics and Prosthetics in Rehabilitation.* Boston, Mass: Butterworth-Heinemann; 2000:569-588.

16. Gailey RS, Roach KE, et al. The amputee mobility predictor: an instrument to assess determinants of the lower-limb amputee's ability to ambulate. *Arch Phys Med Rehab.* 2002;83:613-627.

17. USDA Center for Nutrition Policy and Promotion. Body mass index and health. *Nutrition Insight.* 2000;March.

18. Cutson TM, Bongiorni D, et al. Early management of elderly dysvascular below knee amputees. *Journal of Prosthetics and Orthotics.* 1994;6:62-66.

19. Calianno C. Assessing and preventing pressure ulcers. *Advances in Skin and Wound Care.* 2000;13:244-246.

20. Oatis CA. Mechanics and pathomechanics of muscle activ-
ity at the shoulder complex. In: *Kinesology.* Philadelphia, Pa: Lippincott Williams & Wilkins; 2004:141-176.

21. Ciesla ND. Chest physical therapy for patients in the intensive care unit. *Phys Ther.* 1996;76:609-625.

22. Halbert J, Crotty M, Cameron ID. Evidence for the optimal management of acute and chronic phantom pain: a systematic review. *Clin J Pain.* 2002;18(2):84-92.

23. Oakley DA, Whitman LG, Halligan PW. Hypnotic imagery as a treatment for phantom limb pain: two case reports and a review. *Clin Rehabil.* 2002;16(4):368-377.

24. Gallagher P, Allen D, Maclachlan M. Phantom limb pain and residual limb pain following lower limb amputation: a descriptive analysis. *Disabil Rehabil.* 2001;23(12):522-530.

25. American Physical Therapy Association. Guide to physical therapist practice. 2nd ed. *Phys Ther.* 2001;81:9-744.

26. Dowling JS, May BJ. The diabetic foot. In: May BJ, ed. *Amputations and Prosthetics: A Case Study Approach.* 2nd ed. Philadelphia, Pa: FA Davis Co; 2002.

27. Nadollek H, Brauer S, Isles R. Outcomes after trans-tibial amputation: the relationship between quiet stance ability, strength of hip abductor muscles and gait. *Physiother Res Int.* 2002;7(4):203-214.

28. May BJ. Mobility training for the older adult. *Topics in Geriatric Rehabilitation.* 2003;19(3):191-198.

29. Hubbard WA. Rehabilitation outcomes for elderly lower limb amputees. *Aust J Physiother.* 1989;35:219-224.

30. Gaily RS, Gaily AM. *Stretching and Strengthening for Lower Extremity Amputees.* Miami, Fla: Advanced Rehabilitation Therapy Inc; 1994.

31. Kania A. Integration of massage therapy into amputee rehabilitation and care. *In Motion.* 2004;14(4).

32. Lusardi M, Owens F. Postoperative and preprosthetic care. In: Lusardi M, Nielsen C, eds. *Orthotics and Prosthetics in Rehabilitation.* Woburn, Mass: Butterworth-Heinemann; 2000.

33. Terry M, O'Brien SP, Kerstein MD. Lower-extremity edema: evaluation and diagnosis. *Wounds.* 1998;10(4):118-124.

34. Seymour R. Clinical use of dressings and bandages. In: Seymour R, eds. *Prosthetics and Orthotics.* Baltimore, Md: Williams & Wilkins; 2002.

35. Yigiter K, Sener G, Erbahceci F, Bayar K, Ulger OG, Akdogan S. A comparison of traditional prosthetic training versus proprioceptive neuromuscular facilitation resistive gait training with trans-femoral amputees. *Prosthet Orthot Int.* 2002;26(3):213-217.

36. Jones ME, Bashford GM, Mann JM. Weight bearing and velocity in trans-tibial and trans-femoral amputees. *Prosthet Orthot Int.* 1997;21(3):183-186.

37. Mattes SJ, Martin PE, Royer TD. Walking symmetry and energy cost in persons with unilateral transtibial amputations: matching prosthetic and intact limb inertial properties. *Arch Phys Med Rehabil.* 2000;81(5):561-568.

38. Powers CM, Boyd LA, Fontaine CA, Perry J. The influence of lower-extremity muscle force on gait characteristics in individuals with below-knee amputations secondary to vascular disease. *Phys Ther.* 1996;76(4):369-377; discussion 378-385.

39. Ward KH, Meyers MC. Exercise performance of lower-extremity amputees. *Sports Med.* 1995;20(4):207-214.

40. Psonak R. Transfemoral prosthetics. In: Lusardi M, ed. *Orthotics and Prosthetics in Rehabilitation.* Woburn, Mass:

Butterworth-Heinemann; 2002.

41. Hunter D, Cole E, Murray JM, Murray TD. Energy expenditure of below knee amputees during harness supported treadmill ambulation. *J Orthop Sports Phys Ther.* 1995;21:268-276.

42. Malone JM, Fleming LL, Roberson J. Immediate, early, and late postsurgical management of upper-limb amputation. *J Rehabil Res Dev.* 1984;21:33-41.

43. Pinzur MS, Angelats J, Light TR, Izuierdo R, Pluth T. Functional outcome following traumatic upper limb amputation and prosthetic limb fitting. *Hand Surg (Am).* 1994;19:836-839.

44. Sturup J, Thyregod HC, Jensen JS, et al. Traumatic amputation of the upper limb: the use of body-powered prostheses and employment consequences. *Prosthet Orthot Int.* 1988;12(1):50-52.

45. Gilin M. Above-elbow amputation: a case study in restoring function. *J Hand Ther.* 1998;11:278-283.

46. Petri RP Jr, Aguila E. The military upper extremity amputee. *Phys Med Rehabil Clin N Am.* 2002;13:17-43.

BIBLIOGRAPHY

Shumway-Cook A, Woollacott MH. *Motor Control: Theory and Practical Applications.* 2nd ed. Philadelphia, Pa: Lippincott Williams & Wilkins; 2001.

Sjodahl C, Jarnlo GB, Soderberg B, Persson BM. Kinematic and kinetic gait analysis in the sagittal plane of trans-femoral amputees before and after special gait re-education. *Prosthet Orthot Int.* 2002;26(2):101-112.

WEBSITES OF INTEREST

American Academy of Orthotists and Prosthetists: www.oandp.org
Amputee Coalition of America: www.amputee-coalition.org
Amputee News Service: www.amputee-online.com/amputation
Global Resource for Orthotic and Prosthetic Information: www.oanp.com
International Paralympic Organization: www.paralympic.org

Abbreviations

AAMHR=age-adjusted maximum heart rate
AAROM=active-assistive range of motion
AC=acromioclavicular
ACh=acetylcholine
ACL=anterior cruciate ligament
ADL=activities of daily living
AHC=anterior horn cell
ALL=anterior longitudinal ligament
ANS=autonomic nervous system
A/P=anteroposterior
APL=arcuate popliteal ligament
APTA=American Physical Therapy Association
AROM=active range of motion
ASIS=anterior superior iliac spines
ASO=atherosclerosis
ATP=adenosine triphosphate
AVN=avascular necrosis
BAPS=Biomechanical Ankle Platform System
bid=twice a day
BLE=bilateral lower extremities
BMD=bone mineral density
BMI=body mass index
BOSU=Both Sides Up board
BP=blood pressure
BPTB=bone-patellar tendon-bone
BUE=bilateral upper extremities
CABG=coronary artery bypass graft
CAD=coronary artery disease
CAN=cardiac autonomic neuropathy
CFS=chronic fatigue syndrome
CI=confidence interval
CK=creatinine phosphokinase
CKC=closed-kinetic-chain
CMC=carpometacarpal
CNS=central nervous system
CPM=continuous passive motion
CRF=cardiorespiratory fitness
CROM=cervical range of motion device
CRPS=complex regional pain syndrome
CT=computed tomography
C-T=cervico-thoracic
CVA=cerebrovascular accident
D1=diagonal one
D2=diagonal two
DASH=Disability of the Arm, Shoulder, and Hand questionnaire
DAN=diabetic autonomic neuropathy

DDD=degenerative disc disease
DEXA=dual energy x-ray absorptiometry
DIP=distal interphalangeal
DKA=diabetic ketoacidosis
DIMS=Diabetes Impact Measurement Scale
DM=diabetes mellitus
DMARDs=disease-modifying antirheumatic drugs
DMD=Duchenne muscular dystrophy
DOMS=delayed onset muscle soreness
DQoLS=Diabetes Quality of Life Scale
DP=dorsalis pedis
DTRs=deep tendon reflexes
DVT=deep vein thrombosis
DXA=dual energy x-ray absorptiometry
ECST=extracorporeal shock wave therapy
ECG=electrocardiogram
EMG=electromyography
EMS=electrical muscle stimulation
ER=external rotation
ESR=erythrocyte sedimentation rate
ET=estrogen therapy
FES=functional electrical stimulation
FG=fast, glycolytic
FHP=forward head posture
FOG=fast twitch, oxidative, glycolytic
FS=fibromyalgia syndrome
GAG=glycosaminoglycan
GH=glenohumeral
HHNS=hyperglycemic nonketotic syndrome
HO=heterotopic ossification
HR=heart rate
HT=hormone therapy
HTN=hypertension
HVPC=high-volt pulsed current
IADL=instrumental activities of daily living
IC=ischial containment
ICC=intraclass correlation coefficient
IEP=individualized educational plan
IP=interphalangeal
IR=internal rotation
ISL=interspinous ligament
ITB=iliotibial band
IU=international units
IV=intravenous
K=Kirschner wires
KAT=Kinesthetic Athletic Trainer

LE=left extremity
LF=ligamentum flavum
LLE=left lower extremity
LRTI=ligament reconstruction tendon interposition
LUE=left upper extremity
MC=metacarpal
MCP=metacarpophalangeal
MCV=motor conduction velocities
MHR=maximum heart rate
MMT=manual muscle testing
MNT=medical nutritional therapy
MRE=manual resistive exercise
MRI=magnetic resonance imaging
MT=metatarsal
MTP=metatarsophalangeal
MU=motor unit
MVA=motor vehicle accident
NAFC=National Association for Continence
NCV=nerve conduction velocity
NIH=National Institutes of Health
NMES=neuromuscular electrical stimulation
NPS=numeric pain rating scale
NSAIDs=nonsteroidal anti-inflammatory drugs
NTX= urine N-telopeptide analysis
OA=osteoarthritis
ODQ=Oswestry Low Back Pain Disability Questionnaire
OEE=Outcome Expectations for Exercise
OKC=open-kinetic-chain
ORIF=open reduction internal fixation
OTC=over-the-counter
P/A=posteroanterior
PAIVM=passive accessory intervertebral mobility
PAOD=peripheral arterial occlusive disease
PCA=patient controlled analgesia
PCL=posterior cruciate ligament
pDXA=peripheral dual energy x-ray absorptiometry
PFM=pelvic floor muscles
PFT=pulmonary function test
PG=proteoglycan
PIP=proximal interphalangeal
PLL=posterior longitudinal ligament
PNF=proprioceptive neuromuscular facilitation
PNS=peripheral nervous system
PO=posteroperative
POD=postoperative day
POL=posterior oblique ligament
PPIVM=passive physiological intervertebral mobility
pQCT=peripheral quantitative computed tomography
PRE=progressive resistive exercise
prn=as needed
PROM=passive range of motion
PSIS=posterior superior iliac spines
PSR=physical self-regulation
PT=posterior tibial

PTH=parathyroid hormone
PVD=peripheral vascular disease
q=every
QCT=quantitative computed tomography
qd=once daily
RA=rheumatoid arthritis
RHR=resting heart rate
RLE=right left extremity
RM=repetition maximum
ROM=range of motion
RR=respiratory rate
RROM=resisted range of motion
RSD=reflex sympathetic dystrophy
RUE=right upper extremity
SAID=specific adaptation to imposed demand
SC=sternoclavicular
SCM=sternocleidomastoid
SD=standard deviation
SDS=simple descriptive scale
sEMG=surface electromyography
SH=scapulohumeral
SITS muscles=supraspinatus, infraspinatus, teres minor, and
    subscapularis muscles
SLE=systemic lupus erythematosis
SLR=straight leg raise
SNAP=sensory nerve action potentials
SO=slow twitch, oxidative
SP=spinous process
SSR=supraspinous ligament
ST=scapulothoracic
STM=soft tissue mobilization
SUI=stress urinary incontinence
SXA=single energy x-ray absorptiometry
TENS=transcutaneous electrical nerve stimulation
TFCC=triangular fibrocartilage complex
TFL=tensor fascia latae
THA=total hip arthroplasty
THR=target heart rate
tid=three times a day
TJA=total joint arthroplasty
TKA=total knee arthroplasty
TM=trapeziometacarpal
TMJ=temporomandibular joint
TMT=tarsometatarsal
TSA=total shoulder arthroplasty
UE=upper extremity
ULTT 1=upper limb tension test 1
US=ultrasound
VAS=visual analog scale
VMS=variable muscle stimulation
WFL=within functional limits
WHO=World Health Organization
WNL=within normal limits

Brand Name Drugs and Products

The brand name drugs and products mentioned in this book are listed below, along with their manufacturer information.

DRUGS

Actonel (Proctor & Gamble, Cincinnati, Ohio)
Adriamycin (Pfizer Inc, Cambridge, Mass)
Advil (Wyeth Consumer Healthcare, Richmond, Va)
Aleve (Bayer Healthcare LLC, Morristown, NJ)
Allegra (Aventis, Paris, France)
Calciparine (Sanofi Synthelabo, North Ryde, Australia)
Capoten (Bristol-Myers Squibb Co, New York, NY)
Celebrex (Pfizer Inc, Cambridge, Mass)
Climara (Berlex Inc, Montville, NJ)
Darvocet (Eli Lilly & Co, Indianapolis, Ind)
Darvon (Eli Lilly & Co, Indianapolis, Ind)
Demerol (Sanofi Winthrop, Gentilly, France)
Dilantin (Pfizer Inc, Cambridge, Mass)
Dilaudid (Knoll, Mt. Olive, NJ)
Duragesic (Ortho-McNeill Inc, Titusville, NJ)
Elavil (Stuart Pharmaceuticals, Newark, Del)
Estrace (Warner Chilcott, Rockaway, NJ)
Estraderm (Novartis, Dorval, Quebec)
Estratab (Solvay, Marietta, Ga)
Evista (Eli Lilly & Co, Indianapolis, Ind)
Flovent (GlaxoSmithKline, Brentford, Middlesex, UK)
Forteo (Eli Lilly & Co, Indianapolis, Ind)
Fosamax (Merck, Whitehouse Station, NJ)
Glucophage (Bristol-Myers Squibb Co, New York, NY)
Indocin (Merck, Whitehouse Station, NJ)
Lipitor (Pfizer Inc, Cambridge, Mass)
Liquaemin (Organon USA, Roseland, NJ)
Lopressor (Novartis, Dorval, Quebec)
Medrol (Pfizer Inc, Cambridge, Mass)
Miacalcin (Sandoz, Holzkirchen, Germany)
Motrin (Pfizer Inc, Cambridge, Mass)
Naprosyn (Roche, Basel, Switzerland)
Neurontin (Pfizer Inc, Cambridge, Mass)
Nuprin (Bristol-Myers Squibb Co, New York, NY)

Ogen (Pfizer Inc, Cambridge, Mass)
Orinase (Pfizer Inc, Cambridge, Mass)
Ortho-Est (Ortho, Raritan, NJ)
Paxil (SmithKline Beeacham, Philadelphia, Pa)
Percocet (Endo Pharmaceuticals, Chadds Ford, Pa)
Pegonal (Serono Inc, Rockland, Mass)
Premarin (Wyeth, Madison, NJ)
Questran (Bristol-Myers Squibb Co, New York, NY)
Soma (Wallace, Cranbury, NJ)
Synthroid (Abbott Laboratories, Abbott Park, Ill)
Tylenol (McNeil Consumer, Fort Washington, Pa)
Ultracet (McNeil Consumer, Fort Washington, Pa)
Ultram (McNeil Consumer, Fort Washington, Pa)
Valium (Roche, Basel, Switzerland)
Vicodin (Abbott Laboratories, Abbott Park, Ill)
Vivelle (Novartis, Dorval, Quebec)
Zocor (Merck, Whitehouse Station, NJ)

PRODUCTS

Airdyne bicycle (Pacific Cycle Inc, Madison, Wis)
Airex (SPRI Products, Libertyville, Ill)
Biomechanical Ankle Platform System ([BAPS] CAMP, Jackson, Miss)
Bodyblade (Bodyblade, www.bodyblade.com)
Both Sides Up Balance Trainer ([BOSU] Canton, Ohio)
Cryo Cuff (AirCast, 800-526-8785)
Jamar dynamometer, pinch gauge (Sammons Preston, Bolingbrook, Ill)
Kinesthetic Ability Trainer ([KAT], SportKat, San Diego, Calif)
KT 1000 (MEDMetric Corp, San Diego, Calif)
Metrecom (Faro Technologies Inc, Lake Mary, Fla)
Sportcord (STI, Baton Rouge, La)
Stairmaster (Nautilus, Inc, Vancouver, Wash)

Index

WAIT

...There's More!

SLACK Incorporated's Health Care Books and Journals offers a wide selection of products in the field of Physical Therapy. We are dedicated to providing important works that educate, inform and improve the knowledge of our customers. Don't miss out on our other informative titles that will enhance your collection.

Essentials in Physical Therapy Series

The *Essentials in Physical Therapy* series answers the call to what today's physical therapy students and clinicians are looking for when integrating the *Guide to Physical Therapist Practice* into clinical care.

Essentials in Physical Therapy is led by Series Editor Dr. Marilyn Moffat, who brings together physical therapy's leading professionals to produce the most anticipated series of books in the physical therapy market to cover the four main systems:

- ♦ Musculoskeletal
- ♦ Cardiopulmonary
- ♦ Neuromuscular
- ♦ Integumentary

Written in a similar, user-friendly format, each book inside the *Essentials in Physical Therapy* series not only brings together the conceptual frameworks of the *Guide* language, but also parallels the patterns of the *Guide*.

In each case, where appropriate, a brief review of the pertinent anatomy, physiology, pathophysiology, imaging, and pharmacology is provided. Each pattern then details diversified case studies coinciding with the *Guide* format. The physical therapist examination, including history, systems review, and specific tests and measures for each case, as well as evaluation, diagnosis, prognosis, plan of care, and evidence-based interventions are also addressed.

Series Editor: Marilyn Moffat, PT, DPT, PhD, FAPTA, CSCS, *New York University, New York, NY*

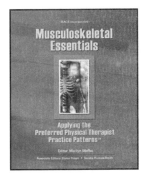
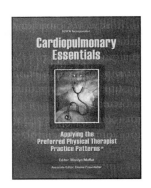
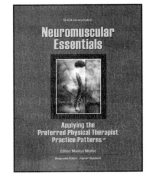
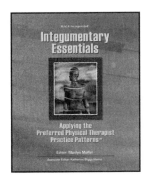

Essentials in Physical Therapy Series

Cardiopulmonary Essentials: Applying the Preferred Physical Therapist Practice Patterns^{SM}
Marilyn Moffat, PT, DPT, PhD, FAPTA, CSCS, *New York University, New York, NY* and Donna Frownfelter, DPT, MA, CCS, FCCP, RRT, *Rosalind Franklin University of Medicine and Science, North Chicago, IL*
400 pp., Soft Cover, February 2007, ISBN 1-55642-668-2, Order #46682, **$58.95**

Neuromuscular Essentials: Applying the Preferred Physical Therapist Practice Patterns^{SM}
Marilyn Moffat, PT, DPT, PhD, FAPTA, CSCS, *New York University, New York, NY* and Joanell Bohmert, PT, MS, *University of Minnesota, Twin Cities, MN*
400 pp., Soft Cover, June 2007, ISBN 1-55642-669-0, Order #46690, **$58.95**

Integumentary Essentials: Applying the Preferred Physical Therapist Practice Patterns^{SM}
Marilyn Moffat, PT, DPT, PhD, FAPTA, CSCS, *New York University, New York, NY* and Katherine Biggs Harris, PT, MS, *Quinnipiac University, Hamden, CT*
160 pp., Soft Cover, June 2006, ISBN 1-55642-670-4, Order #46704, **$50.95**

Musculoskeletal Essentials: Applying the Preferred Physical Therapist Practice Patterns^{SM}
Marilyn Moffat, PT, DPT, PhD, FAPTA, CSCS, *New York University, New York, NY*; Elaine Rosen, PT, DHSc, OCS, FAAOMPT, *Hunter College, New York, NY*, and Sandra Rusnak-Smith, PT, DHSc, OCS, *Queens Physical Therapy Associates, Forest Hills, NY*
448 pp., Soft Cover, June 2006, ISBN 1-55642-667-4, Order #46674, **$58.95**

Please visit

www.slackbooks.com

to order any of these titles!
24 Hours a Day...7 Days a Week!

Attention Industry Partners!
Whether you are interested in buying multiple copies of a book, chapter reprints, or looking for something new and different — we are able to accommodate your needs.

Multiple Copies
At attractive discounts starting for purchases as low as 25 copies for a single title, SLACK Incorporated will be able to meet all your of your needs.

Chapter Reprints
SLACK Incorporated is able to offer the chapters you want in a format that will lead to success. Bound with an attractive cover, use the chapters that are a fit specifically for your company. Available for quantities of 100 or more.

Customize
SLACK Incorporated is able to create a specialized custom version of any of our products specifically for your company.

Please contact the Marketing Manager of the Health Care Books and Journals for further details on multiple copy purchases, chapter reprints or custom printing at 1-800-257-8290 or 1-856-848-1000.

*Please note all conditions are subject to change.

CODE: 328

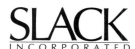

SLACK Incorporated • Health Care Books and Journals
6900 Grove Road • Thorofare, NJ 08086

1-800-257-8290 or 1-856-848-1000

Fax: 1-856-853-5991 • E-mail: orders@slackinc.com • Visit www.slackbooks.com

Date Due
